TEXTBOOK *of*
CLINICAL
ECHOCARDIOGRAPHY

TEXTBOOK *of* CLINICAL ECHOCARDIOGRAPHY

CATHERINE M. OTTO, M.D.

ALAN S. PEARLMAN, M.D.

University of Washington
School of Medicine
Division of Cardiology
Seattle, Washington

W.B. SAUNDERS COMPANY *A Division of Harcourt Brace & Company*
PHILADELPHIA, LONDON, TORONTO, MONTREAL, SYDNEY, TOKYO

W.B. SAUNDERS COMPANY
A Division of Harcourt Brace & Company

The Curtis Center
Independence Square West
Philadelphia, PA 19106

Library of Congress Cataloging-in-Publication Data

Otto, Catherine M.
    Textbook of clinical echocardiography / Catherine M. Otto and Alan
S. Pearlman.—1st ed.
        p. cm.
    Includes bibliographical references and index.
    ISBN 0–7216–6634–5
    1. Echocardiography. I. Pearlman, Alan S. II. Title.
    [DNLM: 1. Heart Diseases—ultrasonography. WG 141.5.E2 091t
1995]
RC683.5.U5087 1995
616.1′207543—dc20
DNLM/DLC   94-6846

TEXTBOOK OF CLINICAL ECHOCARDIOGRAPHY   ISBN 0–7216–6634–5

Printed in the United States of America

Last digit is the print number: 9   8   7   6   5   4   3   2   1

ACKNOWLEDGMENTS

Special thanks go to the cardiac sonographers at the University of Washington Medical Center for acquisition of the echocardiographic figures: Michelle C. Fujioka, RDMS; Carolyn J. Gardner, RDCS; Carol D. Kraft, RDMS; Carolyn Y. Miyake-Hull, RDMS; Rebecca G. Schwaegler, RDMS; and Todd R. Zwink, RDMS. The excellent image quality is due entirely to their skill and dedication. Both our cardiac sonography student, Charles M. Drake, and our cardiology fellow, Robert B. Stewart, MD, also contributed images for figures. In addition to the illustrations, the cardiac sonographers contributed substantially to the text by ongoing discussions of the details of echocardiographic image acquisition, quantitative data analysis, and the echocardiographic examination.

We also wish to thank the following University of Washington faculty: J. David Godwin, MD, generously provided the chest radiographs, aortogram, CT, and MRI illustrations; Dennis D. Reichenbach, MD, photographed the stenotic prosthetic valve; and Douglas K. Stewart, MD, provided coronary angiograms and left ventriculograms. Other individuals kindly gave permission to use previously published figures, including Florence H. Sheehan, MD, Manuel Cerqueira, MD, David T. Linker, MD, and Cornelius Rosse, MD.

Critical review of specific sections of the manuscript was provided by Eric B. Larson, MD, Roy W. Martin, PhD, and J. Geoffrey Stevenson, MD. Their constructive comments were invaluable. The helpful suggestions of our research fellows, Ian G. Burwash, MD, and Malcolm E. Legget, MD, also were appreciated. Nancy L. Healy provided essential "legwork" in locating references and illustrations.

A great deal of thanks is due to Sharon A. Kemp, who bore the burden of typing the entire manuscript (including all those tables), cross-checking references, verifying figure numbers, and proofreading the galleys.

Finally, we wish to thank our families for their constant encouragement, patience and support.

PREFACE

Echocardiography has become an integral part of clinical cardiology with important applications in the initial diagnosis, clinical management, and decision-making in patients with a wide range of cardiovascular diseases. In addition, echocardiographic techniques increasingly are applied not only in the laboratory but also in other clinical settings, such as the operating room and the emergency room, both for diagnosis and for monitoring the effects of therapeutic interventions. It is anticipated that there will be continued expansion of echocardiographic applications given the detailed and precise anatomic and physiologic information that can be obtained with this technique, both at relatively low cost and with minimal risk to the patient.

This textbook on general clinical echocardiography is intended to be read both by individuals new to echocardiography and by those interested in updating their knowledge in this area. The text is aimed primarily at cardiology fellows on their basic echocardiography rotation but also will be of value to residents and fellows in general internal medicine, radiology, anesthesiology, and emergency medicine, as well as to cardiac sonography students. For physicians in practice, this textbook provides a concise and practical update on clinical echocardiography.

After introductory chapters on practical ultrasound physics, normal tomographic views and flow patterns, and indications for echocardiography, the remainder of the book is organized by disease category (for example, cardiomyopathy or valvular stenosis), emphasizing a clinical (rather than technical) approach to echocardiographic diagnosis. In each chapter, basic principles for echocardiographic evaluation of that disease category are reviewed, the echocardiographic approach and differential diagnosis are discussed in detail, limitations and technical considerations are emphasized, and alternate diagnostic approaches are delineated. Schematic diagrams are used to illustrate basic concepts; echocardiographic images and Doppler data show both typical and unusual findings in patients with each disease process. Tables are used frequently to summarize previous studies validating quantitative echocardiographic methods.

At the end of each chapter, a selected list of annotated references is included. These references are suggestions for the individual who is interested in reading more about a particular subject. Additional relevant articles can be found in the suggested readings, or in a reference book on echocardiography. Many individuals will wish to review the most up-to-date articles or to cross-reference key words of interest using an on-line computer database, such as MedLine. An on-line computer medical reference database also is the best way to obtain a comprehensive list of all journal articles on a specific topic.

It should be emphasized that this textbook is only a starting point or frame of reference for learning echocardiography. Appropriate training in echocardiography includes competency in the acquisition and interpretation of echocardiographic and

Doppler data in real-time. Obviously, a textbook cannot replace the experience gained in performing studies, nor can still photographs replace the need for review of real-time data. Clearly defined guidelines for training in echocardiography have been published for both physicians and sonographers, as referenced in Chapter 3. We strongly support these training recommendations. While this textbook cannot replace appropriate training and experience, we hope it will enhance the learning experience of those new to the field and provide a review for those with prior training and experience.

CATHERINE M. OTTO, MD

ALAN S. PEARLMAN, MD

CONTENTS

GLOSSARY

Abbreviations used in figures, tables, and equations

2D = two-dimensional
3D = three-dimensional
A-long = apical long-axis
A-mode = amplitude mode (amplitude versus depth)
A = late (atrial) diastolic velocity peak
A = area (depends on context)
A2C = apical two-chamber
A4C = apical four-chamber
AcT = acceleration time
AF = atrial fibrillation
AMVL = anterior mitral valve leaflet
ant = anterior
Ao = aortic or aorta
AR = aortic regurgitation
AS = aortic stenosis
ASD = atrial septal defect
ASH = asymmetrical septal hypertrophy
ATVL = anterior tricuspid valve leaflet
AV = atrioventricular
AVA = aortic valve area
AVR = aortic valve replacement
BAV = balloon aortic valvuloplasty
BP = blood pressure
BS = Bjork-Shiley tilting-disk mechanical valve
BSA = body surface area
C-TGA = congenitally corrected transposition of the great arteries
C = chordae
c = propagation velocity of sound in tissue
CAD = coronary artery disease
cath = cardiac catheterization
CBV = catheter balloon valvuloplasty
Cm = specific heat of tissue
cm/s = centimeters per second
cm = centimeters
CO = cardiac output
Cont eq = continuity equation valve area
cos = cosine
CS = coronary sinus
CSA = cross-sectional area
CT = computed tomography
CW = continuous wave

Cx = circumflex coronary artery
D = diameter
D1 = first diagonal branch
D2 = second diagonal branch
DA = descending aorta
dB = decibels
dP/dt = rate of change in pressure over time
dT/dt = rate of increase in temperature
dyne•s•cm^{-5} = units of resistance
E = early diastolic peak velocity
ECG = electrocardiogram
echo = echocardiography
ED = end-diastole
EDD = end-diastolic dimension
EDV = end-diastolic volume
EF = ejection fraction
EM-flow = volume flow rate measured by electromagnetic flowmeter
endo = endocardium
EP = electrophysiology
epi = epicardium
EPSS = E-point septal separation
ES = end-systole
ESD = end-systolic dimension
ESPVR = end-systolic pressure-volume relationship
ESV = end-systolic volume
ETT = exercise treadmill test
Δf = frequency shift
f = frequency
FL = false lumen
Fn = near field
Fo = resonance frequency
Fs = scattered frequency
FSV = forward stroke volume
Ft = transmitted frequency
fx = function
Gorlin = Gorlin formula valve area
HCM = hypertrophic cardiomyopathy
HOCM = hypertrophic obstructive cardiomyopathy
HPRF = high pulse repetition frequency
HR = heart rate
HV = hepatic vein

I = intensity of ultrasound exposure
IAS = interatrial septum
ID = indicator dilution
inf = inferior
IV = intravenous
IVC = inferior vena cava
IVCT = isovolumic contraction time
IVRT = isovolumic relaxation time
kHz = kilohertz
L = length
LA = left atrium
LAA = left atrial appendage
LAD = left anterior descending coronary artery
LAE = left atrial enlargement
LAO = left anterior oblique
lat = lateral
LCC = left coronary cusp
LLAT = left lateral
LMCA = left main coronary artery
LPA = left pulmonary artery
LSPV = left superior pulmonary vein
LVE = left ventricular extension branch
LV-EDP = left ventricular end-diastolic pressure
LV = left ventricle
LVE = left ventricular enlargement
LVH = left ventricular hypertrophy
LVI = left ventricular inflow
LVID = left ventricular internal dimension
LVO = left ventricular outflow
LVOT = left ventricular outflow tract
M = myxoma
M-mode = motion display (depth versus time)
MAC = mitral annular calcification
MB = moderator band
MI = myocardial infarction
MR = mitral regurgitation
MRI = magnetic resonance imaging
MS = mitral stenosis
MV = mitral valve
MVA = mitral valve area
MVL = mitral valve leaflet
MVR = mitral valve replacement
n = number of subjects
NBTE = nonbacterial thrombotic endocarditis
NCC = noncoronary cusp
OM1 = first obtuse marginal branch
OM2 = second obtuse marginal branch
ΔP = pressure gradient
P = pressure
PA = pulmonary artery
pAn = pseudoaneurysm
PAP = pulmonary artery pressure
PD = pulsed Doppler
PDA = patent ductus arteriosus ⎫
PDA = posterior descending artery ⎬
  (depends on context) ⎭
PE = pericardial effusion
PEP = preejection period
PET = positron-emission tomography

PISA = proximal isovelocity surface area
PLAX = parasternal long-axis
PM = papillary muscle
PMVL = posterior mitral valve leaflet
post = posterior
PR = pulmonic regurgitation
PRF = pulse repetition frequency
PRFR = peak rapid filling rate
PS = pulmonic stenosis
PSAX = parasternal short-axis
PTCA = percutaneous transluminal coronary angioplasty
PV = pulmonary vein
PVC = premature ventricular contraction
PWT = posterior wall thickness
Q = volume flow rate
Q_p = pulmonic volume flow rate
Q_s = systemic volume flow rate
r = ventricular radius or correlation coefficient (depends on context)
RA = right atrium
RAE = right atrial enlargement
RAM = random access memory
RAO = right anterior oblique
RAP = right atrial pressure
RCA = right coronary artery
RCC = right coronary cusp
Re = Reynolds number
RF = regurgitant fraction
RJ = regurgitant jet
R_o = radius of microbubble
ROA = regurgitant orifice area
RPA = right pulmonary artery
RSPV = right superior pulmonary vein
RSV = regurgitant stroke volume
RV = right ventricle
RVE = right ventricular enlargement
RVH = right ventricular hypertrophy
RVI = right ventricular inflow
RVO = right ventricular outflow
RVOT = right ventricular outflow tract
SAM = systolic anterior motion
SC = subcostal
SEE = standard error of the estimate
SPPA = spatial peak pulse average
SPTA = spatial peak temporal average
SSN = suprasternal notch
ST = septal thickness
STJ = sinotubular junction
STVL = septal tricuspid valve leaflet
SV = stroke volume or sample volume (depends on context)
SVC = superior vena cava
SWMA = segmental wall motion abnormality
$t_{1/2}$ = pressure half-time
T = thrombus
TD = thermodilution
TEE = transesophageal echocardiography
TGA = transposition of the great arteries
TGC = time gain compensation
TL = true lumen
TN = true negatives

TOF = tetralogy of Fallot
TP = true positives
TPV = time to peak velocity
TR = tricuspid regurgitation
TS = tricuspid stenosis
TSV = total stroke volume
TTE = transthoracic echocardiography
TV = tricuspid valve
v = velocity

V = volume or velocity (depends on context)
VAS = ventriculo-atrial septum
Veg = vegetation
V_{max} = maximum velocity
VSD = ventricular septal defect
VTI = velocity-time integral
WPW = Wolff-Parkinson-White syndrome
Z = acoustic impedance

Symbols	Greek Name	Used for
α	alpha	frequency
γ	gamma	viscosity
Δ	delta	difference
θ	theta	angle
λ	lambda	wavelength
μ	mu	micro-
π	pi	mathematical constant (approx. 3.14)
ρ	rho	tissue density
σ	sigma	wall stress
τ	tau	time constant of ventricular relaxation

UNITS OF MEASURE

Variable	Unit	Definition
Amplitude	dB	Decibels = a logarithmic scale describing the amplitude ("loudness") of the sound wave
Angle	degrees	Example: intercept angle
Area	cm²	A two-dimensional measurement (e.g., end-systolic area) or a calculated value (e.g., continuity equation valve area)
Frequency (f)	Hz	Hertz (cycles per second)
	kHz	Kilohertz = 1000 Hz
	MHz	Megahertz = 1,000,000 Hz
Length	cm	Centimeter (1/100 m)
	mm	Millimeter (1/1000 m or 1/10 cm)
Mass	gm	Example: LV mass
Pressure	mmHg	Millimeters of mercury, 1 mmHg = 1333.2 dyne/cm², where dyne measures force in cm•g/s²
Resistance	dyne•s•cm^{-5}	Measure of vascular resistance
Time	s	Second
	ms	Millisecond (1/1000 s)
	μs	Microsecond
Ultrasound intensity	W/cm²	Where watt (W) = joule per second and joule = m²kg/s² (unit of energy)
	mW/cm²	
Velocity (v)	m/s	Meters per second
	cm/s	Centimeters per second
Velocity-time integral (VTI)	cm	Integral of the Doppler velocity curve (cm/s) over time (s), in units of cm

Variable	Unit	Definition
Volume	cm^3	Cubic centimeters
	ml	Milliliter, 1 ml = 1 cm^3
	L	Liter = 1000 ml
Volume flow rate (Q)	L/min	Rate of volume flow across a valve or in cardiac output
	ml/s	L/min = liters per minute
		ml/s = milliliters per second
Wall stress	$dyne/cm^2$	Units of meridional or circumferential wall stress
	$kdyn/cm^2$	Kilodynes per cm^2
	kPa	Kilopascals where 1kPa = 10 $kdyn/cm^2$

CHAPTER

1

PRINCIPLES OF ECHOCARDIOGRAPHIC IMAGE ACQUISITION AND DOPPLER ANALYSIS

INTRODUCTION

An understanding of the basic principles of ultrasound imaging and Doppler echocardiography is essential both during data acquisition and for correct interpretation of the ultrasound information. Although, at times, current instruments provide instantaneous images so clear and detailed that it seems as if we can "see" the heart and blood flow directly, in actuality, we always are looking at images and flow data generated by complex analyses of ultrasound waves reflected and backscattered from the patient's body. Knowledge of the strengths of this technique and, more important, its limitations is critical for correct clinical diagnosis and patient management. On the one hand, echocardiography can be used for decision making with a high degree of accuracy in a variety of clinical settings. On the other hand, if an ultrasound artifact is mistaken for an anatomic abnormality, a patient might undergo needless, expensive, and potentially risky other diagnostic tests or "therapeutic" interventions.

In this chapter, a brief (and necessarily simplified) overview of the basic principles of cardiac ultrasound imaging and flow analysis is presented. The reader is referred to the Suggested Reading at the end of the chapter for more information on these subjects. Since the details of image processing, artifact formation, and Doppler "physics" become more meaningful with experience, some readers may choose to return to this chapter after reading other sections of this book and after participating in some echocardiographic examinations.

BASIC PRINCIPLES OF ULTRASOUND

Ultrasound Waves

Sound waves are mechanical vibrations that induce alternate refractions and compressions of any physical medium through which they pass. Like other waves, sound waves are described in terms of the following (Fig. 1–1):

1. Frequency—cycles per second, or hertz (Hz)
2. Wavelength—millimeters (mm)
3. Amplitude—decibels (dB)
4. Velocity of propagation—which depends on each carrying medium (approximately 1540 m/s in blood)

Humans can hear sound waves with frequencies between 20 Hz and 20 kilohertz (kHz); frequencies higher than this range are termed *ultrasound*. Diagnostic medical ultrasound typically uses transducers with a frequency between 1 million and 20 million Hz or 1 and 20 megahertz (MHz).

Wavelength λ times frequency f equals the propagation velocity c:

$$c = \lambda \cdot f \qquad (1.1)$$

Since the propagation velocity in the heart is constant at 1540 m/s, the wavelength for any transducer frequency can be calculated as

$$\lambda \ (mm) = 1.54/f \ (MHz) \qquad (1.2)$$

as shown in Figure 1–2. Wavelength is important in diagnostic applications for at least two reasons:

1. Image resolution is no greater than 1 to 2 wavelengths (typically about 1 mm).
2. The depth of penetration of the ultrasound wave into the body is directly related to wavelength—shorter wavelengths penetrate a shorter distance than longer wavelengths.

Thus, there is an obvious tradeoff between image resolution (shorter wavelength or higher frequency preferable) and depth penetration (longer wavelength or lower frequency preferable).

The *amplitude* (e.g., "loudness") of an ultrasound wave is described in terms of decibels. Decibels (dB) are logarithmic units based on a ratio of the measured value V of acoustic pressure to a reference value R such that

$$dB = 20 \log (V/R) \qquad (1.3)$$

Thus a ratio of 10,000 to 1 is

$$20 \times \log (10,000) = 20 \times 4 = 80 \ dB$$

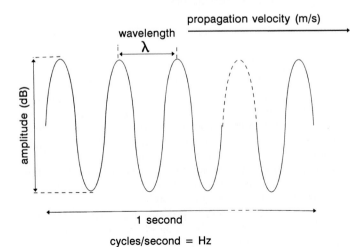

Figure 1–1. Schematic diagram of an ultrasound wave.

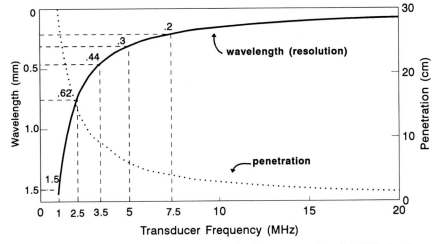

Figure 1–2. Graph of transducer frequency (*horizontal axis*) versus wavelength (*solid line*) and penetration (*dotted line*) of the ultrasound signal in soft tissue. Wavelength has been plotted inversely to show that resolution increases with increasing transducer frequency while penetration decreases. The specific wavelengths for transducer frequencies of 1, 2.5, 3.5, 5, and 7.5 MHz are shown.

a ratio of 1000 to 1 is

$$20 \times \log (1000) = 20 \times 3 = 60 \text{ dB}$$

a ratio of 100 to 1 is

$$20 \times \log (100) = 20 \times 2 = 40 \text{ dB}$$

and a ratio of 2 to 1 is

$$20 \times \log (2) = 20 \times 0.3 = 6 \text{ dB}$$

A simple rule to remember is that a 6-dB change represents a doubling or halving of the signal amplitude (Fig. 1–3). The advantages of use of the decibel scale are that a very large range can be compressed into a smaller number of values and that low-amplitude (weak) signals can be displayed alongside very high amplitude (strong) signals.

Interaction of Ultrasound Waves with Tissues

The interaction of ultrasound waves with the organs and tissues of the body can be described in terms of (1) reflection, (2) scattering, (3) refraction, and (4) attenuation (Fig. 1–4).

Reflection

The basis of ultrasound imaging is *reflection* of the transmitted ultrasound signal from internal structures. Ultrasound is reflected at tissue boundaries and interfaces, with the amount of ultrasound reflected dependent on the relative change in acoustic impedance between the two tissues. Acoustic impedance Z depends on tissue

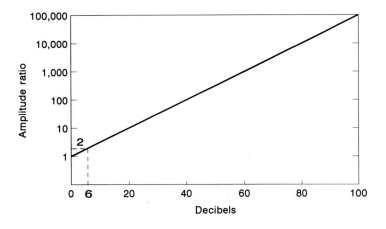

Figure 1–3. Graph of the decibel scale (*horizontal axis*) showing the logarithmic relationship with the amplitude ratio (*vertical axis*). Note that a doubling or halving of the amplitude ratio corresponds to a 6-dB change.

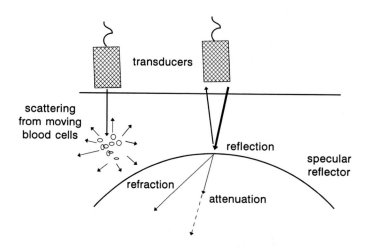

Figure 1–4. Diagram of the interaction between ultrasound and body tissues. Doppler analysis is based on the scattering of ultrasound in all directions from moving blood cells with a resulting change in frequency of the ultrasound received at the transducer. 2D imaging is based on reflection of ultrasound from tissue interfaces (specular reflectors). Attenuation limits the depth of ultrasound penetration. Refraction, a change in direction of the ultrasound wave, results in imaging artifacts.

density p and on the propagation velocity in that tissue c:

$$Z = p \cdot c \qquad (1.4)$$

Differences in acoustic impedance largely relate to differences in tissue density, but the velocity of propagation can differ as well (e.g., bone has a propagation velocity about twice as fast as blood). Smooth tissue boundaries with a lateral dimension greater than the wavelength of the ultrasound beam act as specular, or "mirror-like," reflectors. The amount of ultrasound reflected is constant for a given interface, although the amount received back at the transducer varies with angle because (like light reflected from a mirror) the angle of incidence and reflection is equal. Optimal return of reflected ultrasound occurs at a perpendicular angle (90°). Remembering this fact is crucial for obtaining diagnostic ultrasound images. It also accounts for ultrasound "dropout" in a two-dimensional (2D) image when too little or no reflected ultrasound reaches the transducer due to a parallel alignment between the ultrasound beam and tissue interface.

Scattering

Small structures (<1 wavelength in lateral dimension) result in *scattering* of the ultrasound signal instead of reflection. Unlike a reflected beam, scattered ultrasound energy may be radiated in all directions. Only a small amount of the scattered signal reaches the receiving transducer, and the amplitude of a scattered signal is 100 to 1000 times (40–60 dB) less than the amplitude of the returned signal from a specular reflector. Scattering of ultrasound from moving blood cells is the basis of Doppler echocardiog-

raphy. While some argue that the size of a single red blood cell (7–10 μm) is so much smaller (20 times) than the wavelength of ultrasound (0.2–1.0 mm) that it is unlikely to be an effective scatterer, most investigators consider that detectable scattering occurs due to thousands of blood cells being present in the sound beam. Most evidence suggests that variation in hematocrit over the clinical range has little effect on the Doppler signal as used in clinical applications.

Refraction

Ultrasound waves can be *refracted*—deflected from a straight path—as they pass through a medium with a different acoustic impedance. Refraction of an ultrasound beam is analogous to refraction of light waves as they pass through a curved glass lens (e.g., prescription eyeglasses). Refraction allows enhanced image quality by using acoustic "lenses" to focus the ultrasound beam. However, refraction also occurs in unplanned ways during image formation, resulting in ultrasound artifacts, most notably the "double-image" artifact.

Attenuation

As ultrasound penetrates into the body, signal strength is progressively *attenuated* due to absorption of the ultrasound energy by conversion to heat, as well as by reflection and scattering. Overall attenuation is frequency-dependent such that lower ultrasound frequencies penetrate deeper into the body than higher frequencies. The depth of penetration for adequate imaging tends to be limited to approximately 200 wavelengths. This translates roughly into a penetration depth of 30 cm for a 1-MHz transducer, 6 cm for a 5-MHz transducer, and 1.5 cm for a 20-MHz transducer, although diagnostic images at depths greater than these postulated limits can be obtained with state-of-the-art equipment.

Clinically, attenuation, as much as resolution, dictates the need for a particular transducer frequency in a specific clinical setting. For example, visualization of distal structures from the apical approach in a large adult patient requires a low-frequency transducer. From a transesophageal approach, the same structures can be imaged (at better resolution) with a higher-frequency transducer.

Attenuation also depends on acoustic impedance and on mismatch in impedance between adjacent structures. This factor is important in transducer design so that the signal is not attenuated significantly before it leaves the transducer. It also is important during the examination. Since air has a very high acoustic impedance, any air between the transducer and the cardiac structures of interest results in substantial signal attenuation. This is avoided on transthoracic examinations by use of a water-soluble gel to form an airless contact between the transducer and the skin and on transesophageal examination by maintaining close contact between the transducer and the esophageal wall. The air-filled lungs are avoided by careful patient positioning and the use of acoustic "windows" that allow access of the ultrasound beam to the cardiac structures without intervening lung tissue. Other intrathoracic air (e.g., pneumomediastinum, residual air after cardiac surgery) results in poor ultrasound tissue penetration due to attenuation, resulting in suboptimal image quality.

TRANSDUCERS

Piezoelectric Crystal

Ultrasound transducers use a piezoelectric crystal both to generate and to receive ultrasound waves (Fig. 1–5). A piezoelectric crystal is a material (such as quartz or a titanate ceramic) with the property that an applied electric current results in alignment of polarized particles perpendicular to the face of the crystal with consequent expansion of crystal size. When an alternating electric current is applied, the crystal alternately compresses and expands, generating an ultrasound wave. The frequency that a transducer emits depends on the nature and thickness of the piezoelectric material.

Conversely, when an ultrasound wave impacts the piezoelectric crystal, an electric current is generated. Thus the crystal can serve both as a "receiver" and as a "transmitter." Basically, the ultrasound transducer transmits a brief burst of ultrasound and then switches to the "receive mode" to await the reflected ultrasound signals from the intracardiac acoustic interfaces. This cycle is repeated temporally and spatially to generate ultrasound images. Image formation is based on the *time delay* between ultrasound transmission and return of the reflected signal. Deeper structures have a longer time of flight than shallower structures, with the exact depth calculated based on the speed of sound in blood and the time interval between the transmitted burst of ultrasound and return of the reflected signal.

The burst, or pulse, of ultrasound generated by the piezoelectric crystal is very brief, typically 1 to 6 μs, since a short pulse length results

Figure 1–5. Schematic diagram of an ultrasound transducer. The piezoelectric crystal both produces and receives ultrasound signals, with the electric input/output transmitted to the instrument via the cable. Damping material allows a short pulse length (improved resolution). The shape of the piezoelectric crystal, an acoustic lens, or electronic focusing (with a phased-array transducer) are used to modify the beam geometry. The material of the transducer surface provides impedance matching with the skin. The ultrasound pulse length for 2D imaging is short (1–6 ms), typically consisting of 2 wavelengths (λ). "Ring down"—the decrease in frequency and amplitude in the pulse—depends on damping and determines bandwidth (the range of frequencies in the signal).

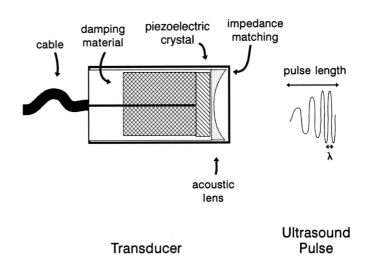

in improved axial (along the length of the beam) resolution. Damping material is used to control the ring-down time of the crystal and, hence, the pulse length. Pulse length also is determined by frequency, since a shorter time is needed for the same number of cycles at higher frequencies.

The range of frequencies contained in the pulse is described as its *frequency bandwidth*. A wider bandwidth allows better axial resolution due to the ability of the system to produce a narrow pulse. Transducer bandwidth also affects the range of frequencies that can be detected by the system. The stated frequency of a transducer represents the center frequency of the pulse.

Types of Transducers

The simplest type of ultrasound transducer is based on a single piezoelectric crystal (Table 1–1). Alternate pulsed transmission and reception periods allow repeated sampling along a single line, with the sampling rate limited only by the time delay needed for return of the reflected ultrasound wave from the depth of interest. Single nonmoving crystal transducers are used for A-mode or M-mode cardiac recordings when a high sampling rate is desirable.

Formation of a tomographic cardiac ultrasound image is based on mechanical or electronic sweeping of the ultrasound beam across the plane of interest. This type of tomographic imaging—*sector scanning*—is used for cardiac ap-

plications, rather than a linear array of parallel ultrasound beams, to allow a faster frame rate (to show cardiac motion) and because the smaller transducer size (aperture or "footprint") fits into the narrow acoustic windows utilized in echocardiography. Mechanical sector scanners actually move the crystal in the transducer either in a rotational fashion or in a "wobble" fashion. Mechanical transducers have the advantage of a high signal-to-noise ratio but the disadvantages of limited Doppler capabilities and potential mechanical malfunction. A phased-array sector scanner consists of a series of ultrasound crystals arranged so that the beam can be electronically "steered" using combinations of the available elements. There are no moving parts prone to malfunction, and all Doppler modalities can be performed. The phased-array transducer currently is the most common type of transducer used for echocardiography.

Continuous-wave Doppler examinations utilize two crystals of a phased-array transducer or two separate crystals in a dedicated nonimaging transducer, with one crystal continuously transmitting and the other continuously receiving the ultrasound waves.

Beam Shape and Focusing

Beam shape and size vary predictably with distance from the transducer. However, the three-dimensional (3D) shape of the ultrasound beam generated by a transducer is complex (Fig. 1–6) and depends on several factors, some of which can be manipulated in the design of the transducer and some of which are inherent to ultrasound physics. For an unfocused beam, the initial segment of the beam is columnar in shape (near field F_n) with a length dependent on the diameter D of the transducer face and wavelength λ:

$$F_n = D^2/4\lambda \qquad (1.5)$$

For a 3.5-MHz transducer with a 5-mm-diameter aperture, this corresponds to a columnar length of 1.4 cm. Beyond this region, the ultrasound beam diverges (far field), with the angle of divergence θ determined as:

$$\sin \theta = 1.22\lambda/D \qquad (1.6)$$

This equation indicates a divergence angle of 6° beyond the near field, resulting in an ultrasound beam width of about 4.4 cm at a depth of 20 cm for this 3.5-MHz transducer. With a 10-mm-diameter aperture, F_n would be 5.7 cm and

---

TABLE 1–1.
ULTRASOUND TRANSDUCERS

Piezoelectric Crystal Arrangements

  Single (or double) crystal
  Mechanical
  Phased array
  Annular array

Types

  Transthoracic
  Transesophageal
  Intravascular

Characteristics

  Frequency
  Focal depth
  Bandwidth
  Aperture ("footprint")
  Power output

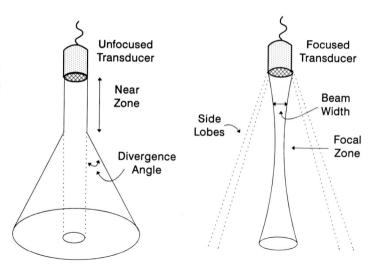

Figure 1–6. Schematic diagram of beam geometry for an unfocused (*left*) and focused (*right*) transducer. The length of the near zone and the divergence angle in the far field depend on transducer frequency and aperture (as shown in Fig. 1–5). The focal zone of a focused transducer can be adjusted, but beam width still depends on depth. Side lobes (and grating lobes with phased-array transducers) occur with both focused and unfocused transducers and, like the central beam, are three-dimensional.

beam width at 20 cm would be about 2.5 cm (Fig. 1–7).

The shape and focal depth (narrowest point) of the primary beam can be altered by making the surface of the piezoelectric crystal concave or by addition of an acoustic lens. This allows generation of a beam with optimal characteristics at the depth of most cardiac structures, but again, divergence of the beam beyond the focal zone occurs. Some transducers allow manipulation of the focal zone during the examination. Even with focusing, the ultrasound beam generated by each transducer has a lateral (azimuthal) and an elevational dimension that depends on the transducer aperture, frequency, and focusing. In addition, beam geometry for phased-array transducers depends on the size, spacing, and arrangement of the piezoelectric crystals in the array.

In addition to the main ultrasound beam, dispersion of ultrasound energy laterally from a single-crystal transducer results in formation of side lobes at an angle θ from the central beam where $\sin \theta = m\lambda/D$, where m is an integer describing sequential side lobes (i.e., 1, 2, 3, and the like) (Fig. 1–8). Reflected or backscattered signals from these side lobes may be received by the transducer, resulting in image or flow artifacts. With phased-array transducers, additional accessory beams termed *grating lobes* also occur as a result of constructive interference of ultrasound wave fronts (Fig. 1–9). Both the side lobes and the grating lobes affect the lateral (azimuthal) resolution of the transducer.

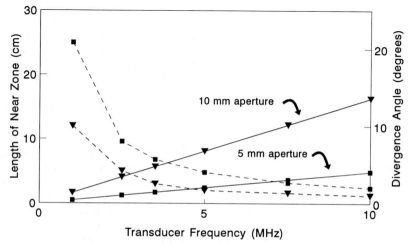

Figure 1–7. Graph of transducer frequency (*horizontal axis*) versus length of the near zone (*solid lines*) and divergence angle (*dashed lines*) for an unfocused 5- and 10-mm-diameter aperture transducer. Equations (1.5) and (1.6) were used to generate these curves.

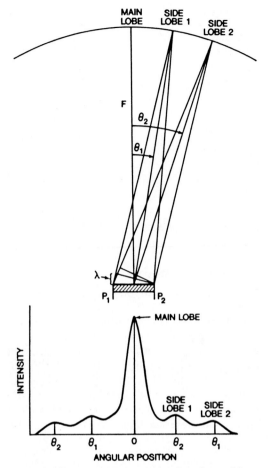

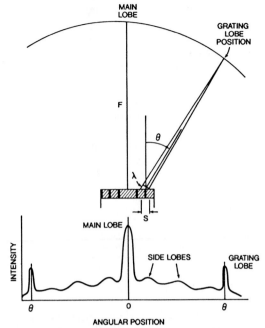

Figure 1–9. (*Above*) Diagram showing the position of grating lobes in phased-array transducers. The position of grating lobes is determined by the spacing between the centers of independent crystal elements in the transducer. At any point where the path length between the two crystal elements differs by one wavelength, a grating lobe is formed. The grating lobe is formed at an angle θ that depends on the wavelength λ of the crystals and the spacing S between the crystal elements. (*Below*) The beam intensity plot formed at focal length F. (*Reprinted with permission from Geiser EA: Chapter 17, in Cardiac Imaging, 3d ed., Philadelphia, W.B. Saunders Co., 1988, p 355.*)

Figure 1–8. (*Above*) Diagram showing the positions at which side lobes will form. Side lobes occur at points at which the distances traversed by the ultrasound pulse from each edge of the crystal face differ by exactly one wavelength. Note that the distance from the left edge of the crystal at point P_1 to the position of side lobe 1 is exactly one wavelength longer than the distance from point P_2 at the extreme right edge of the crystal to the position of side lobe 1. (*Below*) The beam intensity plot formed by sweeping along an arc at focal length F. (*Reprinted with permission from Geiser EA: Chapter 17, in Cardiac Imaging, 3d ed., Philadelphia, W.B. Saunders Co., 1988, p 355.*)

Resolution (Table 1–2)

Image resolution occurs for each of three dimensions: (1) *axial resolution*, that is, along the length of the ultrasound beam, (2) *lateral* or *azimuthal resolution*, that is, the resolution side-to-side across the 2D image, and (3) *elevational resolution*, that is, the thickness of the tomographic "slice."

Of these three, axial resolution is most precise, so quantitative measurements are made most reliably using data derived from a perpendicular alignment between the ultrasound beam and the structure of interest (Fig. 1–10). Axial resolution depends on the transducer frequency, bandwidth, and pulse length. Since the smallest resolvable distance between two specular reflectors with conventional ultrasound is 1 wavelength, higher-frequency (shorter-wavelength) transducers have greater axial resolution. A wider bandwidth also improves resolution by allowing a shorter pulse, thus avoiding overlap between the reflected ultrasound signals from two adjacent reflectors.

Lateral resolution varies with the depth of the specular reflector from the transducer, being most dependent on beam width at each depth. With a narrow beam width in the focal region, lateral resolution may approach axial resolution, and a point target will appear as a point on the 2D image. At greater depths, beam width diverges so that a point target results in a reflected signal as wide as the beam width. The lack of

TABLE 1–2. DETERMINANTS OF RESOLUTION IN 2D IMAGING

Axial Resolution

Transducer frequency
Transducer bandwidth
Pulse length

Lateral (Azimuthal) Resolution

Transducer frequency
Beam width (focusing) at each depth*
Aperture (width) of transducer
Bandwidth
Side and grating lobe levels

Elevational Resolution

Transducer frequency
Beam width in elevational plane
Side lobe and grating lobe levels

*Most important.

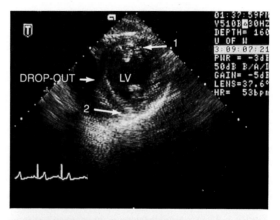

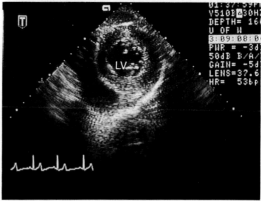

Figure 1–10. 2D echocardiographic view of the left ventricle from a transesophageal approach at end-diastole (*above*) and end-systole (*below*). Even with excellent image quality, as in this example, the effect of beam width can be appreciated by comparing the length of reflections from the endocardium near the transducer (point 1) and more distal reflectors (point 2). Note the relative "dropout" of the epicardium and endocardium when parallel to the ultrasound beam.

lateral resolution at greater depths accounts for the "blurring" of the image in the far field. If the 2D image is examined carefully, progressive widening of the echo signals from similar targets along the ultrasound beam can be appreciated. If this is not recognized, beam width can result in erroneous interpretations. Beam width artifact from a strong specular reflector in the tomographic plane may appear as a linear abnormal structure. Other factors that affect lateral resolution are transducer frequency, aperture, bandwidth, and side and grating lobe levels.

Resolution in the elevational plane is more difficult to recognize on the 2D image but is equally important in the echocardiographic examination. The thickness of the tomographic plane is variable over the 2D image, depending on transducer design and focusing, both of which affect beam width in the elevational plane at each depth. In general, cardiac ultrasound images have a "thickness" of approximately 3 to 10 mm depending on depth and the specific transducer used. The tomographic image generated by the instrument, in effect, includes reflected and backscattered signals from this entire thickness. Strong reflectors adjacent to the image plane may appear to be "in" the image plane due to elevational beam width. Even more distant strong reflectors may appear superimposed on the tomographic plane due to side and grating lobes in the elevational plane. Examples include a calcified aortic valve appearing as a "mass" in the left atrium on apical views or a linear echo in the aortic lumen from adjacent calcified atheroma appearing as a possible dissection flap.

ULTRASOUND INSTRUMENTS AND IMAGING MODALITIES

A Mode/M Mode

Historically, cardiac ultrasound began with a single-crystal transducer display of the amplitude *A* of reflected ultrasound versus depth on an oscilloscope screen. An A-mode display may still be shown on the 2D image screen to aid the examiner in optimal adjustment of the instrument controls. Repeated pulse transmission and receive cycles allow rapid updating of the amplitude versus depth information so that rapidly moving structures, such as the aortic or mitral valve leaflets, can be identified by their characteristic timing and pattern of motion (Fig. 1–11).

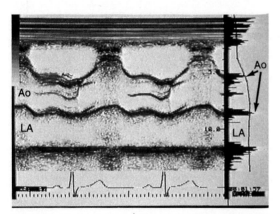

Figure 1–11. An A-mode (along right edge) and M-mode recording of aortic root (Ao), left atrium (LA), and aortic valve motion. On the A-mode recording, the anterior and posterior aortic root (with valve closure in the center) and posterior left atrial wall are clearly identified. The rapid sampling rate of M-mode recording allows visualization of aortic valve motion.

With the time dimension shown explicitly on the horizontal axis and each amplitude signal along the length of the ultrasound beam converted to a corresponding gray scale level, a *motion (M) mode display* is produced. M-mode recordings originally were made by rolling light-sensitive paper under the brightness versus depth display. Now the M-mode data can be recorded on paper or shown on the video monitor either "scrolling" or "sweeping" across the screen at 50 to 100 mm/s. While a single-crystal transducer had to be aligned based on the M-mode output alone, 2D imaging allows guidance of the M-mode beam to ensure an appropriate angle between the M line and the structures of interest.

Because only a single "line of sight" is included in an A-mode or M-mode tracing, the repetition frequency of the pulse transmission and receive phase of the transducer (the pulse repetition frequency) is limited only by the time needed for the ultrasound beam to travel to the maximum depth of interest and back to the transducer. Even a depth of 20 cm requires only 0.26 ms (given a speed of propagation of 1540 m/s), allowing a pulse frequency up to 3850 times per second. In actual practice, sampling rates of about 1800 times per second are used. This extremely high sampling rate is valuable for accurate evaluation of rapid normal intracardiac motion such as valve opening and closing. It also allows detection of high-frequency fluttering of the anterior mitral leaflet in patients with aortic regurgitation and the rapid oscillating motion of valvular vegetations. In addition, continuously moving structures, such as the ventricular endocardium, may be identified more accurately when motion versus time, as well as depth, is displayed clearly on the M-mode recording.

2D Echocardiography

Image Production

A 2D echocardiographic image is generated from the data obtained by mechanically or electronically "sweeping" the ultrasound beam across the tomographic plane. Since a finite time is needed for each scan line of data (depending on the depth of interest), the time needed to acquire all the data for one image frame is directly related to the number of scan lines. Thus there is a tradeoff between scan line density and image frame rate—the number of images per second. For cardiac applications, a high frame rate (≥ 30 frames per second) is desirable for accurate display of cardiac motion. This frame rate allows 33 ms per frame or 128 scan lines per 2D image at a displayed depth of 20 cm.

The reflected ultrasound signals for each scan line are received by the piezoelectric crystal and a small electric signal generated with (1) an amplitude proportional to incident angle and acoustic impedance and (2) timing proportional to distance from the transducer. This signal undergoes complex manipulation to form the final image displayed on the monitor. Typical processing includes signal amplification, time-gain compensation, filtering (to reduce noise), compression, and rectification. Envelope detection generates a bright spot for each signal along the scan line, which then undergoes analog to digital scan conversion, since the original polar coordinate data must be fit to a rectangular matrix with appropriate interpolation for missing matrix elements. This image is subject to further "postprocessing" to enhance the visual appreciation of tomographic anatomy and is displayed in "real time" (nearly simultaneous with data acquisition) on the monitor screen.

Instrument Settings

Many of the elements in the process of image formation are features of a particular instrument that cannot be modified by the operator. Other elements can be manipulated as data are acquired ("preprocessing") or as stored data are reviewed ("postprocessing"). Incorporation of a continuous-loop digital memory to store a series (16–128) of polar images in random access memory (RAM) facilitates the evaluation of the effect of postprocessing options on the displayed image.

Standard imaging controls available in most ultrasound systems include

1. *Power output:* This control adjusts the total ultrasound energy delivered by the transducer in the transmitted bursts, thus resulting in higher-amplitude reflected signals (see "Bioeffects and Safety," below).

2. *Gain:* In contrast to power output, the gain control adjusts the displayed amplitude of the received signals, similar to the volume control in an audio system.

3. *Time-gain compensation (TGC):* The TGC panel allows differential adjustment of gain along the length of the ultrasound beam. Near-field gain can be set lower (since reflected signals are stronger) with a gradually increased gain over the midfield ("ramp" or "slope") and a higher gain in the far field (since reflected signals are weaker). On some instruments, near-field and far-field gain beyond the range of the TGC is adjusted separately.

4. *Depth:* The displayed depth affects the pulse repetition frequency and frame rate of the image as well as allowing maximal display of the area of interest on the screen. Standard depth settings show the entire plane (from the transducer down), while "resolution" or "magnification" modes focus on a specific depth range of interest.

5. *Gray scale/dynamic range:* The number of levels of gray in the image, or *dynamic range*, can be adjusted to provide an image with marked contrast between light and dark areas or a gradation of gray levels between the lightest and darkest areas. A variation of standard gray scale is to use a color intensity for each amplitude value.

Other typical instrument controls include pre- and postprocessing settings that change the appearance of the displayed image. Note that image quality and resolution depend on scan-line density (as well as the factors listed in Table 1–2). Scan-line density (and/or frame rate) can be increased by using a lower depth setting or by narrowing the sector to less than the standard 60° wide image.

Imaging Artifacts (Table 1–3)

Imaging artifacts include (1) extraneous ultrasound signals that result in the appearance of "structures" that are not actually present (at least at that location), (2) failure to visualize structures that are present, and (3) an image of a structure that differs in size and/or shape from its actual appearance. Obviously, recognition of image artifacts is important for both the individual performing the study and the individual interpreting the echocardiographic data.

The most common image "artifact" is *suboptimal image quality* due to poor ultrasound tissue

TABLE 1–3. ULTRASOUND IMAGING ARTIFACTS

ARTIFACT	MECHANISM	EXAMPLE(S)
Suboptimal image quality	Poor ultrasound tissue penetration	Body habitus (obesity, lung disease) Postcardiac surgery
Acoustic shadowing	Reflection of all the ultrasound signal by a strong specular reflector	Prosthetic valve Calcification
Reverberations	Reverberation between two strong parallel reflectors	Prosthetic valve
Beam width	Superimposition of structures within the beam profile (including side lobes) into a signal tomographic image	Aortic valve "in" left atrium Atheroma "in" aortic lumen
Lateral resolution	Displayed width of a point target varies with depth	Excessive width of calcified mass or prosthetic valve
Refraction	Deviation of ultrasound signal from a straight path along the scan line	Double aortic valve or left ventricular image in short-axis view
Range ambiguity	Echo from previous pulse reaches transducer on next cycle	"Herbie" Second, deeper, heart image
Electronic processing	Instrument-specific	Variable

penetration related to the patient's body habitus with interposition of high-impedance tissues (e.g., adipose tissue, lung, or bone) between the transducer and cardiac structures. While, strictly speaking, poor image quality is not an "artifact," a low signal-to-noise ratio makes accurate diagnosis difficult and precludes quantitative measurements.

Acoustic shadowing (Fig. 1–12) occurs when a structure with very high acoustic impedance (prosthetic valve, calcium) blocks transmission of the ultrasound wave beyond that point. The image appears devoid of reflected signals distal to this structure, since no signal penetrates beyond the shadowing structure. The shape of the shadow (like a light shadow) follows the ultrasound path, so a small structure near the transducer casts a large shadow. When shadowing occurs, an alternate acoustic window is needed for evaluation of the area of interest. In some cases, a different transthoracic view will suffice. In other cases (e.g., prosthetic mitral valve), transesophageal imaging may be indicated.

Reverberations (Fig. 1–13) are multiple linear high-amplitude echo signals originating from two strong specular reflectors and resulting in a back-and-forth reflection of the ultrasound signal before it returns to the transducer. On the image, reverberations appear as relatively parallel, irregular, dense lines extending from the structure into the far field. Like acoustic shadowing, prominent reverberations limit evalua-

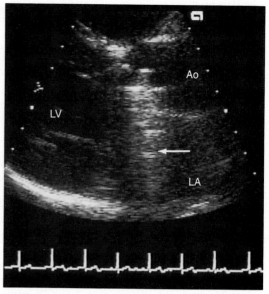

Figure 1–13. Example of reverberations. Parasternal long-axis view of a mechanical aortic valve prosthesis with reverberations obscuring the left atrium.

tion of structures in the far field. In less dramatic cases, reverberations may appear to represent abnormal structures. For example, in the parasternal long-axis view, a linear echo in the aortic root may originate as a reverberation from anterior structures (ribs, etc.) rather than representing a dissection flap.

The term *beam width artifact* is applied to two separate sources of image artifacts. First, remember that all the structures within the 3D volume of the ultrasound beam are displayed in a single tomographic plane. In the focal zone of the beam, the 3D volume is quite small and the

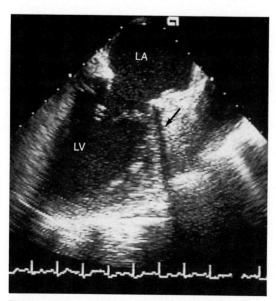

Figure 1–12. Example of acoustic shadowing. Transesophageal view of the left atrium and left ventricle shows shadowing (*arrow*) by mitral annular calcification.

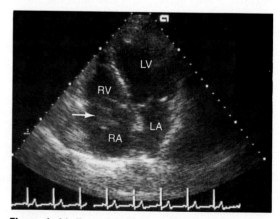

Figure 1–14. Example of beam width artifact. Apparent "mass" in the right atrium in the apical four-chamber view is beam width artifact from a calcified aortic valve.

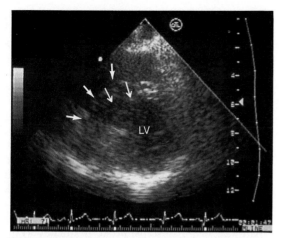

Figure 1–15. Example of refraction. An overlapping double image of the left ventricle is seen in a parasternal short-axis view due to refraction of the ultrasound beam by intervening tissues. The actual and duplicate left ventricular walls are indicated by arrows.

acteristics at that depth and the amplitude of the reflected signal. For example, the struts on a prosthetic valve can appear much longer than their actual dimension due to poor lateral resolution. Sometimes, beam width artifacts can be mistaken for abnormal structures such as a valvular vegetation, an intracardiac mass, or an aortic dissection flap.

The appearance of a side-by-side double image results from ultrasound *refraction* as it passes through a tissue proximal to the structure of interest. This artifact often is seen in parasternal short-axis views of the aortic valve or left ventricle, where a second valve or left ventricle is "seen" medial to and partly overlapping the actual valve or left ventricle (Fig. 1–15). The explanation for this appearance is that the transmitted ultrasound beam is deviated from a straight path (the scan line) by refraction as it passes through a tissue near the transducer. When this refracted beam is reflected by the endocardium back to the transducer, the reflected signal is assumed to have originated from the scan line of the transmitted pulse (see Fig. 1–16) and thus is displayed on the image in the wrong location.

Range ambiguity occurs when echo signals from an earlier pulse cycle reach the transducer on the next "listen cycle" on that scan line, resulting in deep structures appearing closer to the transducer than their actual location. The appearance of an anatomically unexpected echo within a cardiac chamber often is due to range ambiguity (many sonographers call this artifact "Herbie"), as can be demonstrated by the disappearance or a change in position of this artifact when the depth setting (and pulse-repetition frequency) is changed (Fig. 1–17). Another type of

tomographic "slice" is narrow. In the far zone, however, strong reflectors at the edge of a larger beam will be superimposed on structures in the central zone of the beam even though signal intensity falls off at the edges of the beam. In addition, strong reflectors in side lobes of the beam will be displayed in the tomographic section corresponding to the main beam. This type of beam width artifact can result in an image "showing" a calcified aortic valve in the middle of the atrium in an apical four-chamber view (Fig. 1–14).

The second type of beam width artifact is a consequence of varying lateral resolution at different imaging depths. A point target appears as a line whose length depends on the beam char-

Figure 1–16. Schematic diagram showing the mechanism of a double-image artifact on 2D echocardiography. An ultrasound pulse reflected from point 1 of the left ventricular endocardium returns to the transducer and is shown appropriately as a bright spot in the correct position on the 2D image. Later in the scan, an ultrasound pulse is refracted by an intervening tissue so that the beam is reflected back to the transducer from point 2. However, this reflected signal is shown along the *transmission* scan line (point 3), since this is the presumed origin of the reflected signal.

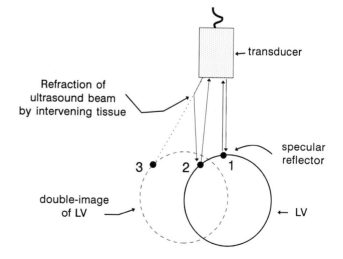

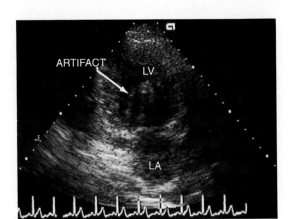

Figure 1–17. Example of range ambiguity artifact ("Herbie") in an apical two-chamber view appearing as an apparent "mass" in the left ventricle. This artifact disappeared with a change in PRF or depth.

range ambiguity is the appearance of an apparent second heart, deep to the actual heart—a double image on the vertical axis. This type of range ambiguity results from echos being re-reflected by a structure close to the transducer (such as a rib), being re-reflected by the cardiac structures and thus received at the transducer at a time *twice* normal. This artifact can be eliminated (or obscured) by decreasing the depth setting or adjusting the transducer position to a better acoustic window.

Electronic processing artifacts can be difficult to identify and vary from instrument to instrument. In addition, other types of artifacts besides those listed here have been described.

Doppler Echocardiography

Doppler Equation

Doppler echocardiography is based on the change in frequency of the backscattered signal

from small moving structures (red blood cells) intercepted by the ultrasound beam. A visual analogy is that Doppler scattering from blood is similar to scattering of light in fog, while imaging is similar to reflections from a mirror. A stationary target, if much smaller than the wavelength, will scatter ultrasound in all directions, with the frequency of the scattered signal being the same as the transmitted frequency when observed from any direction. A moving target, however, will backscatter ultrasound to the transducer so that the frequency observed when the target is moving *toward* the transducer is higher and the frequency observed when the target is moving *away* from the transducer is lower than the original transmitted frequency (Fig. 1–18). This Doppler effect is known to all of us from audio examples of the change in sound of a car horn, siren, or train whistle as it moves toward (higher pitch) and then away (lower pitch) from the observer.

The difference in frequency between the transmitted frequency (F_T) and the scattered signal received back at the transducer (F_S) is the Doppler shift:

$$\text{Doppler shift} = (F_S - F_T) \qquad (1.7)$$

Doppler shifts are in the audible range (0–20 kHz) for intracardiac velocities using diagnostic ultrasound transducer frequencies. The relationship between the Doppler shift and blood flow velocity (v, in m/s) is expressed in the Doppler equation:

$$v = \frac{c(F_S - F_T)}{2F_T\,(\cos\theta)} \qquad (1.8)$$

where c is the speed of sound in blood (1540 m/s), θ is the intercept angle between the ultrasound beam and the direction of blood flow, and 2 is a factor to correct for the transit time both *to* and *from* the scattering source (Fig. 1–19).

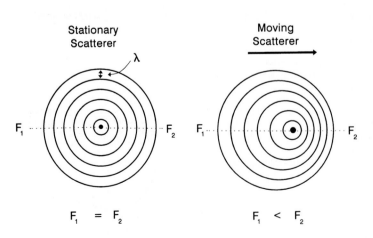

Stationary Scatterer   Moving Scatterer

$F_1 = F_2$ $F_1 < F_2$

Figure 1–18. The Doppler effect. A stationary scatterer (*left*) scatters ultrasound symmetrically in all directions with a wavelength λ identical to the transmitted wavelength and with the same frequency in all directions (no Doppler shift). A moving scatterer (*right*) also scatters ultrasound symmetrically in all directions. However, the frequency will be higher when the scatterer is moving toward the transducer (F_2) than when it is moving away from the transducer (F_1) due to the movement of the scatterer resulting in waves closer together in advance of and further apart behind the moving object.

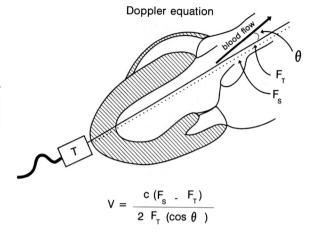

Figure 1–19. The Doppler equation. The velocity V of blood flow can be calculated from the speed of sound in blood c, transducer frequency F_T, backscattered frequency F_S, and the angle θ between the ultrasound beam and direction of blood flow.

$$V = \frac{c\,(F_S - F_T)}{2\,F_T\,(\cos \theta\ )}$$

Note that the intercept angle is critically important in calculation of blood flow velocity. The cosine of an angle of 0 or 180° (parallel toward or away from the transducer) is 1, allowing this term to be ignored when the ultrasound beam is parallel to blood flow direction. However, the cosine of 90° is *zero*, predicting that no Doppler shift will be recorded if blood flow is perpendicular to the ultrasound beam.

In cardiac applications of Doppler ultrasound, the ultrasound beam is aligned as parallel with the direction of blood flow as possible and $\cos \theta$ is assumed to be 1. Since the direction of intracardiac blood flow can be difficult to ascertain and is *not* predictable from the 2D image, especially with abnormal flow conditions, attempts to "correct" for intercept angle may result in significant errors in blood flow velocity calculation. Furthermore, even when blood flow direction is apparent in a 2D plane, direction in the elevational plane remains unknown. Deviation from a parallel intercept angle up to 20° results in only a 6 percent error in blood velocity calculation. However, a 60° intercept angle results in a 50 percent underestimation of flow velocity. The importance of intercept angle is particularly underlined in the setting of abnormal blood flow with high-velocity jets, such as in valvular stenosis. Note that peripheral vascular applications may use angle correction for the presumed direction of blood flow, but this approach is *not* acceptable for cardiac applications.

Spectral Analysis and Doppler Instrument Controls

When the backscattered signal is received at the transducer, the difference between the transmitted and backscattered signal is determined by "comparing" the two waveforms. This is a complex process, since multiple frequencies are present in the backscattered signal. The frequency content of this signal is analyzed by a process known as a *fast Fourier transform* (FFT) that derives the component frequencies of a complex signal. Alternate methods of frequency analysis may be employed, such as the analog Chirp-Z method.

The display generated by this frequency analysis is termed *spectral analysis* (Fig. 1–20). By convention, this display shows time on the horizontal axis, the zero baseline in the center, and frequency shifts toward the transducer above and frequency shifts away from the transducer

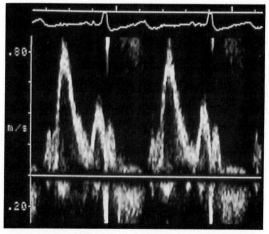

Figure 1–20. Example of a spectral Doppler display generated using a fast Fourier transform. Left ventricular inflow recorded from an apical approach is shown in the standard format. The baseline has been moved from the middle of the vertical axis to display the antegrade flow signal. Velocities toward the transducer are shown above and velocities away from the transducer below the baseline. The velocity range is determined by the Nyquist limit (½ PRF) with pulsed Doppler echo. Velocities are shown in shades of gray corresponding to the amplitude (decibels) of the signal.

below the baseline. Since multiple frequencies exist at any time point, each frequency signal is displayed as a pixel on the vertical axis, with the gray (or color) scale indicating the amplitude (or loudness) of each frequency shift component. The vertical axis represents frequency shift or, using the Doppler equation, blood flow velocity. Thus at each time point the spectral display shows (1) blood flow direction, (2) velocity (or frequency shift), and (3) signal amplitude. Each of these components is displayed at 4-ms intervals (or 250 times per second) simultaneous with data acquisition.

Doppler instrument controls typically include

1. Power output—the electrical energy transmitted to the transducer
2. Receiver gain—the degree of amplification of returning signals
3. "Wall" or high-pass filters—elimination of low-frequency Doppler shifts due to motion of myocardium and valves (allowing only the higher frequencies to pass the filter)
4. Baseline shift—moves the zero line toward the top or bottom of the display
5. Velocity range—expands or compresses the scale (within the limits for each Doppler modality, as discussed below)
6. Postprocessing options—these often include "reject," "compression," and "dynamic range" (i.e., number of shades of gray)

In addition, pulsed Doppler controls include

7. Sample volume depth
8. Sample volume length
9. The number of sample volumes (high pulse repetition frequency Doppler echo)

The Doppler modality may be integrated with 2D imaging for each of the three major Doppler modalities: continuous-wave, pulsed, and color Doppler flow imaging. However, while color Doppler flow imaging is nearly always conjoined with 2D imaging, pulsed Doppler signal quality is optimized when the 2D image is "frozen," and continuous-wave Doppler is optimized using a dedicated, small-footprint transducer with no 2D imaging.

Continuous-Wave Doppler Ultrasound

Continuous-wave Doppler utilizes two ultrasound crystals—one continuously transmits and one continuously receives the ultrasound signal. Thus the advantage of continuous-wave Doppler is that since sampling is continuous, very high frequency shifts (velocities) can be meas-

ured accurately. The potential disadvantage of this Doppler modality is that signals from the entire length of the ultrasound beam are recorded simultaneously. However, even with overlap of flow data, a given signal often is characteristic in timing, shape, and direction, allowing correct identification of the origin of the signal. In some cases, other methods (2D echo, color, pulsed Doppler) must be utilized to determine the depth of origin of the Doppler signal.

Continuous-wave Doppler optimally is performed with a dedicated, nonimaging transducer with two crystals. This type of transducer has a high signal-to-noise ratio and a small footprint, allowing it to fit into small acoustic windows (e.g., between ribs) and to be angled to obtain a parallel intercept angle between the ultrasound beam and the direction of blood flow. Use of a simultaneous imaging transducer may be helpful in some cases but signal quality may be poorer, angulation is more difficult, and the 2D image may distract the operator from optimizing the *flow* signal instead of the anatomic image (which may not coincide).

Careful technique yields a Doppler spectral signal that has a smooth contour with a well-defined edge and maximum velocity, as well as with clearly defined onset and end of flow. The audible signal is tonal and smooth. A continuous-wave Doppler velocity curve is "filled in" because lower-velocity signals proximal and distal to the point of maximum velocity also are recorded. Note that while the maximum frequency shift depends on the intercept angle between the Doppler beam and the flow of interest, amplitude (gray scale intensity), shape, and audible quality are less dependent on intercept angle. Thus a "good quality" Doppler signal may be recorded at a nonparallel intercept angle, resulting in underestimation of flow velocity. The empirical method to ensure a parallel intercept angle is to examine the flow of interest from multiple windows with transducer angulation both in the plane of view and in the elevational plane to discover the highest-frequency shift. The highest value found is then assumed to represent a parallel intercept angle.

Pulsed Doppler Ultrasound

Pulsed Doppler echocardiography allows sampling of blood flow velocities from a specific intracardiac depth. A pulse of ultrasound is transmitted, and then, after a time interval determined by the depth of interest, the transducer briefly "samples" the backscattered sig-

Pulsed Doppler Ultrasound

Figure 1–21. With pulsed Doppler ultrasound, the transducer goes through a repetitive cycle of transmission of an ultrasound pulse at the transducer frequency (F_T), a waiting period determined by the time needed for the signal to travel to and from the depth of interest, and a receive phase when the backscattered signals are sampled. The travel-time duration determines sample volume depth. The duration of the receive phase determines sample volume length.

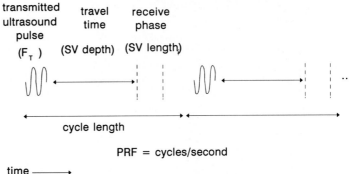

nals. This transducer cycle of transmit–wait–receive is repeated at an interval termed the *pulse-repetition frequency (PRF)* (Fig. 1–21). Since the "wait" interval is determined by the depth of interest—the time it takes ultrasound to travel to and from this depth—each transducer cycle is longer for increasing depths. Thus the pulse-repetition frequency also is depth-dependent, being high at shallow depths and low for more distant sites.

The depth of interest in pulsed Doppler echo is called the *sample volume* because signals from a small volume of blood are sampled, with the width and height of this volume dependent on beam geometry. The length of the sample volume can be varied by adjusting the length of the transducer "receive" interval. Typically, a sample volume length of 5 mm is used to balance range resolution and signal quality, but a longer (up to 20 mm) or shorter (1–2 mm) sample volume may be useful in specific cases.

Because pulsed Doppler echo repeatedly samples the returning signal, there is a maximum limit to the frequency shift (or velocity) that can be measured unambiguously. A waveform must be sampled at least twice in each cycle for accurate determination of wavelength. A visual analogy is a motion picture film of a moving wagon wheel. If the frame rate is at least twice as fast as the rotation of the wheel, the forward rotation of the wheel is "seen." If the frame rate and rotation speed are the same, the wheel will appear to stay still (Fig. 1–22). Even slower frame rates result in the appearance of the wheel going backward. This phenomenon of ambiguity in the speed and/or direction of the sampled signal is known as *signal aliasing*. In order for the frequency of an ultrasound waveform to be correctly identified, it must be sampled at least twice per wavelength. Thus, the maximum de-

tectable frequency shift (the *Nyquist limit*) is one-half the pulse repetition frequency.

If the velocity of interest exceeds the Nyquist limit by a small degree, signal aliasing is seen, with the signal cut off at the edge of the display and the "top" of the waveform appearing in the reverse channel (Fig. 1–23). In these cases, baseline shift (in effect an electronic "cut and paste") restores the expected velocity curve and allows calculation of maximum velocity. When velocities further exceed the Nyquist limit, repeat "wraparound" of the signal occurs first into the reverse channel, then back to the forward channel, and so on. Occasionally, the shape of the waveform can be discerned (Fig. 1–24), but more often only an undifferentiated band of velocity signals can be appreciated (Fig. 1–25). Note that nonlaminar disturbed flow and aliased laminar high-velocity flow will appear (and sound) similar on spectral analysis. Methods that can be employed to resolve aliasing include (1) using continuous-wave Doppler ultrasound, (2) increasing

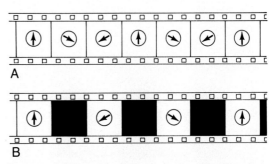

Figure 1–22. Visual analogy for aliasing. The filmstrip in (*A*) shows a wheel rotating clockwise. If the frame rate of the film (or sampling rate) is halved as in (*B*), the wheel will appear to move counterclockwise when the film is played. (*Reprinted with permission from Otto et al., Echocardiography 2:141, 1985.*)

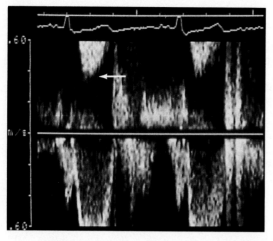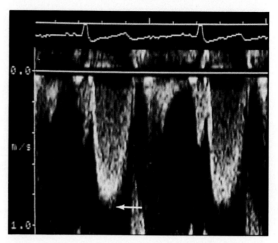

Figure 1–23. The velocity of left ventricular (LV) outflow recorded from an apical approach exceeds the Nyquist limit so that aliasing occurs (*left*) with the appearance of the peak of the outflow curve in the reverse channel (*arrow*). This degree of aliasing can be resolved by shifting the baseline (*right*), in effect an electronic "cut and paste" of the spectral display.

the PRF to the maximum for that depth, (3) increasing the number of sample volumes (high-PRF Doppler), (4) using a lower-frequency transducer, or (5) shifting the baseline. Continuous-wave Doppler is the most reliable approach to resolving aliasing for very high velocities. The other approaches are useful when the aliased velocity exceeds the Nyquist limit by a modest (twice) degree.

High-PRF Doppler is the deliberate use of range ambiguity to increase the maximum velocity that can be measured with pulsed Doppler echo (Fig. 1–26). When a pulse is sent out by the transducer, backscattered signals from the entire length of the ultrasound beam return to the transducer. Range resolution is achieved by sampling only those signals in the short time interval corresponding to the depth of interest. However, signals from exactly twice as far away as the sample volume will reach the transducer during the "receive" phase of the next cycle. Thus signals from "harmonics" at $2\times$, $3\times$, $4\times$, and so on, the sample volume depth, have the potential of being analyzed. Usually, signal strength is low and there are few moving scatterers at these depths, so that this range ambiguity can be ignored. If, instead, the sample volume is placed purposely at one-half the depth of

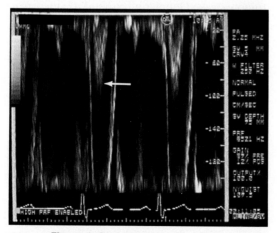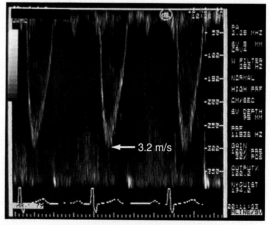

Figure 1–24. In this case, LV outflow velocity exceeds $2\times$ the Nyquist limit so that aliasing persists even after baseline shift (*left*). The "wrapped around" peak velocity is clearly seen (*arrow*). With high-PRF Doppler, the maximum velocity is resolved in this patient with a subaortic membrane (*right*).

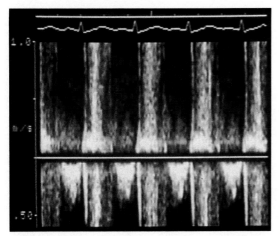

Figure 1–25. Severe aliasing results in a band of frequency shifts due to multiple "wraparounds" of the velocity signal. The maximum velocity cannot be reliably identified unless continuous-wave Doppler ultrasound is used.

interest, backscattered signals from this sample volume (SV_1) and a second sample volume (SV_2) twice as far away (i.e., the depth of interest) will return to the transducer during the "receive" phase (albeit one cycle later). This recording of the signal of interest at a higher PRF allows measurement of higher velocities without signal aliasing. An even higher PRF can be achieved by using additional (three or four) proximal sample volumes. Of course, the limitation of this approach is range ambiguity. The spectral analysis now includes signals from each of the sample volume depths. As with continuous-wave Doppler, the origin of the signal of interest must be determined based on ancillary data.

Color Flow Imaging

Doppler color flow imaging is based on the principles of pulsed Doppler echocardiography. Rather than one sample volume depth along the ultrasound beam, multiple sample volumes (or multigates) are evaluated along each sampling line (Fig. 1–27). By combining data from adjacent lines, a 2D image of intracardiac flow is generated.

Along each scan line, a pulse of ultrasound is transmitted, and then the backscattered signals are received from each "gate" or sample volume along that scan line. In order to calculate accurate velocity data, several bursts along each scan line are used—typically eight—which is known as the *burst length* (Fig. 1–28). The PRF, as for conventional pulsed Doppler, is determined by the maximum depth of the Doppler signals.

Since multiple signals are analyzed along each scan line, an audible output is not helpful. An accurate spectral analysis is not possible, since only a brief sample of the backscattered signal is available for analysis so that signals from the eight sampling lines at each depth are analyzed using mean velocity estimates. Velocities are displayed using a color scale, with flow toward the transducer in red and flow away from the transducer in blue, with the shade of color indicating velocity up to the Nyquist limit. The option of displaying "variance" allows an additional color (usually green) to be added to indicate that the mean velocity for each of the eight bursts had excessive variability. Variance can be seen with nonlaminar disturbed flow or with laminar aliased high-velocity flow.

This process is repeated for each adjacent scan line across the image plane. Each of these processes takes a finite amount of time depending on the speed of sound in tissue. Thus the rapidity with which this image can be updated (the frame rate) depends on the following (Table 1–4):

1. Sector scan width (number of scan lines)
2. Density of scan lines (number of scan lines)
3. Number of bursts per scan line (usually eight to achieve accurate velocity data)
4. Depth of sector (PRF)

During the examination, these variables may be adjusted to optimize frame rate or velocity resolution, as dictated by the specific clinical situation (Fig. 1–29).

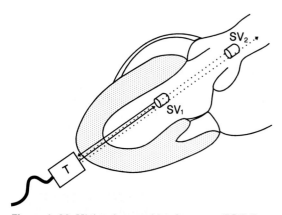

Figure 1–26. High pulse repetition frequency (PRF) Doppler ultrasound. High-PRF Doppler is based on the concept that with a given sample volume depth (SV_1), some ultrasound will penetrate beyond that depth. Backscattered signals from exactly twice the set depth (SV_2) will return to the transducer during the receive phase of the next cycle. Thus signals from both sample volume depths are recorded simultaneously.

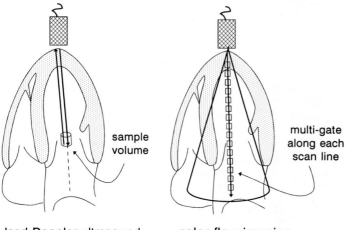

pulsed Doppler ultrasound   color flow imaging

Figure 1–27. With pulsed Doppler, the sample volume depth is determined by the time needed for ultrasound to travel to and from the depth of interest (*left*). With color flow imaging, multiple sample volume "gates" along each scan line are interrogated, with this process repeated for scan lines across the 2D image (*right*).

In addition to depth and sector scan width, color flow instrument settings typically include low-pass filter settings, gain, and power output. Most instruments provide several choices of the color "map" used to display velocity information. Velocity alone, velocity plus variance, or a power-mode display can be used. As for conventional pulsed Doppler, the zero baseline can be shifted and the PRF adjusted to vary the velocity range.

Doppler Artifacts

Spectral Doppler (Continuous Wave and Pulsed) (Table 1–5). Many Doppler artifacts are related to ultrasound physics and beam geometry, analogous to those seen with 2D imaging. Others are specific to Doppler echocardiography.

Clinically, the most important potential artifact is *velocity underestimation* due to a nonparallel intercept angle between the ultrasound beam and the direction of blood flow (Fig. 1–30). Velocity underestimation can occur with either pulsed or continuous-wave Doppler techniques and is of most concern when measuring high-velocity jets due to valve stenosis, regurgitation, or other intracardiac abnormalities. Attention to technical details with interrogation of the flow signal from multiple acoustic windows and careful angulation is needed to avoid velocity underestimation.

With pulsed Doppler echo, *signal aliasing* limits the maximum measurable velocity. If the examiner recognizes that aliasing has occurred, appropriate steps can be taken to resolve the velocity data. Aliasing can be due to nonlaminar disturbed flow as well as to high-velocity laminar flow.

Range ambiguity is inherent to continuous-wave Doppler but can occur with pulsed Doppler as well. With a sample volume positioned close to the transducer, strong signals from twice (or three times) the depth of the sample volume will be received in the next "receive" phase and

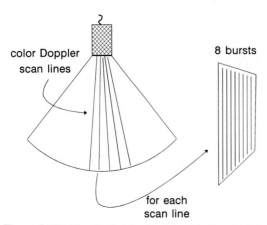

Figure 1–28. Along each color Doppler scan line, several (typically eight) bursts of ultrasound are transmitted and received to allow adequate velocity resolution.

TABLE 1–4. DETERMINANTS OF COLOR FRAME RATE

Depth (PRF)

Sector width

Number of sector lines

Number of ultrasound bursts along each sector line (Burst length)

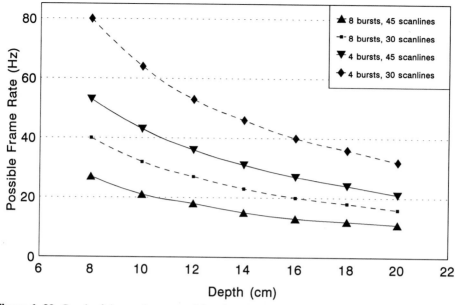

Figure 1–29. Graph of the maximum possible color Doppler frame rate (*y* axis) versus depth (*x* axis) for 8 or 4 bursts per scan line and 30 or 45 scan lines per frame. Note that at a depth of 16 cm, a frame rate 20 or greater can be achieved only by decreasing the burst length to 4 or narrowing the sector to 30 scan lines.

may be misinterpreted as originating from the set sample volume depth. For example, in an apical four-chamber view, placement of a sample volume in the left ventricular apex at half the

TABLE 1–5. SPECTRAL DOPPLER ECHO ARTIFACTS

ARTIFACT	RESULT
Nonparallel intercept angle	Underestimation of velocity
Aliasing	Inability to measure maximum velocity
Range ambiguity	Doppler signals from more than one depth along the ultrasound beam are recorded
Beam width	Overlap of Doppler signals from adjacent flows
Mirror image	Spectral display shows unidirectional flow both above and below the baseline
Electronic interference	Bandlike interference signal obscures Doppler flow
Transit-time effect	Change in the velocity of the ultrasound wave as it passes through a moving media results in slight overestimation of Doppler shifts

distance to the mitral annulus results in a spectral display showing the inflow signal across the mitral valve from the "second" sample volume depth. This phenomenon of range ambiguity is used constructively in the high-PRF Doppler mode.

Beam width (and side or grating lobes) affect the Doppler signal, as occurs with 2D imaging, resulting in superimposition of spatially adjacent flow signals on the spectral display. For example, left ventricular outflow and inflow may be seen on the same recording. Similarly, the left ventricular inflow signal may be seen superimposed on the aortic regurgitant jet (Fig. 1–31).

A *mirror-image artifact* is common with spectral analysis, appearing as a symmetric signal of somewhat less intensity than the actual flow signal in the opposite direction flow channel (Fig. 1–32). Mirroring often can be reduced or eliminated by decreasing the power output or gain of the instrument. Interrogation of a flow signal from a near-perpendicular angle can result in flow signals on both sides of the baseline that must be distinguished from artifact.

Electronic interference appears as a band of signals across the spectral display that may obscure the flow signals. These artifacts are due to inadequate shielding of other electric instruments in the examination environment and are particularly common during studies in the intensive-care unit or operating room.

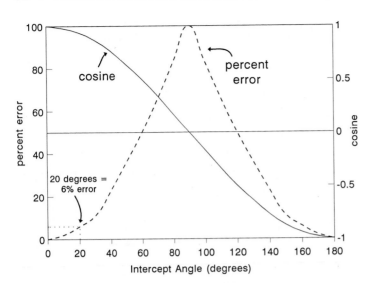

Figure 1–30. The importance of a parallel intercept angle between the ultrasound beam and direction of blood flow is shown. The cosine function (*solid line*) versus intercept angle (*horizontal axis*) varies from 1 at a parallel angle (0 and 180°) to 0 at a perpendicular angle (90°). The percentage error if cos θ is assumed to be 1 in the Doppler equation but, in fact, the intercept angle is *not* parallel; it varies from only 6 percent at a 20° angle to 50 percent at a 60° angle and 100 percent for perpendicular flows. At a perpendicular (90°) intercept angle, no blood flow velocities are recorded.

The *transit-time effect* is the change in propagation speed that occurs as an ultrasound wave passes through a moving medium, such as blood. This phenomenon is separate from the Doppler effect (which affects the backscattered signal) and is the basis of volume flow rate measurement with a transit-time flow probe. On the spectral display, the transit-time effect may result in a slight broadening of the velocity range at a given time point ("blurring" on the vertical axis) which potentially can result in slight overestimation of velocity. Some investigators argue that this should not happen, since the ultrasound signal passes through the moving blood in both directions—out (adding) and back (subtracting). In either case, this effect is insignificant clinically.

Color Doppler Flow Imaging (Table 1–6). Color flow artifacts again relate to the physics of 2D and Doppler flow image generation. *Shadowing* may be prominent distal to strong reflectors with absence of both 2D and flow data within the acoustic shadow.

Ghosting is the appearance of brief (usually 1–2 frames) large color patterns that overlay anatomic structures and do not correspond to underlying flow patterns. This artifact is caused by strong moving reflectors (such as prosthetic valve disks). Typically, this artifact is a uniform red or blue color, but it may be coded with a variance scale depending on the instrument. It is inconsistent from beat to beat.

Color Doppler gain settings have a dramatic effect on the color flow image. Extensive gain settings result in a uniform speckled pattern

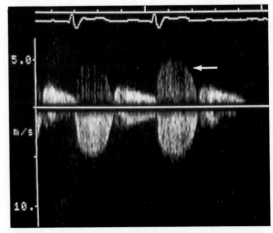

Figure 1–31. Doppler beam width artifact is demonstrated by the simultaneous display of superimposed aortic regurgitation (AR) and LV inflow curves.

Figure 1–32. A mirror-image Doppler artifact with apparent weaker flow signals in the reverse channel (*arrow*).

TABLE 1–6. COLOR DOPPLER ARTIFACTS

ARTIFACT	APPEARANCE
Shadowing	Absence of flow signal distal to strong reflector
Ghosting	Brief flashes of color that overlay anatomic structures and do not correlate with flow patterns
Background noise	Speckled color pattern over 2D sector due to excessive gain
Underestimation of flow signal	Loss of true flow signals due to inadequate gain
Intercept angle	Change in color (or absence at 90°) due to the angle between the flowstream and ultrasound beam across the image plane
Aliasing	"Wraparound" of color display results in a "variance" display even for laminar flow.
Electronic interference	Linear color artifacts or complex artifacts across the 2D image

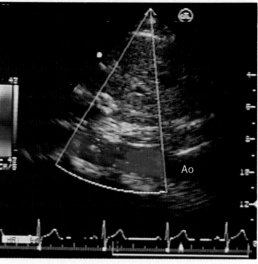

Figure 1–33. Color flow in the proximal abdominal aorta showing the importance of intercept angle on the color display. Although flow in systole goes from right to left across the image plane, flow on the right side of the image appears red (since flow is directed toward the transducer) and flow on the left side of the image appears blue (since flow is directed away from the transducer). In the center, where the direction of flow is perpendicular to the ultrasound beam, no color signal (i.e., black) is seen.

across the 2D image plane due to random *background noise.* Conversely, too low a gain setting results in a smaller displayed flow area than is actually present, an effect colloquially known as "dial-a-jet." Most experienced echocardiographers recommend setting the gain level just below the level of random background noise to optimize the flow signal.

As for any Doppler technique, the *intercept angle* between the ultrasound beam and direction of blood flow *for each scan line* affects the color display in terms of both direction and velocity. Thus a uniform flow velocity traversing the image plane may appear red (toward the transducer) at one side of the sector and blue (away from the transducer) at the other edge of the sector, with a black area in the center where the flow direction is perpendicular to the ultrasound beam (Fig. 1–33).

Flow velocities that exceed the Nyquist limit at any given depth result in *signal aliasing.* Aliasing on color flow results in "wraparound" of the velocity signal, similar to that seen on a spectral display, so that an aliased velocity toward the transducer (should be red) will appear to be trav-

eling away from the transducer (displayed in blue). Aliasing on color flow images is very common; for example, the left ventricular inflow stream appears red and then blue (due to aliasing) in the apical view (Fig. 1–34). Color aliasing can be used to advantage to quantitate flow based on the proximal isovelocity surface area method described in Chapter 10. In some cases, aliasing results in a variance display (due to an apparent range of velocities at that site), emphasizing that a variance display does not always indicate disturbed flow.

Electronic interference on color flow displays is instrument-dependent. As with other electric interference artifacts, it is most likely to occur in settings where numerous other instruments or devices are in use (operating room, intensive-care unit). Sometimes it appears as a linear multicolored band on the image along a few scan lines; sometimes more complex patterns are seen.

RECORDING DEVICES

There are several reasons to record the echocardiographic examination, including (1) later review and/or quantitation, (2) documentation, (3) communication with the patient, referring

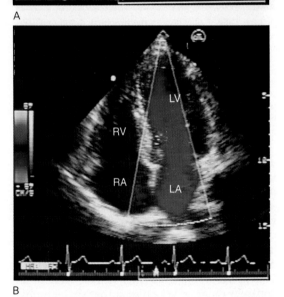

A

B

Figure 1–34. (*A*) A normal LV inflow signal shows aliasing from red to blue at the mitral annulus level, since the velocity exceeds the Nyquist limit of 52 cm/s. (*B*) With an increase in the velocity range (to 69 cm/s), aliasing no longer occurs and the *same* normal flow now appears a uniform red color.

Video recordings are a useful method for recording data with the advantage that a large number of sequential frames can be recorded and replayed in "real time" at low cost. On videotape, the frame rate is 30 frames per second, with each frame consisting of two interlaced "fields" of information. One disadvantage of videotape is that when the tape is stopped, only one field is displayed, resulting in degradation of image quality. Other limitations of videotape are the frame rate (which is less than the achievable 2D frame rate with some ultrasound systems), image degradation in the digital-to-analog recording mode, and the difficulty of rapid access to different data on the same videotape. Recording video data on optical discs may obviate some of these limitations.

Digital recording and storage of echocardiographic data have the advantages of high image quality, rapid access to the data in any order, and the ability to manipulate the data in terms of image processing (such as contrast) and display formats (such as a cine-loop side-by-side display). The major limitation of digital storage is the immense amount of data contained in an echocardiographic examination (10 minutes of videotape at 30 frames per second = 18,000 image frames), which requires a combination of very careful editing of the recorded data, large data storage systems, and compression of the image data (without loss of image quality).

In addition, recording the 3D orientation of the acquired image plane would be ideal, although currently this is not incorporated into clinical echocardiographic instruments.

EXAMINATION TECHNIQUE, EDUCATION, AND TRAINING

The echocardiographic examination is performed by a trained cardiac sonographer under the supervision of a qualified physician. The physician may perform all or part of the examination as well. Guidelines and recommendations for education and training in echocardiography for both sonographers and physicians have been published, as referenced in Chapter 3.

At the time of a transthoracic echocardiographic examination, the patient is positioned comfortably for each view in either a left lateral decubitus or supine position. ECG electrodes are attached for display of a single lead (usually lead II) on the instrument display to aid in timing cardiac events. Specially designed echocardiographic examination stretchers provide apical

physician, and other consultants (e.g., cardiac surgeons), (4) comparison with any future studies in that patient, and (5) clinical research. Since the entire examination may be quite lengthy, depending on the specific findings in each patient, only selected segments of the examination are recorded.

Recordings on paper can be made of M-mode, spectral Doppler, or single 2D or color flow images using a variety of page-printing devices. These recordings are of limited utility for 2D and color flow because only a single frame of information is displayed.

cutouts for optimal transducer positioning at the apex. The transducer is applied to the chest and upper abdomen using a water-soluble gel to obtain good contact without intervening air. The time needed to perform an echocardiographic examination depends on the specific clinical situation—from a few minutes in a critically ill patient to document cardiac tamponade to up to 1½ to 2 hours to quantitate multiple lesions in a patient with complex valvular or congenital heart disease.

An echocardiographic examination is a technically demanding procedure, and most examiners find a significant learning curve in their ability to obtain diagnostic data. The specific examination approaches are detailed in Chapter 2 (for normal anatomy and flows) and throughout this book for specific disease states. The examination also includes appropriate use of the echocardiographic data in patient management, as discussed in Chapter 3 and throughout the text.

BIOEFFECTS AND SAFETY

The use of ultrasound for diagnostic cardiac imaging has no known adverse biologic effects. However, ultrasound waves do have the potential to cause significant bioeffects depending on the intensity of exposure. Thus the physician and cardiac sonographer must be aware of potential bioeffects in assessing the overall safety of the procedure.

Bioeffects

Ultrasound bioeffects can be divided into three basic categories:

1. Thermal effects
2. Cavitation
3. Other (such as torque forces and microstreaming)

Thermal effects predominate with diagnostic ultrasound examinations. As the ultrasound wave passes through a tissue, heating occurs due to absorption of the mechanical energy of the sound wave. The rate of increase in temperature dT/dt depends on the absorption coefficient of the tissue for a given frequency α, the density ρ, and specific heat C_m of the tissue and the intensity I of ultrasound exposure:

$$dT/dt = 2\alpha I/\rho C_m \qquad (1.9)$$

Increases in temperature due to ultrasound exposure are offset by heat loss due to blood flow through the tissue (convective loss) and heat diffusion. More dense tissues (such as bone) heat more rapidly than less dense tissue (such as fat). However, the actual elevation in temperature for a specific tissue is difficult to predict both because of the complexity of the entire biologic system and because it is difficult to assess accurately the intensity of exposure. The rise in temperature in soft tissue with a focused 2- to 5-MHz beam at a typical power output is in the range of 0 to 0.6°C/minute of ultrasound exposure. Since transmission is intermittent, exposure time is far less than total study time. In addition, the actual degree of tissue heating depends on transducer frequency, focus, power output, depth, perfusion, and tissue density.

Cavitation is the creation or vibration of small gas-filled bodies by the ultrasound beam. Cavitation tends to occur only with higher-intensity exposures. Microbubbles resonate (expand and decrease in size) depending on their dimension in relation to the sound wave with a resonance frequency F_o defined by the radius of the microbubble (R_o in microns):

$$F_o = 3260/R_o \qquad (1.10)$$

Microbubbles also can be created by ultrasound by expansion of small cavitation nuclei. Cavitation has not been shown to occur with ultrasound exposure due to diagnostic ultrasound systems.

Other ultrasound bioeffects occur only with much higher exposures than occur with diagnostic ultrasound. These effects include microstreaming, torque forces, and other complex biologic effects.

Safety

The intensity I of ultrasound exposure can be expressed in several ways. The most commonly used unit of measure of intensity is power per area, where power is energy over a specific time interval:

$$I = \text{energy (joules)/time (seconds)/area (cm}^2) \qquad (1.11)$$
$$= \text{watt/cm}^2$$

The maximum overall intensity is then described as the highest exposure within the beam (spatial peak) averaged over the period of exposure (temporal average) and is known as the *spatial peak temporal average (SPTA) intensity*. Another common measure is the *spatial peak pulse average (SPPA)*, defined as the average pulse intensity at the spatial location where the pulse intensity is maximum.

A major limitation of measuring the intensity of ultrasound exposure is that while measuring the *output* of the transducer is straightforward (e.g., in a water bath), estimating the actual tissue *exposure* is more difficult due to attenuation and other interactions with the tissue. Furthermore, tissue exposure is limited to transmission periods only and the time the ultrasound beam dwells at a specific point, both of which are considerably shorter than the total examination time.

The American Institute of Ultrasound in Medicine (AIUM) has proposed guidelines for limits *below* which ultrasound clearly has been demonstrated to be safe. These guidelines include

1. A diagnostic exposure that produces a 1°C or less temperature elevation above normal
2. An exposure intensity less than 100 mW/cm² SPTA for unfocused and less than 1 W/cm² for focused ultrasound beams

Current diagnostic ultrasound systems have outputs ranging from 10 mW/cm² (SPTA) or 250 W/cm² (SPPA) for 2D sector scanning to as high as 1000 mW/cm² (SPTA) or 100 W/cm² (SPPA) for pulsed Doppler ultrasound. There has been no evidence to date to suggest adverse effects of echocardiography at these ultrasonic outputs. Clearly, further characterization of actual tissue exposures and ongoing careful epidemiologic surveys are needed to ensure that diagnostic uses of ultrasound are safe.

While any biologic effect is likely to be small, a prudent approach is to

1. Perform echocardiography only when indicated clinically (see Chap. 3), as part of an approved research protocol, or in appropriate teaching settings.
2. Know the power output and exposure intensity of different modalities (imaging and Doppler) of each instrument.
3. Limit the power output and exposure time as much as possible within the constraints of acquiring the necessary information.
4. Keep up to date on any new scientific findings or data relating to possible adverse effects.

SUGGESTED READING

1. Kremkau FW: Diagnostic Ultrasound: Principles and Instruments (ed 4). Philadelphia, WB Saunders Co, 1993.
Textbook of ultrasound emphasizing basic principles.

2. Geiser EA: Echocardiography: physics and instrumentation. *In* Marcus ML, Skorton DJ, Schelbert HR, Wolf GL (eds): Cardiac Imaging: A Companion to Braunwald's Heart Disease. Philadelphia, WB Saunders Co, 1991.
Advanced chapter on echocardiographic instrumentation with excellent diagrams.

3. Wells PNT (ed): Scientific Basis of Medical Imaging. Edinburgh, Churchill-Livingston, 1982.
Chapter by P.N.T. Wells on ultrasonic imaging provides a concise review of basic principles of ultrasound physics and basic instrumentation.

4. McDicken WN: Diagnostic Ultrasonics: Principles and Use of Instruments (ed 2). New York, John Wiley & Sons, 1981.
Elementary textbook of basic ultrasound principles.

5. Powis RL, Schwartz RA: Practical Doppler Ultrasound for the Clinician. Baltimore, Williams & Williams, 1991.
Detailed but understandable book describing Doppler ultrasound techniques. An introduction to basic ultrasound principles and basic fluid dynamics also is provided.

6. Kremkau FW: Doppler Ultrasound: Principles and Instruments. Philadelphia, WB Saunders Co, 1990.
Detailed discussion of basic principles of ultrasound, hemodynamics, Doppler instruments, and spectral analysis. Excellent discussion of bioeffects and safety of diagnostic ultrasound. Numerous review questions at the end of each chapter, plus a comprehensive 120-question exam (with answers). Ninety references.

7. Hatle L, Angelsen B: Doppler Ultrasound in Cardiology: Physical Principles and Clinical Applications (ed 2). Philadelphia, Lea & Febiger, 1985.
Excellent and detailed presentation of the Doppler effect, the physics of blood flow, Doppler instrumentation, and clinical applications of Doppler echocardiography.

8. Otto CM, Pearlman AS: Measurement of high velocities using pulsed Doppler echocardiography. Echocardiography 1985; 2:141–152.
Review of the use of high pulse repetition frequency Doppler ultrasound for measuring high-velocity intracardiac flow. Emphasizes clinical utility of this approach in mitral stenosis, left ventricular outflow tract flows, and other situations in which partial range resolution is desirable. Limitations of high PRF Doppler in higher-velocity flows (such as aortic stenosis) are discussed.

9. Harris RA, Follett DH, Halliwell M, Wells PNT: Ultimate limits in ultrasonic imaging resolution. Ultrasound Med Biol 1991; 17:547–558.
Detailed review on ultrasound image resolution for readers interested in the technical details of this problem; sixty-one references.

10. Skorton DJ, Collins SM, Greenleaf JF, Meltzer RS, et al: Ultrasound bioeffects and regulatory issues: An introduction for the echocardiographer. J Am Soc Echocardiogr 1988; 1:240–251.
Excellent review of bioeffects and safety prepared by the ASE Committee on Physics and Instrumentation.

11. American Institute of Ultrasound in Medicine Bioeffects Report: Bioeffects consideration for the safety of diagnostic ultrasound. J Ultrasound Med 1988; 7:S1–S38.
AIUM Bioeffects Committee report of ultrasound safety and bioeffects. Detailed document with AIUM safety guidelines

and discussion of thermal mechanisms, cavitation effects, epidemiologic studies, and in vivo biologic effects.

12. Miller DL: Update on safety of diagnostic ultrasonography. J Clin Ultrasound 1991; 19:531–540.
Readable review of ultrasound bioeffects; thirty-nine references.

13. AMA Council on Scientific Affairs: Medical diagnostic ultrasound instrumentation and clinical interpretation: Report of the Ultrasonography Task Force. JAMA 1991; 265:1155–1159.
AMA Council on Scientific Affairs' report on diagnostic ul-

trasound. Review of basic principles of ultrasound with emphasis on ultrasound artifacts.

14. Barnett SB, Kossoff G, Edwards MJ: Is diagnostic ultrasound safe? Current international consensus on the thermal mechanism. Med J Aust 1994; 160:33–37.
Review of the thermal effects of diagnostic ultrasound which concludes that there is no evidence of adverse effects for exposures resulting in temperatures less than 38.5° C.

15. Goldstein A: Overview of the physics of ultrasound. Radiographics 1993; 13:701–704.
Brief review of ultrasound physics for 2D and Doppler modalities.

CHAPTER 2

NORMAL CARDIAC ANATOMY, TOMOGRAPHIC VIEWS, AND INTRACARDIAC FLOW PATTERNS

BASIC IMAGING PRINCIPLES

Tomographic Imaging

Echocardiography provides tomographic images of cardiac structures and blood flow, analogous to a thin "slice" through the heart. In contrast, angiographic techniques provide silhouette-type images; that is, structures at different distances from the imaging device are superimposed onto a single two-dimensional (2D) image. Each approach has specific advantages and disadvantages (Table 2–1). For example, a silhouette technique allows definition of the entire length of a coronary artery in a single image even though the vessel transverses numerous tomographic planes. Conversely, a single-plane right anterior oblique angiogram of the left ventricle allows assessment of regional wall motion only for those segments which form the edge of the silhouette. The lateral wall is superimposed on the opacified chamber and cannot be evaluated.

Tomographic images provide detailed anatomic data in a given image plane. However, complete evaluation of the cardiac chambers and valves requires integration of information from multiple tomographic images. Small structures that transverse numerous tomographic planes (such as the coronary arteries) are difficult to evaluate fully. Another potential problem with tomographic imaging is movement of the heart with respiration and during the cardiac cycle. Respiratory variation in cardiac location is recognized easily by its timing, but movement of the heart during the cardiac cycle is more problematic because it may not be obvious on the 2D image. Cardiac motion relative to surrounding structures is described in three-dimensions as

1. Translation (movement of the heart as a whole in the chest)
2. Rotation (circular motion around the long axis of the left ventricle)

3. Torsion (unequal rotational motion at the apex versus the base of the left ventricle)

Even if the 2D image plane is fixed in position, the location of underlying structures may vary between systole and diastole. For example, in the apical four-chamber view, adjacent segments (which may be supplied by different coronary arteries) of the left ventricle may be seen in systole versus diastole.

Nomenclature of Standard Views
(Table 2–2)

Each tomographic image is defined by its acoustic *window* (the position of the transducer) and *view* (the image plane). The standard three orthogonal echocardiographic image planes are determined by the axis of the heart itself (with the left ventricle as the major point of reference) rather than by skeletal or external body landmarks (Fig. 2–1):

1. *Long-axis plane:* Parallel to the long axis of the left ventricle and defined as an imaginary line drawn through the left ventricular apex and the center of the left ventricular base
2. *Short-axis plane:* Perpendicular to the long-axis view, resulting in circular cross-sectional views of the left ventricle
3. *Four-chamber plane:* Perpendicular to both long- and short-axis views, resulting in an image plane from the apex to the base intersecting the right and left ventricles and atria

Acoustic windows are transducer positions that allow ultrasound access to the cardiac structures. The bony thoracic cage and adjacent air-filled lung limit the possible acoustic windows, making patient positioning and sonographer experience critical factors in obtaining diagnostic images. Transthoracic images typically are obtained from parasternal, apical, subcostal, and suprasternal notch acoustic windows. Transesophageal images are obtained from the esoph-

TABLE 2–1. TOMOGRAPHIC VERSUS SILHOUETTE IMAGING

	TOMOGRAPHIC	SILHOUETTE
Advantages	Detailed anatomic information in a single image plane	Imaging of an entire 3D structure (such as a coronary artery)
Disadvantages	Cardiac motion Need to integrate data from multiple planes	Superimposition of structures

TABLE 2–2. ECHO IMAGE ORIENTATION NOMENCLATURE

Window (Transducer Location)

Parasternal
Apical
Subcostal
Suprasternal
Transesophageal
Transgastric

Image Planes

Transthoracic
   Long-axis
   Short-axis
   Four-chamber
Transesophageal
   Longitudinal
   Transverse

agus (high, middle, low) and from a transgastric position. The transducer motions used to obtain the desired view are described as follows (Figs. 2–2 and 2–3):

1. *Movement* of the transducer to a different position on the chest or in the esophagus
2. *Tilting or pointing* the transducer with a rocking motion to image different structures in the same tomographic plane
3. *Angulation* of the transducer from side to side to obtain different tomographic planes somewhat parallel to the original image plane

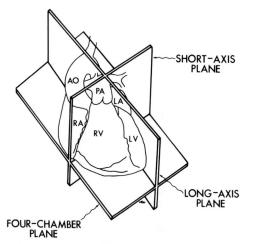

Figure 2–1. Diagram of the three orthogonal imaging planes used in 2D echocardiography. (*Used by permission of the American Society of Echocardiography: Report of the American Society of Echocardiography Committee on Nomenclature and Standards in Two-Dimensional Echocardiography. Circulation 62:212–222, 1980.*)

TILT

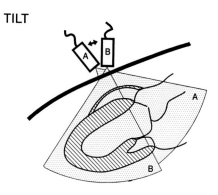

ANGLE

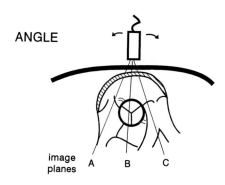

ROTATE

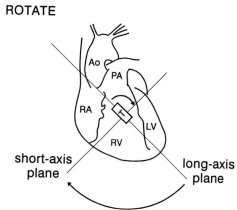

Figure 2–2. Transducer motion at a given acoustic window using the example of a left parasternal transducer position. *Tilt:* The transducer is "rocked" to provide images (*A* or *B*) in the *same* tomographic plane. *Angle:* Different image planes (perpendicular to the plane of the figure at lines *A*, *B*, and *C*) are obtained by angulation of the transducer. *Rotation:* The transducer is "twisted" with a circular motion to provide a different image plane while maintaining the same orientation between the transducer itself and the chest wall.

4. *Rotation* of the image plane at a single position to obtain intersecting tomographic planes either by manual motion of the transducer (on transthoracic imaging) or electronically (with a multiplane transesophageal transducer).

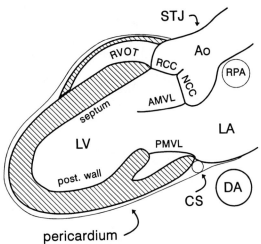

Figure 2–3. Schematic diagram of the parasternal long-axis view in diastole showing the aortic root (Ao), sinotubular junction (STJ), closed right coronary and noncoronary cusps of the aortic valve (RCC and NCC), the open anterior and posterior mitral valve leaflets (AMVL and PMVL), and the left ventricular septum and posterior wall. The medial papillary muscle has been shown for reference, although slight medial angulation is needed to visualize this structure in the long-axis view. The right ventricular outflow tract (RVOT) is anterior, while the coronary sinus (CS) in the atrioventricular groove and the descending aorta (DA) are seen posteriorly. The right pulmonary artery (RPA) lies posterior to the ascending aorta. The position of the pericardium is indicated by the thin line.

Image Orientation

Although some controversy persists regarding appropriate orientation of echocardiographic images, most laboratories follow the American Society of Echocardiography recommendations. The transducer position (narrowest portion of the sector scan) is shown at the top of the screen so that structures nearer to the transducer are at the top and structures farther from the transducer are at the bottom of the screen. This orientation aids in prompt recognition of ultrasound artifacts, shadowing, and reverberations, since the display of the origin of the ultrasound signal is the same for all acoustic windows and image planes.

The lateral (in short-axis views) and superior (in long-axis views) cardiac structures are displayed on the right side of the screen, which is similar to the format used for other tomographic imaging techniques. Short-axis views can be thought of as the observer looking from the apex toward the cardiac base; long-axis views, as the observer looking from the left toward the right side of the heart. The four-chamber plane is displayed with lateral structures on the right side

of the screen and medial structures on the left side (as for the short-axis view).

Technical Quality

Image quality is dependent on the degree of ultrasound tissue penetration as well as on the instrument used, transducer frequency, instrument settings, and sonographer's skill. Acoustic access to the cardiac structures is determined by body habitus, specifically how the heart is positioned in the chest relative to the lungs and chest wall. Conditions that increase the separation between the transducer and the cardiac structures (e.g., adipose tissue), decrease ultrasound penetration (e.g., scar tissue), or interpose air-containing tissues between the transducer and the heart (e.g., chronic lung disease, immediately after cardiac surgery) lead to poor image quality. Transesophageal images tend to show better structure definition because of greater ultrasound penetration given the shorter distance between the transducer and the cardiac structures, the use of a higher-frequency transducer, and the absence of interposed lung. On transthoracic studies, optimal patient positioning for each acoustic window brings the cardiac structures against the chest wall. In addition, respiratory variation can be used to the sonographer's advantage by having the patient suspend respiration briefly in the respiratory phase, which yields the best image quality. Unfortunately, even with careful attention to examination technique, echocardiographic images remain suboptimal in some patients.

Echocardiographic Image Interpretation

The physician uses the tomographic echocardiographic images to build a mental three-dimensional (3D) reconstruction of the cardiac chambers and valves. To do this, an understanding of image planes and orientation and the technical aspects of image acquisition (e.g., in recognizing artifacts) is needed along with a detailed knowledge of cardiac anatomy. (A list of anatomic terminology is shown in Table 2–3.) Recording images as the tomographic plane is moved between standard image planes is important for this analysis and ensures that abnormalities that lie outside or between our arbitrary "standard" views are not missed. In complex cases, the physician may need to perform part of the study to appreciate the 3D relationship of the different image planes. Information obtained

TABLE 2–3. TERMINOLOGY FOR NORMAL ECHOCARDIOGRAPHIC ANATOMY

Aortic root	Sinuses of Valsalva Sinotubular junction Coronary ostia
Aortic valve	Right, left, and noncoronary cusps Nodules of Arantius Lambl's excrescence
Mitral valve	Anterior and posterior leaflets Chordae (primary, secondary, tertiary; basal and marginal) Commissures (medial and lateral)
Left ventricle	Wall segments (see Chap. 6) Septum, free wall Base, apex Medial and lateral papillary muscles
Right ventricle	Inflow segment Moderator band Outflow tract (conus) Supraventricular crest Anterior, posterior, and conus papillary muscles
Tricuspid valve	Anterior, septal, and posterior leaflets Chordae Commissures
Right atrium	Right atrial appendage SVC, IVC junctions Valve of IVC (Chiari network) Crista terminalis Fossa ovalis Patent foramen ovale

Left atrium	Left atrial appendage
	Superior and inferior left pulmonary
	  veins
	Superior and inferior right pulmonary
	  veins
	Ridge at junction of left atrial
	  appendage and left superior
	  pulmonary vein

Pericardium	Oblique sinus Transverse sinus

TABLE 2–4. TRANSTHORACIC ECHO: VIEWS FOR SPECIFIC CARDIAC STRUCTURES

ANATOMIC STRUCTURES	BEST VIEWS
Aortic valve	Parasternal long-axis (PLAX) Parasternal short-axis (PSAX) Apical long-axis Anteriorly angulated apical four-chamber
Mitral valve (MV)	PLAX PSAX–mitral valve level Apical four-chamber Apical long-axis
Pulmonic valve	PSAX (Aortic valve level) RV outflow Subcostal short-axis (Aortic valve level)
Tricuspid valve	Right ventricular (RV) inflow Apical four-chamber Subcostal four-chamber and short-axis

Left ventricle (LV)	PLAX
	PSAX
	Apical four-chamber, two-
	  chamber, long-axis
	Subcostal four-chamber and
	  short-axis

Right ventricle	PLAX (RV outflow tract only) RV inflow PSAX (MV and LV levels) Apical four-chamber Subcostal four-chamber
Left atrium	PLAX PSAX Apical four-chamber, two- chamber, long-axis Subcostal 4-chamber
Right atrium	PSAX (Aortic valve level) Apical four-chamber Subcostal four-chamber and short-axis

Aorta
  Ascending
	High parasternal and standard
	  parasternal long-axis

Arch	Suprasternal notch
Descending thoracic	Suprasternal notch Parasternal with angulation Apical two-chamber with modification Subcostal
Interatrial septum	Parasternal short-axis Subcostal four-chamber

Coronary sinus	Parasternal long-axis to RV
	  inflow view (sweep)
	Apical four-chamber angulated
	  posteriorly

from anatomic 2D imaging then is integrated with physiologic Doppler data and clinical information in the final echocardiographic interpretation.

TRANSTHORACIC TOMOGRAPHIC VIEWS

The normal anatomy as seen on echocardiography is described below for each tomographic view. The best views for specific cardiac structures are indicated in Table 2–4, normal changes with aging are shown in Table 2–5, and normal dimensions are shown in Table 2–6.

Parasternal Window

Long-Axis Views (Figs. 2–3 and 2–4)

With the patient in a left lateral decubitus position and the transducer in the left 3rd or 4th intercostal space, adjacent to the sternum, a long-axis view of the heart is obtained which bisects the long axis of both aortic and mitral valves. The patient position may need adjustment between a steep left lateral and nearly supine position based on the images obtained in each subject.

The *aortic root*, sinuses of Valsalva, sinotubular junction, and proximal 3 to 4 cm of the ascending aorta are seen in long axis. Further segments of the ascending aorta may be visualized by moving the transducer cephalad one or two interspaces. The upper limit of normal for aortic root dimensions in adults is 1.6 cm/m^2 at the annulus and 2.1 cm/m^2 at the aortic leaflet tips in systole.

In the long-axis view, the right coronary cusp of the *aortic valve* is anterior and the noncoronary cusp is posterior (the left coronary cusp is lateral to the image plane). In systole, the thin aortic leaflets open widely, assuming a parallel orientation to the aortic walls. In diastole, the leaflets are closed, with a small obtuse closure angle between the two leaflets. The leaflets appear linear from the closure line to the aortic annulus due to the hemicylindrical shape of the closed leaflets (linear along the length of the cylinder, curved along its short axis). In normal

young individuals, the leaflets are so thin that only the apposed portions at the leaflets' closure line are seen. The 3D anatomy of the attachment line of the aortic leaflets to the aortic root is shaped like a crown with the three commissures attached near the tops of the sinuses of Valsalva and the midportion of each leaflet attached near the base of each sinus (Fig. 2–5). This attachment line often is referred to as the aortic "annulus," although there are no distinct tissue characteristics of this attachment zone. Note that there is fibrous continuity between the aortic root and the anterior mitral leaflet. The absence of intervening myocardium between aortic and mitral valves helps identify the anatomic left ventricle in complex congenital disease.

The anterior and posterior *mitral valve* leaflets appear thin and uniform in echogenicity, with chordal attachments leading toward the medial (or posteromedial) papillary muscle seen in the long-axis view, although the papillary muscle itself is slightly medial to the long-axis plane. The anterior mitral leaflet is longer than the posterior leaflet but has a smaller annular length so that the surface areas of the two leaflets are similar (Fig. 2–6). As the mitral leaflets open in diastole, the tips separate and the anterior leaflet abuts or comes very close to the ventricular septum. In systole, the leaflets coapt, with some overlap between the leaflets (apposition zone) and a slightly obtuse (>180°) angle relative to the mitral annulus plane. The chordae normally remain posterior to the plane of leaflet coaptation in systole. However, some normal individuals have systolic anterior motion of the chordae, due to mild redundancy of chordal tissue, that is not associated with hemodynamic abnormalities. This must be distinguished from the pathologic systolic anterior motion of the mitral leaflets seen in hypertrophic obstructive cardiomyopathy. The mitral annulus (the attachment between the mitral leaflets, left atrium, and left ventricle) is an anatomically well-defined fibrous structure with an elliptical shape. The long-axis view bisects the minor axis of the mitral annulus. (The major axis is seen in the apical four-chamber view.)

The *left atrium* is seen posterior to and, normally, is similar in anteroposterior dimension to the aortic root. The right pulmonary artery lies between the aortic root and superior aspect of the left atrium but may not be well seen on transthoracic images. The *coronary sinus* is seen in the atrioventricular groove posterior to the mitral annulus. Dilation of the coronary sinus due to a persistent left superior vena cava (which can be confirmed by echo-contrast injection in a left arm vein) is an occasional incidental finding

TABLE 2–5. ECHOCARDIOGRAPHIC FINDINGS IN NORMAL ELDERLY PATIENTS

2D echo	Left and right atrial enlargement Mitral annular calcification Aortic valve fibrosis and calcification (usually without significant stenosis) Tortuosity of the aorta Prominent angle between the base of the septum and aortic root appearing as a "septal knuckle"
Doppler echo	LV inflow pattern with $E < A$ and prolonged deceleration slope Pulmonary vein (LA inflow) pattern with reduced antegrade diastolic flow and prominent A wave reversal of flow

TABLE 2–6. SELECTED NORMAL ECHOCARDIOGRAPHIC DIMENSIONS IN ADULTS

	RANGE	RANGE INDEXED TO BSA	UPPER LIMIT OF NORMAL
Aorta			
Annulus diameter (cm)	1.4–2.6	1.3 ± 0.1 cm/m^2	<1.6 cm/m^2 (men and women)
Diameter at leaflet tips (cm)	2.2–3.6	1.7 ± 0.2 cm/m^2	<2.1 cm/m^2 (men and women)
Ascending aorta diameter (cm)	2.1–3.4	1.5 ± 0.2 cm/m^2	
Arch diameter (cm)	2.0–3.6		
Descending thoracic aorta diameter (cm)			
Left ventricle			
Short-axis dimension (cm)			
Diastole	3.5–6.0	2.3–3.1 cm/m^2	
Systole	2.1–4.0	1.4–2.1 cm/m^2	
Long-axis dimension (cm)			
Diastole	6.3–10.3	4.1–5.7 cm/m^2	
Systole	4.6–8.4		
End-diastolic volume (ml)			
Men	96–157	67 ± 9 ml	
Women	59–138	61 ± 13 ml	
End-systolic volume (ml)			
Men	33–68	27 ± 5 ml	
Women	18–65	26 ± 7 ml	
Ejection fraction (%)			
Men	0.59 ± 0.06		
Women	0.58 ± 0.07		
LV-wall thickness (cm) (end-diastole)	0.6–1.1		Men $\leq$ 1.2 cm Women $\leq$ 1.1 cm
LV-mass (g)			
Men	<294 g	109 ± 20 g/m^2	$\leq$150 g/m^2
Women	<198 g	89 ± 15 g/m^2	$\leq$120 g/m^2
Left atrium			
Anterior-posterior dimension (cm)(PLAX)	2.3–4.5	1.6–2.4 cm/m^2	
Medial-lateral dimension (cm)(A4C)	2.5–4.5	1.6–2.4 cm/m^2	
Superior-inferior dimension (cm)(A4C)	3.4–6.1	2.3–3.5 cm/m^2	
Mitral annulus			
End-diastole (cm)	2.7–0.4		
End-systole (cm)	2.9–0.3		
Right ventricle			
Wall thickness (cm)	0.2–0.5	0.2 ± 0.05 cm/m^2	
Minor dimension (cm)	2.2–4.4	1.0–2.8 cm/m^2	
Length			
Diastole (cm)	5.5–9.5	3.8–5.3 cm/m^2	
Systole (cm)	4.2–8.1		
Pulmonary artery			
Annulus diameter (cm)	1.0–2.2		
Main PA (cm)	0.9–2.9		
Inferior vena cava diameter			
(at RA junction)(cm)	1.2–2.3		

Data from:
  Roman et al: AJC 1989; 64:507
  Schnittger et al: JACC 1983; 2:934
  Truiulzi et al: Echo 1984; 1:403
  Levy et al: AJC 1987; 59:956
  Pearlman et al: JAAC 1988; 12:1432
  Pini et al: Circ 1989; 80:915
  Erbel: Dtsch Med Wschr 1982; 107:1872
  Hahn et al: Z. Kardiol 1982; 71:445

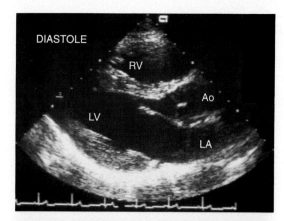

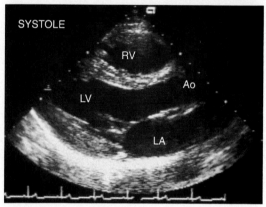

Figure 2–4. Normal parasternal long-axis 2D echo images at end-diastole (*above*) and end-systole (*below*).

tained from this window by rotating the transducer counterclockwise. Note that the oblique sinus of the pericardium lies between the left atrium and the descending thoracic aorta so that a pericardial effusion can be seen between these two structures, while a pleural effusion will be seen only posterior to the descending thoracic aorta.

The *left ventricular* septum and posterior wall are seen at the base and midventricular level in the long-axis view, allowing assessment of wall thickness, chamber dimensions, endocardial motion, and wall thickening of these myocardial segments. From the parasternal window, the left ventricular apex is not seen—the apparent "apex" usually is an oblique image plane through the anterolateral wall.

A portion of the muscular *right ventricular outflow tract* is seen anteriorly. Unlike the symmetrical prolate ellipsoid shape of the left ventricle, the right ventricle does not have an easily defined long or short axis. In effect, the right ventricle is "wrapped around" the left ventricle, with an inflow region, an apical region, and an outflow region forming a somewhat anteroposteriorly flattened U-shaped structure. Most standard image planes result in oblique tomographic sections of the right ventricle, so right ventricular size and systolic function are best evaluated from multiple views, as discussed more fully in Chapter 4.

Right Ventricular Inflow and Outflow Views

In the long-axis plane, the transducer is moved apically and then is angulated medially to obtain a view of the *right atrium, tricuspid*

of no clinical significance that can mimic a left atrial mass.

Posterior to the left atrium, the *descending thoracic aorta* is seen in cross section. A long-axis view of the descending thoracic aorta can be ob-

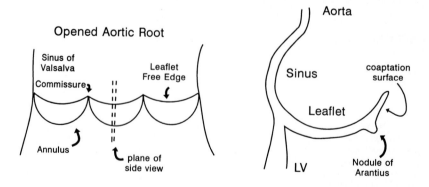

Figure 2–5. Schematic diagram of normal aortic valve anatomy shown in a frontal view (*left*) with the aortic root "opened" between two of the valve leaflets to demonstrate the crown-shaped "annulus." In the side view (*right*), the commissures are near the top of each sinus so that each leaflet-sinus unit has a cuplike shape, as seen from the aortic side of the valve.

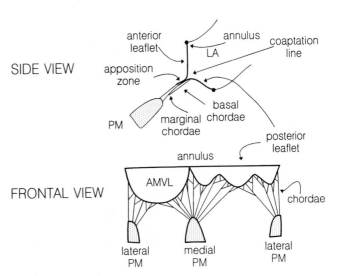

SIDE VIEW

FRONTAL VIEW

Figure 2–6. Schematic diagram of normal mitral valve anatomy. Definition of anatomic structures (*above*) in a long-axis view (*side view*) is shown with attachments of both marginal and basal chordae. The mitral annulus has been opened (*frontal view*) between the anterior and posterior leaflets (bisecting the lateral papillary muscle) to show the relative size and shape of the two leaflets and the chordal attachments of both leaflets to both papillary muscles.

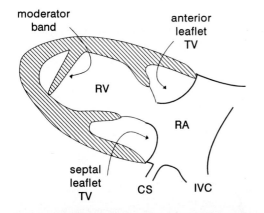

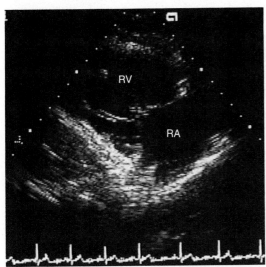

Figure 2–7. Schematic (*above*) and 2D echo images (*below*) in a right ventricular inflow view showing the right ventricle (RV) and atrium (RA), tricuspid valve (TV), and ostia of the coronary sinus (CS) and inferior vena cava (IVC).

valve, and *right ventricle* (Fig. 2–7). In this right ventricular inflow view, the septal and anterior leaflets of the tricuspid valve are well seen. The right ventricular apex is heavily trabeculated, while the outflow tract (supracristal) has a smoother endocardial surface. The moderator band, a prominent muscle trabeculation that traverses the right ventricular apex obliquely and contains the right bundle branch, may be seen in both parasternal and apical views (Fig. 2–8). The papillary muscles are more difficult to identify in the right ventricle than in the left ventricle. Typically, there are two principal papillary muscles (anterior and posterior) with a smaller supracristal (or conus) papillary muscle. The moderator band attaches near the base of the anterior right ventricular papillary muscle.

The *coronary sinus* is identified as it enters the right atrium adjacent to the tricuspid annulus. By slowly scanning back to a left ventricular long-axis view, the coronary sinus can be followed along its length.

The *inferior vena cava* is seen entering the right atrium inferior to the coronary sinus. In some individuals, a prominent Eustachian valve is seen at the junction of the inferior vena cava and right atrium both in this view and from the subcostal window. When a more extensive fenestrated valve is present, it forms a Chiari network extending from the inferior to superior vena cava, attached to the crista terminalis posteriorly and the fossa ovalis medially, with a netlike structure that appears as mobile echos in the right atrium. Both these findings are considered normal variants of no clinical significance.

Another normal anatomic feature of the right atrium (Fig. 2–9) that may be appreciated on echocardiographic imaging is the crista termi-

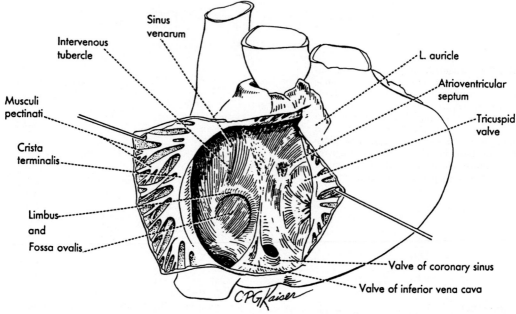

Figure 2–8. The interior of the right atrium seen from the right side. The view is toward the interatrial septum. (*Reprinted with permission from Hollinshead WH, Rosse C: Textbook of Anatomy, 4th ed. Philadelphia, Harper & Row, 1985, p 526.*)

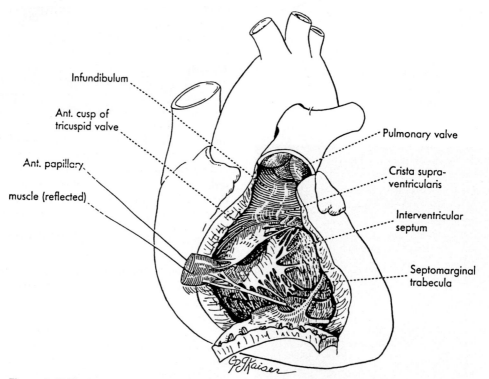

Figure 2–9. The interior of the right ventricle. The crista supraventricularis separates the inflow part of the ventricle from the infundibulum, or conus arteriosus. Note the great distance between the septal leaf of the tricuspid valve and the pulmonary valve. (*Reprinted with permission from Hollinshead WH, Rosse C: Textbook of Anatomy, 4th ed. Philadelphia, Harper & Row, 1985, p 529.*)

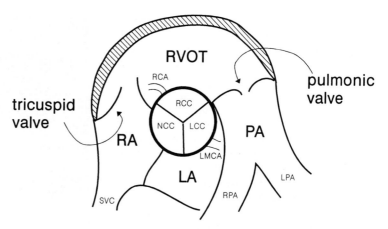

Figure 2–10. Schematic diagram of a parasternal short-axis view at the aortic valve level showing the relationship between the three cusps of the aortic valve—right coronary cusp (RCC), noncoronary cusp (NCC), left coronary cusp (LCC)—and the left atrium (LA), right atrium (RA), right ventricular outflow tract (RVOT), and the pulmonary artery (PA) with right (RPA) and left (LPA) branches. The positions of the right coronary artery (RCA), left main coronary artery (LMCA), pulmonic valve, and tricuspid valve are shown.

nalis, a muscular ridge that courses anteriorly from the superior to inferior vena cava and which divides the trabeculated anterior portion of the right atrium from the posterior, smooth-walled sinus venosus segment. The right atrial appendage is rarely seen on transthoracic imaging but is a trabeculated protrusion of the right atrium extending anterior to the right atrial free wall and base of the aorta.

The interatrial septum is not well seen in the right ventricular inflow view, being just inferior and parallel to the image plane. However, careful angulation between the long-axis and right ventricular inflow views allows examination of the atrial septum with recognition of the thick primum septum at its junction with the central fibrous body, the thin fossa ovalis in the central portion of the atrial septum, the ridgelike limbus located superior to the fossa, and the ridge adjacent to the junction with the coronary sinus.

Moving the transducer toward the base and then angulating laterally, a long-axis view of the right ventricular outflow tract, *pulmonic valve*, and pulmonary artery is obtained. This view is particularly useful for recording flow velocities in the right ventricular outflow tract and pulmonary artery.

Short-Axis Views

Short-axis views are obtained from the parasternal window by rotating the transducer clockwise 90° and then angulating the transducer superiorly or inferiorly to obtain specific image planes.

At the *aortic valve* level (Figs. 2–10 and 2–11), the short-axis view demonstrates all three aortic valve leaflets—right, left, and noncoronary cusps. In systole, the aortic leaflets open to a near-circular orifice. In diastole, the typical Y-

shaped arrangement of the coaptation lines of the leaflets is seen. Identification of the number of aortic valve leaflets is made most accurately in systole, since a bicuspid valve may appear trileaflet in diastole due to a raphe in the position of a normal commissure. Normally, the aortic

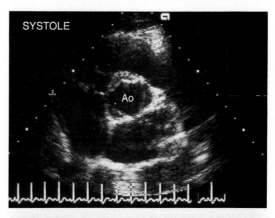

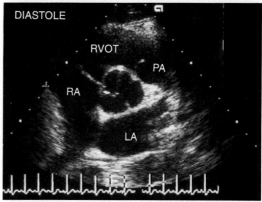

Figure 2–11. Two-dimensional echocardiographic images at the aortic valve level in systole (*above*) and diastole (*below*). Note the three open leaflets of the aortic valve in systole and the normal perpendicular relationship of aortic and pulmonic valves.

valve leaflets are thin at the base with an area of thickening on the ventricular aspect of the middle of the free edge of each cusp which serves to fill the space at the center of the closed valve. These nodules normally enlarge with age (nodules of Arantius) and can have small mobile filaments attached on the ventricular surface (Lambl's excrescences). These small but normal structures may be seen when echocardiographic images are of high quality and should not be mistaken for pathologic conditions. The origins of the left main and right coronary arteries often can be identified in this view.

The aortic and pulmonic valve planes normally lie perpendicular to each other. Thus, when the aortic valve is seen in short axis, the pulmonic valve is seen in long axis. In adults, evaluation of the leaflets of the pulmonic valve is limited; usually only one or two leaflets are seen well, and a short-axis view often is not obtainable.

The close relationship between the aortic valve and other intracardiac structures is apparent in this short-axis view. In addition to the pulmonic valve and right ventricular outflow tract, which are seen anterolaterally adjacent to the left coronary cusp, portions of the tricuspid valve are seen anteriorly and slightly medially, adjacent to the right coronary cusp. The two leaflets of the tricuspid valve seen in this view are the septal and anterior leaflets.

Posteriorly, the right atrium, interatrial septum, and left atrium lie in proximity to the noncoronary cusp of the aortic valve. The left atrial appendage can be better imaged from this view by a slight lateral angulation and superior rotation of the transducer. The central location of the aortic valve illustrates how disease processes can extend from the aortic valve or root into the right ventricular outflow tract, right atrium, or left atrium. Extension of disease processes into the ventricular septum or anterior mitral leaflet also is possible, as evident in the long-axis view.

At the *mitral valve* short-axis level (Fig. 2–12), the thin anterior and posterior mitral leaflets are seen as they open nearly to the full cross-sectional area of the left ventricle in diastole and close in systole. The posterior leaflet consists of three major scallops—medial, central, and lateral—although there is considerable individual variability. The two mitral commissures—the points on the annulus where the anterior and posterior leaflets meet—are located medially and laterally. Note that this parallels the arrangement of the papillary muscles so that chordae from the medial aspects of both anterior and posterior leaflets attach to the medial (or posteromedial) papillary muscle and chordae from the

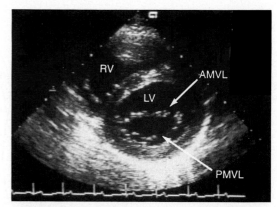

Figure 2–12. Short-axis 2D view at the mitral valve level showing the right ventricle (RV) anteriorly, the circular left ventricle (LV), and the anterior (AMVL) and posterior (PMVL) mitral valve leaflets in middiastole.

lateral aspects of both leaflets attach to the lateral (or anterolateral) papillary muscle. Chordae branch at three levels (primary, secondary, and tertiary) between the papillary muscle tip and mitral leaflet with a progressive decrease in chordal diameter and increase in the number of chordae from approximately 12 at the papillary muscle to 120 at the mitral leaflet. Most chordae attach at the free edge of the leaflets (called *marginal chordae*), but some (called *basal chordae*) attach to the left ventricular surface of the leaflet. Occasionally, aberrant chordae to the ventricular septum or other structures are seen in an otherwise normal individual.

At the *papillary muscle* level short-axis view (Fig. 2–13), the left ventricle is seen in circular cross section. The nomenclature of left ventricular myocardial segments is discussed in Chapter 6, but basically, the ventricle is divided into anterior (septum and free wall), lateral, posterior, and inferior (free wall and septum) segments for consistent descriptors of the location of abnormalities (Fig. 2–14).

The left ventricle typically appears circular in short axis, so that an elliptical appearance of the chamber usually is due to a nonperpendicular orientation relative to the long axis of the left ventricle. Moving the transducer superiorly with apical angulation resolves this problem. Actual distortion of the circular cross section may be seen in patients with ischemic cardiac disease, prior myocardial infarction, and aneurysm formation. The short-axis view at the papillary muscle level allows measurement of wall thickness and internal dimensions of the left ventricle in systole and diastole from either the 2D image or a 2D guided M-mode recording. Rotating the transducer between the long- and

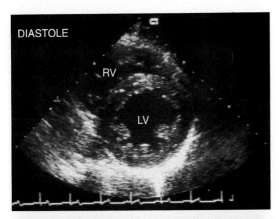

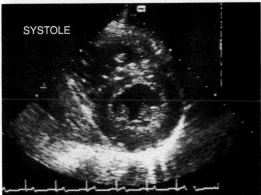

Figure 2–13. Two-dimensional echo short-axis view at the papillary muscle level at end-diastole (*above*) and end-systole (*below*) showing the right ventricle (RV) and the medial and lateral papillary muscles. Note the circular shape of the left ventricle with symmetric wall thickening and inward endocardial motion with contraction.

short-axis views at this level ensures a true short-axis measurement (perpendicular to the long axis). Oblique measurements will result in over-estimation of wall thickness and ventricular dimensions.

This view also allows assessment of endocardial motion and wall thickening at the midventricular level in the distribution of the left anterior descending artery (anterior septum and anterior wall), posterior descending artery (inferior septum and inferior wall), and circumflex artery (lateral and posterior walls) (see Chap. 6). Ventricular septal motion may reflect abnormalities other than coronary disease, including right ventricular volume and/or pressure overload, conduction abnormalities, and the post–cardiac surgery state (see Fig. 4–19).

The medial and lateral papillary muscles are seen in this short-axis plane and serve as landmarks identifying the midventricular level. Rarely, one of the papillary muscles may be bi-

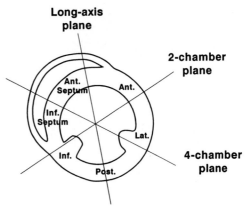

Figure 2–14. Relationship between the short-axis plane, with left ventricular wall segments indicated, and the apical four-chamber, two-chamber, and long-axis image planes (perpendicular to the short-axis plane).

fid, resulting in an appearance of three separate papillary muscles. Note that the apical segments of the left ventricular myocardium are not seen in standard parasternal views. In some patients, a short-axis view of the left ventricle near the apex can be obtained by moving the transducer laterally and angling medially.

Apical Window

The apical window is identified initially by palpation of the left ventricular apex with the patient in a steep left lateral decubitus position. An apical "cutout" in the examination stretcher allows optimal patient positioning and placement of the transducer on the apical impulse. Transducer position then is adjusted as needed to obtain optimal images. The relationship between the three basic apical views and the short-axis plane is shown in Figure 2–14.

Four-Chamber View (Figs. 2–15 and 2–16)

In the apical four-chamber view, the length of the *left ventricle* is seen in a plane perpendicular to both the short-axis and long-axis planes. The lateral wall, apex, and inferior septum lie in this tomographic plane. The left ventricle appears as a truncated ellipse with a longer length than width and a tapered but rounded apex. If the transducer is not positioned at the true apex, the left ventricle will appear foreshortened, with a spherical shape and little tapering of the apex. Foreshortening of the long-axis plane must be distinguished from disease processes, such as chronic aortic regurgitation, which result in in-

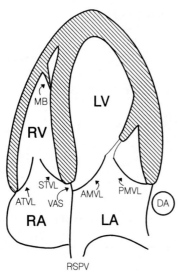

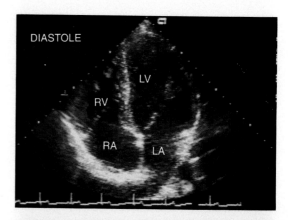

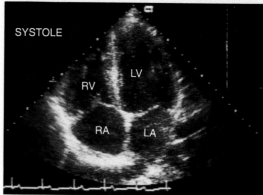

Figure 2–15. Schematic diagram of the apical four-chamber view showing the relationships of the left and right ventricles (LV and RV) and atria (LA and RA). In the left ventricle, the papillary muscle, chordae, and anterior and posterior mitral leaflets (AMVL, PMVL) are seen. The descending aorta (DA) is seen in partial cross section lateral to the left atrium, while the right superior pulmonary vein (RSPV) drains into the left atrium adjacent to the interatrial septum. In the right ventricle, the moderator band (MB) and the anterior and septal tricuspid valve leaflets (ATVL and STVL) are seen. Note the ventriculoatrial septum (VAS) separating the left ventricle from the right atrium in association with the normal, slightly more apical position of the tricuspid compared with the mitral valve annulus.

Figure 2–16. Two-dimensional echo images in an apical four-chamber view at end-diastole (*above*) and end-systole (*below*). Abbreviations as in Figure 2–15.

creased sphericity of the ventricle. Although the right ventricle is more trabeculated than the left ventricle, prominent trabeculation also can be seen at the left ventricular apex and must be distinguished from apical thrombus. When aberrant left ventricular trabeculae transverse the ventricular chamber, a "chord" or "web" is seen on 2D echo.

Medially, the *right ventricle* is triangle-shaped with a cavity about half the area of the left ventricle. The right ventricular apex is less round and more basal than the left ventricular apex. The moderator band often is seen transversing the right ventricle near the apex. The right ventricle can be further evaluated by moving the transducer medially over the right ventricular apex. Considerable individual variability in the shape and wall motion of the right ventricle, particularly at the apex, is seen in normal individuals, so caution is needed in diagnosing an abnormal right ventricle from any single tomographic plane.

The four-chamber view also shows the mitral annulus in its major dimension, the anterior mi-

tral valve leaflet (located adjacent to the septum), and the posterior mitral valve leaflet (adjacent to the lateral wall), along with chordae and attachments to the lateral papillary muscle. The mitral leaflet tips separate widely in diastole, and in systole the closure plane of the leaflets may appear "flat" (a 180° closure angle), but displacement of the leaflets beyond the plane of the mitral annulus is not seen unless the view is foreshortened or mitral valve disease is present.

The tricuspid annulus lies slightly (up to 1.0 cm) closer to the apex than the mitral annulus. The septal and posterior tricuspid leaflets are seen in this view with a wide diastolic opening; thin, uniformly echogenic, leaflets; and normal coaptation in systole.

The left and right atria are distal from the apical transducer position. Although a general assessment of size and shape can be made, ultrasound resolution at this depth is poor, and detailed evaluation of atrial tumors or clots often is not possible. The interatrial septum lies parallel to the ultrasound beam in this view, so "dropout"—absence of reflected signal—from the region of the fossa ovalis is common. This should not be mistaken for an atrial septal defect.

The descending thoracic aorta may be seen lateral to the left atrium. The pulmonary veins enter the left atrium posteriorly but may be difficult to image at this depth in adults. If the transducer is angulated posteriorly from the four-chamber view, more posterior portions of the lateral and inferior septal myocardium are seen. In addition, the length of the coronary sinus comes into view in the atrioventricular groove.

Angulating the transducer anteriorly, the aortic valve and root are seen in an oblique long- or short-axis view. This view is sometimes referred to as the apical "five-chamber" view. More anterior portions of the septum and lateral wall are seen, especially at the base, as the transducer is angulated anteriorly. This view of the anterior mitral leaflet, left ventricular outflow tract, and aortic valve is at an angle approximately 60 to 90° from the long-axis view. In some adults, further anterior angulation of the transducer allows visualization of the pulmonary artery arising from the right ventricle. This view is more easily obtained in young adults and children.

Two-Chamber View (Fig. 2–17)

From the four-chamber view, the transducer is rotated counterclockwise about 60° to obtain the two-chamber view of the left ventricle, mitral valve, and left atrium. The apical two-chamber view is used for evaluation of the anterior left ventricular wall (seen to the right of the screen) and the posterior wall (seen on the left).

Fine adjustments in transducer position may be needed to visualize the anterior wall endocardium due to interference from adjacent lung tissue. To ensure that the proper rotation has been made for a two-chamber view, the transducer is angled posteriorly to intersect both papillary muscles symmetrically. Then the transducer is angled slightly anteriorly so that neither papillary muscle is seen in its long axis in this view. The anterior mitral leaflet is seen *en face*, so the apparent closure plane of the leaflet relative to the annulus can be misleading. The left atrial appendage may be visualized adjacent to the anterior wall. A long-axis view of the descending thoracic aorta can be obtained by angulating posteriorly and rotating counterclockwise from the two-chamber view.

Long-Axis View (Fig. 2–18)

Rotating the transducer another 60° from the two-chamber view (120° from the four-chamber view) yields a long-axis view similar to the parasternal long-axis view. The aortic valve, left ventricular outflow tract, and mitral valve are seen in long axis. The anterior septum and posterior walls are seen. Compared with the parasternal long-axis view, the left ventricular apex now is seen, but the aortic and mitral valves are at a greater image depth (with consequent poorer image resolution).

Other Apical Views

Nonstandard short-axis views of the left ventricular apex using a higher-frequency transducer (5 or 7.5 MHz) are helpful if a left

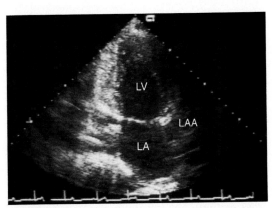

Figure 2–17. Apical two-chamber view showing the inferior and anterior left ventricular walls, the mitral valve, left atrium, and left atrial appendage (LAA).

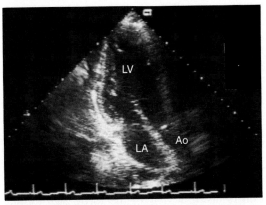

Figure 2–18. Apical long-axis view showing the left ventricle, left atrium, aorta, and aortic and mitral valves. As in the parasternal long-axis view, the posterior and anterior septal left ventricular walls are seen.

ventricular apical thrombus is suspected. One useful view is obtained by sliding the transducer laterally from the left ventricular apex and then angulating medially.

Subcostal Window

With the patient supine and the legs bent at the knees (if necessary) to relax the abdominal wall musculature, subcostal images of the cardiac structures are obtained. A view of all four chambers shows the right ventricular free wall, the midsection of the interventricular septum, and the posterolateral left ventricular wall (Fig. 2–19). In this view, the interatrial septum is perpendicular to the direction of the ultrasound beam, allowing evaluation of atrial septal defects.

A subcostal short-axis view of the left ventricle allows measurements of left ventricular wall thickness and dimensions that are comparable with dimensions obtained from a parasternal short-axis view, albeit at a greater depth and through different myocardial segments. The subcostal window provides a useful alternative for qualitative and quantitative evaluation of the left ventricle when the parasternal window is inadequate.

Rotating the transducer inferiorly from the subcostal four-chamber view, a long-axis view of the inferior vena cava is obtained as it enters the right atrium. Since these 2 to 3 cm of the inferior vena cava are exposed to the negative intrapleural pressures associated with normal respiration, the size and respiratory variation of this vessel can be used to estimate right atrial pressure (see Table 4–6). The hepatic veins, particularly the central hepatic vein, which courses parallel to the ultrasound beam in this view, are helpful in assessing right atrial pressure and for recording right atrial Doppler filling patterns. The proximal abdominal aorta is imaged in long axis medial to the inferior vena cava.

Suprasternal Notch Window

With the patient supine and the neck extended, the transducer is positioned in the suprasternal notch or right supraclavicular position to obtain a view of the aortic arch in long and short axis. The long-axis view (with respect to the aortic arch) shows the ascending aorta, arch, proximal descending thoracic aorta, and

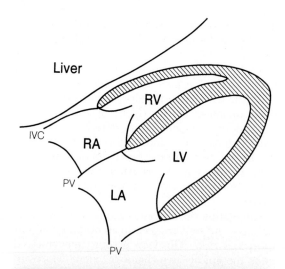

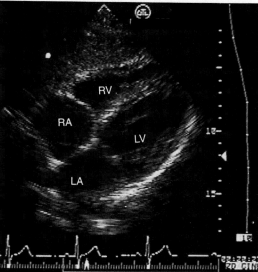

Figure 2–19. Schematic (*above*) and 2D echo (*below*) images from a subcostal approach showing all four cardiac chambers. The interatrial septum is perpendicular to the ultrasound beam from this window, allowing evaluation for atrial septal defects.

the origins of the right brachiocephalic and left common carotid and subclavian arteries (Fig. 2–20). The corresponding veins lie superior to the aortic arch, with the superior vena cava lying adjacent to the ascending aorta. The right pulmonary artery is seen "under" the aortic arch and can be followed to its branch point by rotating the transducer medially.

The short-axis view shows the aortic arch in cross section. The left pulmonary artery can be imaged by rotating slightly laterally. The left atrium lies inferior to the pulmonary arteries in

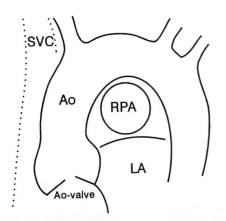

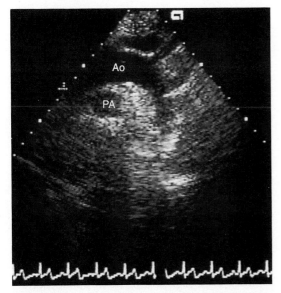

Figure 2–20. Schematic (*above*) and 2D echo (*below*) images of the aorta in a long-axis view from the suprasternal notch window. The ascending aortic (Ao) arch and descending thoracic aorta are seen with the origins of the left carotid and subclavian arteries. The right pulmonary artery (RPA) lies immediately inferior to the arch.

both long- and short-axis views, so it may be possible to evaluate atrial pathology or flow disturbances from this window.

Other Acoustic Windows

In specific cases, other acoustic windows may be needed. For example, a dextropositioned heart would necessitate mirror-image acoustic windows. When a large pleural effusion is present, good-quality images may be obtained in some cases by imaging from the posterior chest

wall through the effusion with the patient in a sitting position.

TRANSESOPHAGEAL TOMOGRAPHIC VIEWS

The exact views obtained on a transesophageal study will vary depending on the relative positions of the heart, esophagus, and diaphragm in each patient. In addition, transesophageal transducers with fixed image planes defined by the axis of the esophageal probe—whether monoplane or biplane—result in oblique image orientations compared with the 3D reference system used for transthoracic images. Transesophageal transducers with multiple possible image planes (multiplane or omniplane) relative to the esophagus allow somewhat more standard image acquisition, although accessible image planes still are limited by the relative positions of the cardiac structures and the esophagus in each patient.

The following section describes representative transesophageal images obtained at different levels (or depths) in the esophagus or the stomach for transverse and longitudinal image planes. The absolute distance of the transducer from the patient's mouth will vary depending on body size and cardiac position. There also will be variability in the exact degree of rotation (with a multiplane transducer) or tilt and angulation (with a biplane probe) needed to obtain the best transverse or longitudinal views. In many cases, short-axis, long-axis, and four-chamber views of the cardiac structures can be obtained. These images then correspond to the anatomy described for the equivalent transthoracic views, with the major difference being image orientation given the transesophageal transducer position.

For transesophageal echocardiograms, transducer motions will be referred to as (1) *repositioning*, defined as movement of the probe up and down in the esophagus, (2) *tilt*, defined as lateral motion of the transducer tip to image different structures in the same image plane (although slight superior motion occurs as well), (3) *angulation*, defined as bending and extending the probe so that the image plane is directed superiorly or inferiorly at an angle to the original image plane, (4) *turning* the entire transducer in the esophagus, to show a medial-lateral change in image plane, and (5) *rotation*, defined as rotating the image plane between longitudinal and transverse planes (using a multiplane probe).

Transverse Plane (Fig. 2–21)

With the image plane oriented perpendicular to the esophageal probe, images are obtained in the transverse plane. Again, note that *transverse* does *not* refer to the axis of the heart but only to the axis of the probe, so images in the *transverse* plane may represent short-axis, long-axis, four-chamber, or oblique views of the cardiac structures.

Great Vessel Level

As the transducer is advanced in the esophagus from the mouth toward the stomach, acoustic access is limited by interposition of the air-filled trachea until the transducer passes the level of the carina. Images obtained just beyond this level show the main pulmonary artery and its bifurcation. Slight further advancement results in an oblique short-axis image of the aortic valve, left atrium, interatrial septum, and right atrium (Fig. 2–22). Visualization of aortic valve anatomy is excellent, showing the three leaflets and sinuses of Valsalva. The origins of both right and left coronary arteries are seen with minor adjustments in the depth and tilt of the image plane. The interatrial septum is well seen, with the fossa ovalis clearly defined. A large portion of the interatrial septum can be examined by slow superior and inferior angulation of the transducer from this position.

By turning the transducer laterally and angulating superiorly, the left atrium appendage is seen (Fig. 2–23). Prominent features include normal trabeculation of the atrial appendage and a variably prominent ridge at the junction of the anteriorly directed left superior pulmonary vein and the left atrial appendage. The laterally directed left inferior pulmonary vein is seen by advancing the transducer and angulating slightly inferiorly.

The right pulmonary veins can be imaged by rotating the transducer medially and withdrawing the transducer cephalad (to see the anteriorly directed superior vein) or by angulating the transducer inferiorly (to see the medially directed inferior vein).

Mitral Valve Level

When the transducer is advanced to a position posterior to the center of the left atrium, the mitral valve is seen. By angulating superiorly, a long-axis type of view of the aortic valve, left ventricular outflow tract, and anterior mitral valve leaflet is obtained. Posterior angulation from this position results in an image of the left atrium and midsegments of the anterior and posterior mitral valve leaflets and a four-chamber type of view of the left ventricle (Fig. 2–24). The inferior septum and lateral walls are seen in this view; however, the apex is often foreshortened. The right ventricle also can be evaluated in this view. The mitral valve is examined from this position by careful, slow angulation from superiorly (aortic valve) to posteriorly (coronary sinus) to image each segment of the mitral apparatus.

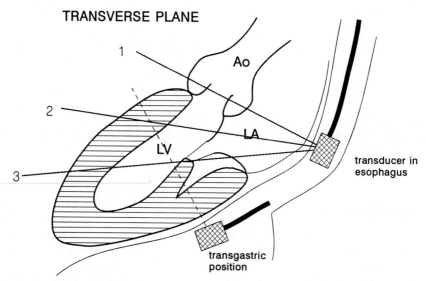

Figure 2–21. Diagram of the transesophageal transverse image planes. With angulation of the transducer (and tilt and repositioning as needed), images can be obtained through the aortic valve (1), left atrium and mitral valve (2), and in a four-chamber view (3). From a transgastric position, a short-axis view of the left ventricle is obtained (*dashed line*).

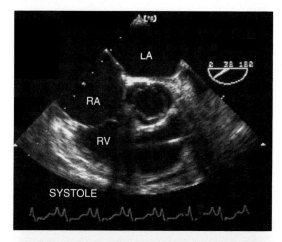

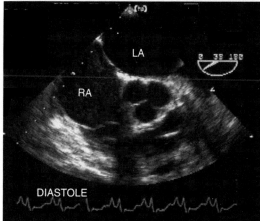

Figure 2–22. Short-axis transesophageal view of the aortic valve in systole (*above*) and diastole (*below*). The left atrium (LA), right atrium (RA), and tricuspid valve (TV) are seen. A Swan-Ganz catheter traverses the right ventricular outflow tract.

Color flow imaging during this image sequence also is helpful if mitral regurgitation is present.

Mid-Left Ventricular Level (Transgastric)

After the transducer is passed into the stomach, superior angulation (flexing the scope) results in a short-axis view of the left ventricle at the papillary muscle level (Fig. 2–25). Depending on the position of the patient's heart with respect to the diaphragm, a short-axis view at the mitral valve level may be obtainable by slight withdrawal of the transducer toward the esophagus. In the transgastric short-axis view, the wall segments are the same as in a transthoracic short-axis view *except* that the entire image has been rotated approximately 180° clockwise (if standard display format is used). Compared with a subcostal short-axis view, the image is rotated 90° clockwise (see Fig. 6–8). In this view,

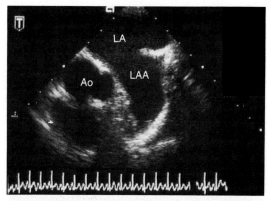

Figure 2–23. Transesophageal view of the left atrial appendage (LAA) showing normal trabecularis, the ridge between the left atrial appendage and the left superior pulmonary vein, and an oblique view of the aortic root (Ao).

global left ventricular systolic function, left ventricular dimensions and wall thickness, and regional left ventricular function can be evaluated. The transgastric short-axis view at the mitral valve level is helpful in precise definition of the mitral valve apparatus anatomy in patients with valve dysfunction.

Transgastric "Apical" View

From the transgastric short-axis view, the transducer is advanced further into the fundus of the stomach. In some individuals an "apical" four-chamber view can be obtained using the transverse image plane of the probe if the left ventricular apex lies on the diaphragm, without intervening lung. Note that the transducer usually does not lie on the true left ventricular apex, so this view typically is foreshortened. How-

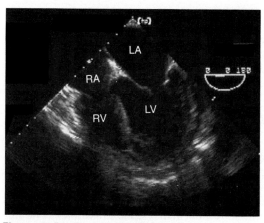

Figure 2–24. Transesophageal four-chamber view obtained in the transverse plane from a high esophageal position by inferior angulation of the transducer.

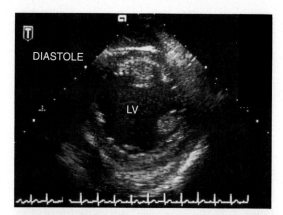

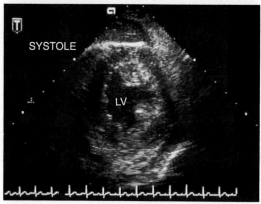

Figure 2–25. Transgastric short-axis view at end-diastole (*above*) and end-systole (*below*) of the left ventricle at the papillary muscle level.

ever, anterior angulation may show the aortic valve, allowing Doppler interrogation of the left ventricular outflow tract and valve at a reasonably parallel intercept angle. Caution still is needed in interpretation of the Doppler data obtained, since unlike a transthoracic examination, a high-velocity signal across the aortic valve cannot be interrogated from multiple windows with careful transducer angulation to ensure that a parallel intercept angle has been obtained. Underestimation of velocities is likely with a transesophageal approach.

Descending Aorta

From the transesophageal position, the transducer is turned (either direction) until the image plane is directed slightly left of the patient's spine, to obtain a short-axis view of the descending thoracic aorta. The aorta appears circular and shows normal systolic pulsations. The descending thoracic aorta can be imaged in sequential short-axis views from its junction with the

arch to its postgastric position. Often the examiner will image the aorta as the transducer is withdrawn in the esophagus. When the transducer reaches the level of the arch, turning the transducer medially, with inferior angulation, allows a long-axis view of the arch itself. The ascending aorta, other than the few centimeters adjacent to the valve seen at the aortic valve level, is not well visualized using a transverse image plane; however, the longitudinal plane provides excellent images of the ascending aorta (also see Chap. 14).

Longitudinal Plane (Fig. 2–26)

From a high transesophageal position, with the probe located posterior to the left atrium, the longitudinal plane of the transducer can be turned from lateral to medial to show (in sequence from left to right) (1) the mitral valve, left atrium, atrial appendage, and left ventricle, (2) the pulmonic valve and right ventricular outflow tract, (3) the aortic root, aortic valve, and left ventricular outflow tract, (4) the right ventricle and tricuspid valve, and (5) the right atrium and superior vena cava. Adjustment of transducer position (advancement and withdrawal) allows imaging of much of the cephalad to caudal extent of the cardiac structures in each of these tomographic planes. With a biplane probe, slight adjustments in transducer tilt (lateral bending of probe tip) and angulation (flexion

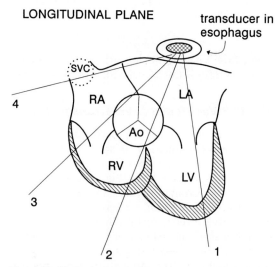

Figure 2–26. In the longitudinal plane, images can be obtained by turning the probe successively from lateral to medial to view the left atrial appendage, left atrium, and left ventricle (1), the aortic root (2), the tricuspid valve and interatrial septum (3), and the superior vena cava and right atrium (4).

and extension of probe tip) or, with a multiplane probe, adjustment in the rotation angle may be needed to optimize each view.

Mitral Valve and Left Ventricle
(Fig. 2–27)

With the longitudinal image plane oriented through the center of the left atrium, mitral valve, and left ventricle, a view similar to a two-chamber view is obtained showing the inferior and anterior left ventricular walls. Slight farther lateral rotation allows visualization of the left atrium appendage in a view approximately perpendicular to that obtained in the transverse plane. The left superior pulmonary vein is seen entering the left atrium.

Pulmonic Valve and Right Ventricular Outflow Tract

The pulmonic valve lies just medial to the left atrial appendage. In this view, a portion of the pulmonic valve is in the far field, with proximal structures including a portion of the left atrium and the ascending aorta. The muscular right ventricular outflow tract, the pulmonic valve, and the main and right pulmonary arteries are seen well.

Aortic Root and Ascending Aorta

By turning the probe medially so that the image plane is directed almost straight anteriorly, a view of the aortic valve, ascending aorta, and left ventricular outflow tract is obtained (Fig. 2–28). The full extent of the ascending aorta is imaged by advancing the transducer and angulating superiorly to show the ascending aorta. Slight adjustment of tilt and angulation may be needed to obtain a long-axis view of the ascending aorta (or rotating the image plane angle to about 120° with a multiplane probe). In this view, the perpendicular relationship between aortic and pulmonic valve planes and the slightly more cephalad position of the pulmonic valve can be appreciated. This view is particularly helpful in evaluating for ascending aortic dissection, subaortic membrane, supracristal ventricular septal defect, sinus of Valsalva aneurysm, and aortic valve endocarditis.

With the probe positioned behind the left atrium, a short-axis view of the aortic valve can be obtained in the longitudinal plane of the probe by adjustment of the transducer tilt or by rotation of the image plane to about 60° from the transverse plane.

Right Ventricle and Tricuspid Valve

Further turning brings the longitudinal plane through a portion of the interatrial septum, the tricuspid valve, and the right ventricle. This view is useful for evaluation of atrial septal defects (particularly sinus venous defects) or a pat-

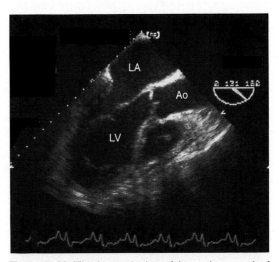

Figure 2–28. This long-axis view of the aortic root, mitral valve, left atrium, and left ventricle is rotated approximately 60° further counterclockwise from the two-chamber view shown in Figure 2–27, and 60° clockwise from the four-chamber view in Figure 2–24. Basically, these TEE image planes are equivalent to transthoracic apical four-chamber, two-chamber, and long-axis views. An important difference is that the true left ventricle apex may be foreshortened or missed on the TEE images.

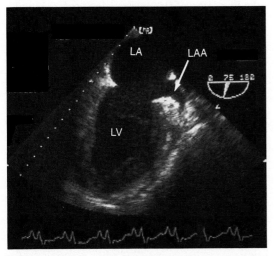

Figure 2–27. The longitudinal image plane results in a two-chamber view of the left atrium (LA), atrial appendage (LAA), mitral valve (MV), and left ventricle (LV). Note that this view is rotated approximately 75° from the four-chamber view in this patient seen in Figure 2–24.

ent foramen ovale and for evaluation of tricuspid valve disease.

Right Atrium and Superior Vena Cava

With the image plane oriented toward the patient's right side, a view of the superior vena cava entering the right atrium is obtained (Fig. 2–29). By advancing the transducer and angulating caudally, the entry of the inferior vena cava into the right atrium is also seen. In some individuals, a Eustachian valve at the caval-atrial junction is seen.

Descending Aorta

Direction of the longitudinal imaging plane slightly to the left of directly posteriorly results in a long-axis view of the descending thoracic aorta. This complements the transverse view of the descending aorta in evaluation of aortic dissections, aneurysms, and atheromas. The use of two orthogonal image planes improves the differentiation of ultrasound artifacts from anatomic abnormalities.

M-MODE RECORDINGS

M-mode recordings are helpful for identifying rapid motion of cardiac structures, since the sampling rate is 1800 per second rather than the 30 frames per second used for 2D imaging.

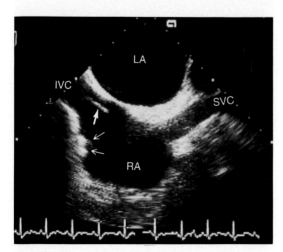

Figure 2–29. Long-axis transesophageal view of the superior vena cava (SVC), right atrium (RA), and inferior vena cava (IVC) with a prominent Eustachian valve (*arrow*). Normal trabeculation of the right atrium is seen (*small arrows*).

The rapid sampling rate also makes identification of thin moving structures, such as the left ventricular endocardium, more accurate and reproducible by showing motion as well as depth of the structure of interest. The potential disadvantage of M-mode data—a nonperpendicular orientation to the structure of interest—can be avoided by utilizing the 2D image in two orthogonal planes to position the M-mode sampling line.

Aortic Valve and Left Atrium
(Fig. 2–30)

An M-mode recording through the aortic root at the leaflet tip level shows the parallel walls of the aorta moving anteriorly in systole and posteriorly in diastole. The left atrium is posterior to the aortic root and shows filling in atrial diastole (ventricular systole) and emptying in atrial systole (ventricular diastole). Left atrial filling is largely responsible for the anterior displacement of the aortic root, so aortic root "motion" on M mode reflects left atrium dimensions. Increased aortic root motion is seen when there is increased left atrial filling and emptying (e.g., with mitral regurgitation). Decreased aortic root motion is seen in low cardiac output states, with corresponding low volumes of atrial filling and emptying.

The aortic leaflet coaptation point is seen as a thin line in diastole. In systole, the leaflets separate rapidly and completely, forming a boxlike appearance on the M-mode recording. Fine systolic fluttering of the aortic valve leaflets may be seen in normal individuals.

Mitral Valve

An M-mode recording at the mitral valve level intercepts the anterior right ventricular wall and chamber, the interventricular septum, the anterior and posterior mitral leaflets, the posterior left ventricular wall, and the pericardium (Fig. 2–31). The coaptation point of the mitral leaflets in systole is seen as a thin line that moves slightly anteriorly during systole, paralleling the motion of the posterior wall. In early diastole, the leaflets separate widely, with the maximum early diastolic motion of the anterior leaflet termed the *E point*. Normally, there is only a small distance between the E point and the maximal posterior motion of the ventricular sep-

Aortic valve and
Left atrial M mode

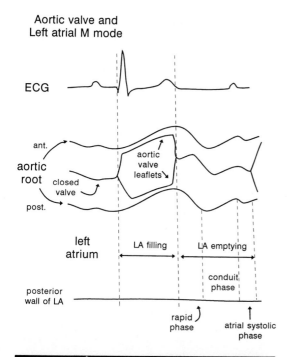

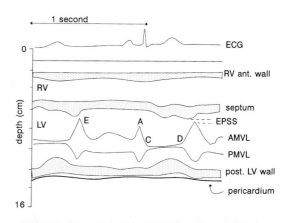

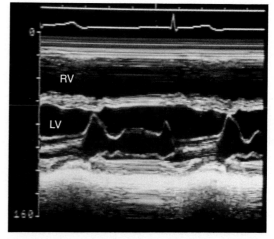

Figure 2–31. Schematic (*above*) and M-mode tracing (*below*) of a normal mitral valve.

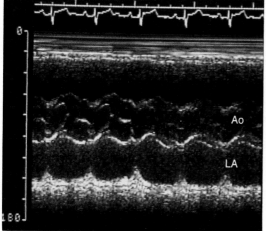

Figure 2–30. Schematic (*above*) and M-mode tracing (*below*) of a normal aortic valve and left atrium.

tum—E-point septal separation (EPSS). In the absence of mitral stenosis, an increased EPSS indicates left ventricular dilation, systolic dysfunction, or aortic regurgitation.

The leaflets move together in middiastole (diastasis) and then separate again with atrial systole, resulting in the late-diastolic peak, the *A point*. The slope of anterior mitral leaflet closure from *A* to the closure point (*C*) is linear unless left ventricular end-diastolic pressure is elevated when a "*B* bump" or "*A–C* shoulder" may be seen on the M-mode recording of mitral valve

motion. Fine fluttering of the anterior mitral leaflet is not seen in normal individuals and usually indicates aortic regurgitation.

Left Ventricle

An M-mode recording perpendicular to the long axis of and through the center of the left ventricle at the papillary muscle level provides standard measurements of systolic and diastolic wall thickness and chamber dimensions (Fig. 2–32). These measurements are limited in that they represent only a single line through the left ventricle and thus do not accurately describe the left ventricle when the disease process is asymmetrical, such as with prior myocardial infarction. However, many disease processes do result in symmetrical changes in the left ventricle (volume overload, hypertrophy), and the accuracy and reproducibility of these measurements make

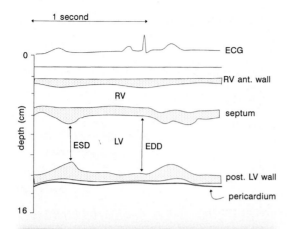

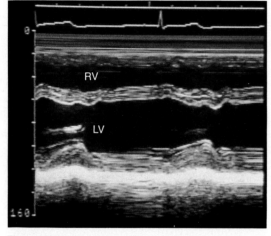

Figure 2–32. Schematic (*above*) and M-mode tracing (*below*) at the left ventricular papillary muscle level.

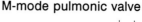

M-mode pulmonic valve

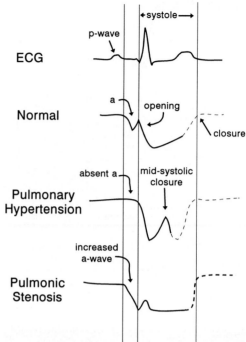

Figure 2–33. Patterns of pulmonic valve motion.

them useful in patient management. Examples of their utility include sequential evaluations of left ventricular end-systolic dimension in patients with chronic asymptomatic aortic regurgitation or assessment of left ventricular hypertrophy in hypertensive patients.

The posterior wall endocardium is identified as the continuous line with the steepest upslope in early systole, taking care to distinguish the endocardium from reflections due to overlying mitral chordal structures. Similarly, the endocardium of the septum is identified as a continuous line with systolic inward motion. Measurements are made (using the ASE recommendations) from the leading edge of the septal endocardial echo to the leading edge of the posterior wall endocardium.

An M-mode recording at this level also may be helpful in timing the motion of the right ventricular free wall when cardiac tamponade is sus-

pected or for detection of a small posterior pericardial effusion.

Other M-Mode Recordings

An M-mode recording through the pulmonic valve is similar to an aortic valve M-mode recording except that usually only one leaflet can be recorded in adults. The slight displacement of the leaflet in diastole (after atrial contraction) is called the *a* wave and is increased (>7 mm) when pulmonic stenosis is present and decreased (<2 mm) when pulmonary hypertension is present. Transient midsystolic closure (or "notching") of the pulmonic valve on M mode may be seen when pulmonary hypertension is present (Fig. 2–33).

An M-mode recording through the tricuspid valve is analogous to a mitral valve recording but rarely is useful clinically.

Use of the M-mode feature is most helpful when guided by the 2D image and used either for (1) timing of rapid cardiac motions, (2) precise measurements of cardiac dimensions, or (3) further evaluation of structures seen on 2D imaging (such as suspected vegetations) to aid in their identification.

NORMAL INTRACARDIAC FLOW PATTERNS

Basic Principles

Laminar versus Disturbed Flow
(Fig. 2–34)

Normal intracardiac flow patterns are characterized by laminar flow. *Laminar flow* is defined as movement of fluid along well-defined parallel stream lines with uniform flow velocities. In three dimensions, laminar flow consists of concentric layers (or lamina) of flow, each with a predictable and uniform direction and velocity.

Steady laminar flow becomes disturbed when the dimensionless Reynolds number exceeds 2000 to 2500. The Reynolds number (Re) is directly related to blood flow velocity V, lumen diameter d, and blood density ρ and inversely related to viscosity γ:

$$\mathrm{Re} = \frac{V \times d \times \rho}{\gamma} \qquad (2.1)$$

When blood flow patterns are disturbed, blood cells move in multiple directions at multiple velocities rather than along uniform, parallel stream lines. *Turbulence*, in fluid dynamic terms, refers to the specific situation in which the flow pattern of a particular fluid element is no longer predictable. While intracardiac flow disturbances rarely exhibit true turbulence, this term is used clinically to denote nonlaminar flow.

Flow-Velocity Profiles

The spatial distribution of velocities in cross section at a specific intracardiac location and at a specific time point in the cardiac cycle is known as the *flow-velocity profile* (Fig. 2–35). If all the parallel stream lines in a laminar flow pattern have the same velocity, then the flow velocity profile is "flat." If velocity is higher in the center of the vessel and lower at the walls of the vessel, the flow profile is "curved" (usually parabolic). While normal flow in peripheral vessels has a curved flow-velocity profile, many intracardiac flows have a relatively flat flow-velocity profile. Factors that tend to equalize the velocity distribution across the cross-sectional area of flow include tapering of the flow stream, acceleration of flow, and an inlet-type geometry. Thus the proximal aorta and pulmonary artery and the mitral and tricuspid annuli have reasonably flat flow-velocity profiles. Downstream, the spatial distribution of flow changes. For example, in the ascending aorta, the flow profile becomes skewed, with higher-velocity flow along the inside curve of the aortic arch and lower velocities along the outer curve. Many Doppler quantitative methods make assumptions about the spatial flow profile at a particular intracardiac site. In some cases, these assump-

Laminar Flow

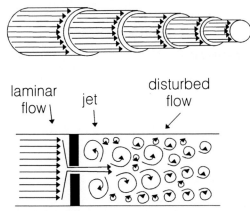

Figure 2–34. Laminar flow is characterized by parallel stream lines at uniform velocities with concentric layers of flow, each with a predictable and uniform direction and velocity (*above*). Disturbed flow occurs downstream from areas of narrowing (stenotic orifice, regurgitant orifice, or intracardiac shunt) with blood flow in multiple directions and velocities (*below*). In the orifice itself, a laminar high-velocity jet occurs.

FLOW VELOCITY PROFILES

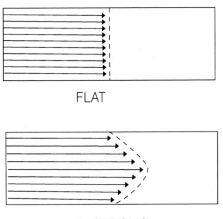

Figure 2–35. In a schematic longitudinal cross section of a flow stream, with the length of each arrow proportional to velocity, the difference between a flat and a parabolic flow velocity profile is shown.

tions can be verified by careful pulsed or color Doppler evaluation.

Clinical Quantitative Doppler Methods

There are three basic principles common to the clinical use of Doppler ultrasound in evaluation of cardiac disease which will be presented briefly here and in more detail, including technical aspects and potential pitfalls, in subsequent chapters as follows: (1) measurement of volume flow in Chapter 4; (2) the relationship between velocity and pressure gradients in Chapter 9; and (3) the concept of the 3D spatial distribution of a flow disturbance in Chapter 10.

Measurement of Volume Flow

When blood flow is laminar with a flat flow-velocity profile, it is intuitive that the instantaneous flow rate can be calculated as cross-sectional area or *CSA* (in cm^2) times flow velocity (in cm/s). Similarly, by integrating flow velocity over the flow period stroke volume, *SV* (in cm^3) can be calculated as

$$SV \text{ (cm}^3) = CSA \text{ (cm}^2) \times VTI \text{ (cm)} \quad (2.2)$$

where *VTI* is the velocity time integral (cm) of the Doppler velocity curve. This method is utilized clinically to measure stroke volume and cardiac output at rest or after physiologic or pharmacologic interventions, to evaluate the severity of valvular regurgitation, as a component in the equation for valve area calculations, and to quantitate the ratio of pulmonary to systemic blood flow in intracardiac shunts.

Velocity-Pressure Relationships

At any area of significant narrowing in the flow stream—whether a stenotic valve, a ventricular septal defect, or a regurgitant orifice—flow velocity increases in relation to the degree of narrowing; the narrower the opening, the faster is the velocity in the narrowing for a given volume flow rate. In most clinical situations, the velocity in this narrow "jet" through the narrowed orifice is related quantitatively to the pressure gradient across the narrowing, as stated in the simplified Bernoulli equation:

$$\Delta P = 4v^2 \quad (2.3)$$

where ΔP is the instantaneous pressure gradient (mmHg), and v is the instantaneous velocity (m/s). This relationship between pressure gradient and velocity is important for quantitation of

valve stenosis severity, noninvasive determination of pulmonary artery pressures, and evaluation of other intracardiac hemodynamics (Table 2–7) using continuous-wave Doppler ultrasound.

Flow Disturbances

Beyond an area of narrowing, disturbed flow patterns are seen. The exact location and timing of the flow disturbance allow diagnosis of valvular regurgitation, intracardiac shunts, and the anatomic level of right or left ventricular outflow obstruction. The spatial extent of the flow disturbance is helpful in evaluation of valve regurgitation. The 3D shape of the flow disturbance may even provide clues as to the etiology of regurgitation.

The presence, location, and extent of an intracardiac flow disturbance can be evaluated with conventional pulsed Doppler ultrasound by sequential repositioning of the sample volume in each tomographic plane. More conveniently, color flow imaging allows real-time demonstrations of the flow disturbance in each tomographic plane.

Normal Antegrade Intracardiac Flows (Table 2–8)

Normal antegrade intracardiac flows can be evaluated with either pulsed or continuous-wave

---

TABLE 2–7. NONINVASIVE HEMODYNAMIC DATA OBTAINED BY ECHOCARDIOGRAPHY

MEASUREMENT	CHAPTER
LV systolic function	
Volume flow rate (SV, CO)	4
LV dP/dt	4
Pulmonary artery systolic	4
pressure	
LV diastolic function	
Filling velocities and volume	5
flow rates	
LV dP/dt	5
LV-EDP	5
Valve stenosis	
Pressure gradients	9
Valve areas	9
Valve regurgitation	
Regurgitant volume, fraction	10
Shunt calculations	15

TABLE 2–8. NORMAL ANTEGRADE DOPPLER FLOW VELOCITIES

	NORMAL RANGE (m/s)
Ascending aorta	1.0–1.7
LV outflow tract	0.7–1.1
LV inflow	
E velocity	0.67–1.3 (0.72 ± 0.14)
Deceleration slope	5.0 ± 1.4 m/s²
A velocity	0.2–0.7 (0.47 ± 0.4)
Pulmonary artery	0.5–1.3
RV inflow	
E velocity	0.3–0.7
RA filling (SVC, HV)	
Systole	0.32–0.69 (0.46 ± 0.08)
Diastole	0.06–0.45 (0.27 ± 0.08)
LA filling (pulm vein)	
Systole	0.56 ± 0.13
Diastole	0.44 ± 0.16
Atrial reversal	0.32 ± 0.07

Data from:
Wilson et al: Br Heart J 1985; 53:451
Hatle and Angelsen: Doppler Ultrasound in Cardiology, 2d ed, Lea & Febiger, Philadelphia, 1985
Van Dam et al: Eur Heart J 1987; 8:1221; 1988; 9:165
Jaffe et al: AJC 1991; 68:550
Appleton et al: JACC 1987; 10:1032

TABLE 2–9. TRANSTHORACIC VIEWS FOR NORMAL ANTEGRADE FLOW VELOCITIES

ANTEGRADE FLOW	VIEW
LV outflow tract	Apical four-chamber (angulated anterior) Apical long-axis
Aorta (ascending)	LV-apex Suprasternal notch (SSN)
Descending aorta (thoracic) (proximal abdominal)	SSN Subcostal
LV inflow (mitral)	Apical four-chamber or long axis
RV outflow tract	RV outflow Poststernal (Ao valve level) Subcostal short-axis
RV inflow (tricuspid)	RV inflow Apical four-chamber
LA inflow (pulmonary vein)	Apical four-chamber
RA inflow	Subcostal (central hepatic vein) SSN (superior vena cava)

Doppler ultrasound. Accurate measurement of antegrade flow velocities is dependent on several technical factors. Most important is a parallel alignment between the ultrasound beam and the direction of blood flow. The ultrasound instrument measures Doppler frequency shifts. The displayed velocities are *calculated* with the Doppler equation based on transducer frequency, the speed of sound in blood, and the angle between the Doppler beam and flow of interest. For intracardiac flows, the 3D direction of flow is difficult to determine, particularly when flow is abnormal, and attempts to "correct" for the presumed intercept angle are likely to increase, rather than decrease, measurement error. Instead, the examiner positions the ultrasound beam as parallel as possible to the flow of interest based on obtaining the highest calculated velocity with careful transducer positioning and angulation (Table 2–9). In the Doppler equation, cos θ = 1 (and therefore can be ignored) when flow is oriented directly away (intercept angle = 0°) or straight toward (intercept angle = 180°) the ultrasound transducer. Small deviations from a parallel intercept angle (up to 20°) result in only a small error (6 percent) in velocity

calculations (See Fig. 1–30). While this approach generally results in accurate velocity data, the possibility of underestimation of intracardiac velocities due to a nonparallel intercept angle always must be considered in an echocardiographic examination. This potential limitation becomes significant when recording high-velocity flows in valvular stenosis, regurgitation, or intracardiac shunts.

Other technical factors pertinent to recording antegrade flow velocities include the use of an appropriate velocity scale, wall filters, and gain settings. The standard velocity format is to display flows toward the transducer above and flows away from the transducer below the zero baseline. The baseline may be shifted to maximize the flow of interest and the velocity scale adjusted so that the velocity curve uses the entire displayed range. Wall filters are set as low as possible, without resulting in excessive noise, to allow accurate measurement of time intervals. Gain settings are adjusted to show the peak velocity and velocity curve clearly without excessive background noise. A sample volume length of 5 to 10 mm typically is used to record antegrade flow velocities because this length provides reasonable intracardiac localization with adequate signal strength.

Signal aliasing (as discussed in Chap. 1) occurs even with normal intracardiac flow velocities. Use of the baseline shift can resolve this problem in most cases. If aliasing persists, use of high pulse repetition frequency or continuous-wave Doppler is needed for unambiguous display of the maximum velocity.

With appropriate instrument setting and attention to technical details, antegrade velocities with pulsed Doppler ultrasound appear as smooth envelopes with a well-defined onset and end of flow, a well-defined maximum velocity, and a thin band of velocities at each time point. The area under the velocity curve is "clear" because the flow velocities at a specific intracardiac site are relatively uniform. Continuous-wave Doppler recordings differ in that the curve is "filled in" due to inclusion of lower velocities along the entire length of the ultrasound beam.

Left Ventricular Outflow (Fig. 2–36)

An apical or suprasternal notch window is used to obtain a parallel intercept angle between the ultrasound beam and direction of blood flow in the left ventricular outflow tract and ascending aorta. Accurate recordings of left ventricular outflow velocities are difficult from a transesophageal approach because of the limited ability to obtain a parallel intercept angle, although a transgastric "apical" approach may be useful in some cases.

With a pulsed Doppler sample volume positioned on the left ventricular side of the aortic valve, an ejection velocity curve is recorded with a steep acceleration slope, a sharply peaked early systolic maximum velocity, and a less steep deceleration slope. Note the narrow band of velocities at any instant in time during acceleration, reflecting the uniformity of blood flow velocity in the outflow tract during acceleration. During deceleration, the range of flow velocities at any instant is slightly wider (spectral broadening) due to instability in the flow pattern during deceleration resulting in slight variation in flow velocities. The aortic valve closing click is seen immediately following end-ejection. Flow recording with pulsed Doppler on the aortic side of the valve appears similar except that the aortic valve opening click is seen, instead of the closing click, and the maximum velocity is slightly higher, by 0.2 to 0.4 m/s, than the outflow tract velocity due to slight narrowing of the cross-sectional area of flow at the aortic leaflet tips.

With continuous-wave Doppler interrogation of the aortic valve, both opening and closing clicks are recorded. The area under the velocity curve is "filled in" with lower-velocity signals be-

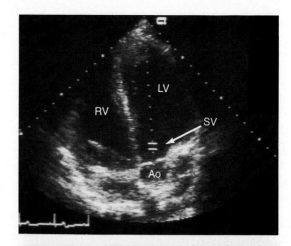

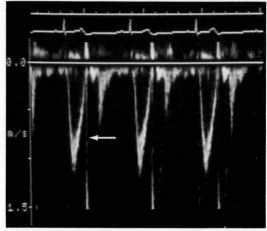

Figure 2–36. Normal left ventricular outflow velocity curve recorded with pulsed Doppler from an anteriorly angulated apical four-chamber view with the sample volume (SV) positioned just proximal to the aortic valve (*above*). The spectral display (*below*) shows a smooth velocity curve with a well-defined peak of 1.3 m/s and a clear closing click (*arrow*).

cause lower-velocity blood flow signals that originate in the left ventricle along the length of the ultrasound beam are displayed as well (Fig. 2–37).

With a normal aortic valve, the area under the velocity curve (the velocity-time integral) reflects stroke volume, which can be calculated by multiplying by cross-sectional area. The normal antegrade maximum velocity across the valve is about 1 to 1.2 m/s and will be the same whether measured by pulsed or continuous-wave Doppler methods. The normal outflow tract velocity typically is 0.8 to 1.0 m/s, corresponding to a velocity "step-up" across the valve or ratio of outflow tract to aortic velocity of 0.7 to 1.0.

The relationship between velocity and pressure gradients across *nonstenotic* valves is somewhat complex and is not described by the

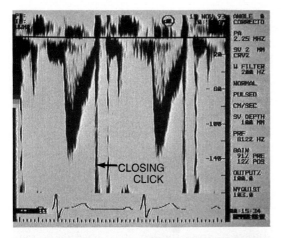

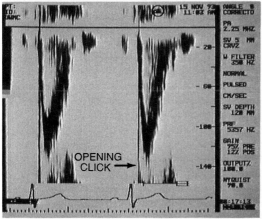

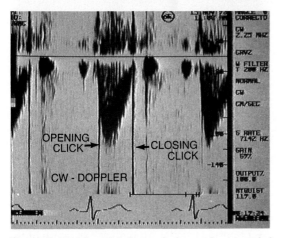

Figure 2–37. Normal left ventricular outflow recorded with pulsed Doppler proximal to the aortic valve (*above*) showing an aortic closing (but not opening) click, distal to the aortic valve (*center*) showing an opening click, and with continuous-wave Doppler (*below*) showing both opening and closing clicks.

Bernoulli equation (which applies to areas of narrowing). The period of acceleration corresponds to a slight pressure gradient from the left ventricle to the aorta, with the maximum pressure gradient corresponding to maximum acceleration. Left ventricular pressure falls below aortic pressure in midsystole, and at this point, deceleration of flow occurs. Thus, for the normal valve, maximum velocity occurs at the pressure crossover point (see Fig. 4–1). During deceleration, aortic pressure remains slightly higher than left ventricular pressure until flow decelerates to zero and the valve closes. At this point, left ventricular pressure continues to decline rapidly. This normal pattern of blood flow contrasts markedly with the pattern seen with a stenotic valve. With stenosis, a positive pressure gradient is present throughout the flow period, and pressure crossover corresponds to valve closure.

Right Ventricular Outflow

The right ventricular outflow tract and pulmonary artery are interrogated from a parasternal short-axis or right ventricular outflow tract view. Transesophageal interrogation may be possible from a high esophageal position in the longitudinal or transverse plane. Occasionally, a subcostal short-axis view from a transthoracic or transesophageal approach allows alignment parallel to blood flow in the pulmonary artery.

In the normal individual, the right ventricular ejection curve is similar to the left ventricular ejection curve except that peak velocity is slightly lower (0.8 to 1.0 m/s), the ejection period is longer, and the velocity curve is more rounded, with the maximum velocity occurring in midsystole. The shapes of the right and left ventricular ejection curves appear to relate to the downstream vascular resistance. The low-resistance pulmonary vasculature results in a slower rate of acceleration of blood flow, with the maximum velocity (and pressure crossover) occurring later in the ejection cycle. When pulmonary vascular resistance is increased, the right ventricular ejection curve resembles left ventricular ejection more closely with a sharper velocity curve and earlier peak velocity.

Left Ventricular Inflow (Fig. 2–38)

Diastolic flow across the mitral valve shows two peaks: an early diastolic peak velocity (*E* wave) reflecting passive early diastolic filling and a late diastolic peak velocity due to atrial contraction (*A* wave). The normal *E* velocity in healthy, young individuals is about 1.0 m/s,

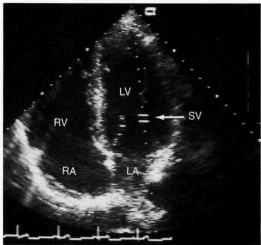

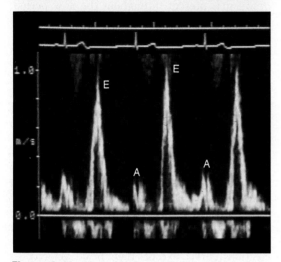

Figure 2–38. Normal left ventricular inflow velocity curve with the pulsed Doppler sample volume (SV) positioned at the mitral leaflet tips in diastole in the apical four-chamber view (*above*). The spectral display shows rapid early diastolic filling (*E*) with a small atrial (*A*) contribution to late diastolic filling.

with an *A* velocity of 0.2 to 0.4 m/s, reflecting the normal small contribution of atrial contraction to left ventricular diastolic filling. If diastole is long enough, a period of no flow, or diastasis, between the two flow curves is seen.

The pattern of left ventricular diastolic filling varies, even in normal individuals, with age, loading conditions, heart rate and PR interval. With age, there is a gradual reduction in *E* velocity, prolongation in the rate of early diastolic deceleration, and increase in *A* velocity such that the ratio of *E* to *A* velocity changes from >1 in young individuals, to about 1 at ages 50 to 60, to <1 in older normal individuals.

Increased preload results in an increase in *E* velocity, while decreased preload has the oppo-

site effect. When diastole is short (i.e., with a rapid heart rate), the *A* velocity becomes superimposed (or summated) onto the downslope of the *E* velocity, resulting in an apparent higher *A* velocity. At very high heart rates, only a single *E/A* peak may be seen. Prolongation of the PR interval has a similar effect. When atrial contraction occurs earlier in diastole, the *A* velocity is added to the downslope of the *E* velocity. These variations in the normal pattern of left ventricular diastolic filling should be recognized to avoid an inappropriate interpretation of an "abnormality."

Typically, left ventricular diastolic filling is recorded from an apical window on transthoracic studies or from the left atrial level on a transesophageal study. In addition to the physiologic variability discussed above, the peak *E* velocity and the ratio of the *E* to *A* peaks may differ depending on whether the sample volume is placed at the mitral annulus or at the mitral leaflet tips. Appropriate positioning of the sample volume depends on whether the Doppler curve is used to evaluate diastolic filling of the left ventricle (leaflet tips probably most useful) or transmitral stroke volume (mitral annular level most useful). Continuous-wave Doppler recordings show the highest velocities wherever they occur along the length of the ultrasound beam. Left ventricular diastolic filling is discussed in more detail in Chapter 5.

Right Ventricular Inflow

Right ventricular inflow can be recorded from an apical approach or from the parasternal right ventricular inflow view. The pattern of right ventricular diastolic filling is similar to left ventricular filling, although peak flow velocities are slightly lower with a normal right ventricular inflow *E* velocity of 0.3 to 0.7 m/s.

Left Atrial Filling

It is technically challenging to record left atrial filling from a transthoracic approach due to suboptimal signal strength at the depth of the pulmonary veins in many adults. However, with careful attention to technical details, this flow curve is obtainable in the right superior pulmonary vein in an apical four-chamber view in the majority of patients. From a transesophageal approach, flow in both right and left pulmonary veins can be recorded, with the clearest flow signals obtained from the left superior pulmonary vein. Atrial contraction results in brief backflow in the pulmonary veins (*a* wave) followed by a biphasic filling pattern with prominent filling of the atrium (x descent) during ventricular systole, a second brief reversal of flow (v wave) following ventricular contraction, and a second atrial filling curve (y descent) during ventricular diastole (see Chap. 5). Abnormalities of left atrial filling can be seen in patients with mitral regurgitation (Chap. 10), constrictive pericarditis (Chap. 8), and restrictive cardiomyopathy (Chap. 7).

Right Atrial Filling

Right atrial filling can be assessed from Doppler recordings of superior vena caval flow (from a suprasternal notch approach) or central hepatic vein flow (which lies parallel to the ultrasound beam from a subcostal window). The pattern of flow again is analogous to the pulsation pattern of the neck veins seen on clinical examination, with an a wave, an x descent reflecting systolic filling, a v wave, and a y descent reflecting diastolic filling of the right atrium.

Descending Aorta

Flow patterns in the descending aorta are important in the evaluation of cardiac disorders because the downstream flow pattern depends on the presence and severity of specific cardiac lesions. Examples include aortic regurgitation, patent ductus arteriosus, and aortic coarctation. Descending thoracic aorta flow can be recorded from a suprasternal notch approach and shows antegrade flow with a systolic velocity curve, a peak velocity of about 1.0 m/s, and brief early diastolic flow reversal. The proximal abdominal aorta recorded from a subcostal approach shows a similar flow pattern.

Normal Color Doppler Flow Patterns

Impact of Color Doppler Physics on Flow Displays

While spectral Doppler (pulsed or continuous) is preferable for accurate measurement of specific intracardiac blood flow velocities, the overall pattern of intracardiac flow is best evaluated with color flow imaging. Unfortunately, although, in theory, normal laminar flow should appear as a uniform red or blue color, in fact, color flow display instrumentation results in more complex patterns.

For example, flow in the left ventricular outflow tract is a uniform red color from a parasternal long-axis view because the direction of flow

is toward the transducer. The same flow is a uniform *blue* color from an apical approach because now it is directed away from the transducer (Fig. 2–39). This same phenomenon can be seen with flows in a single image plane. For example, antegrade flow in the aortic arch from a suprasternal notch view appears red (toward the transducer) in the more proximal segment and blue (away from the transducer) more distally with a small black area in the center of the image where the ultrasound beam is perpendicular to flow. Similarly, in the abdominal aorta from a subcostal approach, antegrade flow appears alternatively red and then blue as it transverses the image plane (see Fig. 1–33). In these examples, the change in color is due to a change in intercept angle between the ultrasound beam and blood flow at the left versus right edge of the sector.

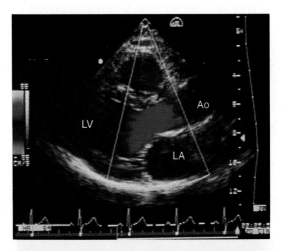

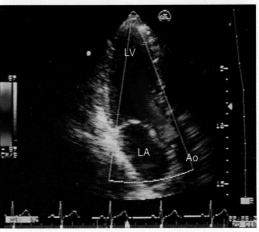

Figure 2–39. Flow in the left ventricular outflow tract recorded from a high parasternal position (*above*) is red (toward the transducer), while the same flow from an apical approach (*below*) is blue (away from the transducer).

Less dramatic changes in intercept angle across the 2D image also result in a complex color flow pattern for laminar normal flow. For example, evaluation of the left ventricular outflow tract in an apical long-axis view may show an apparent higher systolic velocity along the ventricular septum than along the anterior mitral leaflet (Fig. 2–40). This appearance results from a more parallel intercept angle between the Doppler beam and blood flow along the septum than adjacent to the mitral valve. The same actual velocities across the outflow tract result in differing Doppler frequency shifts depending on this intercept angle. Since the instrument assumes that $\cos \theta = 1$ for each signal, a falsely low velocity is calculated for nonparallel intercept angles, with the resulting image showing an apparent increase in velocity across the image plane due to differing intercept angles.

In addition to intercept angle, color flow images also are affected by the phenomenon of signal aliasing. The Nyquist limit, as displayed at the top and bottom of the color scale, typically is 60 to 80 cm/s with a 2- or 3-MHz transducer at depths used for transthoracic cardiac imaging. Since normal intracardiac flow velocities often exceed this limit, signal aliasing occurs. Flow toward the transducer is displayed in red at velocities less than the Nyquist limit, but once aliasing occurs, this same flow signal is displayed in blue. Thus flow toward the transducer is red aliasing to blue, while flow away from the transducer is blue aliasing to red. In fact, multiple aliases can occur with high-velocity flows displayed sequentially as going from red to blue to

red and so on. An example of normal aliasing is seen in the left ventricular inflow pattern on the apical four-chamber view, where the red flow toward the apex turns blue as it exceeds the Nyquist limit (see Fig. 1–34). While confusing at first, patterns of signal aliasing can be used to advantage in quantitation of intracardiac flows using the proximal isovelocity surface area approach discussed in Chapter 10.

Another color image pattern seen even with normal intracardiac flows is *variance*, which often is encoded as green on the color display. While the concept of variance is that a single intracardiac site exhibits multiple flow velocities and directions (such as in a regurgitant jet), from the foregoing discussions of intercept angle and aliasing, it is apparent that a normal flow pattern might meet variance criteria. For example, in a region at the aliasing limit, the instrument may sequentially measure flow toward then away from the transducer due to aliasing and then assign variance to that color pixel. Awareness that a color variance pattern can occur with normal intracardiac flows avoids erroneous interpretations.

Normal Ventricular Outflow Patterns

Color flow imaging of left ventricular outflow can be recorded from an apical approach in either an anteriorly angulated four-chamber view or a long-axis view. Flow is laminar, but aliasing typically occurs at this depth, resulting in a complex color pattern. While measurement of stroke volume proximal to the aortic valve, which *assumes* a flat flow velocity profile, has been validated, it remains controversial whether the appearance of aliasing along the ventricular septum in systole is due to a skewed flow profile or to variations in intercept angle across the color sector.

Note that while accurate measurements of antegrade velocities with pulsed or continuous-wave Doppler require a parallel intercept angle, with color flow imaging, often the spatial pattern of flow is of interest rather than the absolute velocities. Thus views with nonparallel intercept angles can be helpful. For example, left ventricular outflow can be evaluated with color flow imaging in a parasternal long-axis view even though the flow direction is almost perpendicular to the ultrasound beam. As we will see in Chapter 10, this view also is useful for evaluation of abnormal flows in the outflow tract, such as aortic regurgitation. In normal subjects, aortic regurgitation is rarely seen (5 percent of individuals) on color flow imaging.

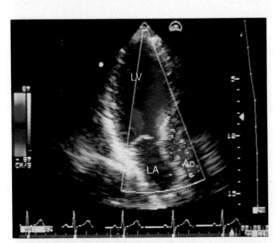

Figure 2–40. Color Doppler of left ventricular outflow from an apical long-axis view shows aliasing proximal to the aortic valve due to either a more parallel intercept angle between the Doppler scan line and direction of blood flow *or* a higher velocity near the septum versus adjacent to the anterior mitral valve leaflet.

Right ventricular outflow can be visualized from a parasternal short-axis view, from the right ventricular outflow view, or from a subcostal short-axis view. Since velocities are slightly lower and the depth of interrogation is less than for left ventricular outflow, the flow pattern away from the transducer typically shows a uniform blue color. Mild pulmonic regurgitation, appearing as a narrow red "flame" in diastole, is an incidental finding (present in 70–80 percent of normal individuals) of no apparent clinical significance.

Normal Ventricular Inflow Patterns

In the apical four-chamber view, left ventricular inflow appears as a broad flow stream extending laterally across the mitral annulus and lengthwise to the left ventricular apex. If the Nyquist limit is exceeded, signal aliasing occurs with a color shift at the aliasing velocity. In real time, the separate flows of early and late diastolic filling may be seen. When ultrasound penetration is optimal, diastolic flow extends from the pulmonary veins to the left ventricular apex. The normal spatial pattern of the left ventricular inflow is directed along the lateral left ventricular wall, in middiastole, with blue flow away from the transducer along the ventricular septum consistent with a "vortex" of flow in the left ventricle in diastole (Fig. 2–41). Interestingly, the normal counterclockwise vortex is reversed in patients after mitral valve replacement.

Right ventricular inflow patterns on color flow imaging are analogous to the patterns seen

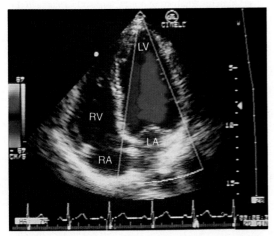

Figure 2–41. Normal pattern of left ventricular filling in middiastole in an apical four-chamber view shows flow toward the apex along the lateral wall simultaneously with flow away from the transducer along the septum.

in the left ventricle, although a diastolic "vortex" is not as prominent.

Normal Atrial Inflow Patterns

Inflow into the left atrium occurs via the four pulmonary veins. On transthoracic imaging, the right superior pulmonary vein is the easiest to visualize in the apical four-chamber view. Color flow imaging showing the biphasic red inflow from this vein allows correct placement of a pulsed Doppler sample volume for recording the spectral Doppler data. All four pulmonary veins can be visualized on transesophageal echo, but again, use of color flow imaging may facilitate identification of each vein. This approach is particularly helpful with right-sided veins, which may be difficult to recognize on 2D imaging alone. With careful examination techniques, a small amount of mitral regurgitation is present in 70–80 percent of normal people.

Inflow into the right atrium occurs via the superior and inferior venae cavae and the coronary sinus. Evaluation may be complicated by some degree of tricuspid regurgitation (present in 80–90 percent of normal subjects and a higher percentage of patients) which typically is directed along the interatrial septum. Flow from the inferior vena cava and coronary sinus may be seen in the right ventricular inflow view as well as in the short-axis view at the aortic valve level and in the apical four-chamber view. Superior vena caval flow is seen from the suprasternal notch approach. On transesophageal imaging, the longitudinal plane allows visualization of the superior vena cava entering the right atrium. In the right atrium, recognition of the several normal inflow patterns is important when an atrial septal defect is suspected. Note that 20 percent of normal subjects have a patent foramen ovale (demonstrable by intravenous echo contrast during a Valsalva maneuver), but color flow evidence for a patent foramen ovale is present in only about 5 percent of normal individuals.

Technical Aspects of Color Flow Imaging

The color flow display is dependent on each specific ultrasound instrument to some extent. However, many parameters are adjustable by the operator, so an optimal examination requires careful attention to instrument settings.

The *color flow map* usually can be varied in terms of (1) the color scale used, (2) the addition of variance to the color scale, and (3) the use of a power scale instead of a color scale. The specific color scale used is a matter of personal preference, with the diagnostic goal being to optimize the display and recognition of abnormal flow patterns.

The *velocity range* of the color flow map is determined by the Nyquist limit, and as for conventional pulsed Doppler, the range can be altered by shifting the zero baseline, changing the pulse repetition frequency, or altering the depth of the displayed image.

Color Doppler power output and *gain* are adjusted so that gain is just below the level at which random background noise appears. "Wall filters" can be varied to exclude low-velocity signals from the color flow display. In addition, many instruments allow variation in the assignment of a returning signal to 2D or Doppler display (depending on signal strength). Another approach to optimizing the color flow display is to reduce the 2D gain, since the instrument does not display flow data on top of "structures" even when the 2D signal is due to excessive gain.

Perhaps the most important technical factor in color flow imaging is optimization of *frame rate*. As discussed in Chapter 1, color flow frame rate depends on sector width, depth, pulse repetition frequency, and the number of samples per sector line. The examiner optimizes frame rate by focusing on the flow of interest, narrowing the sector, and decreasing the depth as much as possible. When frame rate remains inadequate for timing flow abnormalities, a color M-line through the area of interest may be helpful.

THE ECHOCARDIOGRAPHIC EXAMINATION

The specific echocardiographic views and Doppler flow velocities recorded in any individual patient depend on the indication for the study, the abnormalities noted as the examination is in progress, and each laboratory's basic protocol. The next chapter will discuss indications for echocardiography and the echocardiographic examination in detail.

SUGGESTED READING

1. Henry WL, DeMaria A, Gramiak R, et al. and the American Society of Echocardiography, Committee on Nomenclature and Standards: Report on two-dimensional echocardiography. Circulation 1980; 62: 212–222.
   Nomenclature standards for image orientation, imaging planes, and transducer location. Clear schematic drawings.

2. American Society of Echocardiography, Doppler Standards and Nomenclature Committee: Recommendations for Terminology and Display Doppler Echocardiography. Raleigh, NC, American Society of Echocardiography, 1984, pp 1–11.
   Nomenclature standards for Doppler data plus a useful glossary of Doppler terminology.

3. Lentner C (ed): Geigy Scientific Tables, vol 5: Heart and Circulation (ed 8). Basel, Switzerland, Ciba-Geigy, 1990.
   Excellent reference source summarizing normal values for cardiovascular imaging. Includes invasive and noninvasive normal data. Well referenced.

4. Netter FH: The Heart. Basel, Switzerland, Ciba, 1969.
   Clear illustrations of detailed cardiac anatomy with concise accompanying text on pages 2–12. A useful introduction and review of cardiac structure.

5. Thubriker M: The Aortic Valve. Boca Raton, Fla, CRC Press, 1990.
   Monograph on detailed anatomy, structure, and function of the aortic valve.

6. Roberts WC: Morphologic features of the normal and abnormal mitral valve. Am J Cardiol 1983; 51:1005–1028.
   A review of anatomy and function of the mitral valve based on 1010 autopsy cases. Excellent discussion and illustrations of normal mitral valve anatomy, mitral stenosis, and mitral regurgitation. Both photographs and schematic drawings are included.

7. Schnittger I, Gordon EP, Fitzgerald PJ, Popp RL: Standardized intracardiac measurements of two-dimensional echocardiography. J Am Coll Cardiol 1983; 2:934–938.
   Normal 2D echo intracardiac measurements are described in detail for 35 healthy adults.

8. Triulzi M, Gillam LD, Gentile F, et al: Normal adult cross-sectional echocardiographic values: Linear dimensions and chamber areas. Echocardiography 1984; 1:403–426.
   Tabular presentation of normal echo dimensions in 72 normal adults.

9. Pearlman JD, Triulzi MO, King ME, et al: Limits of normal left ventricular dimensions in growth and development: Analysis of dimensions and variance in the two-dimensional echocardiograms of 268 normal healthy subjects. J Am Coll Cardiol 1988; 12:1432–1441.
   Graphic display of normal echo dimensions in 72 adults and 196 children showing relationship of each dimension to body surface area with mean and 90 percent tolerance limits.

10. Roman MJ, Devereux RB, Kramer-Fox R, O'Loughlin J: Two-dimensional echocardiographic aortic root dimensions in normal children and adults. Am J Cardiol 1989; 64:507–512.
    Derivation of gender-specific upper limits of normal (indexed to body size) for aortic root dimensions based on 135 adults and 52 children.

11. Mitchell MM, Sutherland GR, Gussenhoven EJ, et al: Transesophageal echocardiography. J Am Soc Echocardiogr 1988; 1:362–377.
    Review of TEE views and diagnostic applications. Seventy references.

12. Seward JB, Khandheria BK, Edwards WD, et al: Biplanar transesophageal echocardiography: Anatomic correlations, image orientation, and clinical applications. Mayo Clin Proc 1990; 65:1193–1213.

Review of biplane TEE views and experience in 291 patients. Useful schematic drawings, although image orientation is nonstandard.

13. Benjamin EJ, Levy D, Anderson KM, et al: Determinants of Doppler indexes of left ventricular diastolic function in normal subjects (the Framingham Heart Study). Am J Cardiol 1992; 70:508–515.
Detailed study of the relationship between age and Doppler measures of left ventricular diastolic filling in the Framingham population after exclusion of subjects with hypertension, cardiac disease, or other organ system disease (n = 1485). E velocity decreased from 0.71 ± 0.14 m/s at ages 20–29 years to 0.53 ± 0.17 m/s for those ≥70 years of age. A velocity increased from 0.35 ± 0.06 to 0.64 ± 0.14 m/s in the same groups. The E/A ratio was 1.03 ± 0.26 m/s at ages 60–69.

14. Jaffe WM, Dewhurst TA, Otto CM, Pearlman AS: Influence of Doppler sample volume location on ventricular filling velocities. Am J Cardiol 1991; 68:550–552.
Detailed study in 300 subjects showing that E velocity increases from 0.45 ± 0.15 m/s at the annulus to 0.75 ± 0.22 m/s at the leaflet tips, while A velocity increases only from 0.47 ± 0.14 to 0.64 ± 0.28 m/s. This results in differing E/A velocity ratios at the annulus (1.05 ± 0.42) versus the leaflet tips (1.36 ± 0.65).

15. Appleton CP, Hatle LK, Popp RL: Superior vena cava and hepatic vein Doppler echocardiography in healthy adults. J Am Coll Cardiol 1987; 10:1032–1039.
Normal superior vena cava and hepatic vein Doppler flows show a systolic and diastolic antegrade flow with a reduction or reversal in antegrade flow following atrial systole (A wave). Variation with respiration is prominent in normal healthy adults.

16. Basnight MA, Gonzalez MS, Kershenovich SC, Appleton CP: Pulmonary venous flow velocity: Relation to hemodynamics, mitral flow velocity and left atrial volume, and ejection fraction. J Am Soc Echocardiogr 1991; 4:547–558.

17. Klein AL, Tajik AJ: Doppler assessment of pulmonary venous flow in healthy subjects and in patients with heart disease. J Am Soc Echocardiogr 1991; 4:379–392.

18. Bartzokis T, Lee R, Yeoh TK, et al: Transesophageal echo-Doppler echocardiographic assessment of pulmonary venous flow patterns. J Am Soc Echocardiogr 1991; 4:457–464.
Each of these three references (16–18) provide detailed descriptions of normal pulmonary venous flow patterns and the physiologic variables that affect the flow pattern.

CLINICAL INDICATIONS FOR ECHOCARDIOGRAPHY

Clinical indications for echocardiographic examination are best considered within the framework of clinical decision analysis. This chapter provides a brief introduction to this approach, with suggestions for further reading indicated at the end of the chapter.

CLINICAL DECISION ANALYSIS AS THE FRAMEWORK FOR THE DIAGNOSTIC USE OF ECHOCARDIOGRAPHY

Accuracy of a Diagnostic Test

The first level of analysis in evaluating a diagnostic test is to consider its accuracy. The

clinical utility of any diagnostic test, including echocardiography, depends, in large part, on the certainty with which a specific diagnosis can be confirmed or excluded based on the test results (Fig. 3–1). The *sensitivity* of a test is the degree to which it identifies all patients with the disease. *Sensitivity* is defined as the patients with a "true positive" test result divided by all patients with the disease. The *specificity* of a test is the degree to which it identifies all patients *without* the disease. *Specificity* is defined as the patients with a "true negative" test result divided by all patients without the disease. Sensitivity and specificity are related inversely to each other; in general, the higher the sensitivity, the lower is the specificity and vice versa. Whether a higher sensitivity is preferable to a higher specificity depends on the specific clinical question. If the

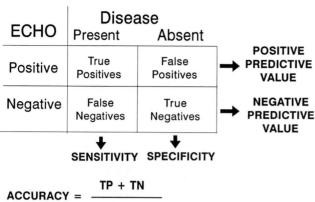

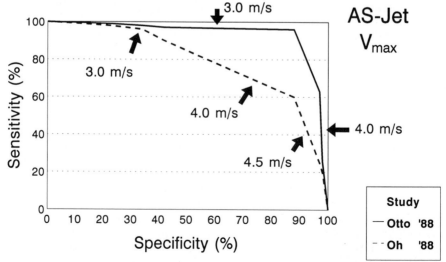

Figure 3–1. Sensitivity and specificity in comparison with positive and negative predictive value. Note that predictive values are dependent on the prevalence of the disease in the study population and thus cannot be extrapolated to other patient groups (TP = true positives; TN = true negatives.)

goal of the test is identification of *all* patients with the disease, a high sensitivity is preferable. If the goal is exclusion of a specific diagnosis in an individual patient, a high specificity is preferable. The relationship between sensitivity and specificity can be evaluated quantitatively for any given diagnostic test using receiver-operator curve (ROC) analysis (Fig. 3–2).

The *accuracy* of a test is defined as the true positives plus the true negatives divided by the total number of tests performed. Accuracy indicates the percentage of patients in whom the test results are correct in identifying the presence or absence of disease.

A major limitation of applying sensitivity/specificity data to an individual patient is the problem of whether a particular patient has a "true" or a "false" test result. At first glance, it might seem that use of positive and negative predictive values would be more useful in the clinical setting. Predictive values indicate the percentage of patients with a positive test result who have the suspected disease (positive predictive value = true positives divided by all positives) and the percentage with a negative test result who do not have the suspected disease (negative predictive value = true negatives divided by all negatives). However, predictive values depend on the *prevalence* of disease in a given population and therefore cannot be extrapolated to other patient groups.

The absolute number of patients with *false-*

Figure 3–2. Graph of sensitivity versus specificity, known as a receiver-operator curve, comparing the studies of Otto and Pearlman[9] and Oh et al.[10] In the first study, a clinical decision rule was proposed for timing of valve replacement in aortic stenosis based on jet velocity breakpoints at 3.0 and 4.0 m/s. In the second study, a single breakpoint at 4.5 m/s was suggested, but the data show that a two-breakpoint approach at 3.0 and 4.5 m/s also would be appropriate. Patients with jet velocities between these breakpoints require calculation of aortic valve area and assessment of coexisting aortic regurgitation.

positive or *false-negative* test results depends on the prevalence of disease in the population studied as well as the sensitivity and specificity of the test. Intuitively, this is obvious comparing the use of echocardiography to "screen" healthy young subjects for endocarditis (many false-positive results due to ultrasound imaging artifacts) versus the same test in patients who have a new murmur, fever, and positive blood cultures. The finding of a valvular vegetation on echocardiography in the latter group has a much higher predictive value for a diagnosis of endocarditis than in the healthy subjects, even though the sensitivity and specificity of echocardiography for diagnosing endocarditis are the same in both groups. Again, the positive or negative predictive value of a test reflects disease prevalence as well as test accuracy.

Integration of Clinical Data and Test Results

A better approach to the use of sensitivity/specificity data in patient management is to integrate relevant clinical data with the test result. The value of a diagnostic test increases when the pretest likelihood of disease is integrated with the test results to derive a posttest likelihood of disease. This approach is known as *Bayesian*

analysis. For example, the pretest likelihood of severe aortic stenosis in an asymptomatic 30-year-old woman with no systolic murmur on careful auscultation is very low. An echocardiogram purporting to show severe aortic stenosis most likely is an erroneous interpretation (a false-positive test result). In this setting, the result does not increase the posttest likelihood of disease very much. In contrast, in an elderly man with a 4/6 aortic stenosis murmur and symptoms of angina, syncope, and heart failure, the diagnosis of severe valvular aortic stenosis can be made with a high level of certainty even before any test is performed. The echocardiogram serves only to confirm the diagnosis and quantitate the severity of obstruction. In general, diagnostic tests are most helpful when the pretest likelihood of disease is intermediate so that the test result will substantially change the posttest likelihood of disease (Fig. 3–3).

The Threshold Approach to Clinical Decision Analysis

The most comprehensive approach to evaluation of a diagnostic test is *clinical decision analysis.* Clinical decision analysis incorporates several rigorous approaches to the problem of clinical prediction, with the method most applicable to a diagnostic test, such as echocardiography, being the threshold approach. The basic tenet of clinical decision analysis as applied to a diagnostic test is that the test results should have an impact on patient care by either (1) prompting a change in therapy or (2) leading to a change in the subsequent diagnostic strategy in that patient. This basic assumption is formalized in the *threshold model* of decision analysis. In this approach, two disease probability thresholds are defined for the diagnostic test: (1) a lower threshold below which the risk of the test is greater than the risk of not treating the patient and (2) an upper threshold above which treating the patient is lower risk than performing the test. The intermediate range—where the risk of treating or not treating the patient is greater than the risk of the diagnostic test—is known as the *testing zone* (Fig. 3–4).

For any *specific* indication, the testing zone for echocardiography generally is wide because of the low risk and high accuracy of this technique. However, both an upper and lower threshold still are definable for echocardiography. The upper threshold is reached in situations in which the diagnosis is clear, and echocardiographic examination would only delay appropriate treat-

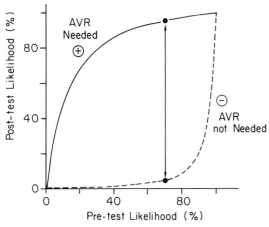

Figure 3–3. Bayesian analysis has been applied to the data from Otto and Pearlman.[9] The posttest likelihood (*y* axis) of need for aortic valve replacement (AVR) was calculated for each hypothetical pretest likelihood (*x* axis). Pretest and corresponding posttest likelihoods for the study population are indicated by the arrow. (*Reprinted with permission from Otto CM, Pearlman AS: Doppler echocardiography in adults with symptomatic aortic stenosis. Arch Intern Med 148:2553–2560, 1988; copyright 1988, American Medical Association.*)

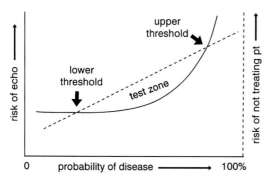

Figure 3–4. Diagram illustrating the threshold approach to clinical decision making. The risk of the diagnostic test—in this case echocardiography—is shown in the solid line (left *y* axis) with the risk of *not* treating the patient for the suspected disease shown in the dashed line (right *y* axis). The probability of disease based on the clinical presentation is shown from 0 to 100 percent on the *x* axis. The lower threshold is the point at which the risk of not treating the patient is greater than the risk of echocardiography. The upper threshold is the point at which the risk of echocardiography (including false-negative results, delay in treatment) is greater than the risk of not treating the patient. The test zone is the pretest likelihood of disease between these two thresholds.

ment. For example, a patient with classic presentation of an ascending aortic dissection (chest pain, wide mediastinum, peripheral pulse loss) requires prompt surgery. Any delay due to unnecessary diagnostic testing could result in additional morbidity or mortality.

It is tempting to assume that there is no lower end to the test zone for echocardiography given the absence of known adverse biologic effects of this procedure. However, the risk of the test also includes costs and, more important, the risks of additional diagnostic tests or even erroneous treatment choices resulting from a false-positive echocardiographic finding. For example, an echocardiogram is not indicated to evaluate for aortic dissection in a young patient with atypical chest pain and a normal physical examination, electrocardiogram, and chest radiograph. If a false-positive diagnosis leads to further evaluation with cardiac catheterization, any complications from the invasive procedure ultimately can be considered a consequence of the echocardiographic results. Thus a lower limit to the test zone *does* exist for echocardiography and can be defined for each specific diagnostic indication by applying decision analysis techniques.

Other clinical decision analysis approaches have been applied to specific clinical problems that utilize echocardiographic data as a branch point in the decision analysis tree. One example is the problem of timing of valve replacement in chronic asymptomatic aortic regurgitation (see Suggested Reading 7).

Cost-Effectiveness

An additional consideration in medical practice is the *cost-effectiveness* of a diagnostic procedure. Note that this term incorporates not only the *cost* of the test (echocardiography compares favorably with other cardiac diagnostic tests) but also the *effectiveness* of the test—that is, test accuracy and its impact on patient management. This type of analysis has been applied to some echocardiographic diagnostic issues, but more widespread use of this approach is needed.

Implications for Diagnostic Use of Echocardiography

As the threshold model for clinical decision analysis indicates, it no longer is acceptable to consider only sensitivity and specificity in deciding whether or not to perform a diagnostic test. The echocardiogram request should indicate an appropriate clinical question (not "evaluate heart") with an estimate of the probability of the diagnosis in that patient. Next, the reliability of echocardiography for that diagnosis is considered, and most important, the likelihood that the echocardiographic results will alter patient management is formulated prior to performing the study. Often it is helpful to consider the specific branch point in the diagnostic/therapeutic plan that the echocardiographic results will be applied to in the clinical decision process.

With these considerations in mind, there are certain situations in which the use of echocardiography clearly changes patient management:

1. Making the correct anatomic diagnosis (e.g., in a patient with heart failure symptoms, differentiation of a pericardial effusion from valvular stenosis or from a cardiomyopathy)

2. Providing important prognostic data in a patient with a known anatomic diagnosis (e.g., vegetation size in endocarditis, left ventricular ejection fraction in cardiomyopathy, sequential changes in left ventricular chamber size in chronic valvular regurgitation)

3. Identifying complications of a known diagnosis (e.g., paravalvular abscess in endocarditis, left ventricular thrombus in cardiomyopathy)

In addition, there are numerous other settings in which echocardiography is considered to be clinically indicated. Whether all these situations meet the strict criteria of the clinical threshold model requires ongoing appraisal.

Throughout this text, the accuracy (sensitivity and specificity) of echocardiography for each specific diagnosis will be indicated, if known. Critical evaluations of the diagnostic utility of echocardiography in specific patient populations and clinical settings will be highlighted, including symptomatic adults with aortic stenosis (Chap. 9), asymptomatic chronic aortic regurgitation (Chap. 10), evaluation of chest pain in the emergency room (Chap. 6), intraoperative assessment of mitral valve repair (Chap. 10), and the diagnosis and prognosis of endocarditis (Chap. 12).

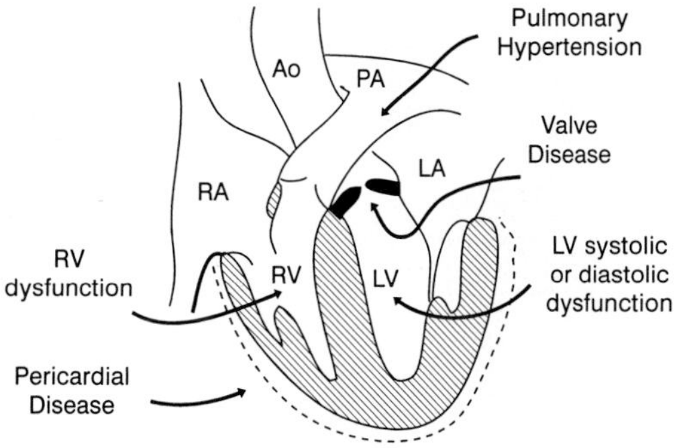

INDICATIONS FOR ECHOCARDIOGRAPHY

Transthoracic Echocardiography

By Clinical Signs and Symptoms

An echocardiogram often is requested to evaluate a specific clinical sign or symptom such as chest pain, heart failure symptoms (Fig. 3–5), a murmur, or cardiomegaly on chest radiography (Fig. 3–6). When the echocardiographer evaluates a patient with one of these indications, it is important that the differential diagnosis be considered and each possibility excluded or confirmed during the course of the examination. For example, a patient with a systolic murmur may have valvular aortic stenosis, a subaortic membrane, hypertrophic cardiomyopathy, mitral regurgitation, a ventricular septal defect, pulmonic stenosis, or tricuspid regurgitation. With two-dimensional (2D) imaging and Doppler evaluation, each of these possible diagnoses can be evaluated. If a careful examination reveals none of these abnormalities, it may be concluded that the murmur is a benign "flow" murmur (Fig. 3–7).

Similarly, in the echocardiographic examination of a patient with chest pain, even if the referring physician has made a presumptive diagnosis of coronary artery disease, the echocardiographer should be alert to any findings suggesting other causes for chest pain such as left ventricular outflow obstruction (valvular aortic stenosis or hypertrophic cardiomyopathy), aortic dissection, or pericarditis. The echocardiographic differential diagnosis for common symptoms is shown in Table 3–1 and for common physical signs in Table 3–2. These examples are not meant to be an exhaustive list of the possibilities but rather represent an illustration of the types of conditions the echocardiographer should consider in performing and interpreting the examination.

Figure 3–5. Diagram illustrating some of the more common causes of heart failure that should be actively excluded or confirmed during echocardiographic examination.

By Anatomic Diagnosis

In many patients referred for echocardiography, a definite or presumptive anatomic diagnosis has been made. In these patients, the echocardiographer needs to be aware of the information that can be obtained by echocardiography, the limitations of echocardiography, and alternative diagnostic approaches.

For example, in a patient with a systolic mur-

TABLE 3–1. DIFFERENTIAL DIAGNOSIS FOR THE ECHOCARDIOGRAPHER: COMMON SYMPTOMS

"REASON FOR ECHO"	DIFFERENTIAL DIAGNOSIS
Chest pain	Coronary artery disease: acute myocardial infarction or angina Aortic dissection Pericarditis Valvular aortic stenosis Hypertrophic cardiomyopathy
Heart failure	Left ventricular systolic dysfunction (global or segmental) Valvular heart disease Left ventricular diastolic dysfunction Pericardial disease Right ventricular dysfunction
Palpitations	Left ventricular systolic dysfunction Mitral valve disease Congenital heart disease (e.g., ASD, Ebstein's anomaly) Pericarditis No structural cardiac disease

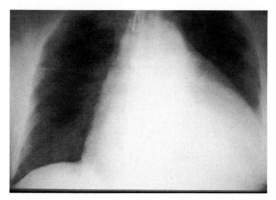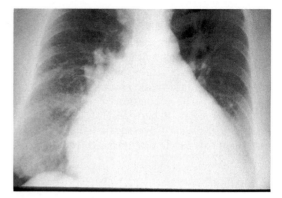

Figure 3–6. Chest radiographs demonstrating cardiomegaly due to a large pericardial effusion (*left*) and cardiomegaly due to multivalve disease with four-chamber enlargement (*right*).

mur known to be due to valvular aortic stenosis, the echocardiogram may be requested to evaluate the severity of obstruction, the degree of co-existing aortic regurgitation, the presence of left ventricular hypertrophy, and the status of left ventricular systolic function, as well as to detect any associated valvular abnormalities (e.g., mitral regurgitation). Usually echocardiography provides all the needed information for clinical decision making other than coronary artery anatomy, but the echocardiographer must acknowledge that stenosis severity may have been underestimated if there was a nonparallel intercept angle between the direction of the aortic jet and the ultrasound beam. In cases where the echocardiographic results appear to be discordant with the clinical impression, alternate diagnostic tests such as cardiac catheterization may be needed.

Echocardiography in a patient with endocarditis is a second, more complex example. On the one hand, echocardiography can detect valvular vegetations, identify the specific valves involved, evaluate the presence and degree of valve dysfunction, and quantitate associated chamber enlargement. Both left and right ventricular systolic function can be qualitatively and quantitatively evaluated. In addition, abscess formation may be identified. While the potential prognostic value of measuring vegetation size remains controversial, many clinicians find this information of clinical value. On the other hand, endocarditis is a clinical and bacteriologic diagnosis and cannot be excluded by echocardiography. The sensitivity of echocardiography for detection of valvular vegetations varies with image quality; conversely, a healed valvular vegetation may persist after a previous episode of endocarditis. Transesophageal echocardiography is more sensitive for diagnosing valvular

vegetations and should be considered if the clinical suspicion of endocarditis is high and the transthoracic study is nondiagnostic. Transesophageal echocardiography also is much more sensitive for the diagnosis of paravalvular abscesses and for evaluation of prosthetic valve endocarditis.

TABLE 3–2. DIFFERENTIAL DIAGNOSIS FOR THE ECHOCARDIOGRAPHER: COMMON SIGNS

"REASON FOR ECHO"	DIFFERENTIAL DIAGNOSIS: COMMON SIGNS
Cardiac murmur	
Systolic	Flow murmur (no valve abnormality)
	Aortic stenosis, subaortic obstruction, hypertrophic obstructive cardiomyopathy
	Mitral regurgitation
	Ventricular septal defect
	Pulmonic stenosis
	Tricuspid regurgitation
Diastolic	Mitral stenosis
	Aortic regurgitation
	Pulmonic regurgitation
	Tricuspid stenosis
Cardiomegaly on chest radiography	Pericardial effusion
	Dilated cardiomyopathy
	Specific chamber enlargement (e.g., left ventricle in chronic aortic regurgitation)
Systemic embolic event	Left ventricular systolic function and segmental wall motion abnormalities (aneurysms)
	Left ventricular thrombus
	Aortic valve disease
	Mitral valve disease
	Left atrial thrombus (TTE has low sensitivity)
	Patent foramen ovale

In Table 3–3, the key echocardiographic findings, limitations of echocardiography, and alternate diagnostic approaches for several anatomic diagnoses are indicated. Each of these topics is covered in detail in subsequent chapters.

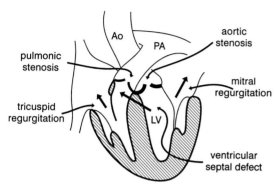

Figure 3–7. Diagram illustrating the more common etiologies for a systolic murmur. If an echocardiogram is requested for this indication, the sonographer should focus the examination toward confirmation or exclusion of each of these possibilities.

By Clinical Setting (Table 3–4)

The third category of indications for echocardiography is the examination requested because the patient is a member of a clinical group in whom "routine" echocardiographic studies are thought to be clinically valuable. These examinations fall into one of four categories: (1) *screening* examinations to detect cardiac abnormalities in a group of patients with a high prevalence of disease, (2) *monitoring* examinations performed as part of a therapeutic procedure, (3) *evaluation* before and after a therapeutic intervention to assess the effect of the intervention and detect possible complications, and (4) *baseline* studies performed in patients at risk for subsequent cardiac disease or progression of preexisting cardiac disease.

Screening examinations are performed in first-degree family members of patients with genetically transmitted cardiac diseases, such as Marfan's syndrome or hypertrophic cardiomyopathy, to detect possible cardiac involvement in those individuals. In patients with positive blood cultures and/or a fever of unexplained etiology, an echocardiogram may be ordered to detect possible endocarditis. Similarly, in patients with cerebrovascular events that may be embolic in origin, an echocardiogram is requested to identify any potential cardiac sources of emboli. The value of echocardiography for the last two "indications" is low if the prevalence of disease in the population is low. A potential cardiac source of emboli is unlikely to be found in patients with a known noncardiac cause of the neurologic disorder. Conversely, the likelihood of identifying a potential source of embolus is high in younger patients (age <45 years) or in those with a cardiac history (e.g., left ventricular apical thrombus in a patient with prior myocardial infarction) or pertinent physical findings (e.g., mitral valve disease). Furthermore, the value of the test is directly related to the impact of the test results on the patient's subsequent medical treatment. If the results of the echocardiogram will not alter therapy or the subsequent diagnostic strategy, then the echocardiogram is of little value.

Screening examinations often are requested in patients with cardiac arrhythmias to identify underlying structural abnormalities. For supraventricular arrhythmias without other evidence of underlying heart disease or a family history of a genetic disorder, the likelihood of a structural abnormality is low. Although most patients with ventricular arrhythmias will have significant structural disease, including left ventricular systolic dysfunction and/or segmental wall motion abnormalities, these diagnoses usually are known on clinical grounds or on the basis of other diagnostic tests prior to echocardiography.

The use of echocardiography as a low-yield screening examination can have a major negative impact on the diagnostic utility of this technique if only a limited number of echocardiographic studies can be performed (depending on the number of instruments, sonographers, and physicians available). In this situation, unnecessary examinations may delay or prevent diagnosis and subsequent therapy in patients with higher-priority indications for echocardiography. For example, an inpatient echocardiogram performed urgently for "source of embolus" in a patient with a low likelihood of disease may delay scheduling of an "elective" outpatient study in a patient with suspected valvular aortic stenosis. Delay in diagnosis and treatment of a patient with symptomatic severe aortic stenosis may result in an adverse medical outcome. Use of practice guidelines, as suggested by the American College of Cardiology and the American Heart Association (Suggested Reading 12) or triage of requested studies based on diagnostic yield and urgency, as suggested in Table 3–5, helps to formalize the process of prioritizing requests for echocardiographic examinations.

Monitoring examinations may be performed sequentially over brief or prolonged periods of time. Intraoperative monitoring of left ventric-

TABLE 3-3. INDICATIONS FOR ECHOCARDIOGRAPHY

CLINICAL DIAGNOSIS	KEY ECHO FINDINGS	LIMITATIONS OF ECHO	ALTERNATE APPROACHES
Valvular Heart Disease			
Valve stenosis	Etiology of stenosis, valve anatomy Transvalvular ΔP, valve area Chamber enlargement and hypertrophy LV and RV systolic function Associated valvular regurgitation	Possible underestimation of stenosis severity Possible coexisting coronary artery disease	Cardiac cath
Valve regurgitation	Mechanism and etiology of regurgitation Severity of regurgitation Chamber enlargement LV and RV systolic function PA pressure estimate	TEE may be needed to evaluate mitral regurgitant severity and valve anatomy (esp. before MV repair)	Cardiac cath
Prosthetic valve function	Evidence for stenosis Detection of regurgitation Chamber enlargement Ventricular function PA pressure estimate	Imaging prosthetic valves is limited by shadowing and reverberations TEE is needed for suspected prosthetic MR due to "masking" of the LA on TTE	Cardiac cath
Endocarditis	Detection of vegetations (TTE sensitivity 70–85%) Presence and degree of valve dysfunction Chamber enlargement and function Detection of abscess Possible prognostic implications	TEE more sensitive for detection of vegetations (>90%) Endocarditis is a clinical diagnosis and cannot be excluded by echo TEE more sensitive for abscess detection	Blood cultures and clinical exam form the basis for diagnosis of endocarditis
Coronary Artery Disease			
Acute myocardial infarction	Segmental wall motion abnormality reflects "myocardium at risk" Global LV function (EF) Complications: Acute MR vs. VSD Pericarditis LV thrombus, aneurysm RV infarct	Coronary artery anatomy itself not directly visualized	Coronary angio Radionuclide LV angio Cardiac cath
Angina	Global and segmental LV systolic function Exclude other causes of angina (e.g., AS, HOCM)	Resting wall motion may be normal despite significant CAD Stress echo needed to induce ischemia and wall motion abnormality	Coronary angio Stress thallium ETT
Pre-/post-revascularization	Assess wall thickness and endocardial motion at baseline Improvement in segmental function postprocedure	Viable but nonfunctioning myocardium cannot be identified	PET Thallium ETT

TABLE 3–3. INDICATIONS FOR ECHOCARDIOGRAPHY *Continued*

CLINICAL DIAGNOSIS	KEY ECHO FINDINGS	LIMITATIONS OF ECHO	ALTERNATE APPROACHES
End-stage ischemic disease	Overall LV systolic function (EF) PA pressures Associated MR LV thrombus RV systolic function		Coronary angio Radionuclide EF
Cardiomyopathy			
Dilated	Chamber dilation (all four) LV and RV systolic function (qualitative and EF) Coexisting atrioventricular valve regurgitation PA systolic pressure LV thrombus	No direct measure of LVEDP Accurate EF may be difficult if image quality poor	Radionuclide EF LV and RV angiography
Restrictive	LV wall thickness LV systolic function Pattern of LV diastolic filling and LA filling via pulmonary veins PA systolic pressure	Diastolic dysfunction is difficult to assess Must be distinguished from constrictive pericarditis	Cardiac cath with direct, simultaneous RV and LV pressure measurement after volume loading
Hypertrophic	Pattern and extent of LV hypertrophy Dynamic LVOT obstruction (imaging and Doppler) Coexisting MR Diastolic LV dysfunction		
Hypertension	LV wall thickness and internal dimensions LV mass LV systolic function Aortic root dilation, AR		
Pericardial Disease	Pericardial thickening Detection, size, and location of PE 2D signs of tamponade physiology Doppler signs of tamponade physiology	Diagnosis of tamponade is a hemodynamic and clinical diagnosis Constrictive pericarditis is a difficult diagnosis Not all patients with pericarditis have an effusion	Intracardiac pressure measurements for tamponade or constriction MRI or CT to detect pericardial thickening
Aortic Disease			
Aortic root dilation	Etiology of aortic dilation Accurate aortic root diameter measurements Anatomy of sinuses of Valsalva (esp. Marfan's syndrome) Associated aortic regurgitation		CT, MRI Aortography

Table continued on following page

TABLE 3–3. INDICATIONS FOR ECHOCARDIOGRAPHY *Continued*

CLINICAL DIAGNOSIS	KEY ECHO FINDINGS	LIMITATIONS OF ECHO	ALTERNATE APPROACHES
Aortic dissection	2D images of ascending aorta (PLAX, PSAX), aortic arch (SSN), descending thoracic (A2C), and proximal abdominal (SC) aorta Imaging of dissection "flap" Associated aortic regurgitation Ventricular function	TEE more sensitive (97%) and specific (100%) Cannot assess distal vascular beds	Aortography CT MRI TEE
Cardiac Masses			
LV thrombus	High sensitivity and specificity for diagnosis of LV thrombus Suspect with apical wall motion abnormality or diffuse LV systolic dysfunction	Technical artifacts can be misleading 5-MHz transducer and angulated apical views often needed	LV thrombus may not be recognized on radionuclide or contrast angiography
LA thrombus	Low sensitivity for detection of LA thrombus, although specificity is high Suspect with LA enlargement, MV disease	TEE is needed to detect LA thrombus reliability	TEE
Cardiac tumors	Size, location, and physiologic consequences of tumor mass	Extracardiac involvement not well seen Cannot distinguish benign from malignant, or tumor from thrombus	TEE, CT, MRI (with cardiac gating)
Pulmonary Hypertension			
	Estimate of PA pressure Evidence of left-sided heart disease to account for increased PA pressures RV size and systolic function (cor pulmonale) Associated TR	Indirect PA pressure measurement Unable to determine pulmonary vascular resistance accurately	Cardiac cath
Congenital Heart Disease			
	Detection and assessment of anatomic abnormalities Quantitation of physiologic abnormalities Chamber enlargement Ventricular function	No direct intracardiac pressure measurements Complicated anatomy may be difficult to evaluate if image quality is poor (TEE helpful)	MRI with cardiac gating and realignment of images Cardiac cath

A2C = apical two-chamber; Angio = angiography; AS = aortic stenosis; CAD = coronary artery disease; Cath = catheterization; CT = computed tomography; EF = ejection fraction; ETT = exercise treadmill test; HOCM = hypertrophic obstructive cardiomyopathy; LA = left atrial; LV = left ventricular; LVEDP = left ventricular end-diastolic pressure; LVOT = left ventricular outflow tract; MHz = megaHertz; MR = mitral regurgitation; MRI = magnetic resonance imaging; MV = mitral valve; ΔP = pressure gradient; PA = pulmonary artery; PE = pericardial effusion; PET = positron emission tomography; PLAX = parasternal long-axis; PSAX = parasternal short-axis; RV = right ventricular; SC = subcostal; SSN = suprasternal notch; 2D = two-dimensional; TEE = transesophageal echocardiography; TR = tricuspid regurgitation; TTE = transthoracic echocardiography; VSD = ventricular septal defect.

TABLE 3–4. OTHER CLINICAL SETTINGS IN WHICH ECHOCARDIOGRAPHY OFTEN IS INDICATED

Screening Examinations

First-degree relatives of patients with genetic cardiovascular diseases
Patients with fevers, positive blood cultures, and suspected endocarditis
Patients with cerebrovascular events for possible cardiac "source of embolus"
Arrhythmia patients

Monitoring Studies

Intraoperative evaluation of LV function in high-risk patients
LV size and systolic function in patients with chronic valvular regurgitation
LV hypertrophy in hypertensives

Pre-/Postintervention Echocardiography

Possible procedural complications
    Electrophysiologic studies
    Endomyocardial biopsy
Effect of intervention
    Revascularization (wall motion and thickening)
    Pharmacologic therapy (heart failure, hypertension, HOCM)
    Valve repair or commissurotomy

Baseline Studies

After valve replacement
Before chemotherapy (cardiotoxic)

TABLE 3–5. AN EXAMPLE OF HOW THE PRIORITY OF REQUESTED ECHOCARDIOGRAPHIC STUDIES MIGHT BE GROUPED

1. *High diagnostic yield, emergency indications*
   Hypotension—suspected pericardial tamponade
   Chest pain—suspected acute aortic dissection or acute myocardial infarction (nondiagnostic ECG)
   Heart failure—severe, unknown etiology
   Complications of acute MI
   Complications of endocarditis—new murmur, heart failure, prolonged PR-interval
   Decompensated congenital heart disease
2. *High diagnostic yield, nonemergency*
   Cardiac murmur—stable patient with suspected significant valvular disease
   Clinical diagnosis of endocarditis—stable patient with definite clinical criteria for endocarditis
   Congestive heart failure—stable patient with new diagnosis of heart failure or change in clinical status
   Suspected prosthetic valve dysfunction—currently stable patient with suspected valve dysfunction
   Congenital heart disease—patient with new diagnosis or prior surgery
   Coronary artery disease—stress echo for diagnosis or follow-up
   Chronic aortic root dilation
   Pulmonary heart disease or recurrent pulmonary emboli
3. *High diagnostic yield but can be scheduled electively*
   Known valvular heart disease—follow-up studies for ventricular size and systolic function with no interim change in clinical symptoms
   Preoperative assessment for elective surgery of patients with suspected cardiac dysfunction
   Baseline studies after cardiac surgery or valve replacement
   "Source of embolus" evaluation in patient < 45 years old or in patients with suspected cardiac disease
   Family history of inherited cardiac disease
   Suspected cardiac mass
   Hypertension
4. *Moderate to low diagnostic yield*
   Cardiac "source of embolus" in patient > 45 years of age with no evidence of cardiac disease
   "Screening" examinations in arrhythmia patients, organ-transplant donors or recipients, or "routine" preoperative patients

ular size and systolic function by transesophageal echocardiography is useful in cardiac patients undergoing noncardiac surgery to optimize ventricular preload and for early identification of ischemia, thus preventing perioperative myocardial infarction. Monitoring of left ventricular size and systolic function over many years is performed in patients with chronic valvular regurgitation to determine the optimal timing of surgical intervention. In hypertensive patients, monitoring of left ventricular wall thickness and mass allows assessment of the effect of long-term antihypertensive therapy on end-organ damage (in this case, the left ventricle).

Pre- and postintervention echocardiography may be utilized to detect possible procedural complications (e.g., pericardial effusion after electrophysiologic catheter studies or after endomyocardial biopsy). In addition, echocardiography may be used to assess the effect of the intervention by comparing pre- and postprocedure studies (e.g., in patients undergoing coronary revascularization procedures, percutaneous mitral balloon commissurotomy, or surgical mitral valve repair). The effects of pharmacologic therapy on a specific endpoint of interest also may be evaluated. Examples include the changes in stroke volume with vasodilator therapy in a patient with dilated cardiomyopathy or changes in the pattern of left ventricular diastolic filling after beta blockade in a patient with hypertrophic cardiomyopathy.

Baseline echocardiographic studies serve as a reference point in patients with a high likelihood of subsequent cardiac dysfunction. In a patient with a prosthetic valve, a baseline study performed when the patient is asymptomatic and clinically stable provides the normal antegrade velocity across the valve in that individual; the degree of normal prosthetic valve regurgitation; the state of the left ventricle with respect to residual dilation, hypertrophy, or systolic dysfunction; and an estimate of postoperative pulmonary artery pressure. If the patient subsequently presents with suspected valve dysfunction, a more complete and sensitive assessment is possible by comparison with the baseline study than if no previous examination were available. Another example of the value of a baseline study is assessment of left ventricular systolic function prior to starting a potentially cardiotoxic chemotherapeutic regimen. A baseline study allows differentiation of subtle early systolic dysfunction due to chemotherapy from mild dysfunction that may be at the lower limits of the normal range.

Stress Echocardiography (Table 3–6)

In many cardiac conditions, abnormalities of cardiac function are manifested only when increased oxygen consumption results in increased cardiac demands that cannot be met by the usual compensatory changes. This basic concept has led to the widespread use of stress testing in patients with cardiovascular disease. Increased cardiac demand can be induced by exercise or with appropriate pharmacologic interventions. The risk of this approach is related to the risk of stress testing with no significant additive effect of echocardiographic imaging.

Exercise echocardiography can be performed by recording images of the left ventricle immediately before and immediately after treadmill exercise testing or by recording images during supine or upright bicycle exercise. The most common indication for exercise echocardiography is suspected or known coronary artery disease. At rest, left ventricular endocardial motion and wall thickening are normal, even if significant coronary disease is present, unless there has been prior myocardial infarction. Increased myocardial oxygen demands, such as with exercise, result in ischemia when significant stenosis of an epicardial coronary artery is present. This results sequentially in myocardial metabolic changes, decreased wall thickening and endocardial motion, electrocardiographic changes, and angina, in that order. Echocardiographic images recorded *during* ischemia show abnormalities of wall motion, allowing detection of significant coronary artery disease (Fig. 3–8). The specific coronary arteries involved can be identified by the anatomic pattern of induced wall motion abnormalities. Exercise echocardiography, as discussed in detail in Chapter 6, has been found to be more sensitive than exercise electrocardiography (and as sensitive as thallium imaging) for detection of significant coronary artery disease. Exercise echocardiography is particularly helpful in patients with an abnormal resting electrocardiogram (such as bundle branch block or left ventricular hypertrophy). It also has been used to assess the extent of disease, to document functional improvement after re-

TABLE 3–6. INDICATIONS FOR STRESS ECHOCARDIOGRAPHY

Exercise Echocardiography

Coronary artery disease
    Diagnosis
    Extent of disease and vessels involved
    After revascularization
Valvular heart disease
    PA pressures in mitral stenosis patients
Congenital disease
    Aortic coarctation

Pharmacologic Stress Echo

Same indications as exercise echocardiography
    In patients unable to exercise due to:
        Peripheral vascular disease
        Musculoskeletal limitations
    Or as an alternate to exercise stress
Image acquisition during therapeutic pharmacologic
    intervention

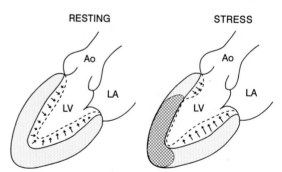

RESTING   STRESS

Figure 3–8. Diagram illustrating the concept of stress echocardiography in a patient with a 70 percent stenosis in the proximal third of the left anterior descending (LAD) coronary artery. At rest (*left*), endocardial motion and wall thickening are normal. After stress (*right*), either exercise or pharmacologic, the middle and apical segments of the anterior wall become ischemic, showing reduced endocardial wall motion and wall thickening. If the LAD extends around the apex, the apical segment of the posterior wall also will be affected, as shown here. The normal segment of the posterior wall shows compensatory hyperkinesis.

vascularization, and to detect restenosis after angioplasty.

In addition to changes in segmental wall motion with exercise stress testing, parameters of global ventricular function, including ventricular volumes, ejection fraction, and the Doppler left ventricular ejection velocity curve, can be evaluated. Other Doppler parameters may be helpful in specific settings. For example, a patient with mitral stenosis will show an excessive rise in pulmonary artery systolic pressure (estimated from the tricuspid regurgitant jet) with exercise. In a patient with aortic coarctation, the increase in gradient across the coarctation with exercise can be demonstrated with Doppler recordings.

Pharmacologic stress echocardiography replaces exercise testing when the patient is unable to exercise (e.g., peripheral vascular disease, musculoskeletal limitations). It also is an attractive alternate to exercise testing when recording of 2D and Doppler data at sequential stages of increased cardiac demand provides useful clinical data. In fact, it can be argued that pharmacologic stress testing is preferable in that the patient can be monitored carefully by echocardiography as the dose is increased, allowing termination of the "stress" as soon as a wall motion abnormality is seen. Pharmacologic stress agents include dobutamine, which increases myocardial contractility, myocardial oxygen demands, and peripheral vasodilation; and adenosine, which vasodilates normal coronary vessels "stealing" blood from stenosed vessels resulting in ischemia.

Contrast Echocardiography
(Table 3–7)

Intravenous injection of microbubbles formed by agitating saline or by using a commercially available product results in a marked increase in echogenicity of the right-sided cardiac chambers—an echocardiographic "contrast" effect (Fig. 3–9). Depending on the size of the microbubbles relative to the lung capillary diameter, the microbubbles are trapped in the pulmonary capillaries so that no contrast material is seen in the left side of the heart in the absence of an intracardiac right-to-left communication. Clinically, right-sided echo contrast studies are performed to document an atrial septal defect (Chap. 15) or patent foramen ovale (Chap. 13) or to increase the signal strength of the tricuspid regurgitant jet (Chap. 4) to allow a more accurate estimate of pulmonary artery pressure.

TABLE 3–7. INDICATIONS FOR CONTRAST ECHOCARDIOGRAPHY

IV contrast (clinical)
  Detection of atrial septal defects and patent foramen ovale
  Enhancement of TR-jet signal
Intracoronary contrast (research)
  Opacification of myocardium perfused by injected vessel
  Detection of myocardial ischemia
IV contrast with pulmonary transit (research)
  Enhancement of contrast between LV chamber and endocardium (improved border recognition)
  Myocardial perfusion

Potential future uses of echo contrast include injection in a coronary artery to opacify the area of myocardium perfused by the injected vessel (Fig. 3–10) and to detect ischemia during intracoronary procedures. Further development of contrast agents that can be injected intravenously but appear in the left side of the heart as well (small enough to pass through the pulmonary capillary bed) may allow improved endocardial border recognition for wall motion analysis or calculation of left ventricular volumes and, ultimately, may provide a clinical method for assessing myocardial perfusion.

Transesophageal Echocardiography

Procedure and Potential Complications

Transesophageal echocardiography is performed by a physician skilled in both echocardiography and the endoscopy procedure, as detailed in published guidelines for physician training. A cardiac sonographer assists the phy-

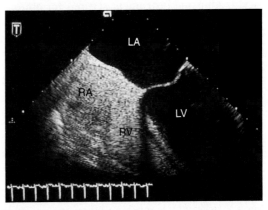

Figure 3–9. Transesophageal view showing dense opacification of the right atrium following a peripheral venous injection of agitated saline.

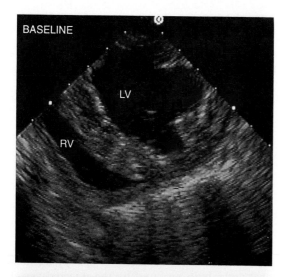

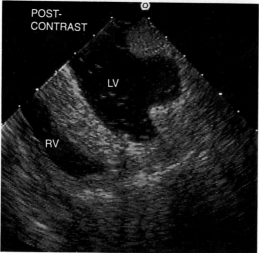

Figure 3–10. Epicardial images of the left ventricle in an experimental model showing myocardial opacification after injection of echo contrast material in the aortic root.

The risk of aspiration is minimized by having the patient fast for several hours prior to the procedure and use of a left lateral decubitus position. Esophageal trauma or perforation is unlikely in the absence of a history of esophageal disease or swallowing difficulty, both of which can be ascertained by clinical history. Bleeding complications are rare and usually mild. Initial concern that transesophageal imaging might increase the risk of endocarditis has been alleviated by several studies showing the absence of bacteremia following this procedure. Other reported complications include bronchospasm, arrhythmias, hypoxia, and hypotension, with a total complication rate serious enough to interrupt the procedure of less than 1 percent. The reported mortality rate is fewer than 1 in 10,000 patients.

Indications

The indications for transesophageal echocardiography are based on its superior image quality compared with transthoracic imaging, particularly of posterior cardiac structures (Table 3–8). Several definite indications for transesophageal echocardiography are apparent when the limitations of transthoracic imaging are considered. In Table 3–3, situations in which transesophageal echocardiography is helpful are indicated. The improved sensitivity of transesophageal versus transthoracic echocardiography for detection of paravalvular abscess in pa-

sician, adjusting instrument settings for optimal image quality and data acquisition. Many echocardiographers use mild general sedation, in addition to local anesthesia of the pharynx, to minimize discomfort and improve patient tolerance. A designated, qualified individual (often a nurse) monitors the patient's blood pressure, heart rate, respiratory rate, and symptoms and provides suction of oral secretions as needed during the procedure (see Suggested Reading 14).

Transesophageal echocardiography has a very low incidence of complications when performed by trained individuals with appropriate patient monitoring. However, this procedure does have known risks which must be taken into consideration in deciding whether the potential information obtained justifies use of this procedure.

TABLE 3–8. INDICATIONS FOR TRANSESOPHAGEAL ECHOCARDIOGRAPHY

Definite

Endocarditis with suspected paravalvular abscess
Suspected prosthetic (esp. mitral) valve dysfunction
Perioperative evaluation of mitral valve anatomy and function pre- and post-MV repair
Evaluation of posterior structures (e.g., interatrial baffle, sinus venosus ASD) in congenital heart disease
Suspected aortic dissection
Detection of left atrial thrombus (e.g., before catheter balloon mitral commissurotomy)

Probable

Search for cardiac "source of embolus" (including patent foramen ovale) in patients with an unexplained systemic embolic event
Whenever transthoracic images are nondiagnostic and echocardiography is indicated (e.g., LV function post-cardiac surgery)
Suspected endocarditis when TTE nondiagnostic

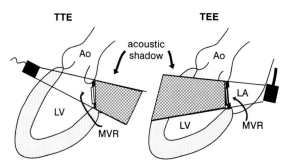

TTE   **TEE**

acoustic shadow

Ao   Ao

LA

LV   LV   MVR

MVR

Figure 3–11. Diagram illustrating the problem of acoustic shadowing from a prosthetic mitral valve. On the left, with transthoracic echocardiography (TTE), the acoustic shadow obscures the left atrium, limiting assessment of valvular incompetence by Doppler techniques. On the right, with transesophageal echocardiography (TEE), the left atrium now can be evaluated for valvular incompetence. However, the acoustic shadow now obscures the left ventricular outflow tract.

tients with endocarditis has been demonstrated convincingly (Chap. 12). Transesophageal echocardiography clearly is indicated for evaluation of prosthetic mitral valve dysfunction, since the shadows and reverberations from the prosthetic valve no longer obscure the left atrium from this approach as they do on transthoracic images (Fig. 3–11) (see also Chap. 11). Abnormalities of the posterior aspect of a prosthetic aortic valve also will be seen well with the transesophageal approach, although the anterior portion of the paravalvular region will be shadowed by the posterior aspect of the prosthetic valve.

Improved evaluation of mitral valve anatomy and the degree of mitral regurgitation are especially useful in the perioperative evaluation of patients undergoing surgical mitral valve repair (Chap. 10). In patients with congenital heart disease, transesophageal imaging improves diagnostic certainty, particularly in evaluation of posterior structures such as an interatrial baffle surgical repair or a sinus venosus atrial septal defect. The sensitivity of transesophageal echocardiography for detection of left atrial thrombus far exceeds transthoracic imaging. Finally, excellent images of the thoracic aorta, arch, and ascending aorta allow accurate diagnosis of aortic dissection by transesophageal echocardiography.

Other potential indications for transesophageal echocardiography are less firmly established. While often performed to detect a potential cardiac "source of embolus," including a patent foramen ovale, in patients with a systemic embolic event, the diagnostic utility of this test, that is, how it affects patient management, has not been critically evaluated in this

patient population. Transesophageal imaging to exclude a diagnosis of endocarditis is of little utility when the pretest likelihood of disease is low. Some echocardiographers advocate the use of transesophageal imaging whenever transthoracic images are nondiagnostic. However, given that the threshold approach to clinical testing predicts a narrower test window as the risk of the test increases, it is appropriate to consider transesophageal studies somewhat more critically. The indications for a transesophageal study should be discussed with the referring physician on a case-by-case basis to determine if the information potentially obtainable justifies the slight but definite risk of the transesophageal approach.

Intravascular Ultrasound

Intravascular ultrasound has focused on detailed evaluation of intraarterial atherosclerotic disease. This application of ultrasound requires an "invasive" approach in the cardiac catheterization laboratory and will not be addressed in this textbook. Introductory readings on this topic are included in the suggested readings.

APPROACH TO THE ECHOCARDIOGRAPHIC EXAMINATION

Basic Format

The echocardiographic examination should be directed toward the specific clinical question in each individual patient. In addition, as the study is in progress, the examination should be modified to fully pursue any observed abnormalities. Most laboratories find that structuring the examination around a basic set of 2D views and Doppler recordings facilitates a directed examination while ensuring that the most important aspects of cardiac anatomy and function are examined in a systematic manner. While this "basic" examination may differ from laboratory to laboratory and may be more or less "comprehensive," it should be noted that the large number of possible imaging planes, Doppler recordings, and quantitative measurements make a truly comprehensive examination impractical in terms of examination time. An examination that includes every view and every Doppler recording without regard to the underlying pathology rarely is useful for appropriate clinical decision making, although an extensive directed examination may be needed in patients with multiple or complex cardiac lesions.

The need to focus the examination on the specific clinical question and at the same time ensure that significant abnormalities are not missed highlights the necessity for appropriate training of both the physician responsible for the examination and the sonographer performing the study, as well as for close interaction between these two individuals during the performance and interpretation of the study. Furthermore, close interaction with the referring physician is needed both before the examination is performed to clarify the differential diagnosis and clinical questions and after the examination to integrate the pretest likelihood with the echocardiographic findings and estimate the probability of any remaining diagnostic problems.

The basic echocardiographic examination should include evaluation of the following areas:

1. Left ventricle: Internal dimensions, wall thickness, segmental wall motion abnormalities, and global systolic function, with an ejection fraction estimated visually or calculated from endocardial border tracings

2. Aortic valve and root: Aortic root dimension and appearance, aortic valve anatomy, and evidence for regurgitation or stenosis

3. Mitral valve and left atrium: Mitral valve anatomy and motion, evidence for stenosis or regurgitation, left atrial size

4. Right side of the heart: Right ventricular size and systolic function (qualitative), right atrial size, tricuspid and pulmonic valve anatomy and function, and estimate of pulmonary artery pressure

5. Pericardium: Evidence for thickening or effusion

This evaluation can be performed using the following 2D views and Doppler recordings:

1. Parasternal window
   a. 2D views:
      Long-axis view
      Short axis at aortic valve, mitral valve, and papillary muscle levels
      Right ventricular inflow and outflow views
      Measurements (2D or 2D-guided M-mode):
      Left ventricle wall thickness and internal dimensions
      Aortic root and left atrial dimensions
   b. Doppler recordings:
      Pulsed Doppler of pulmonary artery flow

Continuous-wave Doppler of tricuspid regurgitant jet
Color flow imaging of aortic, mitral, tricuspid and pulmonic valves
Measurements:
PA peak flow velocity
Time-to-peak velocity in PA

2. Apical window
   a. 2D views:
      Apical four-chamber view with anterior and posterior angulation
      Apical two-chamber view
      Apical long-axis view
      Measurements:
      Biplane end-systolic and end-diastolic left ventricular endocardial borders for left ventricular volumes and ejection fraction
   b. Doppler recordings:
      Pulsed Doppler of left ventricular inflow and outflow
      Color flow imaging of mitral, aortic, and tricuspid valves
      Continuous-wave Doppler of tricuspid regurgitation and of aortic and mitral antegrade flow
      Measurements:
      Left ventricular inflow E and A velocities
      Left ventricular outflow velocity distal to the aortic valve (continuous wave)
      Tricuspid regurgitant jet

3. Subcostal window
   a. 2D views:
      Subcostal four-chamber and short-axis views
      Inferior vena cava and abdominal aorta

4. Suprasternal notch window
   a. 2D views: Long- and short-axis views of aortic arch

Starting from this basic format, a more detailed examination of the specific abnormalities in each patient and an evaluation directed toward the specific clinical question may be needed. In a patient with no abnormalities noted on this basic examination and no other specific clinical questions (e.g., suspicion of an intracardiac shunt), further evaluation may not be necessary.

Focusing the Examination

As the basic examination is in progress, the study is tailored toward the specific abnormalities noted. For example, if the aortic valve leaflets appear abnormal, attention is focused first on the precise valve anatomy—bicuspid, degenerative changes, rheumatic—and then on the function of the valve. The degree of stenosis is quantitated from the maximum aortic jet velocity (see Chap. 9), and the degree of regurgitation is evaluated with pulsed Doppler, color flow imaging, and continuous-wave Doppler techniques (see Chap. 10). Next, the left ventricular response to the pressure and/or volume load imposed by the abnormal aortic valve is assessed qualitatively (dilation, hypertrophy, overall systolic function) and quantitatively (ejection fraction, wall thickness, mass).

Another example is evaluation of a patient after myocardial infarction. In this case, attention is focused on the extent and distribution of left ventricular segmental wall motion abnormalities (see Chap. 6). If apical akinesis or dyskinesis is noted, a diligent search for an apical thrombus is indicated (see Chap. 13). If the patient has a new murmur, careful evaluation is performed to evaluate the possibility of mitral regurgitation due to papillary muscle dysfunction or the possibility of a postinfarction ventricular septal defect. Overall left ventricular systolic function is evaluated, as is right ventricular function.

Even if no obvious abnormalities are noted during the basic examination, the study may be focused toward the specific clinical question in that patient. For example, if endocarditis is suspected (see Chap. 12), more attention to valvular anatomy is needed, with careful transducer angulation and nonstandard views to optimize visualization of possible valvular vegetations. Although endocarditis cannot be excluded by echocardiography, a careful and thorough negative examination does decrease the likelihood of disease.

Close interaction between the referring physician, cardiac sonographer, and cardiologist is needed to ensure that an appropriate and complete examination is performed in each patient. Subsequent chapters detail the examination sequence and findings in each disease category.

Education and Training Guidelines

As these examples show, the sonographer must be familiar with patterns of disease in clinical cardiology as well as with the technical aspects of performing the examination. Conversely, the physician must have expertise in the technical aspects of the examination, as well as

the expected findings in each disease state, in order to guide the sonographer in optimizing data quality and to interpret the recorded data correctly. Details such as transducer frequency, gain controls, processing curves, and depth settings significantly affect 2D image quality. The appropriate choice of Doppler modality for the flow of interest—pulsed, color flow, or continuous-wave Doppler—affects the data obtained. Factors such as wall filters, gain, sample volume size, and color sector width also significantly affect data collection. Knowledge of how these factors affect data quality and knowledge of which views and approaches yield optimal data allow the physician to assess the reliability of recorded data, to suspect abnormalities that may not have been noted explicitly during the examination, to recognize imaging and flow artifacts, and to direct the sonographer in optimal data acquisition. Detailed guidelines for physician training and for education and training of cardiac sonographers have been published and should be followed.

Echocardiographic Interpretation

The interpretation session provides an opportunity for the sonographer to relay technical concerns to the physician and to direct attention to abnormalities noted during the examination. The physician can give feedback to the sonographer about the completeness and quality of data recorded and offer suggestions for future patient studies. If review suggests that additional echocardiographic recordings are needed, the patient may be asked to return for further examination.

The echocardiographic report serves at least two purposes: (1) it conveys the results of the test to the referring physician, and (2) it serves as a narrative summary of the echocardiographic examination for comparison with future studies. Given the wide variety of views and flows that can be recorded, it is helpful for the report to document which structures were imaged (even if normal), which flow signals were evaluated, the different Doppler modalities used, and the overall quality of the study. Any areas of limitation in the study is noted.

In each patient, the various echocardiographic findings then are integrated with each other in the final interpretation. For example, a report describing mitral regurgitation also would include a clear description of valve anatomy with an indication of the most likely etiology of regurgitation or the differential diagnosis if the etiology is unclear. Mitral regurgitant severity is estimated and the method(s) used to generate this estimate are indicated. In addition, the degrees of left atrial and left ventricular dilation are described, with attention to serial changes if previous studies are available. Left ventricular systolic function is quantitated, and the degree of pulmonary hypertension is estimated. All these findings fit together physiologically and thus can be reported in a logical integration of the data: For example, significant mitral regurgitation results in left ventricular and left atrial enlargement due to volume overload, while the chronically elevated left atrial pressure leads to pulmonary hypertension.

Finally, these findings are reviewed in the context of the patient's clinical presentation, potential implications of the findings are discussed with the referring physician, and additional diagnostic tests or follow-up studies are recommended as clinically indicated. If principles of clinical decision analysis are being utilized in patient management, the pretest and posttest likelihood of disease can be estimated. Ideally, the overall impact of the echocardiographic findings on the patient's therapy or subsequent diagnostic evaluation is reviewed with the referring physician both before and after the examination.

SUGGESTED READING

1. Sox HC Jr, Blatt MA, Higgins MC, Martin KI: Medical Decision Making. Stoneham, Mass, Butterworth-Heinemann, 1988.
   A readable concise textbook summarizing the entire spectrum of medical decision making from sensitivity/specificity to cost-benefit analysis.

2. Diamond GA, Forrester JS: Analysis of probability as an aid in the clinical diagnosis of coronary-artery disease. N Engl J Med 1979; 300:1350–1358.
   Classic article on use of Bayes' theorem to determine posttest likelihood based on pretest likelihood and test results using the example of exercise electrocardiography for diagnosis of coronary artery disease.

3. Patterson RE, Horowitz SF: Importance of epidemiology and biostatistics in deciding clinical strategies for using diagnostic tests: A simplified approach using examples from coronary artery disease. J Am Coll Cardiol 1989; 13:1653–1665.
   Emphasizes integration of test results in overall patient management.

4. Wasson JH, Sox HC, Neff RK, Goldman L: Clinical prediction rules. Applications and methodological standards. N Engl J Med 1985; 313:793–799.
   Defines approach to developing and validating new clinical prediction rules. This article will be of particular value to individuals proposing new diagnostic approaches based on echocardiographic data.

5. Pauker SG, Kassirer JP: The threshold approach to clinical decision making. N Engl J Med 1980; 302:1109–1117.
   Clear and concise discussion of the concepts of decision analysis focusing on the threshold approach.

6. Pauker SG, Kassirer JP: Decision analysis. N Engl J Med 1987; 316:250–258.
   Review of decision analysis including Bayes' rule, decision trees, and outcome measures. Fifty-two references.

7. Biem HJ, Detsky AS, Armstrong PW: Management of asymptomatic chronic aortic regurgitation with left ventricular dysfunction. A decision analysis. J Gen Intern Med 1990; 5:394–401.
   Example of the application of clinical decision methods to a clinical problem (timing of valve replacement in chronic aortic regurgitation) in which echocardiographic data (left ventricular size and systolic function) are critical to patient management.

8. Detsky AS, Naglie IG: A clinician's guide to cost-effectiveness analysis. Ann Intern Med 1990; 113:147–154.
   Outlines simplified models for cost-effectiveness analysis that should be applicable to comparisons of the use of different diagnostic tests in a specific clinical setting. Provides guidelines for setting priorities within a health care organization based on cost-effectiveness analysis.

9. Otto CM, Pearlman AS: Doppler echocardiography in adults with symptomatic aortic stenosis. Arch Intern Med 1988; 148:2553–2560.
   An example of development and validation of a clinical prediction rule for timing of valve replacement in symptomatic aortic stenosis based on Doppler echo data. Maximum aortic jet velocity (V_{max}) breakpoints are proposed at (1) >4.0 m/s (valve replacement indicated), (2) <3.0 m/s (valve replacement not needed), and (3) between 3.0 and 4.0 m/s (evaluation of valve area and coexisting aortic regurgitation needed). Simple cost analysis compares noninvasive with invasive diagnostic approach.

10. Oh JK, Taliercio CP, Holmes DR Jr, et al: Prediction of the severity of aortic stenosis by Doppler aortic valve area determination: Prospective Doppler-catheterization correlation in 100 patients. J Am Coll Cardiol 1988; 11:1227–1234.
    Evaluation of Doppler data for diagnosis of severe aortic stenosis. Proposed single maximum aortic jet velocity breakpoint at 4.5 m/s with a sensitivity of 44 percent and a specificity of 93 percent for diagnosis of severe stenosis.

11. Popp RL: Echocardiography (2 parts). N Engl J Med 1990; 323:101–109, 165–172.
    Review article, directed toward the general internist, summarizes major accepted indications for echocardiography. One-hundred and fifty-one references.

12. ACC/AHA Task Force Report: ACC/AHA Guidelines for the Clinical Application of Echocardiography: A Report of the American College of Cardiology/American Heart Association Task Force on Assessment of Diagnostic and Therapeutic Cardiovascular Procedures (Subcommittee to Develop Guidelines for the Clinical Application of Echocardiography). J Am Coll Cardiol 1990; 16:1505–1528.
    Task force guidelines on indications for echocardiography divided into class I indications (general agreement that echocardiography is important), class II (divergence of opinions), and class III (not appropriate).

13. Schiller NB, Maurer G, Ritter SB, et al: Transesophageal echocardiography. J Am Soc Echocardiogr 1989; 2:354–357.
    ASE position paper on utility of transesophageal echo.

14. Fisher EA, Stahl JA, Budd JH, Goldman ME: Transesophageal echocardiography: Procedures and clinical application. J Am Coll Cardiol 1991; 18:1333–1348.

Review of methodology, examination technique, and indications for TEE.

15. Pearlman AS, Gardin JM, Martin RP, et al: Guidelines for physician training in transesophageal echocardiography: Recommendations of the American Society of Echocardiography Committee for Physician Training in Echocardiography. J Am Soc Echocardiogr 1992; 5:187–194.
    Recommendations for physician training in transthoracic echocardiography.

16. ACC Echocardiography Committee Position Statement: Transesophageal echocardiography. J Am Coll Cardiol 1992; 20:506.
    Recommendations for physician training in transesophageal echocardiography.

17. Guidelines and Essentials for Education of the Diagnostic Medical Sonographer (JRC-DMS). Chicago, Joint Review Committee for Diagnostic Medical Sonography, 1987.
    Criteria for accreditation of programs offering training in diagnostic medical sonography (including echocardiography).

18. Tubis JM, Yock PG (eds): Intravascular Ultrasound Imaging. New York, Churchill-Livingstone, 1992.
    Comprehensive, multiauthor textbook of intravascular ultrasound.

19. Kaul S: Clinical applications of myocardial contrast echocardiography. Am J Cardiol 1992; 69:46H-55H.
    Review article on the current utility of myocardial contrast echocardiography. The need for a method to opacify myocardium from a venous injection of contrast is emphasized.

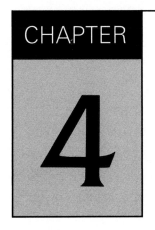

CHAPTER 4

ECHOCARDIOGRAPHIC EVALUATION OF LEFT AND RIGHT VENTRICULAR SYSTOLIC FUNCTION

INTRODUCTION

The degree of left ventricular systolic dysfunction is a potent predictor of clinical outcome for a wide range of cardiovascular disease, including ischemic cardiac disease, cardiomyopathies, valvular heart disease, and congenital heart disease. Echocardiography provides both qualitative and quantitative measures of systolic function. Visual estimates of global and regional function from two-dimensional (2D) echocardiographic images, quantitative ventricular volumes and ejection fractions based on endocardial border tracing, and Doppler echocardiographic ejection phase indices all are valuable clinical tools.

Evaluation of ventricular systolic function is the most important application of echocardiography, and even when evaluation of ventricular systolic function is not the focus of the examination, it plays a key role in every study. For research applications, echocardiographic measures of left ventricular systolic function provide important baseline data and sensitive and reliable endpoints of disease severity.

BASIC PRINCIPLES

Cardiac Cycle (Fig. 4–1)

Systole typically is defined as the segment of the cardiac cycle from mitral valve closure to aortic valve closure. The onset of systole is defined by ECG as ventricular depolarization (QRS complex), with the end of systole occurring after repolarization (end of T wave). In terms of ventricular pressure and volume curves over time, systole begins when left ventricular diastolic pressure exceeds left atrial pressure, resulting in closure of the mitral valve. Mitral valve closure is followed by isovolumic contraction, during which the cardiac muscle depolarizes, calcium influx and myosin-actin shortening occur, and ventricular pressure rises rapidly at a constant ventricular volume (although shape changes may occur). When ventricular pressure exceeds aortic pressure, the aortic valve opens. During ejection (aortic valve opening to closing), left ventricular volume falls rapidly as blood flows from the left ventricle to the aorta. Left ventricular pressure exceeds aortic pressure for approximately the first half of systole, corresponding to rapid acceleration of blood flow and a small pressure difference from the ventricle to the aorta. In the normal heart, pressure crossover occurs in midsystole, so during the second half of systole, aortic pressure exceeds left ventricular pressure, resulting in continued forward blood flow but at progressively slower velocities (deceleration). Aortic valve closure occurs at the dicrotic notch of the aortic pressure tracing, immediately following end-ejection. In sum, sys-

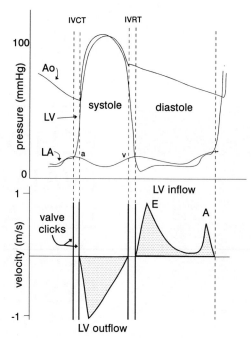

Figure 4–1. The cardiac cycle. Left ventricular (LV), aortic (Ao), and left atrial (LA) pressures are shown with the corresponding Doppler left ventricular outflow and inflow velocity curves. The isovolumic contraction time (IVCT) represents the time between mitral valve closure and aortic valve opening, while the isovolumic relaxation time (IVRT) represents the time between aortic valve closure and mitral valve opening.

tole includes isovolumic contraction and ventricular ejection (acceleration and deceleration phases). Ventricular volume ranges from a maximum at end-diastole (or onset of systole) to a minimum at end-systole.

Physiology of Systolic Function

Fundamentally, ventricular systolic function is best described by *contractility:* the basic ability of the myocardium to contract. However, contractility is affected by several physiologic parameters, including heart rate, coupling interval, metabolic factors, and pharmacologic agents. In addition, for a given degree of contractility, ventricular function can vary depending on *preload* (initial ventricular volume or pressure) and *afterload* (aortic resistance/impedance or end-systolic wall stress). Evaluation of contractility itself thus requires measurement under different loading conditions. Experimentally, contractility often is described by the slope of the end-systolic pressure-volume relationship (E_{max}). To derive this value, left ventricular pressure is

Pressure-Volume Loop

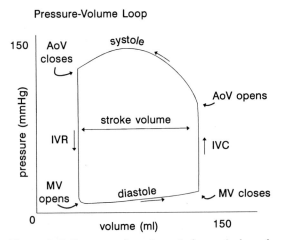

Figure 4–2. Pressure-volume loop. Left ventricular volume is graphed on the horizontal axis, with pressure on the vertical axis. The direction of pressure-volume changes is shown by the arrows. During diastole, volume increases with little rise in pressure. After mitral valve (MV) closure, isovolumic contraction (IVC) results in a rapid rise in pressure with no change in volume. At the onset of ejection, the aortic valve (AoV) opens with a rapid decrease in left ventricular volume during systole. Aortic valve closure is followed by isovolumic relaxation (IVR).

ESPVR

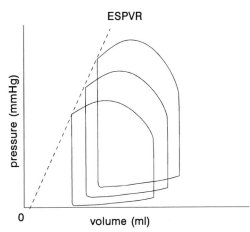

Figure 4–3. Pressure-volume loops at different loading conditions (e.g., increasing end-diastolic volumes) are used to derive a line describing end-systolic pressure-volume relationship (ESPVR). This measure of left ventricular contractility is insensitive to changes in loading conditions.

graphed on the horizontal axis, with volume on the vertical axis, rather than graphing both as a function of time (Fig. 4–2). A pressure-volume "loop" then represents a single cardiac cycle, with different pressure-volume loops for the same ventricle representing different loading conditions (such as increasing or decreasing ventricular end-diastolic volume). E_{max} is the slope of the line that intersects the end-systolic pressure-volume point for each curve (Fig. 4–3).

The effect of preload on ventricular function is summarized by the Frank-Starling curve showing ventricular end-diastolic volume (or pressure) on the horizontal axis and stroke volume on the vertical axis (Fig. 4–4A). For a given degree of contractility, there is a curvilinear relationship between these variables such that increasing end-diastolic volume results in a greater stroke volume. An increase in contractility shifts this curve up and to the left; a decrease in contractility shifts it downward and to the right.

Afterload, defined by resistance or impedance, has an inverse relationship with stroke volume such that increasing vascular resistance results in a decreased stroke volume (Fig. 4–4). An increase in contractility shifts this curve downward and to the left; a decrease in contractility shifts it to the right.

Measurement of left ventricular systolic function independent of loading conditions is diffi-

PRELOAD

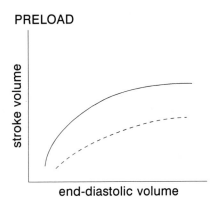

AFTERLOAD

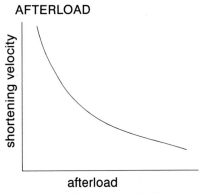

Figure 4–4. (*Above*) The relationship between end-diastolic volume and stroke volume is shown for a normal (*solid line*) and failing (*dashed line*) left ventricle. (*Below*) The inverse relationship between afterload and left ventricular myocardial shortening velocity is shown.

cult using echocardiographic or other clinical approaches. It rarely is possible to construct pressure-volume loops under different loading conditions due to the problem of measuring instantaneous left ventricular volume and the potential risk of altering loading conditions in ill patients. Thus clinical evaluation of ventricular function has focused on measurements of cardiac output and ejection fraction, even though the load dependence of these measures is a clearly acknowledged limitation.

Ventricular Volumes and Geometry

The normal shape of the left ventricle is symmetrical with two relatively equal short axes and with the long axis running from the base (mitral annulus) to the apex. In long-axis views, the apex is slightly rounded, so the apical half of the ventricle resembles a hemiellipse. The basal half of the ventricle is more cylindrical, so the ventricle appears circular in short-axis views. Various assumptions about left ventricular shape have been used to derive formulas for calculating ventricular volumes. Of course, all these formulas are simplifications to greater or lesser degrees, and there is variability among patients in the shape of the ventricle. It is plausible that left ventricular volumes would be measured most accurately in individual patients by complete three-dimensional (3D) reconstruction of the endocardial surface at end-diastole and end-systole, an approach that rarely is clinically feasible.

While ventricular volumes instantaneously throughout the cardiac cycle are of interest, usually only end-diastolic volume (EDV) and end-systolic volume (ESV) are measured in the clinical setting. Ejection fraction (EF) is

$$EF(\%) = (SV/EDV) \times 100\% \qquad (4.1)$$

where stroke volume (SV) is calculated as

$$SV = EDV - ESV \qquad (4.2)$$

with cardiac output obtained by multiplying stroke volume by heart rate.

Other useful parameters of ventricular function include (1) left ventricular mass—the total weight of the myocardium, derived by multiplying the volume of myocardium times the specific density of cardiac muscle—and (2) wall stress. Wall stress is the force per unit area exerted on the myocardium. Wall stress is dependent on cavity dimensions, pressure, and wall thickness. Wall stress can be described in three dimensions as circumferential, meridional (longitudinal), or radial. Typically, end-systolic calculations of circumferential and meridional wall stress are used clinically.

Cardiac Output

The basic function of the heart is as a pump, and measurements of cardiac output are useful in routine day-to-day patient management. *Cardiac output* is the volume of blood pumped by the heart per minute, with *stroke volume* being the amount pumped on a single beat. While cardiac output can be derived from ventricular volumes, as described above, a variety of other approaches to measurement are available, including indicator dilation methods (Fick, thermodilution), Doppler velocity data, ventricular impedance, and radionuclide methods.

Response to Exercise

Ventricular systolic function and cardiac output are dynamic, responding rapidly to the metabolic demands of the individual. Cardiac output increases from a resting mean of 6 liters/min with exercise to 18 liters/min in young, healthy adults. Most of the increase in cardiac output is mediated by an increase in heart rate. With supine exercise, there is only a minimal increase in stroke volume (about 10 percent), but with upright exercise, the increase in stroke volume is approximately 20 to 35 percent. With exercise, end-diastolic volume is unchanged or slightly decreased, but ejection fraction increases and end-systolic volume decreases. With imaging techniques, endocardial motion and myocardial wall thickening are augmented with an appearance of "hypercontractility" during and immediately following exercise.

2D AND M-MODE EVALUATION OF LEFT VENTRICULAR SYSTOLIC FUNCTION

M-Mode Echocardiography

Dimensions and Fractional Shortening

M-mode echocardiography allows measurement of ventricular internal dimensions and wall thickness throughout the cardiac cycle. The major advantage of M-mode echo is high time resolution, which facilitates recognition of the endocardial borders. Left ventricular measurements are made with the M-mode beam positioned just beyond the mitral leaflet tips (mitral chordal level), perpendicular to the long axis of the ventricle, and centered in the short-axis view. The left ventricular posterior wall endocardium is identified on the M-mode recording as the most continuous line with the steepest systolic motion. The posterior wall epicardium is identified as the echo reflection immediately anterior to the pericardium. The septal endocardium again is identified as the steepest motion in systole with a continuous reflection through the cycle. On the right ventricular side of the septum, it is important to exclude any reflections due to right ventricular trabeculations. Conversely, a dark "midseptal" stripe often is noted and should not be confused with the endocardial borders. Left ventricular wall thickness and dimensions are measured from leading edge to leading edge (American Society of Echocardiography [ASE] recommendations), with normal values for these measurements indicated in Table 2–6.

In addition to left ventricular wall thickness and internal dimensions (LVID) at end-diastole (d) and end-systole (s), fractional shortening can be calculated as

Fractional shortening (%)
$$= \frac{\mathrm{LVID_d - LVID_s}}{\mathrm{LVID_d}} \times 100\% \quad (4.3)$$

Fractional shortening is a rough measurement of left ventricular systolic function, with the normal range being 25 to 45 percent (95 percent confidence limits).

A potential disadvantage of M-mode dimensions is that overestimation will occur if the beam is oblique with respect to the long or short axis of the ventricle. Underestimation can occur if the M-line is not centered in the ventricular chamber. Both these potential errors can be avoided by using 2D imaging in both long- and short-axis planes to verify the M-mode beam orientation. With nonsymmetrical disease processes (ischemic cardiac disease) or with alterations in left ventricular shape (dilated cardiomyopathy), M-mode measurements at the base may not be representative of overall left ventricular dimensions or function.

Left Ventricular Mass and Volumes

Left ventricular mass can be estimated from M-mode dimensions of septal thickness (ST), posterior wall thickness (PWT), and left ventricular internal dimensions (LVID) at end-diastole. Note that the original description of this method

by Reichek and Devereux used PENN convention measurements with the endocardial echos included in wall thickness and excluded from chamber dimensions (rather than leading edge to leading edge). If ASE recommendation measurements are used, a correction factor is needed. The formula then is

Left ventricular mass $= 0.80 \times 1.05 \times$
$$[(\mathrm{ST + PWT + LVID^3)} - \mathrm{LVID^3]} \quad (4.4)$$

Left Ventricular Wall Stress

Estimates of left ventricular wall stress can be calculated from M-mode data in combination with pressure data. Meridional stress σ_m is

$$\sigma_m = 0.334P(\mathrm{LVID})/[\mathrm{PWT} \times (1 + \mathrm{PWT/LVID})] \quad (4.5)$$

where P = left ventricular pressure, LVID = left ventricular internal dimensions, and PWT = posterior wall thickness. A simpler approach to estimating wall stress is to calculate the relative wall thickness (RWT):

$$\mathrm{RWT} = \frac{2 \times \mathrm{PWT}}{\mathrm{LVID}} \quad (4.6)$$

which is a useful index for evaluation of patients with left ventricular hypertrophy.

Other M-Mode Measures

Other M-mode signs of left ventricular systolic function are (1) the separation between the maximum anterior motion of the mitral leaflet and maximum posterior motion of the ventricular septum (E-point septal separation) and (2) the degree of anteroposterior motion of the aortic root (see Fig. 7–3). With normal systolic function, the anterior mitral leaflet opens to nearly fill the ventricular chamber resulting in little (0–5 mm) E-point septal separation. With systolic dysfunction, this distance is increased due to a combination of left ventricular dilation and reduced motion of the mitral valve as a result of low transmitral volume flow. Similarly, left ventricular systolic dysfunction results in reduced left atrial filling and emptying (low cardiac output), seen on M-mode as reduced anteroposterior motion of the aortic root.

Because of the limitations of M-mode echocardiography, it usually is preferable to utilize 2D images for measurement of left ventricular volumes and mass and for calculation of circumferential wall stress.

2D Echocardiography

Quantitative Evaluation of Systolic Function

Both global and regional ventricular function can be evaluated with 2D echocardiography on a semiquantitative scale by an experienced observer. Overall left ventricular systolic function is evaluated best from multiple tomographic planes, typically parasternal long- and short-axis views and apical four-chamber, two-chamber, and long-axis views. Attention to image acquisition is needed to obtain adequate endocardial definition. The echocardiographer then integrates the degree of endocardial motion and wall thickening from these views to classify overall systolic function as normal, mildly reduced, moderately reduced, or severely reduced. Some experienced observers can estimate ejection fraction visually from 2D images with a reasonable correlation with ejection fractions measured quantitatively by echocardiography or other techniques. Typically, ejection fraction is estimated in intervals of 5 to 10 percent (i.e., 20, 30, 40 percent, etc.) or an estimated ejection fraction range is reported (e.g., 20 to 30 percent).

Qualitative evaluation of systolic function is a simple and highly predictive index that is of great clinical utility. On the other hand, several factors can limit the usefulness of this evaluation. First, the accuracy of the estimated ejection fraction is dependent on the experience of each observer. Second, inadequate endocardial definition can result in incorrect estimates of systolic function. Third, integration of data from multiple tomographic images can be difficult when the pattern of contraction is asynchronous (with conduction defects, pacers, postoperative septal motion) or when the pattern of contraction is asymmetrical (with prior myocardial infarction or with ischemia), especially when dyskinesis is present. To some extent, these limitations are minimized by an experienced observer, optimal endocardial definition, and integration of data from multiple views. However, when possible, it is preferable to avoid the limitations of estimates of systolic function by performing quantitative measurements.

Regional ventricular function also can be evaluated by imaging in multiple tomographic planes. Most often, regional function is evaluated qualitatively by dividing the ventricle into segments corresponding to the coronary artery anatomy and then grading wall motion on a 1 to 4 scale as normal (score = 1), hypokinetic (score = 2), akinetic (score = 3), or dyskinetic (score

= 4). In some cases, hyperkinesis—that is, a compensatory increase in wall motion in regions remote from an acute myocardial infarction or the normal increase seen with exercise—also is scored. Evaluation of segmental wall motion is discussed in detail in Chapter 6.

Quantitative Evaluation of Left Ventricular Systolic Function

Quantitative evaluation of left ventricular systolic function is based on endocardial (and sometimes epicardial) border tracing at end-diastole and end-systole in one or more tomographic planes. Prerequisites for quantitative evaluation are (1) nonoblique standard image planes or image planes of known orientation relative to the long and short axis of the left ventricle, (2) adequate endocardial definition, and (3) accurate identification of the endocardial borders. In some patients, image quality is inadequate for endocardial definition. In addition, manual tracing of endocardial borders by a trained echocardiographer is time-consuming and tedious, which is a major barrier to routine quantitation of left ventricular systolic function by echocardiography.

Since echocardiography is a tomographic technique, left ventricular volume calculations are based on geometric assumptions about the shape of the left ventricle. Obviously, accuracy in individual patients will be highest with methods that have the fewest geometric assumptions and that utilize data from multiple tomographic images. The greatest accuracy would be expected with 3D reconstructions that use data from multiple tomographic images of known orientation and make no geometric assumptions. However, 3D methods are limited by the need for 3D localization of the image plane and the need for endocardial border tracing in multiple views. Simpler methods, based on one to three image planes, provide reasonably accurate information with less time-consuming data collection. These simpler methods are the current standard for clinical practice.

The geometric assumptions for calculating left ventricular volumes from tomographic data range from a simple ellipsoid shape to complex hemicylindrical hemiellipsoid shapes (Fig. 4–5). For each approach, left ventricular end-diastolic and end-systolic volumes are calculated from the corresponding tracings at that phase of the cardiac cycle. Methods that use a single dimension *D* clearly provide only a rough approximation of left ventricular volumes but can be useful in some situations. The "cubed" method assumes

Biplane apical

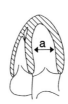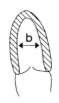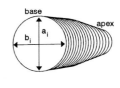

Single-plane ellipsoid

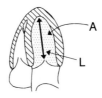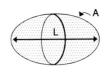

Hemisphere-cylinder

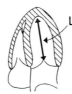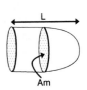

Figure 4–5. Examples of three formulas for left ventricular volume calculations showing the 2D echocardiographic views and measurements on the left and the geometric model on the right. For the biplane apical method, endocardial borders are traced in apical four-chamber and two-chamber views which are used to define a series of orthogonal diameters (*a* and *b*). A "Simpson's rule" assumption based on stacked disks is used to calculate volume. The single-plane ellipsoid method uses the 2D area A and length L in a single (usually apical four-chamber) view. The hemisphere-cylinder method uses a short-axis endocardial area at the midventricular level A_m and a long-axis length L. For each method, both end-diastolic and end-systolic measurements are needed for calculation of end-diastolic and end-systolic volumes, respectively, and for ejection fraction determination.

that the major axis of the left ventricle is equal to twice the short-axis dimension. Then, volume V can be approximated from a single short-axis dimension as

$$V = D^3 \quad \text{Cubed formula} \quad (4.7)$$

The single-plane ellipsoid method uses the length L and 2D area A of a single long-axis view. Left ventricular volume is calculated assuming an ellipsoid shape as

$$V = \frac{8A^2}{3\pi L} \quad \text{Single plane ellipsoid} \quad (4.8)$$

This formula also can be written as

$$V = 0.85A^2/L \quad (4.9)$$

or

$$\text{Area-length method}$$
$$V = (5/6A^2)/L \quad (4.10)$$

The biplane ellipsoid model uses a long-axis view only for length L and area A_L and incorporates an orthogonal short-axis diameter D and area A_s:

$$\text{Biplane ellipsoid}$$
$$V = \frac{\pi L}{6}\left(\frac{4A_s}{\pi D}\right)\left(\frac{4A_L}{\pi L}\right) \quad (4.11)$$

or

$$V = \frac{\pi}{6}D_1 D_2 L \quad (4.12)$$

where D_1 and D_2 are orthogonal short-axis diameters. The hemicylindrical hemiellipsoid model assumes that the base of the ventricle is approximated by a cylinder and the apex by an ellipsoid. Volume is calculated from a long-axis length L and the cross-sectional area A_m of an orthogonal short-axis view at the midpapillary level:

$$\text{Hemisphere cylinder}$$
$$V = (A_m)\frac{L}{2} + \frac{2}{3}(A_m)\frac{L}{2} \quad (4.13)$$

or

$$V = 5/6AL \quad \text{"Bullet" formula} \quad (4.14)$$

In the presence of regional wall motion abnormalities, all these methods will be less accurate, since if the region of abnormal wall motion is included in the dimension or area measurements, volumes will be overestimated. Apical biplane methods are more robust in this setting, using summation of a series of disks from apex to base (often called *Simpson's rule*):

$$V = \sum_{n=20} (\text{area} \cdot \frac{L}{20}) \quad \text{Simpson's rule} \quad (4.15)$$

or a modified Simpson's rule approximation, which uses three parallel "slices" of the ventricle to obtain volume:

Modified Simpson's rule

$$V = (A_1 + A_2)b + \frac{A_3 b}{2} + \frac{\pi b^3}{6} \quad (4.16)$$

where $b = L/3$, A_1 = mitral valve short-axis area, A_2 = papillary muscle level area, and A_3 = apex short-axis area.

For each of these formulas, end-diastolic volume is calculated from end-diastolic images and end-systolic volumes from end-systolic images. Stroke volume, then, is the difference between EDV and ESV [Eq. (4.2)], while ejection fraction (EF) is calculated with Eq. (4.1).

Other modifications and simplifications of left ventricular volume formulas have been suggested (see Table 4–1 and Suggested Reading). The American Society of Echocardiography recommends use of biplane apical views with a modified Simpson's rule approach:

Biplane apical volume

$$V = \frac{\pi}{4} \sum_{i=1}^{20} a_i b_i \times \frac{L}{20} \quad (4.17)$$

where the length L of the ventricle is divided into 20 disks ($i = 1$ to $i = 20$) from base to apex with a diameter of each disk determined in two apical views (a and b). The recommended alternate approach (when two views are not available) is the single-plane ellipsoid formula, Eq. (4.9). An example of the 2D images needed for left ventricular volume calculation is shown in Figure 4–6.

Left Ventricular Mass

Left ventricular mass theoretically can be determined by tracing epicardial borders to calculate the total ventricular volume (walls plus chamber), subtracting the volumes determined from endocardial border tracing, and then multiplying by the specific density of myocardium:

$$\text{LV mass} = 1.05(\text{total volume} - \text{chamber volume}) \quad (4.18)$$

However, epicardial definition rarely is adequate for this approach. Instead, mean wall thickness is calculated from epicardial (A_1) and endocardial (A_2) cross-sectional areas in a short-axis view at the papillary muscle level. The short-axis radius b is calculated as

$$b = \sqrt{\frac{A_2}{\pi}} \quad (4.19)$$

Mean wall thickness t, then, is

$$t = \sqrt{\frac{A_1}{\pi}} - b \quad (4.20)$$

and the cross-sectional area of the myocardium (A_m) in this short-axis view is

$$A_m = A_1 - A_2 \quad (4.21)$$

Myocardial mass is calculated from these measurements plus the left ventricular length L from the level of the short-axis plane to the base d and to the apex a such that $d + a = L$. Using a truncated ellipsoid formula,

$$\text{LV mass} = 1.05\pi \left\{ (b + t)^2 \left[2/3 \right. \right.$$
$$\left. (a + t) + d - \frac{d^3}{3(a + t)^2} \right] \quad (4.22)$$
$$\left. - b^2 \left[2/3a + d - \frac{d^3}{3a^2} \right] \right\}$$

or using an area-length formula, as

$$\text{LV mass} = 1.05 \{ [5/6 A_1 (a + d + t)] \quad (4.23)$$
$$- [5/2 A_2 (a + d)] \}$$

The images needed for LV mass calculation are shown in Figure 4–7.

Left Ventricular Wall Stress

Both meridional and circumferential stress can be calculated from 2D echocardiographic images in combination with ventricular pressure measurements. Meridional wall stress σ_m is calculated from left ventricular peak pressure P, the myocardial area A_m, and cavity area A_c in a short-axis view at the papillary muscle level as (Fig. 4–8):

$$\sigma_m = 1.33 P(A_c/A_m) \times 10^3 \text{ dyn/cm}^2 \quad (4.24)$$

Circumferential stress σ_c can be calculated using these variables plus ventricular length L from an apical four-chamber view as

$$\sigma_c = \frac{(1.33)P\sqrt{A_c}}{\sqrt{A_m + A_c} - \sqrt{A_c}} \times$$
$$\left(1 - \frac{4A_c \sqrt{A_c}/\pi L^2}{\sqrt{A_m + A_c} + \sqrt{A_c}} \right) \text{kdyn/cm}^2 \quad (4.25)$$

TABLE 4–1. SELECTED STUDIES VALIDATING 2D ECHOCARDIOGRAPHIC LEFT VENTRICULAR VOLUME MEASUREMENTS

FIRST AUTHOR/ YEAR	VOLUME/METHOD	n	r	REGRESSION EQUATION	SEE	STANDARD OF REFERENCE
Teichholz/74	Ejection fraction $V = [7.0/(2.4 + D)] \times D^3$	25	0.87	Echo = 0.61 angio + 0.01 ml		Biplane LV-angio
Schiller/79	Modified Simpson's rule	30				Biplane angio
	Diastolic volume		0.80	Echo = 0.7 angio − 1 ml	15 ml	
	Systolic volume		0.90	Echo = 0.7 angio = 2 ml	8.5 ml	
	Ejection fraction		0.87	Echo = angio + 5	7.6%	
Folland/79	Modified Simpson's rule	35				
	Ejection fraction		0.78	Angio = 1.01 echo + 0.04	9.7%	Single-plane angio
	Ejection fraction		0.75	Radionuclide = 0.75 echo + 0.07	8.7%	Radionuclide
Parisi/79	Modified Simpson's rule	50				Single-plane angio
	Diastolic volume		0.82	Angio = 1.08 echo + 30 ml	39 ml	
	Systolic volume		0.90		29 ml	
	Ejection fraction		0.80		9%	
Gueret/80	Modified Simpson's rule	11				Cineangiography in closed-chest dogs
	Diastolic volume		0.89	Cine = 0.88 echo + 22 ml	10 ml	1 h S/P LAD occlusion
	Systolic volume		0.86	Cine = 0.95 echo + 11 ml	9 ml	
	Ejection fraction		0.92	Cine = 1.13 echo − 7.5%	5%	
Silverman/80	Biplane area-length	20				Biplane angio
	Diastolic volume		0.96	Echo = 1.05 angio − 3.64		
	Systolic volume		0.91	Echo = 1.37 angio − 1.37		
	Ejection fraction		0.82	Echo = 0.87 angio + 0		
Wyatt/80	Modified Simpson's rule	21	0.98	Echo = 1.0x − 0.7 ml	6.6 ml	Directly measured fluid volume in fixed hearts
	2/3 area-length		0.97	Echo = 1.0x − 8.9 ml	8.6 ml	
	Area-length (cylinder)		0.97	Echo = 1.49x − 13.4 ml	12.8 ml	
	Hemiellipsoid (bullet)		0.97	Echo = 1.25x − 11.1 ml	10.9 ml	
Starling/81	Simpson's rule	70				Single or biplane (n = 30) LV angio
	Diastolic rule		0.80	Echo = 0.66 angio + 42 ml	34 ml	
	Systolic volume		0.88	Echo = 0.72 angio + 18 ml	27 ml	
	Ejection fraction		0.90	Echo = 0.76 angio + 12%	7%	
Quinones/81	Simplified method	55				
	Ejection fraction		0.93		6.7%	Radionuclide
			0.91		7.4%	Angio
Tortoledo/83	Simplified method	52				Single-plane angio
	Diastolic volume		0.88	Angio = 1.07 echo − 7.3 ml	28 ml	
	Systolic volume		0.94	Angio = 1.0 echo + 1.3 ml	19 ml	
	Ejection fraction		0.92	Angio = 0.93 echo + 3.5 ml	7%	
Weiss/83	Modified Simpson's rule (15–19 "slices")	52	0.97		6.6% (mean % error)	Direct volume measurement in isolated ejecting dog hearts
Erbel/85	Simpson's rule	46				Single-plane LV-angio
	Diastolic volume		0.91	Echo = 0.66 angio + 0.8 ml	26 ml	
	Systolic volume		0.94	Echo = 0.57 angio + 18 ml	19 ml	
	Ejection fraction		0.80	Echo = 0.61 angio + 13%	9%	
Zoghbi/90	Echo-tilt method	24				Biplane angio
	Diastolic volume		0.92	Angio = 0.80 echo + 37 ml	23 ml	
	Systolic volume		0.96	Angio = 0.97 echo − 1 ml	16 ml	
	Ejection fraction		0.82	Angio = 1.17 echo − 4	10%	
Smith/92	TEE Simpson's rule	36				LV angio (single-plane)
	Diastolic volume		0.85	Echo = 0.75 angio + 0.2 ml	42 ml	
	Systolic volume		0.94	Echo = 0.78 angio − 3.5 ml	22 ml	
	Ejection fraction		0.85	Echo = 0.82 angio + 9.0 ml	8%	
Zile/92	Prolate ellipsoid using constant long-axis/ short-axis ratio	25				LV angio in dog model
	Diastolic volume		0.96	Echo = 1.0 angio − 1.8 ml		
	Systolic volume		0.95	Echo = 0.98 angio − 0.65 ml		

Data from Teichholz LE, et al: NEJM 291:1220–26, 1974; Schiller NB, et al: Circ 60:547–555, 1979; Folland ED, et al: Circ 60:760–766, 1979; Parisi AF, et al: Clin Cardiol 2:257–263, 1979; Gueret P, et al: Circ 62:1308–1318, 1980; Silverman NH, et al: Circ 62:548–557, 1980; Wyatt HL, et al: Circ 61:1119–1125, 1980; Kan et al: Eur Heart J 2:337, 1981; Starling MR, et al: Circ 63:1075–1084, 1981; Quinones MA, et al: Circ 64:744–753, 1981; Tortoledo FA, et al. Circ 67:579–584, 1983; Weiss JL, et al: Circ 67:889–895, 1983; Erbel R, et al: Circ 67:205–215, 1983; Zoghbi WA, et al: JACC 15:610–617, 1990; Smith MD, et al: JACC 19:1213–1222, 1992; Zile MR, et al: JACC 20:986–993, 1992. SEE = standard error of the estimate.

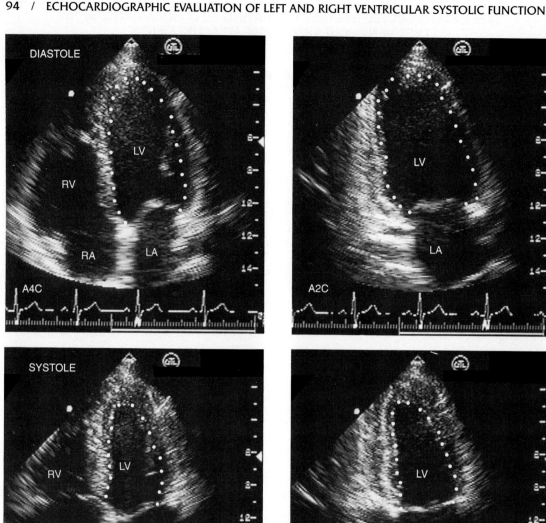

Figure 4–6. Examples of apical four-chamber (*left*) and two-chamber (*right*) views at end-diastole (*above*) and end-systole (*below*) showing the traced endocardial borders for calculation of ventricular volumes.

Measures of wall stress are most useful in ventricular pressure or volume overall states (such as hypertension, aortic stenosis, aortic or mitral regurgitation) to evaluate left ventricular systolic function.

Other 2D Measures of Left Ventricular Systolic Function

There are several other semiquantitative 2D measures of LV systolic function. The mitral an-

nulus moves toward the ventricular apex in systole, with the magnitude of this motion proportional to the extent of shortening in ventricular length—a useful measure of overall left ventricular systolic function. Normal subjects have motion of the mitral annulus toward the apex ≥ 8 mm, with a mean value of 12 ± 2 mm in both four- and two-chamber views. The sensitivity of mitral annulus motion < 8 mm is 98 percent with a specificity of 82 percent for identification of an ejection fraction < 50 percent.

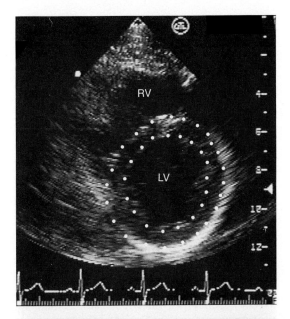

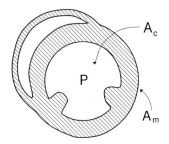

$$\sigma_m = 1.33P(A_c/A_m) \times 10^3 \text{ dynes/cm}^2$$

Figure 4–8. Schematic diagram of the measurements needed for calculation of meridional wall stress σ_m. In a short-axis view at the papillary muscle level, the cavity area A_c and myocardial area A_m at end-systole are measured in combination with left ventricular pressure P.

Limitations of 2D Evaluation of Left Ventricular Systolic Function

Endocardial Definition

Image quality remains a major potential limitation of 2D echocardiographic evaluation of left ventricular systolic function (Table 4–2). Endocardial definition is affected by the physics of ultrasound instrumentation, by anatomic factors, and by technical factors, including the skill of the sonographer. The endocardial-ventricular cavity interface is curved from any imaging window, so the endocardium appears as a thin, bright line where it is perpendicular to the ultrasound beam (axial resolution) but as a broad, "blurred" line where the beam is less perpendicular or parallel to the endocardial-ventricular

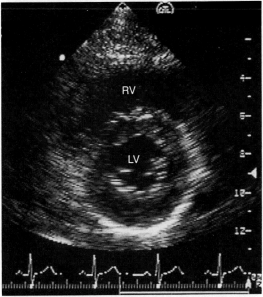

Figure 4–7. Parasternal short-axis view at the papillary muscle level. Epicardial and endocardial borders are traced at end-diastole for calculation of left ventricular mass, in combination with a left ventricular length measurement from an apical approach.

In addition, the overall shape of the left ventricle provides important data. As ventricular dilation occurs, the normal elliptical shape of the apex changes to a rounded shape, and the ventricular chamber becomes spherical. The ratio of long- to short-axis dimensions (or the sphericity index) provides a semiquantitative measure of the degree of abnormality.

TABLE 4–2. OPTIMIZATION OF 2D ECHO ENDOCARDIAL DEFINITION

---

1. Position the patient to bring the cardiac structures in contact with the chest wall (often a steep left lateral decubitus position).
2. Have the patient suspend respiration where image quality is optimal.
3. Adjust the transducer position on the chest to improve acoustic access while maintaining the correct tomographic plane.
4. Adjust gain and gray-scale settings to enhance identification of the endocardium.
5. Use the highest transducer frequency that provides adequate penetration.
6. Adjust the focal depth of the ultrasound beam to the depth of interest.
7. Use the cine-loop function to ensure optimal endocardial definition at end-diastole and at end-systole.
8. Have the sonographer who records the data be responsible for tracing the endocardial borders.

---

cavity interface (lateral resolution). As for other ultrasound targets, lateral resolution is depth-dependent. In addition, there may be "dropout" of signals due to attenuation, a perpendicular intercept angle, acoustic shadowing, or reverberations.

Anatomically, the endocardium is not a smooth surface but has numerous trabeculations that are most prominent at the left ventricular apex. The ultrasound beam is reflected from the inner edge of these trabeculations so that the "endocardium" identified by echocardiography differs from the "endocardium" identified by contrast ventriculography, in which contrast material fills these trabeculations, outlining their outer edge.

Several technical factors affect endocardial definition during image acquisition, and meticulous examination technique is needed for optimal image quality. First, acoustic access can be optimizing by (1) patient positioning so that the cardiac structures are in contact with the chest wall, (2) having the patient suspend respiration at the point in the cycle where image quality is optimal, and (3) careful adjustment of transducer position while maintaining the correct tomographic plane.

Instrument settings can dramatically affect image quality, most notably gain and gray-scale settings, but other instrument parameters (pre- and postprocessing, TGC curve, etc.) also may affect endocardial definition. A higher-frequency transducer is used for optimal image quality, provided penetration is adequate, and when available, the focal depth of the transducer can be adjusted to the depth of interest. The cine-loop function is utilized to ensure that endocardial definition is clear on freeze-frame images at end-diastole and end-systole. Finally, the individual who acquires the images should be responsible for tracing the endocardial borders. In some patients, even with careful attention to imaging technique, ultrasound tissue penetration is poor, precluding adequate endocardial definition.

The trained human observer remains the most accurate means for endocardial border tracing, limiting the wide application of quantitative methods because manual tracing of endocardial borders at end-diastole and end-systole in at least two views remains a tedious and time-consuming task. In many cases, identification of the endocardium requires analysis of the moving image using both the cine-loop and frame-by-frame features of the system to assist in identification of the border as the bright linear echo reflection that moves with the cardiac cycle and is spatially continuous. In the future, automatic edge-detection programs or other approaches to determination of area changes (such as acoustic quantification) may alleviate this problem.

Geometric Assumptions

In addition to the geometric assumptions of the mathematical models themselves, quantitation of left ventricular volumes depends on accurate measurement of ventricular lengths, diameters, and cross-sectional areas. 2D echo views that foreshorten the left ventricle will result in underestimation of left ventricular length, while oblique short-axis views will overestimate the cross-sectional area of the chamber. Adequate apical views require a steep left lateral decubitus position with an apical cutout in the echo-stretcher mattress to obtain the true long axis of the chamber. Short-axis views should appear circular if perpendicular to the long axis of the left ventricle. In the future, 3D volume calculations may circumvent these geometric assumptions (Table 4–3).

Cardiac motion during the cardiac cycle and with respiratory motion further confounds the geometric assumptions of left ventricular volume calculations. The effect of respiratory motion of the heart relative to the transducer can be avoided by measuring beats at the same phase of respiration or by having the patient briefly suspend respiration during data acquisition. It is more difficult to correct for the motion of the heart itself using a tomographic imaging procedure. Cardiac translation (movement of the heart in the chest), rotation (movement around the long axis of the heart), and torsion (unequal rotational motion of the heart) can result in images of different segments of the left ventricle during systole and diastole, even with a fixed image plane. While cardiac motion has only a limited effect on the accuracy of left ventricular volume calculations, it can have a pronounced effect on quantitative evaluation of regional ventricular function, as discussed in Chapter 6.

Accuracy and Reproducibility

Qualitative comparison of left ventricular systolic function from different studies on the same patient is facilitated by a cine-loop side-by-side format. With this approach, a single high-quality beat is captured in digital format (either the entire cardiac cycle or just the systolic phase). The study to be compared is captured similarly with the same number of frames in the cine-loop

TABLE 4–3. SELECTED STUDIES VALIDATING 3D ECHOCARDIOGRAPHIC LEFT VENTRICULAR VOLUME MEASUREMENTS

FIRST AUTHOR/ YEAR	METHOD	*n*	*r*	REGRESSION EQUATION	SEE	STANDARD OF REFERENCE
Nessly/91	Dog model, 3D reconstruction	33	0.86	Echo = 0.83 RN + 4 ml	6 ml	Radionuclide (RN)
Kuroda/91	Balloons in water bath					True volume by weight
	Pull-back reconstruction		0.99	Echo = 1.1x − 10 ml	5.8 ml	
	Rotational reconstruction		0.99	Echo = 1.0x − 7 ml	6.5 ml	
Handschumacher/93	Ventricular phantoms and gel-filled excised ventricles		0.99	Echo = 0.96x + 2.2 ml	2.7 ml	Direct volumes
			0.99	Echo = 0.99x + 0.11 ml	5.9 ml	
Gopal/93	Normal adults, 6–8 nonparallel, nonintersecting short-axis planes	15				Magnetic resonance imaging (MRI)
	End-diastolic volume		0.92	Echo = 0.84 MRI + 22 ml	7 ml	
	End-systolic volume		0.81	Echo = 0.51 MRI + 18 ml	4 ml	
Sui/93	Canine model, spark-gap 3D location	84	0.98	Echo = 1.0x − 0.8 ml	3.6 ml	Direct volumes
		19	0.94	Echo = 0.96x + 1.3 ml	4.3 ml	Doppler stroke volume
Sapin/93	Excised porcine hearts	25	0.99	y = 1.02 Echo + 3.7 ml	7.1 ml	Direct volumes

Data from Nessly ML, et al: J Cardiothorac Vasc Anesthesiol 5:40–45, 1991; Kuroda T, et al: Echocardiography 4:475–484, 1991; Handschumacher MD, et al: JACC 21:743–753, 1993; Gopal AS, et al: JACC 22:258–270, 1993; Sui, et al: Circ 88(I):1715, 1993; Sapin, et al: JACC 22:1530, 1993.

so that when the images are played side by side, heart rates are "matched." The advantage of this approach is that the same view can be examined as long as is needed for careful qualitative (or quantitative) evaluation. This approach is particularly useful for evaluation of regional ventricular function. Of course, the influence of loading conditions on left ventricular systolic function still must be considered when comparing studies performed at different time points in a patient's clinical course.

In most reported series, intraobserver variability for left ventricular volumes ranges from 5 to 10 percent. Interobserver variability is greater, ranging from 7 to 25 percent for ventricular volumes. Since ejection fraction is a calculated percentage, reproducibility is better, with variability of about 10 percent. These values are similar to reported variability for ventricular volumes and ejection fraction determined by contrast or radionuclide ventriculography. Note that variability between studies in an individual patient includes (1) physiologic variability (load-

ing condition, heart rate, volume states), (2) variability in image acquisition (endocardial definition, image orientation), and (3) variability in tracing the endothelial borders. In a careful study designed to assess measurement variability for 2D echo left ventricular volumes, it was concluded that a significant change between studies is a change in ejection fraction > 2 percent, end-diastolic volume > 2 percent, and end-systolic volume > 5 percent (Suggested Reading #7).

DOPPLER EVALUATION OF LEFT VENTRICULAR SYSTOLIC FUNCTION

Stroke Volume Calculation

Doppler echocardiographic evaluation of left ventricular systolic function usually is based on

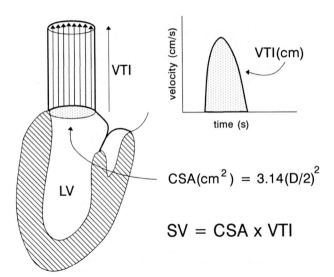

$$CSA(cm^2) = 3.14(D/2)^2$$

$$SV = CSA \times VTI$$

Figure 4–9. Doppler stroke volume calculation. The cross-sectional area (CSA) of flow is calculated as a circle based on a 2D echo diameter D measurement. The length of the cylinder of blood ejected through this cross-sectional area on a single beat is the velocity-time integral (VTI) of the Doppler curve. Stroke volume (SV) then is calculated as CSA $\times$ VTI.

calculation of stroke volume and cardiac output. Using Doppler and 2D echo data, stroke volume (SV) is calculated as cross-sectional area (CSA) times the velocity-time integral (VTI) of flow through that region:

$$SV = CSA \times VTI \qquad (4.26)$$

Conceptually, the left ventricle ejects a volume of blood into the cylindrical aorta on each beat (Fig. 4–9). The base of this cylinder is the systolic cross-sectional area of the aorta, while its height is the distance the average blood cell traveled during ejection for that beat. This distance is expressed as the integral of the Doppler systolic velocity-time curve, since velocity is the first derivative of distance. This distance also can be thought of as mean velocity (cm/s) multiplied by ejection duration (s). Again, since the volume of a cylinder is base times height, stroke volume is cross-sectional area multiplied by the velocity-time integral.

This approach to stroke volume calculation depends on several basic assumptions (Table 4–4). First, the cross-sectional area must be measured accurately. Typically, diameter is measured and 2D area calculated as $\pi(D/2)^2$ based on the assumption of a circular geometry. Deviations from a circular geometry or changes in cross-sectional area during the flow period will result in inaccuracies unless appropriate corrections are included in the calculations. Of note, small errors in 2D diameter measurements become large errors in cross-sectional area calculations because of the quadratic relationship between these variables. Using a transducer orientation and instrument settings that maximize image quality, performing measurements based on axial (rather than lateral) resolution, performing diameter measurements in two orthogonal planes (when possible), and averaging several beats can help minimize this source of error.

Second, the pattern of flow is assumed to be laminar, and (in most clinical applications) the spatial flow profile across the flowstream is assumed to be relatively flat. These assumptions ensure that the velocity curve represents the spatial (as well as temporal) average flow in that region. The assumption of laminar flow is justified in the great vessels and across normal cardiac valves and can be verified by demonstration of a narrow band of velocities and smooth spectral signal on pulsed Doppler echo recordings. A flat flow profile also is a reasonable assumption at the inlet to the great vessels and across the valve planes due to the effects of geometric convergence and acceleration. A flat flow velocity profile can be confirmed by moving the sample volume across the flowstream in two orthogonal views to demonstrate uniform velocities at the center and the edges of the flowstream.

Third, the Doppler signal is assumed to have been recorded at a parallel intercept angle to

---

TABLE 4–4. ASSUMPTIONS FOR ACCURATE VOLUME FLOW MEASUREMENT BY DOPPLER ECHO

- Accurate cross-sectional flow area measurement
- Laminar flow
- Spatially "flat" flow velocity profile
- Parallel intercept angle between Doppler beam and direction of blood flow
- Velocity and diameter measurements are made at the same anatomic site

---

flow, resulting in an accurate velocity measurement (based on a cos θ = 1 in the Doppler equation). In practical terms, the sonographer aligns the Doppler beam in the presumed direction of flow and then carefully moves the ultrasound beam across the image plane and in the elevational plane to obtain the highest-velocity signal, indicating the most parallel alignment with flow. Note that the optimal window for Doppler interrogation is when the ultrasound beam and flowstream are parallel, while the optimal window for diameter measurement is when the ultrasound beam and tissue-blood interfaces are perpendicular.

Fourth, it is crucial that the diameter and velocity measurements be made *at the same anatomic site*. Of course, the cross-sectional area and flow velocity curves must be temporally and spatially congruent for accurate volume flow rate calculations. As the cross-sectional area of flow narrows or expands, flow velocity will increase or decrease correspondingly so that conjoining information from two different anatomic sites will result in erroneous stroke volume data. Similarly, dynamic changes in stroke volume occur with changes in heart rate, loading conditions, exercise, etc. so that measurements made at disparate times cannot be combined. In clinical practice, diameter and velocity recordings are made in close sequence and are repeated if there is any question of an interval physiologic change.

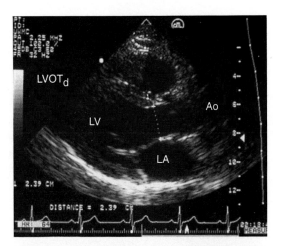

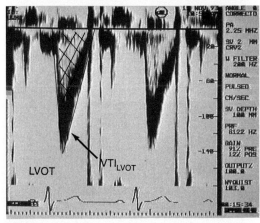

Figure 4–10. Examples of left ventricular outflow tract diameter measurement for a parasternal long-axis view (*above*) and the pulsed Doppler left ventricular outflow just proximal to the aortic valve from an apical approach (*below*) for stroke volume calculation.

Sites for Stroke Volume Measurement

Stroke volume can be measured by this approach at any intracardiac site where both cross-sectional area and the flow velocity integral can be recorded given the assumptions of laminar flow and a flat flow profile.

Left Ventricular Outflow (Fig. 4–10)

Left ventricular stroke volume can be measured in the aorta either at the aortic valve leaflet tips or in the ascending aorta. While some would argue which anatomic level (ascending aorta or leaflet tips) should be used, measurements at each of these levels can be accurate provided that diameter and flow velocity are measured at the same anatomic site. Ascending aortic diameter is measured from a parasternal long-axis view, and the flow velocity curve is recorded from either an apical or a suprasternal notch window. If continuous-wave Doppler ultrasound is used,

the highest velocities along the path of the beam will be recorded, so the narrowest segment of the aorta (the sinotubular junction) should be used for diameter measurements. Alternatively, a circular orifice area can be calculated from an M-mode diameter of aortic leaflet opening, and pulsed Doppler can be used to record the flow velocity in the aortic orifice itself. Note that if aortic valve disease is present, stroke volume measurement in the ascending aorta will be inaccurate due to nonlaminar flow distal to the valve.

Measurement of stroke volume in the left ventricular outflow tract, at the aortic annulus just proximal to the valve leaflets, offers the advantages that (1) flow remains laminar proximal to a stenosis (allowing transaortic stroke volume calculations in patients with aortic valve disease) and (2) the needed data can be recorded in nearly all patients. Left ventricular outflow tract diameter is measured from a parasternal long-axis view, in midsystole, from the septal endocardium to the leading edge of the anterior mitral leaflet parallel and immediately adjacent to the aortic valve. Pulsed Doppler is used from an apical approach to record the velocity curve, using the closing click of the aortic valve to ensure that the sample volume is located at the annulus (the same site as the diameter measurement). The small region of flow convergence proximal to a narrowed aortic valve is avoided by moving the sample volume slightly apically until a narrow spectral width is seen at maximum velocity.

Mitral Valve (Fig. 4–11)

Transmitral stroke volume can be calculated by one of two basic approaches. Given the complex motion of the mitral leaflets in diastole, the first approach utilizes a "mean" mitral orifice area derived from the maximal 2D opening of the mitral valve in early diastole multiplied by the ratio of the mean degree of leaflet separation throughout diastole as recorded by M-mode echo (six measurements) divided by the maximum opening:

$$\text{Maximum orifice} \times \frac{\text{mean}}{\text{max}} \quad (4.27)$$
$$= \text{average mitral valve orifice}$$

Transmitral flow then is recorded with pulsed Doppler at the leaflet tips. Although accurate, this approach is tedious to perform in the clinical setting. The alternate approach to transmitral stroke volume determination postulates that the mitral annulus is the limiting cross-sectional flow area, with the leaflets moving passively in response to the flowstream. This approach multiplies cross-sectional annulus area by the velocity-time integral of flow recorded at the mitral

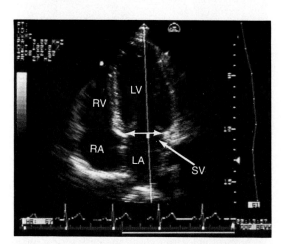

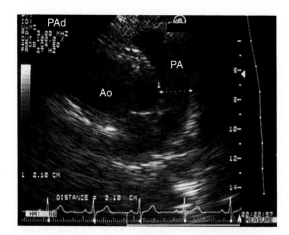

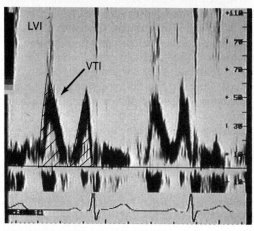

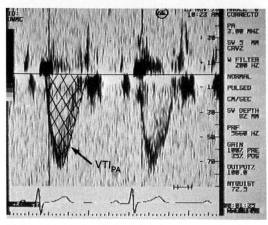

Figure 4–11. (*Above*) Example of mitral annulus diameter measurement (*arrow*) in an apical four-chamber view with the sample volume (SV) positioned at the mitral annulus. (*Below*) The pulsed Doppler left ventricular inflow signal is recorded for transmitral stroke volume calculation.

Figure 4–12. Examples of pulmonary artery diameter measurement in a parasternal right ventricular outflow view (*above*) and pulsed Doppler pulmonary artery flow recorded from a parasternal approach (*below*) for transpulmonic stroke volume calculation.

annulus level. The mitral annulus is assumed to be circular, using a parasternal long-axis diameter, or, more accurately, elliptical, using an apical four-chamber view for the major axis of the ellipse and the long-axis view for the minor axis.

Right Side of the Heart (Fig. 4–12)

In the right side of the heart, stroke volume can be calculated by analogous methods in the pulmonary artery or across the tricuspid valve. In adult patients, use of the pulmonary artery site may be limited by poor image quality resulting in unobtainable or inaccurate pulmonary artery diameter measurements. However, from a transesophageal echocardiography approach, pulmonary artery flow and diameter often can be measured.

Differences in Transvalvular Volume Flow Rates

In a normal heart, stroke volume across each of the four valves will be equal, and measurement at more than one site only serves as an internal accuracy check. However, in the presence of valvular regurgitation or an intracardiac shunt, calculation of stroke volume at two intracardiac sites allows quantitation of the degree of regurgitation or pulmonic-to-systemic shunt ratio, as detailed in Chapters 10 and 15.

Other Doppler Measures of Left Ventricular Systolic Function

Acceleration Times

In addition to stroke volume calculations, the shape of the Doppler ejection curve may provide information about ventricular function. When systolic function is normal, the isovolumic contraction period is short, and the rate of pressure rise in early systole is rapid. These features are reflected in the Doppler velocity curve, which shows a short isovolumic contraction time, a rapid acceleration of blood in early systole, and a short time interval from the onset of flow to maximum velocity. With impaired left ventricular systolic function, the isovolumic contraction time (also known as the *preejection period*) becomes progressively longer, the rate of acceleration diminishes, and the time to maximum velocity prolongs, with all these changes mirrored in the Doppler velocity curve (Fig. 4–13). In addition to measuring these variables at rest, some centers have found evaluation of aortic

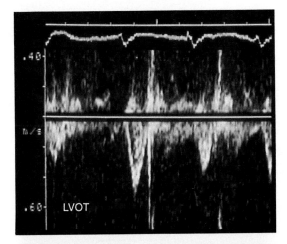

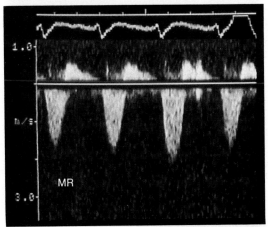

Figure 4–13. In a patient with severely reduced left ventricular systolic function, the left ventricular outflow velocity (*above*) shows a delayed time to peak and low peak velocity (compare with Fig. 4–10). The mitral regurgitant jet (*below*) is low velocity with a depressed rate of velocity rise in early systole.

ejection curves with exercise useful in detection of left ventricular systolic dysfunction.

dP/dt

When mitral regurgitation is present, the continuous-wave Doppler velocity curve indicates the instantaneous pressure difference between the left ventricle and the left atrium in systole, assuming a constant intercept angle between the mitral regurgitant jet and the ultrasound beam. Given the rapid rate of rise of left ventricular pressure with normal systolic function (and the low left atrial pressure), mitral regurgitation typically shows a rapid rise to maximum velocity as per the Bernoulli equation. If the rate of rise in ventricular pressure is reduced due to left ventricular systolic dysfunction, the rate of increase in velocity of the mitral regurgitant jet also is reduced. For example, in patients with premature ventricular beats, the altered contractility of the premature beat will be evidenced by a marked difference in the rate of velocity increase of the mitral regurgitant jet. The slope of the mitral regurgitant jet can be quantitated as *dP/dt* by measuring the time interval between the mitral regurgitant jet velocity at 1 and at 3 m/s (Fig. 4–14). At each velocity, the corresponding pressure gradient is $4v^2$ per the Bernoulli equation. Then,

$$dP/dt = \frac{[4(3)^2] - [4(1)^2]}{\text{time interval}} \quad (4.28)$$
$$= \frac{32 \text{ mmHg}}{\text{time interval}}$$

Thus a longer time interval indicates a depressed *dP/dt*, and vice versa. Of course, the calculation of *dP/dt* can be performed only when a recordable mitral regurgitant jet is present and assumes a constant (and parallel) intercept angle between the mitral regurgitant jet and the ultrasound beam throughout the cardiac cycle.

Limitations/Technical Considerations

The major limitation of Doppler evaluation of left ventricular systolic function in adults is accurate diameter measurement for cross-sectional area calculations. While the Doppler velocity curves can be recorded consistently with little interobserver measurement variability (2 to 5 percent), the variability of 2D diameter measurements is significantly greater (8 to 12 percent). Again, measurement variability includes (1) technical differences in *recording* the data (such as intercept angle, image quality, tomographic plane), (2) variability in *measuring* the recorded data, and (3) *physiologic* variability occurring between the time of repeat data recording. For Doppler velocity data, the major source of measurement variability is data recording, given the critical importance of obtaining a parallel intercept angle between the ultrasound beam and the flow of interest. For 2D diameters, the major source of variability is measuring the 2D images, particularly when image quality is suboptimal or when lateral resolution limits accurate border recognition. Despite these potential limitations, Doppler measurement of stroke volume has been well validated in a variety of clinical and research settings (Table 4–5).

Measurement of *dP/dt* is limited by the need for enough mitral regurgitation to generate a Doppler signal with a well-defined velocity curve. Changes during ejection in the intercept angle between the ultrasound beam and the regurgitant jet will result in an erroneous measurement, since the assumption that cos θ = 1 in the Doppler equation will not be valid.

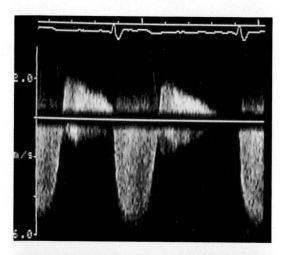

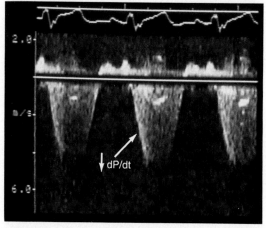

Figure 4–14. Left ventricular *dP/dt* can be calculated from the mitral regurgitant jet. Continous wave Doppler mitral regurgitation curves are consistent with normal (*above*) and severely reduced (*below*) left ventricular systolic function.

Alternate Approaches

Thermodilution cardiac outputs, measured with an indwelling right-sided heart catheter, are the standard approach to evaluation of cardiac output both in the catheterization laboratory and in the coronary care unit. Thermodilution outputs offer the advantages that measurements can be repeated frequently by the

TABLE 4–5. SELECTED STUDIES VALIDATING DOPPLER VOLUME FLOW MEASUREMENT

FIRST AUTHOR/YEAR	VOLUME FLOW SITE/METHOD	n	r	REGRESSION EQUATION	SEE	STANDARD OF REFERENCE
Huntsman/83	Ascending aorta	100	0.94	$DOP = 0.95x + 0.38$	0.58 L/min	TD-CO
Fisher/83	Mitral leaflets	52	0.97	$DOP = 0.98x + 0.02$	0.23 L/min	Roller pump
Meijboom/83	Mitral leaflets	26	0.99	$DOP = 0.97x + 0.07$	0.13 L/min	EM flow and roller pump
	RVOT	26	0.99	$DOP = 0.96x + 0.11$	0.16 L/min	Roller pump
Lewis/84	Mitral annulus	35	0.96	$TD = 0.91x + 5.1$	5.9 ml	TD-SV
	LVOT	39	0.95	$TD = 0.91x + 7.8$	6.4 ml	TD-SV
Stewart/85	Mitral leaflets	29	0.97	$DOP = 0.98x + 0.3$	0.3 L/min	Roller pump
	Aortic annulus	33	0.98	$DOP = 1.06x + 0.2$	0.3 L/min	Roller pump
	Pulmonary annulus	30	0.93	$DOP = 0.89x + 0.4$	0.5 L/min	Roller pump
Bouchard/87	Aortic leaflets	41	0.95	$DOP = 0.97x + 1.7$	7 ml	TD-SV
Dittmann/87	Mitral annulus	40	0.86	$DOP = 0.88 + 1.75$	0.80 L/min	TD-CO
	LVOT (M-mode)	40	0.93	$DOP = 0.94x + 0.44$	0.59 L/min	TD-CO
DeZuttere/88	Mitral orifice (instantaneous)	30	0.91	$DOP = 0.92x + 0.35$	0.53 L/min	TD-CO
Hoit/88	Mitral leaflets	48	0.93	$DOP = 1.1x - 0.45$	0.36 L/min	TD-CO
Otto/88	LVOT (proximal to stenotic aortic valve)	52	0.91	$DOP = 1.0x + 0.03$	0.25 L/min	EM flow and timed collection
Burwash/93	LVOT (proximal to aortic stenosis)	75	0.86	$Inv\text{-}CO = 0.92\ COP + 0.26$	0.50 L/min	Transit-time flow probe

Data from Huntsman, et al: Circ 67:593–601, 1983; Fisher, et al: Circ 67:872–877, 1983; Meijboom, et al: Circ 68:437–445, 1983; Lewis, et al: Circ 70:425–431, 1984; Stewart, et al: JACC 6:653–662, 1985; Bouchard, et al: JACC 9:75–83, 1987; Dittman, et al: JACC 10:818–823, 1987; DeZuttere, et al: JACC 11:343–350, 1988; Hoit, et al: AJC 62:131–135, 1988; Otto, et al: Circ 78:435–441, 1988; Burwash, et al: Am J Physiol 265 (Heart Circ Physiol 34):1734, 1993.

nurse caring for the patient and pulmonary artery pressures can be monitored continuously as well. Disadvantages of this approach are that it is invasive (risks, discomfort) and it provides only a volumetric flow rate, without direct visualization of ventricular function. Stroke volume can be maintained despite a low ejection fraction due to compensatory left ventricular dilation. For example, the same stroke volume of 60 ml may result from an ejection fraction of 20 percent with a left ventricular end-diastolic volume of 300 ml or from a normal ejection fraction (60 percent) with a smaller left ventricular end-diastolic volume (100 ml).

Available alternate approaches to measurement of left ventricular volumes and ejection fraction are contrast angiography in the cardiac catheterization laboratory (Fig. 4–15) and radionuclide ventriculography (Fig. 4–16). Both computed tomography and magnetic resonance imaging are capable of left ventricular volume calculation, although they may not be available routinely. The choice of imaging technique in an individual patient will depend on what other clinical questions are present (e.g., possible valvular disease) as well as availability and cost.

ECHO APPROACH TO RIGHT VENTRICULAR SYSTOLIC FUNCTION

2D/M-Mode

Qualitative

The right ventricle is evaluated qualitatively by 2D evaluation from several different windows: parasternal long- and short-axis, right ventricular inflow, apical four-chamber, and subcostal four-chamber views (Fig. 4–17). In each view, the area of the right ventricular chamber (relative to the left ventricular chamber), the shape of the right ventricular cavity, right ventricular wall thickness, the degree of motion of the right ventricular free wall, and the pattern of ventricular septal motion are evaluated.

The *normal shape* of the right ventricle is complex in three dimensions, with the inflow segment located medial to the left ventricle, the body and apex located anterior to the left ventricle, and the right ventricular outflow tract located superior to the left ventricle and aortic valve. There is no simple geometric shape that

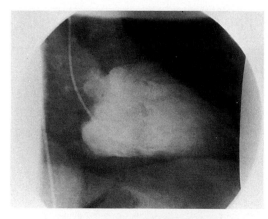

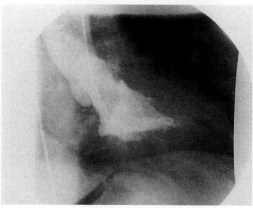

Figure 4–15. Left ventricular angiography is an alternate approach to evaluation of left ventricular systolic function, which is performed most often in patients undergoing cardiac catheterization for other indications, such as coronary artery disease. End-diastolic (*above*) and end-systolic (*below*) frames are shown.

approximates the right ventricular chamber; rather, it is "wrapped around" the left ventricle in a U-shaped fashion. Since echocardiographic long- and short-axis views are oriented with respect to the left ventricle, the right ventricle may appear abnormal in some individuals due to the position of the right ventricle relative to the image plane. This occurs most often in parasternal views, where the right ventricle may be imaged in an oblique orientation. Both subcostal and apical four-chamber windows tend to offer more consistent views of the right ventricle, with the right ventricle appearing somewhat triangular in shape with a broad base and narrow apex. The right ventricular apex is slightly closer to the base than the left ventricular apex in normal individuals.

With right ventricular dilation, the right ventricular outflow tract may be enlarged in the parasternal long-axis view. On apical and subcostal views, the right ventricular chamber will

be larger and the right ventricular apex is either closer to or encompasses the left ventricular apex. The degree of right ventricular dilation is described as mild (enlarged but a 2D area < left ventricular area), moderate (right ventricular = left ventricular area), or severe (right ventricular > left ventricular area) using the combination of multiple image planes in this overall assessment. Right ventricular dilation is the normal response of the ventricle to volume overload, and its presence mandates a careful search for etiology, such as an atrial septal defect, tricuspid regurgitation, or pulmonic regurgitation. Long-standing pressure overload of the right ventricle also can lead to dilation.

Right ventricular hypertrophy is manifested as increased thickness of the right ventricular free wall as seen on 2D images or by M-mode, with a wall thickness > 0.5 cm being abnormal in adults. The presence of right ventricular hypertrophy suggests right ventricular pressure overload and should prompt a search for evidence of elevated pulmonary pressures or pulmonic valve stenosis. Increased thickness of the right ventricular free wall also may be seen in some infiltrative cardiomyopathies or in hypertrophic cardiomyopathy.

Quantitative

Quantitative evaluation of right ventricular systolic function by 2D/M-mode echo is difficult. Standard geometric formulas for volume calculations have only limited applicability given the shape of the right ventricle, and while 3D reconstructions have been shown to be accurate, the need for tedious endocardial border tracing and extensive data analysis has restricted its use to the research setting. In most cases, qualitative evaluation is sufficient for clinical decision making.

Technical Considerations/ Alternate Approaches

Evaluation of right ventricular systolic function may be limited by poor ultrasound tissue penetration in some individuals. With careful patient positioning and a search from multiple windows, the right ventricle usually can be visualized, but endocardial definition may be suboptimal. If clinically indicated, transesophageal echo offers superior images of the right ventricle both in the high esophageal four-chamber view and from a transgastric approach.

Right ventricular contrast angiography can be performed at catheterization, but there is wide

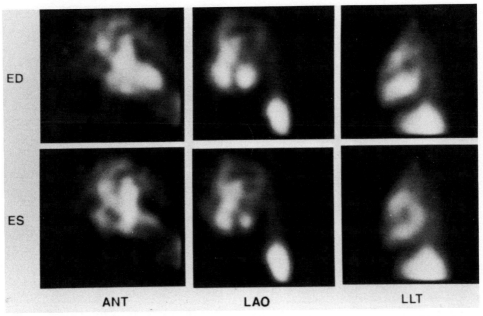

Figure 4–16. A radionuclide ventriculogram. Standard view radionuclide ventriculographic images at end-diastole (ED) and end-systole (ES) in a patient with normal cardiac chamber size and global function of both ventricles (ANT = anterior; LAO = left anterior oblique; LLT = left lateral). (*Reprinted from Cerqueira M (ed.). Nuclear Cardiology. Blackwell Scientific Publications, 1993.*)

variability in the appearance of the normal right ventricle. Radionuclide ventriculography can be used to derive a right ventricular ejection fraction by identifying an "area of interest" over the right ventricle. The right ventricle also can be imaged on computed tomography or magnetic resonance imaging scanning, and cine-views may be helpful, when available, for evaluation of systolic function.

Patterns of Ventricular Septal Motion

The interventricular septum functions as part of the left ventricle in the normal heart. During diastole, the left ventricle is circular in a short-axis view, with the normal septal curvature convex toward the right ventricle and concave toward the left ventricle. With the onset of systole, the septal myocardium thickens, and the septal endocardium moves toward the center of the left ventricle such that at end systole the short-axis image shows a circular left ventricular chamber.

A number of cardiac disorders alter the pattern of ventricular septal motion, the most prominent being right ventricular pressure and volume overload. The basic principle underlying the pattern of septal motion with right ven-

tricular dilation or hypertrophy is that the septum moves toward the center of mass of the entire heart. Normally, the center of cardiac mass coincides with the center of the left ventricle. When right and left ventricular masses are equal, septal motion will be "flat" (on M-mode) or minimal (on 2D echo). When right ventricular mass exceeds left ventricular mass, the septum moves "paradoxically" anterior in systole (on M-mode) and flattens or reverses its curvature in diastole (on 2D echo). Thus, with isolated pressure overload of the right ventricle (increased mass due to increased wall thickness with a non-dilated chamber), the pattern of septal motion is anterior in systole, despite normal septal thickening and flattening of motion in diastole (Fig. 4–18).

With increased right ventricular mass due to volume overload, the additional factor of increased right ventricular filling and emptying accentuates the diastolic reverse motion of the septum (due to rapid right ventricular diastolic filling), resulting in a D shape of the left ventricular chamber in diastole. Anterior motion with systole may appear less prominent than with isolated pressure overload as the septum moves from its abnormal diastolic position back toward the center of the heart, resulting in a more convex curve relative to the right ventricular chamber. Often, the observation of abnormal septal

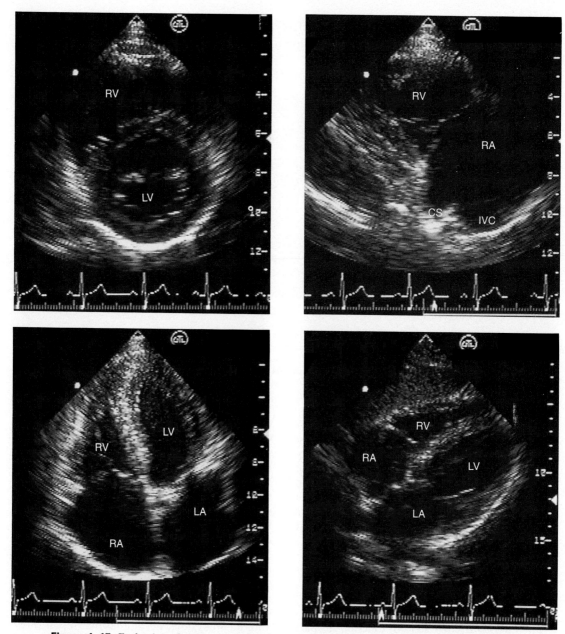

Figure 4–17. Evaluation of right ventricular size and systolic function is based on multiple image planes including parasternal short-axis (*above, left*), right ventricular inflow (*above, right*), apical four-chamber (*below, left*), and subcostal four-chamber (*below, right*) views. CS = coronary sinus; IVC = inferior vena cava.

motion during the examination is the first clue of right ventricular pressure and/or volume overload.

Other abnormalities that affect the pattern of ventricular septal motion are summarized in Figure 4–19. Conduction defects affect the pattern of motion by altering the sequence of right and left ventricular contraction. Valvular disease can affect the timing of right ventricular versus left ventricular diastolic filling, particularly in early diastole. Pericardial tamponade or constriction results in a fixed total cardiac volume so that respiratory changes in right ventricular filling result in respiratory shifts in the pattern of septal motion.

An abnormal pattern of septal motion may be appreciated on 2D imaging, but M-mode echo offers more detailed time resolution for studying the pattern of motion. Abnormal septal motion rarely is diagnostic in and of itself, but it may

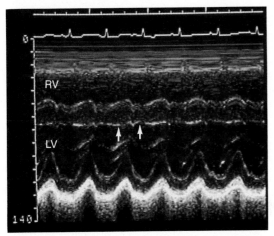

Figure 4–18. Abnormal septal motion on M-mode in a patient after cardiac bypass surgery. In systole, the septum moves anteriorly but thickens normally. (For septal motion with right ventricular volume overload, see Fig. 15–17.)

raise a diagnostic possibility that had not been considered previously or may support a suspected diagnosis. For example, a pattern of paradoxical septal motion in association with right ventricular and right atrial enlargement suggests the possibility of an atrial septal defect. This possibility then can be specifically excluded (or confirmed) during the echocardiographic examination. In contrast, in a patient with a pericardial effusion and suspected tamponade physiology, a changing pattern of septal motion with respiration supports the diagnosis. There are no alternate imaging techniques that offer such a detailed analysis of ventricular septal motion.

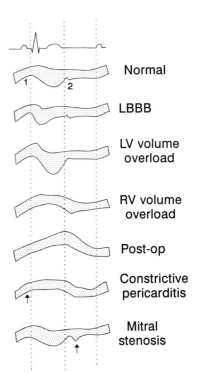

Figure 4–19. Schematic diagram of different patterns of septal motion on M-mode echocardiography. The normal pattern is characterized by systolic brief anterior motion (1) followed by posterior motion and myocardial thickening. In diastole, a small diastolic dip (2) following mitral valve opening may be seen. Left bundle branch block (LBBB) is characterized by systolic rapid downward septal motion. Left ventricular (LV) volume overload results in exaggerated septal (and posterior wall) motion. Right ventricular (RV) volume overload results in paradoxical anterior motion of the septum in systole. A similar pattern is seen in patients after cardiac surgery (postop). Constrictive pericarditis is characterized by anterior motion of the septum with atrial filling (before the QRS), while mitral stenosis typically shows a prominent early diastolic dip.

Pulmonary Artery Pressure Estimates

Clinically, one of the most important quantitative parameters of right ventricular systolic function is an estimate of pulmonary artery pressures. Pulmonary hypertension often occurs in response to chronic left-sided heart diseases, such as mitral stenosis, mitral regurgitation, cardiomyopathy, and ischemic cardiac disease. Knowledge of the degree of pulmonary pressure elevation is critical in patient management (Tables 4–6 and 4–7).

Tricuspid Regurgitant Jet Plus Right Atrial Pressure

The most reliable method for estimating pulmonary artery pressures noninvasively is based on measurement of the velocity in the tricuspid regurgitant jet. This velocity V_{TR} reflects the right ventricular (RV) to right atrial (RA) pressure difference ΔP, as stated in the Bernoulli equation (Fig. 4–20):

$$\Delta P_{RV-RA} = 4(V_{TR})^2 \qquad (4.29)$$

When added to an estimate of right atrial pressure, right ventricular systolic pressure (RVP) is obtained:

$$RVP = \Delta P_{RV-RA} + RAP \qquad (4.30)$$

In the absence of pulmonic stenosis (which is rare in adults), right ventricular systolic pressure equals pulmonary artery systolic pressure, so that

$$PAP_{systolic} = 4(V_{TR})^2 + RAP \qquad (4.31)$$

as diagrammed in Figure 4–21.

TABLE 4–6. DOPPLER ECHO METHODS FOR PULMONARY ARTERY PRESSURE ESTIMATION

METHOD	ADVANTAGES	POTENTIAL LIMITATIONS
$4(V_{TR})^2 + RAP$	Accurate Measurable in a high percentage of patients overall (90%)	Nonparallel intercept angle between jet and ultrasound beam Misidentification of jet signal Right atrial pressure estimate (not available in ventilated patients) Presence of pulmonic stenosis Inadequate signal in patients with chronic lung disease (recordable in only about 30%)
TPV in pulmonary artery (see Table 4–7)	Readily measured in nearly all patients, including patients with chronic lung disease Estimates *mean* pulmonary artery pressure	Skewed flow profile in pulmonary artery Measurement variability
RV-IVRT	Alternate approach	Difficulty in recording tricuspid and pulmonic valve closure in adults Measurement variability

This method has been shown to be highly accurate compared with invasive measurements of pulmonary artery pressure over a wide range of values. Of course, the reliability of this approach is dependent on obtaining a parallel intercept angle between the tricuspid regurgitant jet and the ultrasound beam. Most often the apical or right ventricular inflow view yields the highest-velocity signal given careful angulation of the ultrasound beam in three dimensions. Occasionally, the highest-velocity tricuspid regurgitant jet is recorded from a subcostal approach.

TABLE 4–7. SELECTED STUDIES VALIDATING NONINVASIVE PULMONARY ARTERY PRESSURE MEASUREMENT

FIRST AUTHOR/ YEAR	METHOD	n	r	REGRESSION EQUATION	SEE
Kitabatake/83	Time to peak flow (RVOT)	33	−0.88	Log (mean PAP) = 0.0068(AcT) + 2.1 mmHg	—
Stevenson/84	IVRT (Burstin method, in sedated patients)	95	0.97	Doppler mean PAP = 0.97(cath) + 1.7 mmHg	6.4 mmHg
Isobe/86	PEP/AcT	45	0.89	PEP/AcT = 0.023 mean PAP + 0.48 mmHg	—
Stevenson/89	TR-jet Time to peak flow (PA) IVRT Pulmonic regurgitation	50	0.96 0.63 0.97 0.96		6.9 mmHg 16.4 mmHg 5 mmHg 4.5 mmHg
Yock/84	TR-jet	62	0.95	Doppler RV-RA ΔP = 1.03 ΔP + 0.71 mmHg	7 mmHg
Berger/85	TR-jet	69	0.97	Systolic PAP = 1.23 (Doppler ΔP) − 0.09 mmHg	4.9 mmHg
Currie/85	TR-jet	127	0.96	Doppler RV-RA ΔP = 0.88 ΔP + 2.2 mmHg	7 mmHg
Lee/89	Pulmonic regurgitation	29	0.94	Diastolic PAP (echo) = 0.95(cath) − 1.0 mmHg	Mean diff: 3.3 ± 2.2 mmHg

Kitabatake A, et al: Circ 68:302–309, 1983; Stevenson JG, et al: JACC 4:1021–1027, 1984; Isobe M, et al: AJC 57:316–332, 1986; Stevenson JG, et al: JASE 2:157–171, 1989; Yock PG, Popp RL: Circ 70:657–662, 1984; Berger M, et al: JACC 6:359–365, 1985; Currie PJ, et al: JACC 6:750–756, 1985; Lee RT, et al: AJC 64:1366–1370, 1989.

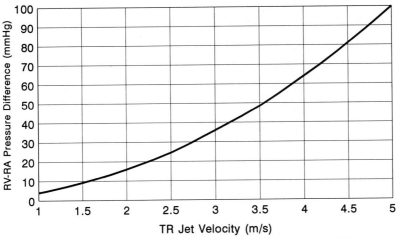

Figure 4–20. Relationship between the velocity in the tricuspid regurgitant (TR) jet and the right ventricular–right atrial (RV-RA) pressure difference as calculated with the simplified Bernoulli relationship.

Although this method requires the presence of tricuspid regurgitation, this rarely is a limitation, since about 90 percent of normal individuals and patients have some degree of tricuspid regurgitation (Fig. 4–22).

The same concept can be applied to the pulmonic regurgitant velocity curve. The end-diastolic pulmonic regurgitant velocity reflects the pulmonary artery to right ventricular end-diastolic pressure gradient per the Bernoulli equation. When added to an estimate of right atrial pressure, this provides a noninvasive estimate of diastolic pulmonary artery pressure.

Right atrial pressure is best estimated from evaluation of the inferior vena cava during respiration (Fig. 4–23). From a subcostal window, this segment of the inferior vena cava is imaged during quiet respiration (see also Chapter 5, section on right atrial pressure). If the inferior vena cava diameter is normal (1.2 to 2.3 cm) and the segment adjacent to the right atrium collapses by at least 50 percent with respiration, then right atrial pressure is equal to normal intrathoracic pressures (i.e., 5 to 10 mmHg). Failure to collapse with respiration and/or dilation of the inferior vena cava and hepatic veins is associated with higher right atrial pressures (Table 4–8). When no response is noted with normal respiration, the patient is asked to "sniff." This gen-

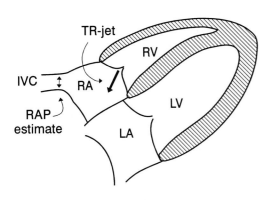

$$\Delta P_{RV-RA} = 4(TR\text{-jet})^2$$

$$PAP = \Delta P_{RV-RA} + RAP$$

Figure 4–21. Pulmonary artery pressure (PAP) can be calculated noninvasively based on the velocity in the tricuspid regurgitant (TR) jet and the respiratory variation in inferior vena cava (IVC) size as an estimate of right atrial pressure (RAP).

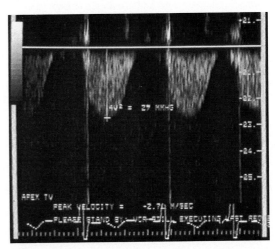

Figure 4–22. Tricuspid regurgitant jet in a patient with normal pulmonary pressures and a maximum jet velocity of 2.7 m/s.

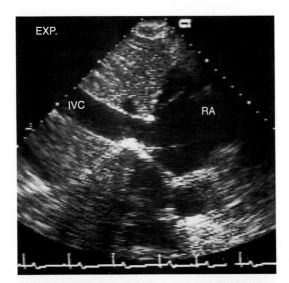

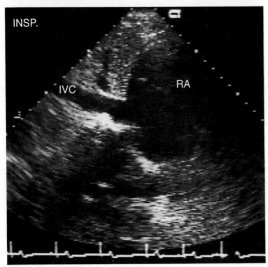

Figure 4–23. Subcostal view of the junction between the inferior vena cava (IVC) and the right atrium (RA) during normal expiration (*above*) and inspiration (*below*).

erates a sudden decrease in intrathoracic pressure, resulting in a change in inferior vena cava diameter.

An alternate approach to estimation of right atrial pressure is clinical examination of the degree of jugular venous distension. However, while this approach is reliable in distinguishing changes (increases or decreases) over time in filling pressures in an individual patient, it is less accurate in determining the absolute right atrial pressure.

Pulmonary Artery Velocity Curve

Another approach to estimating pulmonary pressure is based on the shape of the pulmonary artery Doppler velocity curve. Comparison of the normal left ventricular and right ventricular ejection curves reveals that left ventricular ejection shows very rapid acceleration with a short time from flow onset to maximum velocity, whereas right ventricular ejection shows a slower acceleration, a longer time from onset of flow to peak flow, and a more "rounded" velocity curve (see Figs. 4–10 and 4–12). As pulmonary vascular resistance increases, the shape of the right ventricular ejection curve more closely approximates the left ventricular ejection curve, suggesting that the shapes of these velocity curves are related to the downstream resistance or impedance. A log relationship between the time from onset of flow to peak velocity and mean pulmonary artery pressure has been described, as shown in Table 4–6 and Figure 4–24.

The time to peak velocity estimates of pulmonary artery pressure are not as reliable as tricuspid regurgitant jet estimates for two reasons. First, this method depends on measurement of a relatively short time interval, so measurement

TABLE 4–8. ESTIMATION OF RIGHT ATRIAL PRESSURE

IVC	CHANGE WITH RESPIRATION OR "SNIFF"	ESTIMATED RIGHT ATRIAL PRESSURE
Small (<1.5 cm)	Collapse	0–5 mmHg
Normal (1.5–2.5 cm)	Decrease by ≥ 50%	5–10 mmHg
Normal	Decrease by < 50%	10–15 mmHg
Dilated (>2.5 cm)	Decrease < 50%	15–20 mmHg
Dilated with dilated hepatic veins	No change	>20 mmHg

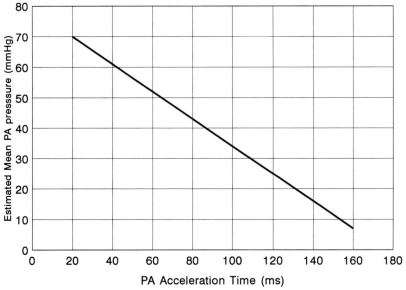

Figure 4–24. Graph of the relationship between mean pulmonary artery pressure and the pulmonary artery acceleration time or time to peak velocity (TPV).

error is high and reproducibility is low. Second, the spatial flow velocity profile in the pulmonary artery is skewed, with higher acceleration and velocity along the inner edge of the curvature. Even when the sample volume appears positioned in the center of the vessel, it may be near the inner wall in the elevational plane, since this curvature is three-dimensional. Thus the shape of the pulmonary artery velocity curve is most helpful when it is normal. An apparent short time to peak velocity can be due to measurement variability or to the nonuniform spatial flow velocity distribution in the vessel.

Isovolumic Relaxation Time

Pulmonary hypertension is associated with prolongation of the right ventricular isovolumic relaxation time (IVRT). This time can be measured as the interval between pulmonic valve closure and tricuspid valve opening, recorded either with M-mode echocardiography (showing leaflet closure) or Doppler echo (showing the valve "clicks"). Nomograms relating the right ventricular IVRT to the degree of pulmonary hypertension have been shown to be accurate in pediatric populations. In adults, this approach is rarely used because of the difficulty in recording pulmonic valve closure given suboptimal acoustic access in many patients. In addition, like the time to peak velocity in the pulmonary artery velocity curve, the IVRT is a

short interval that is subject to considerable measurement variability.

Limitations/Technical Considerations/Alternate Approaches

Tricuspid regurgitant jet velocities are recorded with continuous-wave Doppler from an apical or parasternal approach. As noted above, the determination of pulmonary artery systolic pressure derived from the tricuspid regurgitant jet velocity is only as accurate as the primary data. Underestimation of tricuspid regurgitant jet velocity due to a nonparallel intercept angle between the jet and the ultrasound beam results in underestimation of pulmonary artery pressures. Overestimation of pulmonary artery pressures can occur if the mitral regurgitant jet is mistaken for tricuspid regurgitation. Although both signals occur in systole and are directed away from the left ventricular apex, the duration of tricuspid regurgitation is slightly longer than mitral regurgitation (when right and left ventricular systolic function are normal) due to a slightly longer right ventricular systolic ejection period (Fig. 4–25). The shapes of the velocity curves tend to differ as well, with tricuspid regurgitation having a slower upstroke and a peak later in systole, although the shapes of both velocity curves are affected by changes in ventric-

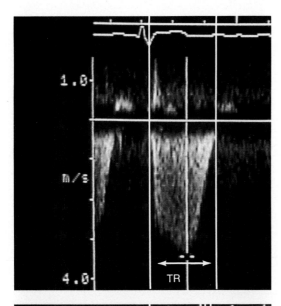

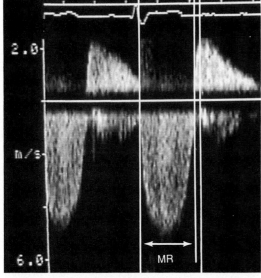

Figure 4–25. Comparison of the flow duration typically shows that tricuspid regurgitation (*above*) is slightly longer than mitral regurgitation (*below*).

valve—and regurgitant jet *velocity*—which reflects the instantaneous *pressure gradient* across the valve.

The tricuspid regurgitant jet can be used to estimate pulmonary artery pressure when right ventricular and pulmonary artery systolic pressures are equal, specifically in the absence of pulmonic stenosis. When pulmonic stenosis is present, pulmonary pressures can be estimated by subtracting the right ventricle to pulmonary artery pressure difference derived from the pulmonic stenotic jet from the estimated right ventricular systolic pressure:

$$PAP = [4(V_{TR})^2 + RAP] - [4(V_{PS})^2] \quad (4.32)$$

The estimate of right atrial pressure from the appearance of the inferior vena cava also can affect the accuracy of Doppler echo pulmonary artery pressure estimates. The importance of this source of error is greatest at intermediate tricuspid regurgitant jet velocities: A tricuspid regurgitant jet velocity of 2.5 m/s with a right atrial pressure of 5 mmHg indicates a pulmonary artery pressure of only 30 mmHg (normal to mildly elevated), but if right atrial pressure is 20 mmHg, then pulmonary artery pressure is 45 mmHg (moderate pulmonary hypertension). At the extreme (i.e., a tricuspid regurgitant jet of 5 m/s), pulmonary hypertension clearly is severe regardless of the right atrial pressure estimate.

If images of the inferior vena cava are suboptimal, or if the degree of change with respiration is equivocal, it is appropriate to report the range of possible pulmonary artery pressures or to indicate that the right ventricle to right atrial pressure gradient should be added to a clinical estimate of right atrial pressure. Evaluation of respiratory variation in inferior vena cava diameter can be confounded by respiratory motion in the position of the inferior vena cava such that the center of the vessel moves in and out of the image plane. Of course, evaluation of inferior vena cava size and respiratory variation is not helpful in patients on positive-pressure ventilation, since intrathoracic pressures are abnormal.

The time to peak velocity in the pulmonary artery can appear short when the Doppler sample volume is positioned along the inner curve of the pulmonary artery. Conversely, impaired right ventricular systolic function may result in an apparently normal time to peak velocity even in the presence of pulmonary hypertension.

The alternative to noninvasive Doppler echo estimate of pulmonary artery pressures is direct measurement in the coronary care unit or cardiac catheterization laboratory with a Swan-Ganz catheter. This approach has the advantages of precision, a high degree of accuracy (as-

ular function or atrial pressure. Note that the velocity of mitral regurgitation always is high, since it reflects the systolic left ventricular (approximately 100 mmHg) to left atrial (approximately 10 mmHg) pressure difference. With normal pulmonary artery pressures, tricuspid regurgitant jet velocity is 2 to 2.5 m/s. With pulmonary hypertension, pulmonary pressure may approach systemic pressures, with a corresponding tricuspid regurgitant jet velocity in the range of 5 m/s.

It is important conceptually to keep separate the grading of regurgitant *severity*—which is a measure of the *volume* of reverse flow across the suming appropriate transducer calibration and balancing), and the ability to continuously record measurements over a period of several days. Disadvantages are its costs, potential complications of line placement, and the difficulty of performing repeat measures over longer time intervals.

SUGGESTED READING

1. American Society of Echocardiography Committee on Standards, Subcommittee on Quantitation of Two-Dimensional Echocardiograms: Recommendations for quantitation of the left ventricle by two-dimensional echocardiography. J Am Soc Echocardiogr 2:361–367, 1989.
   Clear description of methods for quantitating left ventricular systolic function by 2D echocardiography as recommended by the American Society of Echocardiography. Technical details of image acquisition, diagrams illustrating quantitative techniques, and tables of normal values are included.

2. Folland ED, Parisi AF, Moynihan PF, et al: Assessment of left ventricular ejection fraction and volumes by real-time, two-dimensional echocardiography. A comparison of cineangiographic and radionuclide techniques. Circulation 60:760–766, 1979.
   Key paper comparing five different algorithms for determining left ventricular volumes by 2D echocardiography in comparison with both radionuclide ventriculography and contrast angiography.

3. Tortoledo FA, Quinones MA, Fernandez GC, et al: Quantification of left ventricular volumes by two-dimensional echocardiography: A simplified and accurate approach. Circulation 67:579–584, 1983.
   Proposed simplified approach to calculation of left ventricular volumes that does not require planimetry. End-diastolic area (EDA) is calculated from the largest minor axis diameter (D_{max}) and major axis length (L_{max}) as

$$EDA = D_{max} \times L_{max} \times \pi/4$$

Ejection fraction calculations are based on the percentage change in the average minor axis dimensions (%ΔD) based on end-diastolic (D_{ed}) and end-systolic (D_{es}) minor axis dimensions, where

$$\%\Delta D = (D_{ed}^2 - D_{es}^2)/D_{ed}^2$$

and the percentage change in the long axis dimension (%ΔL) is estimated from the pattern of apical wall motion as 0.15 (normal), 0.05 (hypokinesis), 0 (akinesis), and −0.05 (dyskinesis). Then, ejection fraction (EF) is calculated as

$$EF = (\%\Delta D^2) + [(1 - \%\Delta D^2)(\%\Delta L)]$$

This method requires acquisition of three views (parasternal long-axis, apical four-chamber and two-chamber views) with measurement of several minor axis dimensions (two in parasternal, three in each apical view) and one long-axis dimension in either apical view.

4. Zile MR, Tanaka R, Lindrith JR, et al: Left ventricular volume determined echocardiographically by assuming a constant left ventricular epicardial long-axis/short-axis dimension ratio throughout the cardiac cycle. J Am Coll Cardiol 20:986–993, 1992.
   Simplified approach to left ventricular volume calculations based on the assumption of a constant epicardial long-axis to short-axis dimension ratio. Volumes (V) are calculated from the left ventricular endocardial short-axis dimension (D_{endo}) and length (L_{endo}):

$$V = \pi \frac{(D_{endo})^2}{6} L_{endo}$$

where minor axis dimension is measured throughout the cardiac cycle, but length is measured only once. The long-axis to short-axis ratio (Z) is calculated at end-diastole as

$$Z = \frac{L_{endo} + (0.4)b}{D_{endo} + 2b}$$

where b = wall thickness. Using Z calculated at end-diastole, L_{endo} at end-systole is calculated by rearranging this equation.

5. Zoghbi WA, Buckey JC, Massey MA, Blomqvist CG: Determination of left ventricular volumes with use of a new nongeometric echocardiographic method: Clinical validation and potential application. J Am Coll Cardiol 15:610–617, 1990.
   Calculations of left ventricular volumes based on a single transducer position with angulation of the image plane through the ventricle. Volume is calculated by a nongeometric mathematical model. Advantages of this approach are acquisition of images from the window providing optimal acoustic access, data allowing a 3D reconstruction of the ventricle, and the absence of geometric assumptions. However, precise measurement of the transducer angle (using a custom designed transducer holder) is necessary.

6. Smith MD, MacPhail B, Harrison MR, et al: Value and limitations of transesophageal echocardiography in determination of left ventricular volumes and ejection fraction. J Am Coll Cardiol 19:1213–1222, 1992.
   Calculation of left ventricular volumes using a modified Simpson's rule can be made from transesophageal images using short-axis views at the mitral valve, papillary muscle, and apical levels plus left ventricular length measured in the four-chamber view. Underestimation of left ventricular length on TEE images results in smaller calculated left ventricular volumes than angiographic measurements.

7. Gordon EP, Schnittger I, Fitzgerald PJ, et al: Reproducibility of left ventricular volumes by two-dimensional echocardiography. J Am Coll Cardiol 2:506–513, 1983.
   Repeat recordings and measurement of left ventricular volumes by 2D echocardiography showed 95 percent confidence limits for individual subjects' measurements of ±15 percent for end-diastolic volume, ±25 percent for end-systolic volume, and ±10 percent for ejection fraction.

8. Nessly ML, Bashein G, Detmer PR, et al: Left ventricular ejection fraction: Single-plane and multiplanar transesophageal echocardiography versus equilibrium gated-pool scintigraphy. J Cardiothorac Vasc Anesthesiol 5:40–45, 1991.
   Left ventricular ejection fraction was calculated from a 3D reconstruction of the ventricle generated using acquisition of multiple nonparallel short-axis views of known orientation. Accuracy and precision were greater for 3D than for 2D echocardiographic estimates of ejection fraction in this animal model.

9. Handschumacher MD, Lethor J-P, Siu SC, et al: A new integrated system for three-dimensional echocardiographic reconstruction: Development and validation for ventricular volume with application in human subjects. J Am Coll Cardiol 21:743–753, 1993.
   A 3D reconstruction of the left ventricle was performed using transthoracic images of known orientation (using a spark gap locating device). Volumes were calculated for ventricular phantoms (balloons) and for excised, nonbeating hearts in a water bath.

10. Gopal AS, Keller AM, Rigling R, et al: Left ventricular volume and endocardial surface area by three-dimensional echocardiography: Comparison with two-dimensional echocardiography and nuclear magnetic resonance imaging in normal subjects. J Am Coll Cardiol 22:258–270, 1993.
    A 3D spatial acoustic locator was used to acquire nonparallel short-axis images in 15 normal subjects. 3D volume calculation showed little interobserver (5 to 8 percent) variability and compared well (r = 0.81 to 0.92) with volume from MRI images.

11. Gorsan J III, Romand JA, Mandarino WA, et al: Assessment of left ventricular performance by on-line pressure-area relations using echocardiographic automated border detection. J Am Coll Cardiol 23:242–252, 1994.
    Echocardiographic images of the left ventricle were analyzed using automated border detection to derive ventricular areas from short axis images throughout the cardiac cycle. Using directly measured ventricular pressure, pressure-area loops were generated and used to calculate stroke area, stroke force, end-systolic elastance, and pre-load recruitable stroke force.

12. Simonson JS, Schiller NB: Descent of the base of the left ventricle: An echocardiographic index of left ventricular function. J Am Soc Echocardiogr 2:25–35, 1989.
    The motion of the mitral annulus toward the ventricular apex in systole (lengthwise ventricular shortening) provides a simple method for quantitation of left ventricular systolic function. Average motion in normal individuals was 12 ± 2 mm, with motion < 8 mm sensitive (98 percent) and specific (82 percent) for diagnosis of an ejection fraction of less than 50 percent.

13. Douglas PS, Reichek N, Plappert T, et al: Comparison of echocardiographic methods for assessment of left ventricular shortening and wall stress. J Am Coll Cardiol 9:945–951, 1987.
    2D echocardiography allows calculation of circumferential as well as meridional stress. In pressure overload (such as valvular aortic stenosis), left ventricular circumferential stress is elevated. Cardiomyopathic hearts (more spherical) have a meridional to circumferential stress ratio closer to 1.

14. Vandenberg BF, Rath LS, Stuhlmuller P, et al: Estimation of left ventricular cavity area with an on-line, semiautomated echocardiographic edge detection system. Circulation 86:159–166, 1992.
    Description of one approach to real-time automated endocardial edge detection.

15. Chen C, Rodriguez L, Guerrero JL, et al: Noninvasive estimation of the instantaneous first derivative of left ventricular pressure using continuous-wave Doppler echocardiography. Circulation 83:2101–2110, 1991.
    The rate of ventricular pressure rise in early systole (dP/dt) can be calculated from the mitral regurgitant jet velocity curve. Both dP/dt$_{max}$ and − dP/dt$_{max}$ also can be determined accurately and reliably.

16. Chung N, Nishimura RA, Holmes DR Jr, Tajik AJ: Measurement of left ventricular dP/dt by simultaneous Doppler echocardiography and cardiac catheterization. J Am Soc Echocardiogr 5:147–152, 1992.
    Doppler measurement of left ventricular dP/dt from the mitral regurgitant velocity curve was most accurate using the time interval from 1 to 3 m/s on the velocity curve.

17. Bouchard A, Blumlein S, Schiller NB, et al: Measurement of left ventricular stroke volume using continuous-wave Doppler echocardiography of the ascending aorta and M-mode echocardiography of the aortic valve. J Am Coll Cardiol 9:75–83, 1987.
    Description of stroke volume measurement based on a continuous-wave Doppler recording of ascending aortic flow and an M-mode tracing of the aortic valve (assuming a circular systolic orifice).

18. Lewis JF, Kuo LC, Nelson JG, et al: Pulsed Doppler echocardiographic determination of stroke volume and cardiac output: Clinical validation of two new methods using the apical window. Circulation 70:425–431, 1984.
    Description of left ventricular outflow tract and mitral annulus methods for stroke volume calculation. Validation in 39 patients versus thermodilution cardiac output and application of Doppler stroke volume measurement at two intracardiac sites to calculation of regurgitant volume is described. Interobserver variability for stroke volume or cardiac output (mean percentage error ± 1 SD) was 16.4 ± 13.8 percent for the mitral annulus method and 6.8 ± 5.0 percent for the left ventricular outflow method.

19. Otto CM, Pearlman AS, Gardner CL, et al: Experimental validation of Doppler echocardiographic measurement of volume flow through the stenotic aortic valve. Circulation 78:435–441, 1988.
    Validation of left ventricular outflow tract method for measurement of stroke volume proximal to a stenotic aortic valve. Repeat measurement of left ventricular outflow tract diameter showed a mean coefficient of variation of 2 percent.

20. Sjoberg BJ, Ask P, Loyd D, Eng D, and Wranne B: Subaortic flow profiles in aortic valve disease: A two-dimensional color Doppler study. J Am Soc Echocardiog 7:276–285, 1994.
    Using time-corrected quantitative color Doppler echocardiography, the spatial flow velocity profile proximal to the aortic valve was examined. In 10 patients with aortic stenosis, the flow profile was fairly flat; however, deviations from a flat flow profile were observed in 5 healthy control subjects.

21. Jiang L, Siu SC, Handschumacher MD, et al: Three-dimensional echocardiography: In vivo validation for right ventricular volume and function. Circulation 89:2342–2350, 1994.
    Echocardiographic three-dimensional reconstructions of the right ventricle (using epicardial image acquisition with a spark-gap locater system) were performed during 20 hemodynamic states in 5 dogs. Both end-diastolic (r = 0.99, y = 1.0x − 3.4, SEE = 1.8 ml) and end-systolic (r = 0.98, y = 1.0x + 2.0, SEE = 2.5 ml) echocardiographic volumes correlated well with actual volumes measured using an intracavity balloon connected to an external calibrated column.

22. Yock PG, Popp RL: Noninvasive estimation of right ventricular systolic pressure by Doppler ultrasound in patients with tricuspid regurgitation. Circulation 70:657–662, 1984.
    Description and validation of calculating the right ventricular to right atrial maximum systolic pressure difference from the maximum tricuspid regurgitant jet velocity using the simplified Bernoulli equation. While the Doppler and invasive pressure gradient correlated well (r = 0.95), clinical estimates of right atrial pressure from the degree of jugular venous distension correlated only modestly with measured right atrial pressure (r = 0.80).

23. Currie PJ, Seward JB, Chan K-L, et al: Continuous-wave Doppler determination of right ventricular pressure: A simultaneous Doppler-catheterization study in 127 patients. J Am Coll Cardiol 6:750–756, 1985.
    Further validation of the use of tricuspid regurgitant jet velocity to estimate right ventricular systolic pressure in a

larger series of patients. An adequate tricuspid regurgitant jet velocity signal was obtained in 111 of 127 (87 percent) of patients. The average coefficient of variation for measurement of maximum velocity was 2.8 percent (range 0 to 18 percent).

24. Kitabatake A, Inoue M, Asao M, et al: Noninvasive evaluation of pulmonary hypertension by a pulsed Doppler technique. Circulation 58:302–309, 1983.
   Estimation of pulmonary artery mean pressure from the shape of the right ventricular outflow tract velocity curve; specifically the time interval from onset of flow to maximum velocity is described (see Fig. 4–24).

25. Stevenson JG: Comparison of several noninvasive methods for estimation of pulmonary artery pressure. J Am Soc Echocardiogr 2:157–171, 1989.
   In a pediatric population, noninvasive methods for estimation of pulmonary artery pressure were compared. Both the Burstin method (pulmonic valve closure to tricuspid opening) and the tricuspid regurgitant jet method were highly accurate (r = 0.97 and 0.96, respectively) and could be recorded in nearly all subjects (82 to 89 percent). The right ventricular output tract time to peak velocity (TPV) correlated better (r = 0.94) with directly measured pulmonary artery pressure than did TPV from the pulmonary artery velocity curve (r = 0.63).

26. Lee RT, Lord CP, Plappert T, St. John Sutton M: Prospective Doppler echocardiographic evaluation of pulmonary artery diastolic pressure in the medical intensive care unit. Am J Cardiol 64:1366–1370, 1989.
   Estimation of pulmonary artery diastolic pressure from the pulmonic regurgitant velocity curve was possible in 17 of 29 (59 percent) of ICU patients. The pulmonary artery to right ventricular diastolic pressure difference was calculated at $4V^2$, where V is the end-diastolic pulmonic regurgitant jet velocity, and then added to a clinical estimate of right atrial pressure. Correlation with invasively measured pulmonary artery pressure was excellent (r = 0.94, mean absolute difference = 3.3 mmHg).

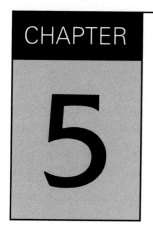

CHAPTER 5

ECHOCARDIOGRAPHIC EVALUATION OF VENTRICULAR DIASTOLIC FILLING AND FUNCTION

INTRODUCTION

There has been increasing recognition that *diastolic* ventricular function often plays a key role in the clinical manifestations of disease in pa-

tients with a wide range of cardiac disorders. For example, many patients with clinical heart failure have normal systolic function with predominant diastolic dysfunction. Diastolic dysfunction may be an early sign of cardiac diseases (as in hypertension), often antedating clinical or echocardiographic evidence of systolic dysfunction. In addition, the degree of diastolic dysfunction may explain the difference in clinical symptoms between patients with similar degrees of systolic dysfunction.

Echocardiographic techniques allow evaluation of right and left ventricular diastolic filling patterns and right and left atrial filling patterns. The relationship between these noninvasive measures and ventricular diastolic function and the utility of these measures in patient evaluation are discussed in this chapter.

BASIC PRINCIPLES

Phases of Diastole

Although several different definitions of diastole have been proposed, the most widely accepted clinical definition is the interval from aortic valve closure (end-systole) to mitral valve closure (end-diastole) (Fig. 5–1). The isovolumic

contraction period, from mitral valve closure to aortic valve opening, typically is considered to be part of systole.

Diastole can be divided into four phases: (1) isovolumic relaxation, (2) the early rapid diastolic filling phase, (3) diastasis, and (4) late diastolic filling due to atrial contraction. During the isovolumic relaxation interval, left ventricular pressure falls rapidly following aortic valve closure. At the point where left ventricular pressure falls below left atrial pressure, the mitral valve opens, ending the isovolumic relaxation period. With mitral valve opening, blood flows from the left atrium to the left ventricle, with the rate and time course of flow being determined by several factors, including the pressure difference along the flow path, ventricular relaxation, and the relative compliances of the two chambers. Maximal opening of the mitral leaflets typically occurs rapidly, within 100 ± 10 ms of valve opening, in normal individuals.

As the ventricle fills, pressures between the atrium and ventricle equalize, resulting in a period of *diastasis*, during which there is little movement of blood between the chambers and the mitral leaflets remain in a semiopen position. The duration of diastasis is heart rate–dependent, being longer at slow heart rates and entirely absent at faster heart rates. With atrial contraction, left atrial pressure again exceeds left ventricular pressure, resulting in mitral leaflet opening and a second pulse of left ventricular filling. In normal individuals, the atrial contribution to ventricular filling typically is small, comprising only about 20 percent of total ventricular filling (Fig. 5–2).

The phases of diastole for the right ventricle are analogous to those described for the left ventricle, with the difference that the total duration of diastole is slightly shorter in normal individuals due to a slightly longer right ventricular systolic ejection period.

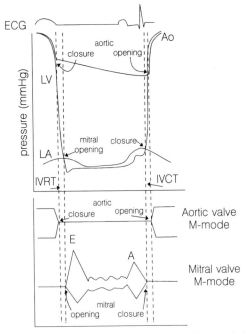

Figure 5–1. The relationship between left ventricular (LV), left atrial (LA), and aortic (Ao) pressures and M-mode tracings of the aortic and mitral valve is shown. The isovolumic relaxation time (IVRT) is the interval from aortic valve closure to mitral valve opening. During this interval, left ventricular pressure declines rapidly. A rapid rise in left ventricular pressure occurs during the isovolumic contraction time (IVCT), the interval between mitral valve closure and aortic valve opening.

Parameters of Diastolic Function

There are several physiologic parameters that can be used to describe different aspects of diastolic function, but there is no single measure of overall diastolic function. The most clinically relevant parameters identified to date include ventricular relaxation, myocardial compliance, and chamber compliance. Additional parameters of interest include elastic recoil of the ventricle and the effect of pericardial constraint, but the importance of these factors in normal diastolic ventricular function remains controversial.

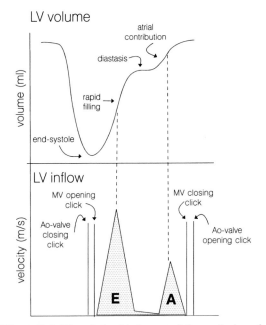

Figure 5–2. The relationship between left ventricular volume and the diastolic left ventricular Doppler filling pattern is shown. Early rapid filling coincides with the *E* velocity, followed by diastasis, with little or no flow from left atrium to left ventricle, and atrial contraction, which coincides with the late diastolic *A* velocity. The Doppler velocity curve, in effect, is the first derivative of the left ventricular volume curve.

Ventricular Relaxation

Left ventricular relaxation, occurring during isovolumic relaxation and the early diastolic filling period, is an active process involving utilization of energy by the myocardium. Factors affecting isovolumic relaxation include internal loading forces (cardiac fiber), external loading conditions (wall stress, arterial impedance), inactivation of myocardial contraction (metabolic, neurohumoral, and pharmacologic), and nonuniformity in the spatial and temporal patterns of these factors. Abnormal relaxation results in prolongation of the isovolumic relaxation time, a slower rate of decline in ventricular pressure, and a consequent reduction in the early peak filling rate (due to a smaller pressure difference between the atrium and the ventricle when the atrioventricular valve opens). Measures of left ventricular relaxation include the isovolumic relaxation time (IVRT), the maximum rate of pressure decline ($-dP/dt$), and the time constant of relaxation (tau or τ). There are several different mathematical approaches to calculation of tau, but basically it reflects the rate of pressure decline from the point of maximum $-dP/dt$ to mitral valve opening. While peak rapid filling

rate is affected by ventricular relaxation, it is only an indirect measure of this physiologic parameter, since several other factors also affect peak filling (Fig. 5–3).

Ventricular Compliance

Compliance is the ratio of change in volume to change in pressure (dV/dP). Stiffness is the inverse of compliance: the ratio of change in pressure to change in volume (dP/dV). Conceptually, compliance can be divided into myocardial (the characteristics of the isolated myocardium) and chamber (the characteristics of the entire chamber) components. Chamber compliance is influenced by ventricular size and shape, as well as by the characteristics of the myocardium. Extrinsic factors also may affect measurement of compliance, including the pericardium, right ventricular volume, and pleural pressure. Evaluation of ventricular compliance is based on pressure-volume curves showing the degree to which pressure and volume change in relation to each other over the physiologic range of pressures and volumes (Fig. 5–4).

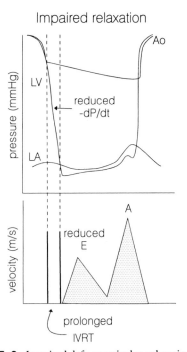

Figure 5–3. Impaired left ventricular relaxation is described by a reduced $-dP/dt$, and a prolonged time constant of relaxation. The Doppler velocity curve shows a prolonged IVRT, reduced *E* velocity (corresponding to a low left atrial–left ventricular gradient at mitral valve opening), and an increased *A* velocity.

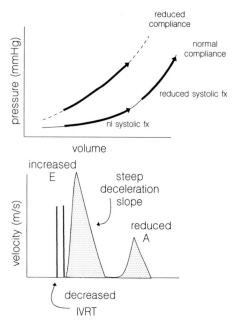

Figure 5–4. Reduced diastolic compliance is described by a steeper passive pressure-volume relationship of the left ventricle. As left ventricular volume increases in diastole, pressure rises rapidly, resulting in an initial high left atrial–left ventricular pressure gradient with a rapid decrease in the filling gradient during diastole. The Doppler velocity curve shows a decreased IVRT, steep deceleration slope, and reduced *A* velocity. Note that even with normal compliance, reduced systolic function results in a rightward shift along the normal pressure-volume relationship, resulting in a similar pattern of diastolic filling.

Ventricular Diastolic Pressures

Clinically, evaluation of diastolic pressures alone often is utilized in patient management. Measurement of left ventricular end-diastolic pressure (or its surrogate, pulmonary artery wedge pressure) is the most commonly available measure of diastolic "function," although its limitations as a descriptor of diastole are well recognized.

Ventricular Diastolic Filling (Volume) Curves

Another clinically available measure related to diastolic function is the time course of ventricular filling: the ventricular diastolic filling curve. Experimentally, filling curves can be derived on a beat-to-beat basis from implanted sonocrystal-derived ventricular dimensions or from impedance catheter data. Clinically, filling curves can be generated for an individual cardiac cycle from frame-by-frame measurements of ventric-

ular volumes using angiographic, computed tomography, magnetic resonance, or echocardiographic images or from high-temporal-resolution radionuclide studies. Doppler echocardiography offers the ability to measure left ventricular diastolic filling, noninvasively, on a beat-to-beat basis.

Unfortunately, while ventricular diastolic *function* is one of the major factors affecting the pattern of diastolic *filling*, these two concepts are not identical. Several physiologic parameters other than diastolic function affect diastolic filling. Given no change in diastolic function (i.e., relaxation, compliance, etc.), the peak early diastolic filling rate will be affected by (1) changes in the pressure difference between the ventricle and the atrium (the *opening pressure*) due to changes in preload (e.g., increased with volume loading, decreased with volume depletion), (2) a change in transmitral volume flow rate (e.g., increased with coexisting mitral regurgitation), or (3) a change in atrial pressure (e.g., elevated left ventricular end-diastolic pressure or a *v* wave due to mitral regurgitation).

Late diastolic filling is affected by cardiac rhythm, atrial contractile function, ventricular end-diastolic pressure, heart rate, and the timing of atrial contraction (PR interval), as well as by ventricular diastolic function. In addition, it is obvious that the utility of ventricular diastolic filling patterns for assessing diastolic function is valid only in the absence of obstruction at the atrioventricular valve level (i.e., mitral stenosis). The importance of considering the influence of these factors on the pattern of diastolic filling as assessed by Doppler echocardiography will be discussed in more detail below.

Atrial Pressures and Filling Curves

Another somewhat indirect approach to evaluation of ventricular diastolic function is measurement of atrial filling patterns and pressures. This approach is conceptually sound given that elevations in ventricular diastolic pressures will be reflected in elevated pressures in the atrium. Atrial filling patterns obviously are closely linked with diastolic ventricular function, especially in early diastole, when the atrioventricular valve is open, since the atrium serves as a "conduit" for flow from the venous circulation to the ventricle (Fig. 5–5).

Right atrial pressures normally are quite low (0 to 5 mmHg), with only small increases in pressure following atrial contraction (*a* wave) and following ventricular contraction (*v* wave). Right atrial filling is characterized by (1) a small reversal of flow following atrial contraction (*a*

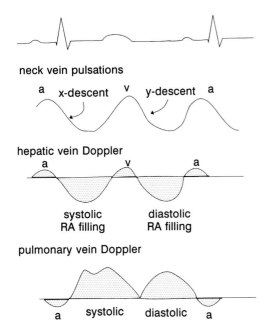

neck vein pulsations

a x-descent v y-descent a

hepatic vein Doppler

a   v   a

systolic   diastolic
RA filling   RA filling

pulmonary vein Doppler

a   systolic   diastolic   a

Figure 5–5. Schematic diagram of right atrial (hepatic vein) and left atrial (pulmonary vein) filling patterns and the close correspondence with the pattern of jugular venous pulsations. Pulmonary and hepatic vein patterns appear "opposite" in direction, since the direction of flow in the hepatic vein is away from the transducer (into the right atrium), while the direction of flow from a transthoracic view of the pulmonary vein is toward the transducer (into the left atrium).

wave), (2) a systolic phase (which is effectively "diastole" for the atrium) when blood flows from the superior and inferior vena cava into the atrium, (3) a small reversal of flow at end-systole (v wave), and (4) a diastolic filling phase when the atrium serves as a conduit for flow from the systemic venous return to the right ventricle. These filling phases are reflected in the patterns of jugular venous pulsation familiar to the clinician: the a wave following atrial contraction, the x descent corresponding to atrial systolic filling, the v wave with ventricular contraction, and the y descent corresponding to atrial diastolic filling. Disease processes affect the jugular venous pulsations and the Doppler pattern of right atrial filling in similar ways.

Left atrial filling from the pulmonary veins also is characterized by (1) a small reversal of flow following atrial contraction (a wave), (2) a systolic filling phase, (3) a blunting of flow or brief reversal at end-systole, and (4) a diastolic filling phase. In normal individuals, the systolic and diastolic filling phases are approximately equal in volume. Normal left atrial pressure is low (5 to 10 mmHg), corresponding to the normal left ventricular end-diastolic pressure, with slight increases in pressure following atrial (a wave) and ventricular (v wave) contraction.

Normal Respiratory Changes

The patterns of right and left ventricular diastolic filling show normal respiratory variation. With inspiration, negative intrapleural pressure results in an increase in systemic venous return into the thorax and, thus, into the right atrium. This increased right atrial volume and pressure results in a transient increase in right ventricular diastolic filling volumes and velocities, with the magnitude of increase up to 20 percent compared with end-expiratory values.

Left atrium filling does *not* increase with inspiration, since pulmonary venous return is entirely intrathoracic and thus not affected significantly by respiratory changes in intrathoracic pressure. In fact, left atrial and, consequently, left ventricular diastolic filling is slightly higher at end-expiration than during inspiration. The mechanism of the observation remains controversial. Some postulate a delay in transit of the increased right ventricular filling to the left side of the heart. Others suggest a decrease in left atrial filling during inspiration due to an increased volume (or "pooling") in the pulmonary venous bed. Less likely, in normal individuals, is impaired left ventricular diastolic filling due to an increase in right ventricular diastolic volume within a fixed-volume pericardium. This last mechanism may become important in patients with pericardial disease (constriction, tamponade) and may partly account for the exaggerated respiratory changes in right ventricular and left ventricular diastolic filling seen in these conditions.

Clinical Etiologies of Diastolic Dysfunction

While diastolic dysfunction can be seen with a wide range of cardiac disorders, there are three basic mechanisms of disease that lead to diastolic dysfunction. First, diseases that affect the ventricular myocardium with preserved contractile (systolic) function present with "isolated" diastolic dysfunction. Examples include left ventricular hypertrophy due to hypertension, hypertrophic cardiomyopathy, ischemic disease without prior myocardial infarction, and restrictive cardiomyopathy. Second, pericardial disease (tamponade, constriction) results in impaired cardiac filling due to extrinsic compression of the heart. Third, diastolic dysfunction often accompanies systolic dysfunction of the left ventricle (e.g., in dilated cardiomyopathy or end-stage ischemic disease).

ECHOCARDIOGRAPHIC APPROACH TO LEFT VENTRICULAR DIASTOLIC FUNCTION

2D/M-Mode Evaluation

Evaluation of ventricular chamber dimensions and wall thickness is an integral part of the echocardiographic evaluation of diastolic function. In a patient with clinical heart failure, the findings of increased wall thickness with a nondilated chamber and normal systolic function suggest that diastolic dysfunction may be the etiology of "heart failure." Of course, this finding is neither sensitive nor specific for the diagnosis of diastolic dysfunction. Diastolic dysfunction can be present concurrently with systolic dysfunction (e.g., in dilated cardiomyopathy) and may be absent despite ventricular hypertrophy in some situations, such as physiologic hypertrophy in an athlete. On M-mode echocardiography, early studies suggested that the degree and rate of motion of the posterior left ventricular wall might provide a useful measure of diastolic function. In practical terms, the magnitude of these changes is too small to be measured reliably. Other findings on two-dimensional (2D) or M-mode echocardiography that raise the question of diastolic dysfunction include pericardial thickening (as in constrictive pericarditis), the pattern of ventricular septal motion with respiration (especially with tamponade physiology), and dilation of the inferior vena cava and hepatic veins (consistent with elevated right atrial pressures). Tissue characterization of the myocardium using ultrasound techniques may prove to be useful in evaluation of patients with suspected diastolic dysfunction, but further studies are needed. Thus direct evaluation of ventricular diastolic function by 2D or M-mode techniques is limited. Instead, attention has focused on the utility of Doppler echocardiography for evaluation of diastolic function.

Doppler Evaluation of Left Ventricular Filling

Description of Left Ventricular Filling by Doppler Echo

Doppler recordings of left ventricular diastolic filling velocities correspond closely with ventricular filling parameters measured by other techniques (Fig. 5–6). The normal Doppler ventricular inflow pattern is characterized by a brief time interval between aortic valve closure and the onset of ventricular filling (the isovolumic relaxation time). Immediately following mitral valve opening, there is rapid acceleration of blood flow from the left atrium to the ventricle with an early peak filling velocity of 0.6 to 0.8 m/s occurring 90 to 110 ms after the onset of flow in young, healthy individuals. This early maximum filling velocity (E velocity) occurs simultaneously with the maximum pressure gradient between the atrium and ventricle. After this maximum velocity, flow decelerates rapidly (i.e., with a steep slope) in normal individuals with a normal deceleration slope of 4.3 to 6.7 m/s². Early diastolic filling is followed by a variable period of minimal flow (diastasis), depend-

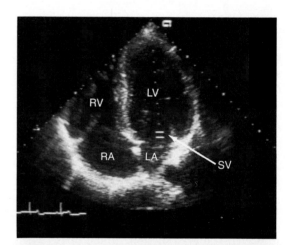

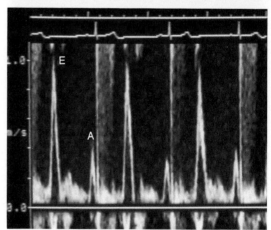

Figure 5–6. Normal pattern of left ventricular diastolic filling recorded with pulsed Doppler in an apical four-chamber view. The A velocity is low in this normal individual. (The systolic flow signal represents normal left ventricular outflow since the sample volume is on the left ventricular side of the mitral valve in systole.)

ing on the total duration of diastole. With atrial contraction, left atrial pressure again exceeds ventricular pressure, resulting in a second velocity peak (late diastolic or atrial velocity) which typically ranges from 0.19 to 0.35 m/s in young, normal individuals.

Quantitative Velocity and Time Interval Measurements

Quantitative measurements that can be made from the Doppler velocity curve include (Table 5–1 and Fig. 5–7)

1. *Maximum velocities:* The *E* velocity, the *A* velocity, and their ratio (*E/A* ratio).
2. *Velocity-time integrals:* Total, early diastolic, atrial contribution, first third or half of diastole, and their ratios.
3. *Time intervals:* The isovolumic relaxation period, the total duration of diastole, the rapid filling period, the length of diastasis, and the atrial filling period.
4. *Measures of acceleration and deceleration:* The time from onset of flow to the *E* velocity, the maximum rate of rise in velocity, and the slope of early diastolic deceleration.

Instead of deceleration slope, some centers measure the deceleration *pressure half-time*, as is used in evaluation of mitral stenosis. The *half-time* is defined as the time interval from the maximum *E* velocity to the point where the maximum pressure gradient has fallen to half its initial value (see Chap. 9). When assessing dia-

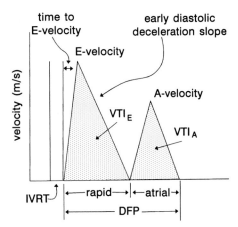

Figure 5–7. Schematic diagram of quantitative measurements that can be made from the Doppler left ventricular filling curve.

stolic dysfunction (which presumes the absence of mitral stenosis), use of the deceleration time is preferable, since the half-time depends on both this slope and the maximum *E* velocity.

Volumetric Flow Rates

In order to convert the Doppler ventricular inflow *velocity* curve to a *volume* curve, the cross-sectional area of flow must be taken into account. As described in Chapter 3, volumetric flow rates can be calculated as the product of velocity and cross-sectional area in regions where flow is laminar with a spatially symmetrical flow pattern. Thus the instantaneous volume flow rate across the mitral valve can be calculated as instantaneous velocity times the flow cross-sectional area (CSA). Similarly, transmitral stroke volume (SV) can be determined from the integral of the flow velocity curve (VTI) over the diastolic filling period:

$$SV_{transmitral} = VTI \times CSA$$

Two basic approaches to determining the cross-sectional area of flow across the mitral valve have been described. One approach is to measure the maximal opening area of the mitral leaflets and, since this area changes markedly during diastole, approximate a temporal mean area by correcting for leaflet motion from the M-mode recording of mitral leaflet motion. Temporal averaging theoretically also is feasible by frame-by-frame tracing of the mitral opening area, although this method is tedious and possibly inaccurate due to the relatively slow frame rate of 2D echo compared with the rapid motion of the mitral valve.

TABLE 5–1. DOPPLER MEASURES OF LEFT VENTRICULAR DIASTOLIC FILLING

Velocities
  E velocity
  A velocity
  E/A ratio

Intervals
  Isovolumic relaxation time (IVRT)
  Rapid filling period
  Diastasis
  Atrial filling period

Acceleration/deceleration
  Time from mitral valve opening to *E* velocity
  Maximal acceleration
  Early diastolic deceleration slope (or half-time)

Filling rates/volumes
  Peak rapid filling rate
  Peak atrial filling rate
  Stroke volume
  Fractional filling rates (first third)

A simpler approach is to calculate the cross-sectional area of flow at the mitral annulus level. Motion of the mitral leaflets is a passive process, with the degree of motion reflecting flow across the valve (in the absence of mitral stenosis). Although there is some tapering of the flow area from the annulus to the leaflet tips, the more rigid mitral annulus may be a preferable site for flow measurement rather than the flexible, mobile leaflets. The shape of the mitral annulus is best described as an ellipse, with its long axis in the apical four-chamber view and its short axis in a parasternal long-axis view; however, a circular assumption is a reasonable approximation in most clinical situations (Fig. 5–8).

Combining Doppler left ventricular inflow velocity data with the cross-sectional area of the mitral annulus, additional filling parameters that can be calculated include

1. *Peak filling rates:* Peak rapid filling rate, atrial peak filling rate, and their ratio
2. *Stroke volume*
3. *Fractional filling rates:* For example, first third filling fraction or the ratio of early to late filling

For each of these parameters, the filling rate is calculated by multiplying the appropriate velocity or velocity-time integral by cross-sectional area. For example, peak rapid filling rate (PRFR) is

$$PRFR \text{ (ml/s)} = E \text{ velocity (cm/s)} \times CSA \text{ (cm}^2)$$

Of course, these measurements are accurate only when velocities and diameters are measured at the same anatomic location, so when an-nular diameters are used, the Doppler velocity should be recorded at the annulus level.

Doppler Data Recording

Left ventricular inflow can be recorded in nearly all patients from an apical approach in either a four- or two-chamber view. This window allows parallel alignment between the ultrasound beam and the direction of left ventricular filling. On transesophageal echocardiography, left ventricular inflow can be recorded from a high esophageal position, taking care to align the Doppler beam parallel to the inflow stream (Fig. 5–9). In some patients, a transgastric apical view also may allow recording of left ventricular inflow, although caution is needed to avoid foreshortening of the ventricle and a nonparallel intercept angle (with resultant underestimation of velocities) from this window.

Inflow velocities can be recorded with pulsed or continuous-wave Doppler modalities. With continuous-wave ultrasound, signals from the entire length of the ultrasound beam are recorded so that the maximal velocities—wherever they occur in relation to the mitral leaflet tips and annulus—are recorded. This lack of range resolution may lead to errors in calculation of volumetric flow rates in some individuals, since the site of cross-sectional area measurement may not correspond to the site of maximal velocity.

With pulsed Doppler ultrasound, the sample volume depth can be placed at the mitral annulus level or can be moved slowly along the length of the ultrasound beam to identify the site of maximal velocity, usually at the mitral leaflet tip level. The normal increase in velocities seen between the annulus and leaflet tips is consistent with some tapering of the flowstream area, although there is marked individual variation. If volumetric flow rates will be calculated using the

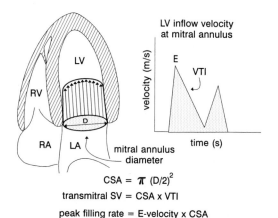

Figure 5–8. Calculation of volumetric flow rates across the mitral annulus.

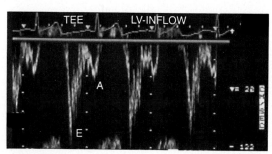

Figure 5–9. Transesophageal recording of left ventricular filling. Flow is directed away from the transducer from this approach.

annulus diameter, velocities should be recorded at the annulus level. Conversely, many of the studies using velocity, time interval, or deceleration slope data to describe left ventricular filling patterns are based on maximal inflow velocities (without calculation of volumetric flow rates). Since even the pattern of inflow (e.g., *E/A* ratio)—not just the absolute velocities—can vary between the annulus and leaflet tips, this inconsistency in methodology has led to a dilemma for the clinician echocardiographer. One approach is to record left ventricular inflow both at the annulus and leaflet tips in each patient so that volumetric flow rates can be calculated if indicated. Alternatively, if volumetric flow rates are not needed, recording left ventricular inflow at the leaflet tips may be adequate for patient management.

Optimal recordings of left ventricular inflow velocities are dependent on careful patient positioning and transducer angulation both to obtain a parallel intercept angle between the direction of flow and the ultrasound beam and to enhance the signal-to-noise ratio. Typically, with pulsed Doppler, a sample volume size of 5 mm is used with the velocity range adjusted to maximize the display of the velocity of interest. Wall filters are reduced (as allowed by signal quality) so that the velocities approach the baseline, allowing accurate time interval measurements. While normal left ventricular filling shows slight respiratory variation, care is needed to ensure that apparent velocity changes are not simply due to respiratory changes in the intercept angle between the ultrasound beam (which is held still) and the inflow stream (which moves with the heart during respiration).

Color Doppler flow imaging of left ventricular filling provides a spatial display of the flow pattern but is less useful for evaluation of left ventricular diastolic function. The normal pattern seen with color Doppler imaging is laminar inflow rapidly filling the ventricular chamber from base to apex, with flow predominantly along the posterior lateral wall. Inflow is associated with flow within the ventricle away from the transducer along the anteroseptal walls (often referred to as a *vortex*) in middiastole. Situations in which the normal color inflow pattern are disturbed include left ventricular systolic dysfunction (with lower velocity "puffs" of inflow and an abnormal apical flow pattern) and prosthetic mitral valves (with inflow along the anteromedial wall instead of the posterolateral wall); however, specific abnormalities on color flow imaging have not been described for diastolic dysfunction. Possibly, methods that allow

quantitation of the color flow data will lead to further insight into diastolic filling.

Factors That Affect Doppler Left Ventricular Filling Velocities
(Table 5–2)

Normal Variations

As discussed above, there may be normal slight variation (<20 percent) in ventricular inflow velocities with respiration. In addition, the pattern of left ventricular inflow is affected by heart rate and the timing of atrial versus ventricular contraction. At higher heart rates, diastole is shorter—particularly the period of diastasis—so that the *A* velocity more closely succeeds the *E* velocity. When overlap of these two velocity curves occurs, the *A* velocity, in effect, is "added" to the *E*-velocity curve, resulting in a higher *A* velocity and lower *E/A* ratio (Fig. 5–10). Similarly, a longer PR interval results in an *A* velocity earlier in diastole that may become superimposed on the *E* velocity curve. At very high heart rates (short diastolic filling periods), the *E* and *A* velocity curves become merged into a single *E/A* velocity. Evaluation of a patient with complete heart block but intact atrial contraction often demonstrates this nicely, with the location of the *A* velocity relative to the *E* velocity affecting its magnitude accordingly (Fig. 5–11).

TABLE 5–2. DIASTOLIC FILLING ≠ DIASTOLIC FUNCTION: FACTORS THAT MAY AFFECT THE DOPPLER LEFT VENTRICULAR FILLING PATTERN

Technical
   Sample volume location
   Doppler modality
   Intercept angle

Normal variations
   Respiration
   Heart rate
   Age
   PR interval

Physiologic
   Preload (LA pressure)
   Volume flow rate (MR)
   Left ventricular systolic function
     (LV-ESV)
   Atrial contractile function
   Diastolic "function"
     Relaxation
     Compliance/stiffness

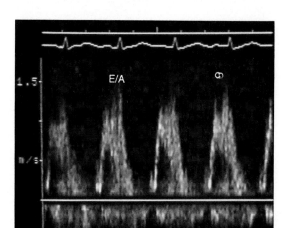

Figure 5–10. Overlap or "summation" of *A* velocity with *E* velocity at a rapid heart rate.

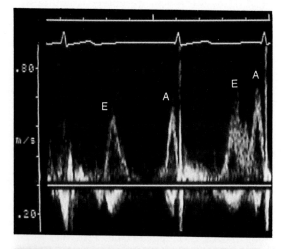

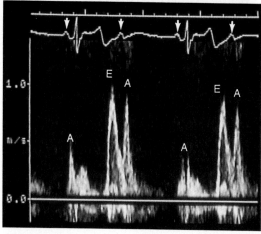

Figure 5–11. Left ventricular filling in a patient with an atrial arrhythmia showing the effect of a shorter diastolic interval on the *E/A* pattern (*above*) and in a patient with second-degree heart block showing two *a* waves for each diastole.

Diastolic left ventricular inflow patterns also are affected by patient age. In children and young adults, the majority of ventricular filling occurs in early diastole, with a prominent *E* velocity and only a small contribution to ventricular filling due to atrial contraction (20 percent of total left ventricular volume). With age, the *E* velocity diminishes, and the atrial contribution becomes more prominent, with equalization of *E* and *A* velocities at approximately age 60 years and reversal of the *E/A* ratio after that age in normal individuals. Early diastolic deceleration time also is progressively prolonged with age. Presumably the mechanism of the changes in left ventricular filling patterns with age is a gradual reduction in the rate of early diastolic relaxation.

Physiologic Factors

Several physiologic variables other than left ventricular diastolic function also affect the pattern of left ventricular diastolic filling. While it is clear that Doppler velocity recordings accurately represent left ventricular filling patterns, it should be emphasized again that left ventricular *filling* is not equivalent to left ventricular diastolic *function*.

Left atrial pressure, *preload*, dramatically affects the pattern of left ventricular filling (Fig. 5–12). Increased preload results in an increase in the *E* velocity, a shortened IVRT, and steeper deceleration slope of early diastolic filling. As the left ventricle fills rapidly in early diastole, left ventricular diastolic pressure rises, so atrial contraction results in only a small pressure gradient between the left atrium and the left ventricle and a small *A* velocity. Examples of elevated preload include volume infusion or an elevated left atrial pressure due to elevation of left ventricular end-diastolic pressure.

Mitral regurgitation also results in an increase in *E* velocity both via the mechanism of an elevated left atrial pressure and because of the increased volume flow rate across the mitral valve. Again, the *A* velocity tends to be reduced (Fig. 5–13).

Situations with a reduced left atrial pressure have a reduced *E* velocity due to a smaller gradient between the left atrium and left ventricle at mitral valve opening. Thus hypovolemia or use of a venodilator (such as nitroglycerin) results in a decrease in the *E* velocity. Reduced preload is unlikely to affect atrial contraction, so the *A*-velocity peak is either unaffected or enhanced if left ventricular diastolic pressure remains low at the time of atrial contraction.

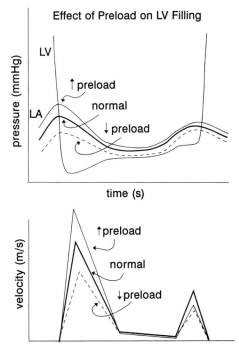

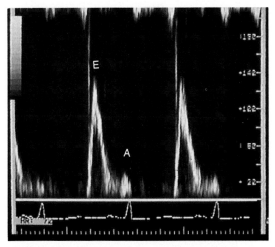

Figure 5–13. Left ventricular inflow in a patient with severe mitral regurgitation showing a high *E* velocity due to increased volume flow across the mitral valve and an increased left atrial pressure.

Figure 5–12. Effect of preload on left ventricular filling pattern. With increased preload, an increased pressure gradient from the left atrium to the left ventricle at the time of mitral valve opening results in a higher *E* velocity. The *A* velocity remains the same or is reduced if a high end-diastolic pressure results in a smaller left atrial to left ventricular pressure gradient following atrial contraction. The opposite changes occur with decreased preload.

Left ventricular systolic function affects the pattern of diastolic filling in that for a given diastolic pressure-volume curve, an increased end-systolic volume results in a shift to a steeper portion of the pressure-volume curve. Diastolic filling then occurs with a greater increase in pressure for a given increase in volume. This results in an increased *E* velocity and reduced *A* velocity, similar to the pattern seen with decreased compliance due to a shift to a different diastolic pressure-volume curve (see Fig. 5–4).

Atrial contractile function, although not always recognized clinically, can affect the pattern of left ventricular diastolic filling. This is obvious in the case of atrial fibrillation, when no atrial contribution to ventricular filling is seen (Fig. 5–14), or with atrial flutter, when small "flutter" waves in the inflow velocity pattern may be noted, but is less obvious in sinus rhythm with ineffective atrial contraction, which may result in a small *A* velocity.

Despite the potential influence of all these factors on the pattern of left ventricular diastolic filling, the Doppler velocity data still can provide useful information on diastolic dysfunction

if carefully interpreted. The two parameters of diastolic function that are most readily evaluated with Doppler velocity data are ventricular relaxation and ventricular compliance.

Left Ventricular Relaxation

Impaired ventricular relaxation results in the classic pattern of diastolic dysfunction with impaired early diastolic filling and an increased atrial contraction to total left ventricular filling. Impaired relaxation is associated with a reduced *E* velocity, a lengthened IVRT, a prolonged

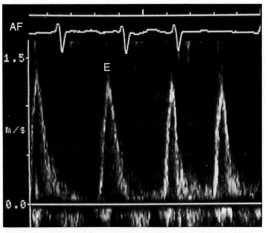

Figure 5–14. Left ventricular inflow in a patient with atrial fibrillation shows a single velocity peak and no *A* velocity.

early diastolic deceleration time, and an E/A ratio < 1 (Figs. 5–3 and 5–15).

Left Ventricular Compliance

Abnormal ventricular compliance results in rapid early diastolic filling following mitral valve opening with a short IVRT and rapid acceleration time. As the ventricle fills, left ventricular diastolic pressure rises rapidly, so a high E velocity is followed by a steep deceleration slope. The atrial contribution to filling is relatively small, since left ventricular end-diastolic pressure is elevated with only a small left atrium to left ventricle pressure gradient following atrial contraction (see Fig. 5–4).

Clinical Implications

In the clinical setting, evaluation of diastolic ventricular function is complicated by the coexistence of more than one of the factors that affect diastolic filling. For example, patients with reduced compliance also may have an elevated preload. Thus an elderly patient with reduced compliance may have a pattern of left ventricular filling similar to a younger patient with normal diastolic function (a pattern referred to as *pseudonormalization*). A patient with impaired relaxation may have coexisting mitral regurgitation. As these examples illustrate, sorting out the relative contribution of diastolic dysfunction from other physiologic parameters can be difficult in an individual patient. Furthermore, the factors that affect diastolic filling are not independent. A change in one physiologic parameter (such as left atrial pressure) may affect other parameters (such as atrial compliance and left ventricular contractility). The interdependence of these physiologic parameters complicates not only our ability to evaluate individual patients but also our understanding of the physiology of diastolic filling. Elegant in vitro studies by Dr. Thomas and colleagues provide insight into the interdependence of these relationships (see Suggested Reading 4).

RIGHT VENTRICULAR DIASTOLIC FUNCTION

Right Ventricular Filling

The pattern of right ventricular diastolic filling is similar to left ventricular diastolic filling except that maximal velocities are lower (because the tricuspid annulus is larger) and the diastolic filling period is slightly shorter. Although few studies have addressed right ventricular diastolic filling, the same measurements described for left ventricular diastolic filling are applicable.

Doppler Data Recording

On transthoracic echocardiography, right ventricular inflow can be recorded from the parasternal right ventricular inflow view or from the apical four-chamber view (Fig. 5–16). Either pulsed or continuous-wave ultrasound can be used with the same technical considerations as apply to recording left ventricular inflow veloc-

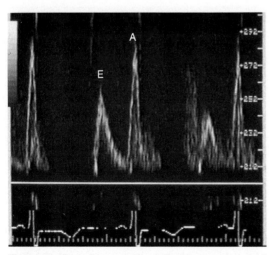

Figure 5–15. Left ventricular inflow in a patient with amyloidosis showing a pattern consistent with impaired relaxation.

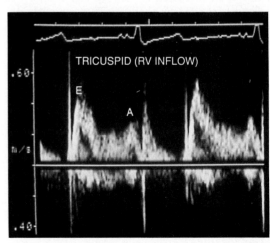

Figure 5–16. Doppler right ventricular inflow shows an E velocity and A velocity similar to left ventricular inflow.

ities. Again, evaluation of respiratory variation on inflow velocities is complicated by the respiratory motion of the heart, so care must be taken to ensure a parallel intercept angle between the ultrasound beam and inflow stream throughout the respiratory cycle. This can be accomplished in most patients by using a window where 2D echo shows little respiratory variation in the image plane itself or in the Doppler beam orientation relative to the 2D image.

Physiologic Factors That Affect Right Ventricular Filling

Right ventricular filling appears to be affected by all the same physiologic parameters that affect left ventricular filling, although less attention has been directed toward right ventricular inflow patterns. Again, the major differences between right ventricular and left ventricular filling are (1) timing, (2) reciprocal respiratory variation (as described earlier), and (3) absolute velocities, which are lower for right ventricular inflow because the tricuspid annulus is larger than the mitral annulus.

LEFT ATRIAL FILLING

Doppler Assessment

Left Atrial Filling Curves

Left atrial filling is evaluated by Doppler recordings of pulmonary vein flow either from a transesophageal or a transthoracic approach. Again, the Doppler pattern of velocities parallels the normal filling curves, with inflow into the left atrium in two phases—systolic and diastolic—and with a small reversal of flow after atrial contraction and flow deceleration following ventricular contraction (Fig. 5–17). On transesophageal recordings, the systolic inflow pattern is biphasic in most patients, with an early systolic peak related to atrial relaxation and a second late systolic peak related to displacement of the mitral annulus toward the left ventricular apex. Respiratory variation in flow may be seen in left-sided heart filling patterns (atrial and ventricular) but is less prominent than the variation seen in right-sided heart filling *and* is directionally opposite: Left-sided heart filling diminishes slightly with inspiration. Both the pulmonary veins and the left atrium are intrathoracic in their entirety, so negative intrathoracic pressure does not result in a pressure

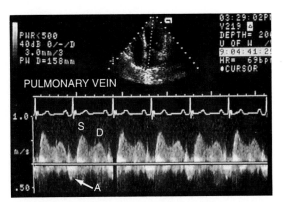

Figure 5–17. Normal pattern of left atrial inflow recorded in the right superior pulmonary vein from a transthoracic apical four-chamber view. Note the systolic (S) and diastolic (D) filling phases with a slight flow reversal following atrial contraction (A).

gradient between them. Instead, atrial filling may diminish during inspiration as blood "pools" briefly in the expanded pulmonary veins, which then empty during expiration.

Left Atrial Pressure

Accurate noninvasive assessment of left ventricular end-diastolic pressure has been an elusive goal, but several promising approaches to this problem have been proposed. One approach is to utilize the end-diastolic velocity of the aortic regurgitant velocity curve, recorded with continuous-wave Doppler, to calculate the end-diastolic pressure gradient between the aorta and left ventricle using the Bernoulli equation. Diastolic blood pressure then is subtracted from this pressure gradient to obtain left ventricular end-diastolic pressure (LV-EDP). For example, if the end-diastolic aortic regurgitant velocity is 3.9 m/s, then the aortic to left ventricular gradient is $4(3.9)^2$, or 61 mmHg. With a diastolic blood pressure of 72 mmHg, left ventricular end-diastolic pressure would be $(72 - 61) = 11$ mmHg. While conceptually sound, this approach is limited by (1) the need for a recordable aortic regurgitant jet, (2) dependence on an accurate cuff diastolic blood pressure measurement, and (3) derivation of a small number (LV-EDP) from two larger numbers, so small errors in either measured variable lead to large errors in the calculated result.

Another proposed approach is based on the pattern of pulmonary venous inflow. The ratio of flow in systole relative to total flow is inversely related to the left ventricular end-diastolic pressure. The higher the left ventricular end-diastolic pressure, the lower is the contribution of systolic filling to total pulmonary venous flow (i.e., "blunting" of the systolic flow signal). Using velocity-time integrals (VTI), a ratio of the systolic VTI to total left atrial-filling VTI that is greater than 55 percent is predictive of a left atrial pressure of 15 mmHg or less with a sensitivity of 91 percent and a specificity of 87 percent.

A more complicated approach is based on the pattern of left ventricular diastolic filling. The variables most closely correlated with left ventricular end-diastolic pressure are the IVRT and the atrial filling fraction. A regression equation incorporating these measures plus deceleration time, the E/A ratio, and the time interval from the end of mitral flow to the R wave has been proposed (see Suggested Reading 22).

Further evaluation of these methods is needed to verify their accuracy in the clinical setting.

Doppler Data Recording

From a transesophageal approach, left atrial inflow patterns can be easily recorded in each of the four pulmonary veins in the transverse plane. Careful positioning and angulation are needed to ensure that the pulsed Doppler sample volume is located in the pulmonary vein itself rather than in the adjacent left atrium. A sample volume size of 5 mm typically is used with wall filters lowered to show the low-velocity components associated with atrial and ventricular contraction. The flow pattern varies somewhat with distance from the pulmonary vein orifice. A distance of 0.5 to 1.0 cm from the orifice provides optimal signal strength with the most consistent inflow pattern.

The left superior pulmonary vein is most easily visualized adjacent to the left atrial appendage, directed somewhat anteriorly. The left inferior pulmonary vein can be visualized by advancing the transducer a short distance to see the inflow pattern from this horizontally directed vein. The right pulmonary veins can be imaged by turning the transducer medially to identify the superior right pulmonary vein (again anteriorly directed) and advancing the probe slightly to image the horizontally positioned right inferior pulmonary vein (Fig. 5–18).

From a transthoracic approach, recording pulmonary venous flow patterns is more challenging. Most echocardiographers utilize the apical four-chamber view, which allows a parallel alignment between the right superior pulmonary vein flowstream and the ultrasound beam.

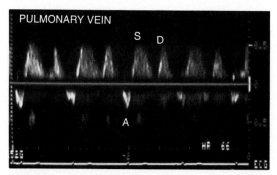

Figure 5–18. Normal pattern of left atrial inflow recorded in the left superior pulmonary vein from a transesophageal approach.

Signal strength may be a limiting factor at this depth of interrogation (typically about 14 cm), so careful attention to sample volume position, wall filters, and gain settings is needed to optimize the velocity data. Sample volume positioning may be facilitated by the use of color flow imaging to identify the flowstream from the pulmonary vein into the left atrium. Again, the sample volume should be positioned *in* the pulmonary vein within 0.5 to 1.0 cm of the orifice. Of note, the biphasic pattern of systolic inflow and atrial reversal may be more difficult to demonstrate on transthoracic compared with transesophageal imaging due to a lower signal-to-noise ratio. In addition, the flow pattern in the left upper pulmonary vein (on transesophageal echocardiography) shows a more laminar flow pattern than the right upper pulmonary vein (on transesophageal or transthoracic echocardiography). Alternate transthoracic windows that may allow recording of pulmonary vein flow in some individuals include subcostal and parasternal short axis views at the aortic valve level or suprasternal notch views of the left atrium and pulmonary viens. However, intercept angle tends to be suboptimal from these windows.

Physiologic Factors That Affect Left Atrial Filling (Table 5–3)

Left atrial filling is affected by many of the same variables that affect left ventricular diastolic filling. Higher heart rates result in merging of the systolic and diastolic phases of left atrial filling, while lower heart rates result in clearer separation between them. Changes in left atrial inflow with aging have been described, including a reduction in the diastolic filling phase, a compensatory increase in the systolic filling

TABLE 5–3. FACTORS THAT AFFECT LEFT ATRIAL FILLING PATTERNS

Systolic atrial filling
   Age
   Left atrial size
   Left atrial pressure
   Atrial contractile function

Diastolic atrial filling
   Gradient from pulmonary veins to left ventricle
   Left ventricular diastolic relaxation
   Left atrial compliance
   Left ventricular compliance

Reversal following atrial contraction
   Atrial contraction function
   Left atrial compliance
   Left ventricular compliance
   Cardiac rhythm

phase, and a more prominent atrial reversal in subjects over age 50.

Since, during diastole, the flowstream is continuous from the pulmonary veins to the left ventricle, the diastolic flow pattern is affected mostly by the pressure gradient from the pulmonary veins to the left ventricle, left ventricular relaxation, and left atrial and left ventricular compliance.

The systolic phase of atrial filling is most affected by left atrial size, pressure, compliance, and atrial contractile function.

Atrial reversal is dependent on left atrial contraction/relaxation, left atrial and left ventricular compliance, and cardiac rhythm. Increases in preload will augment the diastolic filling phase by augmenting the pressure gradient along this flowstream.

With impaired left ventricular relaxation, the pulmonary venous pattern is expected to show a prominent atrial reversal and blunting of the diastolic filling phase corresponding to the low E/A ratio seen on the left ventricular inflow pattern. With reduced left ventricular compliance, the pulmonary venous flow pattern is expected to show prominent diastolic inflow. Atrial reversal is prominent as well, since a high left ventricular diastolic pressure reduces late diastolic left ventricular filling so that atrial contraction results in reversal of flow in the pulmonary veins. Note that these pulmonary venous flow patterns allow differentiation of a high E/A ratio with normal diastolic function (normal pulmonary venous flow pattern) from a high E/A ratio due to "pseudonormalization" with reduced ventricular compliance (pulmonary venous flow pattern with prominent diastolic phase and atrial flow reversal).

RIGHT ATRIAL FILLING

Doppler Assessment

Right Atrial Filling Curves

Doppler velocity curves of right atrial filling can be recorded in the superior vena cava (from a suprasternal notch approach) or the central hepatic vein (from a subcostal approach), since these central veins empty directly into the right atrium without intervening venous valves. The pattern of right atrial filling recorded by Doppler parallels the jugular venous pressure curves seen clinically (Fig. 5–19). However, the Doppler data represent a more reliable approach, since evaluation of jugular venous patterns is difficult in some patients due to body habitus and interpretation is subjective (with no recorded data).

Again, right atrial filling patterns show respiratory variation in normal individuals with augmentation of right atrial inflow during inspiration, as is seen in the right ventricular inflow pattern. A plausible explanation for these observations is that the negative intrathoracic pressure with voluntary inspiration (but not with mechanical ventilation) results in an extra- to intrathoracic pressure gradient from the great veins into the right atrium, leading to increased blood flow into the right side of the heart.

Right Atrial Pressure

Right atrial pressure can be estimated by echocardiographic evaluation (from the subcostal window) of the inferior vena cava as it enters the right atrium (see Table 4–8). First, the *size* of the inferior vena cava reflects the intraluminal

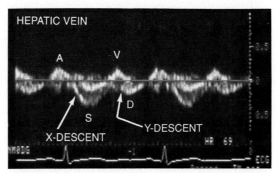

Figure 5–19. Normal pattern of right atrial inflow recorded in the central hepatic vein from a subcostal approach. Again, systolic (S) and diastolic (D) antegrade filling with slight flow reversal following atrial (A) contraction is seen.

volume, resulting in dilation with elevated right atrial pressures and a reduction in size with low atrial pressures. Second, the segment of the thin-wall vessel immediately adjacent to the atrium responds to the changes in right atrial pressure and volume that are seen with the normal changes in intrathoracic pressure with spontaneous respiration. As the right atrium fills more rapidly during inspiration, the inferior vena cava partially "collapses" due to flow from the inferior vena cava into the right atrium when inferior vena cava and right atrial pressures are low. Thus a low right atrial pressure (0 to 5 mmHg) is present when the inferior vena cava is small (<1.5 cm diameter) with respiratory "collapse" to ≥50 percent of the original diameter. Right atrial pressure is normal (5 to 10 mmHg) when the inferior vena cava size is normal (1.5 to 2.5 cm diameter) with ≥50 percent collapse of the proximal segment with normal respiration (or a "sniff"). When inferior vena cava size is normal but respiratory collapse is <50 percent, estimated right atrial pressure is 10 to 15 mmHg. Elevated right atrial pressure (15 to 20 mmHg) is manifested by inferior vena cava dilation with little respiratory variation. More severe elevations in right atrial pressure (>20 mmHg) tend to be associated with dilation of the hepatic veins as well. The validity of this approach to right atrial pressure estimation has been well established, with reported sensitivities and specificities of 87 and 82 percent, respectively, for detection of elevated right atrial pressures (≥10 mmHg). Of course, this approach is not valid in patients on mechanical ventilation, since the changes in intrathoracic pressure are not physiologic in this situation.

Doppler Data Recording

Right atrial filling is most often evaluated from the subcostal window. After the long-axis view of the inferior vena cava is obtained, the transducer is rotated and angulated to visualize the central hepatic vein, which tends to be directed toward the transducer in this view, allowing a parallel intercept angle between the pulsed Doppler beam and hepatic vein flow. Hepatic vein flow is assumed to be representative of inferior vena caval flow, since both enter into the right atrium without intervening venous valves. Direct interrogation of inferior vena caval flow is limited by a nearly perpendicular intercept angle.

Right atrial inflow also can be recorded in the superior vena cava from the suprasternal notch

window. From the standard aortic arch view, the transducer is angulated toward the patient's right to visualize the superior vena cava adjacent and slightly anterior to the ascending aorta. The pulsed Doppler sample volume is positioned in the superior vena cava, with adjustment of transducer angle and sample volume depth to obtain a well-defined velocity curve. As for other inflow patterns, wall filters are minimized (as allowed by signal-to-noise ratio) to demonstrate the low-velocity flows associated with atrial filling.

Limitations

From both the superior vena cava and hepatic vein recordings it is important to distinguish respiratory variation in the Doppler curves due to (1) respiratory variation in the angle between the ultrasound beam and blood flow direction from (2) true variations in atrial filling volumes. The hepatic vein is small, so several positions often need to be tried to find one that maintains the sample volume in the hepatic vein throughout the respiratory cycle.

The physiologic factors that affect left atrial filling also affect right atrial filling, although (as for ventricular filling) less attention has been focused on physiologic parameters affecting the right side of the heart. Respiratory variation in right atrial filling typically is much more prominent than the respiratory variation seen in left atrial filling.

ALTERNATE APPROACHES TO EVALUATION OF DIASTOLIC DYSFUNCTION

Despite the numerous potential shortcomings of Doppler echocardiographic evaluation of diastolic filling, it has great promise as a repeatable, noninvasive, widely available method for evaluation of diastolic function (Table 5–4). Techniques used in the research laboratory (time constant of relaxation, pressure-volume curves, etc.) rarely are applicable to clinical patient management. The other available clinical modalities for evaluation of diastolic function include

1. Direct intracardiac pressure measurements
2. Contrast angiographic filling curves based on frame-by-frame volume calculations
3. Radionuclide high-resolution time-activity curves

CLINICAL UTILITY

The four major disease categories that affect left ventricular diastolic function are secondary hypertrophy, cardiomyopathies, ischemic cardiac diseases, and pericardial disease. These categories include examples of diastolic dysfunction per se, including (1) abnormal relaxation, (2) reduced compliance, and (3) pericardial restraint, as well as the confounding effects of other physiologic variables on the pattern of left ventricular filling (Table 5–4).

Left Ventricular Hypertrophy

The "classic" pattern of left ventricular diastolic dysfunction is seen with left ventricular hypertrophy due to hypertension or to valvular aortic stenosis. The predominant abnormality is impaired relaxation, resulting in a pattern of reduced early diastolic filling and an enhanced atrial contribution to filling. The Doppler velocity curve typically shows a prolonged IVRT, reduced acceleration to a reduced E velocity, prolonged early diastolic deceleration slope, an increased A velocity, and an E/A ratio < 1. When left ventricular systolic dysfunction supervenes, the elevated left ventricular end-diastolic pressure and elevated left atrial pressure may result in "pseudonormalization" of this pattern with an enhanced E velocity (related to a higher mitral valve opening gradient) and reduced A velocity (due to the elevated left ven-

tricular end-diastolic pressure). Coexisting mitral regurgitation also can lead to a "paradoxical" higher E velocity despite impaired ventricular relaxation.

Cardiomyopathy

Patients with hypertrophic cardiomyopathy often have a pattern of left ventricular diastolic filling consistent with impaired relaxation. Some studies have suggested that Doppler evaluation of left ventricular diastolic filling can be used to assess the effects of medical therapy (e.g., beta blockers or calcium channel blockers) on diastolic function in this disease.

A variety of diastolic filling patterns can be seen in patients with dilated cardiomyopathy (see Chapter 7). Preliminary evidence suggests that differences in diastolic function may explain differences in clinical symptoms between patients with similar degrees of systolic dysfunction. When systolic dysfunction is present, the elevated end-systolic volume results in a shift along the pressure-volume curve to a steeper segment. This means that for a given diastolic pressure-volume relationship, compliance is reduced at higher left ventricular volumes (see Fig. 5–4). Thus the expected pattern of diastolic filling in dilated cardiomyopathy is that of reduced compliance: a high E velocity, rapid deceleration slope, low A velocity, and an E/A ratio > 1. Keeping in mind that E velocity and E/A ratio usually decrease with age, the finding of a "normal" left ventricular filling pattern in a patient older than 50 years of age should raise the question of abnormal ventricular compliance.

In cardiac amyloidosis, a specific example of restrictive cardiomyopathy, the patterns of left ventricular diastolic filling and the change in these patterns during the disease course are particularly instructive. With amyloid infiltration of the myocardium, the first change is impaired relaxation, resulting in the classic pattern of diastolic dysfunction with a reduced E velocity and increased A velocity. As the disease progresses, compliance also becomes abnormal, resulting in a shift from $E/A < 1$ to an $E/A > 1$, with all the other findings of reduced compliance. This "pseudonormalized" pattern can be distinguished from normal (if the patient is seen at only one point in the disease course) by the pattern of pulmonary venous inflow, which shows a diastolic component greater than the systolic component with an enhanced atrial reversal. To some extent, this description oversimplifies the changes seen in amyloid heart disease,

---

TABLE 5–4. SELECTED NORMAL PARAMETERS OF DIASTOLIC FUNCTION

Time intervals	
IVRT	63 ± 11 ms
Derived measures	
Tau	33 ± 6 ms
$-dP/dt$	2048 ± 335 mmHg/s
Filling rates	
Peak filling rate	288 ± 66 ml/s
Peak filling rate normalized to LV-EDV	2.9 ± 1.0 s^{-1}
Atrial filling rate	229 ± 83 ml/s
Ratio of early to atrial FV1	1.71 ± 0.43
Velocities	
E/A ratio	1.32 ± 0.42
Deceleration slope	5.0 ± 1.4 m/s^2

References: Tebbe, et al: Clin Cardiol 3:19, 1980; Shapiro and McKenna: Br Heart J 51:637, 1984; Pearson, et al: Am Heart J 113: 1417, 1987; Snider R, et al: Am J Cardiol 56:921, 1985.

since concurrent changes in left ventricular systolic function, the degree of mitral regurgitation, and left atrial filling pressures also occur, all of which affect the pattern of left ventricular diastolic filling. However, it does serve as a useful framework for understanding the complex changes that occur with diastolic dysfunction.

Pericardial Disease

With both pericardial tamponade and pericardial constriction, cardiac filling is impaired by pericardial "restraint." In the case of tamponade physiology, filling is impaired in both early and late diastole, with an accentuation of the normal variation seen in right and left ventricular filling with respiration. With constrictive pericarditis, early diastolic filling tends to be normal, with marked impairment of filling late in diastole when the heart has expanded to the maximum allowed by the fibrotic pericardial encasement. Both these conditions are discussed in more detail in Chapter 8.

Ischemic Cardiac Disease

In patients with coronary artery disease and no prior myocardial infarction, induction of ischemia results in diastolic dysfunction prior to systolic dysfunction (see Chapter 6). Diastolic filling curves with ischemia induced by balloon inflation during percutaneous transluminal angioplasty show rapid onset of a reduced E velocity, with resolution of these changes as ischemia is relieved. In acute myocardial infarction, a pattern of delayed relaxation is seen acutely. At follow-up, one of several patterns of left ventricular filling may be observed: (1) With successful reperfusion with little myocardial damage, left ventricular diastolic filling returns to normal. (2) With an infarction but preserved left ventricular systolic function, the pattern of impaired relaxation often persists. (3) With a large infarction and significant left ventricular systolic dysfunction, the "pseudonormalized" pattern of a high E velocity and low A velocity due to a combination of reduced compliance, a high left ventricular end-diastolic pressure, and a shift along the diastolic pressure volume curve (increased end-systolic volume) can be seen. Thus an apparent "normal" pattern of left ventricular filling late after myocardial infarction may be due to normal left ventricular diastolic and systolic function or to impaired diastolic and systolic function. As for cardiomyopathy patients, these

two groups can be distinguished by a higher E/A ratio, shorter IVRT, and steeper deceleration slope than normal and by the pattern of pulmonary venous flow.

SUGGESTED READING

1. Bonow RO, Udelson JE: Left ventricular diastolic dysfunction as a cause of congestive heart failure: Mechanisms and management. Ann Intern Med 117: 502–510, 1992.
   Review of mechanisms of diastolic dysfunction and the effects of physiologic changes (heart rate, loading conditions) and aging on diastolic filling. The diagnosis and management of heart failure due to diastolic dysfunction are also reviewed. Eighty-five references.

2. Harizi RC, Bianco JA, Alpert JS: Diastolic function of the heart in clinical cardiology. Arch Intern Med 148:99–109, 1988.
   Review of the physiology of diastole, indexes of diastolic function, and clinical correlates of diastolic dysfunction. Ninety-nine references.

3. Nishimura RA, Abel MD, Hatle LK, Tajik AJ: Assessment of diastolic function of the heart: Background and current applications of Doppler echocardiography: II. Clinical studies. Mayo Clin Proc 64: 181–204, 1989.
   Review emphasizing the Doppler evaluation of diastolic function with examples of venous inflow patterns, as well as ventricular inflow patterns, in normal and abnormal subjects. One hundred and ten references.

4. Thomas JD, Weyman AE: Echocardiographic Doppler evaluation of left ventricular diastolic function: Physics and physiology. Circulation 84:977–990, 1991.
   Detailed mathematical approach to left ventricular diastolic filling with excellent diagrams showing the effects of changes in specific parameters on the pattern of diastolic filling.

5. Spirito P, Maron BJ, Bonow RO: Noninvasive assessment of left ventricular diastolic function: Comparative analysis of Doppler echocardiographic and radionuclide angiographic techniques. J Am Coll Cardiol 7:518–526, 1986.
   Comparison of Doppler and radionuclide angiographic evaluation of diastolic filling in 12 normal subjects and 25 patients with cardiac disease. Good correlations were noted between Doppler and radionuclide measures of the ratio of early to late diastolic filling (r = 0.76), the time interval from end-systole to end of early rapid filling (r = 0.83), and the slope of the early flow velocity peak versus peak filling rate (r = 0.79).

6. Friedman BJ, Drinkovic N, Miles H, et al: Assessment of left ventricular diastolic function: Comparison of Doppler echocardiography and gated blood pool scintigraphy. J Am Coll Cardiol 8:1348–1354, 1986.
   Comparison of Doppler and radionuclide measures of diastolic filling in 25 patients showed excellent correlations for fractional filling in early diastole (r = 0.84), atrial systolic filling (r = −0.85), their ratio (r = 0.83), and the diastolic filling period (r = 0.94).

7. Rokey R, Kuo LC, Zoghbi WA, et al: Determination of parameters of left ventricular diastolic filling with pulsed Doppler echocardiography: Comparison with cineangiography. Circulation 71:543-550, 1985.

Comparison of Doppler and cineangiographic measures of left ventricular diastolic filling in 30 patients showed that the Doppler curve resembles the first derivative of the angiographic volume curve. Doppler and angiographic peak filling rate (r = 0.87) and normalized peak filling rate (r = 0.83) correlated well.

8. Flachskampf FA, Weyman AE, Guerrero JL, Thomas JD: Calculation of atrioventricular compliance from the mitral flow profile: Analytic and in vitro study. J Am Coll Cardiol 19:998–1004, 1992.
Net compliance C_n of the left ventricle can be calculated as

$$C_n = -[A/\rho(dv/dt)]$$

where A = effective mitral valve area, ρ = blood density, and dv/dt = deceleration rate. The shape of the early deceleration curve depends on the time course of net compliance.

9. Chen C, Rodriguez L, Levine RA, et al: Noninvasive measurement of the time constant of left ventricular relaxation using the continuous-wave Doppler velocity profile of mitral regurgitation. Circulation 86:272–278, 1992.
The time constant of relaxation can be calculated from the Doppler mitral regurgitant velocity curve by exponential regression with correction for left atrial pressure. Assuming a left atrial pressure of 10 mmHg, the Doppler mitral regurgitant velocity curve yields estimates with an accuracy of ± 15 percent.

10. Chen C, Rodriguez L, Lethor JP, et al. Continuous wave Doppler echocardiography for non-invasive assessment of left ventricular dP/dt and relaxation time constant from mitral regurgitant spectra in patients. J Am Coll Cardiol 23:970–976, 1994.
In 12 patients with mitral regurgitation, Doppler-derived measures correlated well with invasive data for maximum +dP/dt (r = 0.91), maximum −dP/dt (r = 0.89), and tau (r = 0.93).

11. Bowman LK, Lee FA, Jaffe CC, et al: Peak filling rate normalized to mitral stroke volume: A new Doppler echocardiographic filling index validated by radionuclide angiographic techniques. J Am Coll Cardiol 12:937–943, 1988.
Normalization of Doppler peak filling rate to transmitral stroke volume avoids errors due to geometric assumptions, diameter measurements, and sample volume position. Normalization then simply is early peak filling velocity divided by the velocity time integral of mitral inflow. This measure correlated well (r = 0.91) with radionuclide peak filling rate in 30 patients.

12. Berk MR, Xie G, Kwan OL, et al: Reduction of left ventricular preload by lower body negative pressure alters Doppler transmitral filling patterns. J Am Coll Cardiol 16:1387–1392, 1990.
To avoid confounding effects of pharmacologic intervention, preload was reduced by lower body negative pressure. Decreased preload resulted in a reduced E velocity, no change in A velocity, a reduced E/A ratio, and a reduction in mean acceleration and deceleration with a corresponding prolongation of the pressure half-time.

13. Stoddard MF, Pearson AC, Kern MJ, et al: Influence of alteration in preload on the pattern of left ventricular diastolic filling as assessed by Doppler echocardiography in humans. Circulation 79:1226–1236, 1989.
Preload reduction with nitroglycerin in 50 patients resulted in a reduced left ventricular end-diastolic pressure, peak early filling velocity, and E/A ratio. Relaxation and chamber stiffness were unchanged. The importance of preload in

the Doppler patterns of left ventricular diastolic filling is emphasized.

14. Thomas JD, Choong CYP, Flachskampf FA, Weyman AE: Analysis of the early transmitral Doppler velocity curve: Effect of primary physiologic changes and compensatory preload adjustment. J Am Coll Cardiol 16:644–655, 1990.
Elegant description of early diastolic filling with mathematical explanations (for the mathematically inclined) and clear diagrams showing the effects of changes in each parameter (for the rest of us).

15. Appleton CP: Influence of incremental changes in heart rate on mitral flow velocity: Assessment in lightly sedated, conscious dogs. J Am Coll Cardiol 17:227–236, 1991.
Progressive increases in heart rate (shortening of diastole) induced by atrial pacing, isoproterenol, or atropine result in little change in early diastolic filling but an increase in A velocity, causing a decrease in the E/A ratio. At very high heart rates, the E and A velocities become "fused".

16. Zoghbi WA, Bolli R: The increasing complexity of assessing diastolic function from ventricular filling dynamics. J Am Coll Cardiol 17:238–248, 1991.
Editorial comment on Suggested Reading 14 emphasizing the clinical importance of the confounding effect of heart rate on left ventricular diastolic filling patterns.

17. Harrison MR, Clifton GD, Pennell AT, DeMaria AN: Effect of heart rate on left ventricular diastolic transmitral flow velocity patterns assessed by Doppler echocardiography in normal subjects. Am J Cardiol 67:622–627, 1991.
In 20 adult volunteers, heart rate was varied by transesophageal atrial pacing. Although E velocity was unchanged, A velocity increased from 0.37 ± 0.06 m/s at a heart rate of 70 bpm to 0.50 ± 0.07 m/s at a heart rate of 88 bpm (p < 0.003), demonstrating the significant effects of minor changes in heart rate on left ventricular filling.

18. Otto CM, Pearlman AS, Amsler LC: Doppler echocardiographic evaluation of left ventricular diastolic filling in isolated valvular aortic stenosis. Am J Cardiol 63:313–316, 1989.
In 49 adults with isolated valvular aortic stenosis, an increased A velocity was associated with the presence of left ventricular hypertrophy. In patients with aortic stenosis, left ventricular systolic dysfunction, compared with normal systolic function, was associated with a higher E velocity, lower A velocity, higher E/A ratio, and steeper deceleration slope.

19. Appleton CP, Hatle LK, Popp RL: Demonstration of restrictive ventricular physiology by Doppler echocardiography. J Am Coll Cardiol 11:757–768, 1988.
In 14 patients with a clinical diagnosis of restrictive cardiomyopathy, the pattern of left ventricular diastolic filling was characterized by a shortened deceleration time and a reduced A velocity. The venous inflow pattern (SVC, HV) showed reduced systolic inflow and a prominent atrial reversal.

20. Snow FR, Gorcsan J, Lewis SA, et al: Doppler echocardiographic evaluation of left ventricular diastolic function after percutaneous transluminal coronary angioplasty for unstable angina pectoris or acute myocardial infarction. Am J Cardiol 65:840–844, 1990.
In 42 patients with ischemia, Doppler echo left ventricular inflow 8 ± 5 h before PTCA showed a prolonged IVRT and deceleration time, decreased E/A ratio, and increased atrial filling fraction. Repeat study 2 ± 1 days after PTCA showed an increase in E/A ratio, a decrease in atrial filling

function, and a reduction in the IVRT and deceleration time. These findings suggest improved left ventricular diastolic filling following revascularization.

21. Johannessen K-A, Cerqueira MD, Stratton JR: Influence of myocardial infarction size on radionuclide and Doppler echocardiographic measurements of diastolic function. Am J Cardiol 65:692–697, 1990.
    In 83 patients studied 8 to 12 weeks after acute myocardial infarction, infarct size measured by thallium-201 tomography was inversely correlated with peak A velocity and directly correlated with peak E velocity, deceleration slope, and E/A ratio.

22. Kuecherer HF, Muhiudeen IA, Kusumoto FM, et al: Estimation of mean left atrial pressure from transesophageal pulsed Doppler echocardiography of pulmonary venous flow. Circulation 82:1127–1139, 1990.
    In 47 patients undergoing cardiovascular surgery, the systolic fraction of pulmonary venous inflow correlated with mean left atrial pressure (r = −0.88). A systolic fraction <55 percent had a sensitivity of 91 percent and a specificity of 87 percent for detection of a left atrial pressure ≤15 mmHg.

23. Mulvagh S, Quinones MA, Kleiman NS, et al: Estimation of left ventricular end-diastolic pressure from Doppler transmitral flow velocity in cardiac patients independent of systolic performance. J Am Coll Cardiol 20:112–119, 1992.
    A combined approach to estimates of left ventricular end-diastolic pressure (LV-EDP) is proposed:

$$\text{LV-EDP} = 46 - (0.22\text{IVRT}) - (0.10\text{AFF}) - (0.03\text{DT}) - (2 \div \text{E/A}) + (0.05\text{MAR})$$

where IVRT = isovolumic relaxation time, in ms, AFF = atrial filling fraction, DT = deceleration time, E/A = E to A velocity ratio, and MAR = time from end of mitral flow to R wave. In the test group, this equation was 90 percent sensitive and specific for detection of an LV-EDP > 15 mmHg.

24. Castello R, Pearson AC, Lenzen P, Labovitz AJ: Evaluation of pulmonary venous flow by transesophageal echocardiography in subjects with a normal heart: Comparison with transthoracic echocardiography. J Am Coll Cardiol 18:65–71, 1991.
    Pulmonary venous flow consists of four phases: two antegrade flows in systole (due to atrial relaxation and ventricular contraction), antegrade flow in diastole, and flow reversal during atrial contraction. Flows are more clearly demonstrated on TEE, particularly in the left superior pul-

monary vein at a depth of 0.5 to 1.0 cm from entry into the left atrium.

25. Simonson JS, Schiller NB: Sonospirometry: A new method for noninvasive estimation of mean right atrial pressure based on two-dimensional echographic measurements of the inferior vena cava during measured inspiration. J Am Coll Cardiol 11:557–564, 1988.
    Dimension and respiratory variations in size of the inferior vena cava are related to right atrial pressure. Respiratory variation in inferior vena cava size is due to a close relationship between mean right atrial pressure and inspiratory pressure. The authors propose that the thin-walled inferior vena cava "collapses" on inspiration due to increased right atrial filling and (consequent emptying of the inferior vena cava) with the negative intrathoracic pressure of normal breathing.

26. Kircher BJ, Himelman RB, Schiller NB: Noninvasive estimation of right atrial pressure from the inspiratory collapse of the inferior vena cava. Am J Cardiol 66:493–496, 1990.
    The inferior vena cava (IVC) size and respiratory motion are related to right atrial pressure such that a 50 percent respiratory collapse in IVC diameter has a sensitivity of 87 percent and specificity of 82 percent for detection of a right atrial pressure of ≥ or < 10 mmHg.

27. Kono T, Sabbah HN, Rosman H, et al: Divergent effects of intravenous dobutamine and nitroprusside on left atrial contribution to ventricular filling in dogs with chronic heart failure. Am Heart J 127:874–880, 1994.
    In seven dogs with chronic heart failure, dobutamine infusion did not affect the atrial contribution to LV filling but it did increase LV filling pressure, LV end-diastolic wall stress, and stiffness. In contrast, nitroprusside infusion increased the atrial contribution to LV filling from 12 + 2% to 17 + 2% (p < 0.01) in association with decreased LV filling pressure, end-diastolic wall stress, and stiffness. These potential pharmcologic effects should be considered in the clinical setting.

28. Marino P, Prioli AM, Destro G, et al: The left atrial volume curve can be assessed from pulmonary vein and mitral valve velocity tracings. Am Heart J 127:886–898, 1994.
    A novel approach to derviation of the left atrial volume curve from the instantaneous transmitral volume flow rate (annular area × mitral velocity) and the right upper pulmonary vein flow curve as described. Left atrial volumes by 2D echocardiography correlated well (r = 0.95, SEE − 11.9 ml). Further evaluation of this new approach is needed.

THE UTILITY OF ECHOCARDIOGRAPHY IN PATIENTS WITH ISCHEMIC CARDIAC DISEASE

INTRODUCTION

Given the high prevalence of coronary artery disease, evaluation of patients with suspected or documented ischemic disease is one of the most common indications for echocardiography. Echocardiographic evaluation focuses on the functional outcome of coronary artery disease—specifically systolic wall thickening and endocardial motion—rather than on direct imaging of the coronary arteries. While the proximal left main and right coronary arteries often can be identified, even on transthoracic images, tomographic imaging techniques currently do not provide the detailed knowledge of distal vessel anatomy or the location and severity of coronary artery narrowings that is needed for patient management. Coronary angiography remains the procedure of choice for direct assessment of coronary artery anatomy.

However, echocardiography offers detailed functional assessment of segmental and global left ventricular systolic function both at rest and after interventions to induce ischemia (Table 6–1). In many cases, this functional assessment provides critical data for patient management. For example, stress echocardiography is a reliable approach for the initial diagnosis of coronary artery disease, especially in patients with a nondiagnostic stress electrocardiogram. Early diagnosis of acute myocardial infarction in the emergency room may be possible in patients with an equivocal electrocardiogram. The central role of echocardiography in evaluation for complications of acute myocardial infarction has long been recognized. In addition, echocardiography often provides important prognostic data in patients with coronary artery disease.

TABLE 6–1. ECHOCARDIOGRAPHY FOR CORONARY ARTERY DISEASE

1. Myocardial ischemia

   Diagnosis of coronary artery disease
   Severity of disease (number of vessels involved, extent of myocardium at risk)
   Overall LV systolic function
   Diastolic LV function

2. Myocardial infarction

   Early diagnosis in emergency room
   Definition of area of myocardium at risk (if performed before or soon after administration of thrombolytic therapy)
   Assessment of results after intervention
   Evaluation of recurrent ischemia after myocardial infarction
   Assessment of overall LV systolic function

3. Complications of acute myocardial infarction

   LV systolic dysfunction
   LV thrombus
   Aneurysm formation
   Acute mitral regurgitation
   Acute ventricular septal defect
   LV rupture
   Pericardial effusion

4. End-stage ischemic disease

   LV and RV systolic dysfunction
   Associated mitral regurgitation
   Pulmonary artery pressures
   LV thrombus

BASIC PRINCIPLES

Relationship Between Coronary Artery Anatomy and Segmental Wall Motion by Echocardiography

While coronary anatomy varies to some degree from patient to patient, the overall pattern of coronary artery branching is relatively uniform (Fig. 6–1). The left main coronary artery arises from the superior aspect of the left coronary sinus of Valsalva and divides into (1) the left anterior descending artery, which extends via the interventricular groove down the anterior wall to (and sometimes around) the left ventricular apex, and (2) the circumflex artery, which continues laterally in the atrioventricular groove. The right coronary artery arises from the superior aspect of the right coronary sinus of Valsalva and extends inferomedially following the atrioventricular groove. Approximately 80 percent of patients have a *right-dominant* coronary circulation; the right coronary gives rise to the posterior descending artery, which lies in the inferior interventricular groove supplying both the inferior aspect of the ventricular septum and the inferior free wall (Figs. 6–2 and 6–3). In about 20 percent of patients, the coronary circulation is *left-dominant*; the circumflex artery gives rise to the posterior descending artery.

The posterior left ventricular wall may be supplied by extension branches from the right coronary artery or by obtuse marginal branches

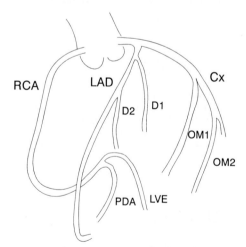

Figure 6–1. Schematic drawing of coronary artery anatomy showing the left anterior descending (LAD) artery with diagonal (D1 and D2) branches, the circumflex artery (Cx) with obtuse marginal branches (OM1 and OM2), and the right coronary artery (RCA) giving rise to the posterior descending artery (PDA) and left ventricular extension (LVE) branch.

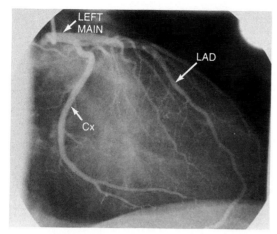

Figure 6–2. Normal left coronary artery in a right anterior oblique (RAO) projection showing the left anterior descending (LAD) and circumflex (Cx) coronary arteries.

of the circumflex arteries. The lateral wall is supplied by obtuse marginal branches of the circumflex artery. The left anterior descending artery supplies the anterior portion of the interventricular septum via septal perforating branches and the anterior wall via diagonal branches. There is marked individual variability in the blood supply to the left ventricular apex. In some cases, the left anterior descending artery extends around the apex to supply the apical segment of the inferior wall. In other cases, the posterior descending artery extends around the apex to supply the apical segment of the anterior wall. More commonly, the blood supply to the apex arises from both the left anterior descending and the posterior descending coronary arteries.

Segmental wall motion abnormalities seen by echocardiography correspond closely with the coronary artery blood supply to the myocardium. Several different schemes for reporting the location of wall motion abnormalities on echocardiography have been proposed. These approaches differ mainly in the number of segments into which the left ventricle is divided; all are similar in the use of nomenclature that corresponds both to coronary anatomy and to the application of these terms for other cardiac imaging modalities.

From base to apex, the left ventricle typically is divided into three segments—base, midventricular, and apical—to correspond to proximal, middle, and apical lesions of the coronary arteries. In a short-axis view, both at the basal (mitral valve) and mid–left ventricular (papillary muscle) levels, the ventricle is divided clockwise, beginning with the interventricular groove, into the anterior wall, the lateral wall, the posterior wall, and the inferior wall (Fig. 6–4). The ventricular septum is divided into at least two segments (inferior and anterior), since it receives blood flow from both the posterior descending and the left anterior descending arteries. The apical region often is divided into only three or four segments (instead of five to eight segments at the base) because of the normal tapering of the ventricle toward the apex. Depending on the exact scheme used, this results in between 15 and 20 myocardial segments. While a more elaborate segmental system may be needed for research purposes, for routine patient evaluation a 15-segment scheme provides sufficient detail for clinical correlation between coronary anatomy and echocardiographic findings. The location of wall motion abnormalities can be reported descriptively, using a series of drawings showing different echocardiographic views, using a target diagram with the apex in the center and the base around the circumference (Fig. 6–5), or using more quantitative display formats (Fig. 6–6).

The segmental wall motion abnormalities seen with ischemia or infarction correspond to the coronary anatomy as follows:

1. Left anterior descending artery disease results in wall motion abnormalities of the anterior septum, anterior free wall, and anterior left ventricular apex. Depending on the degree to which diagonal branches supply the lateral wall, abnormalities may be seen for these segments as well. If the left anterior descending artery extends around the apex, apical segments of the inferior and posterolateral walls may be affected. The location of the lesion along the length of the coronary artery obviously affects

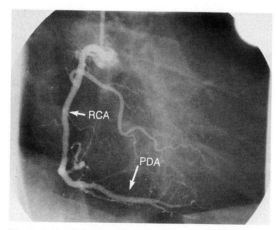

Figure 6–3. Normal right coronary anatomy with the posterior descending artery (PDA) seen in a right anterior oblique (RAO) projection.

Echo Views for Wall Motion

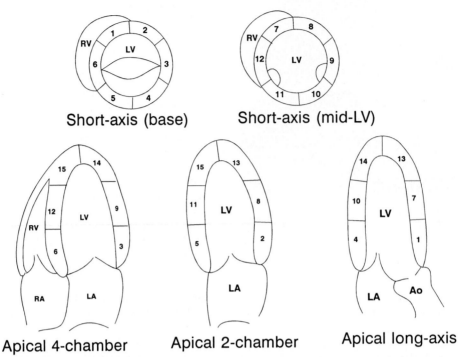

Short-axis (base)   Short-axis (mid-LV)

Apical 4-chamber   Apical 2-chamber   Apical long-axis

Figure 6–4. Echocardiographic views for wall motion evaluation. In the short-axis view, at the base and midventricular levels, the left ventricle is divided into anterior septum (1, 7) and free wall (2, 8), lateral (3, 9), posterior (4, 10), inferior free wall (5, 11) and inferior septal (6, 12) segments. These same wall segments are seen in apical views as indicated, plus the anterior (13), inferior (15), and posterolateral (14) apical segments are seen.

the pattern of wall motion. A lesion in the distal third of the vessel affects only the apex, a lesion in the midsegment of the vessel affects the midventricular and apical segments, while a proximal lesion affects the entire wall including the basal segments.

2. Circumflex artery disease affects wall motion of the lateral and posterior left ventricular walls. Again, the extent of segmental wall motion is related to the exact coronary anatomy in an individual patient. Echocardiography is particularly helpful in patients with circumflex disease because this myocardial region often is "silent" electrocardiographically and is not well seen on a single-plane right anterior–oblique left ventricular angiogram.

3. Posterior descending artery disease results in abnormal wall motion in the inferior septum, inferior free wall, and posterior left ventricular segments. If the posterior descending artery is a short vessel, the apex will not be affected, while extensive wall motion abnormalities of the apex may be seen if it is supplied by the posterior descending artery.

Other patterns of abnormal wall motion are seen with lesions of the branches of the three major coronary arteries. For example, isolated disease in a diagonal branch of the left anterior

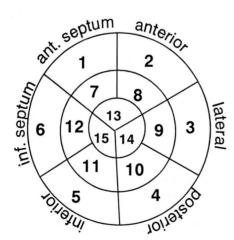

Figure 6–5. "Target" diagram for reporting left ventricular segmental wall motion with the apex in the center of the circle and the base around the circumference. Segment numbers correspond to those shown in Figure 6–4.

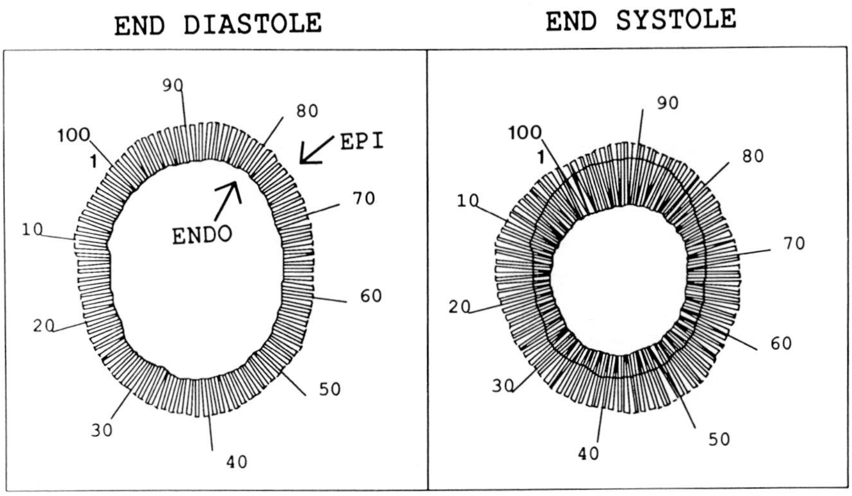

END DIASTOLE

END SYSTOLE

Figure 6–6. Measurement of wall thickening by the centerwall method. The epicardial (EPI) and endocardial (ENDO) contours of the left ventricular wall are displayed at end-diastole (*left*) and at end-systole (*right*). Thickness is measured as the length of each of 100 chords constructed perpendicular to and evenly spaced along a line in the center of the myocardial wall (not shown), midway between the epicardial and endocardial contours. The end-diastolic endocardial contour is reproduced on the end-systolic plot to illustrate the extent of endocardial wall motion. (*From Sheehan FS, Feneley MP, DeBruijn NP, et al: Quantitative analysis of regional wall thickening by transesophageal echocardiography. J Thorac Cardiovasc Surg 103:347, 1992.*)

descending artery results in a discrete wall motion abnormality in the portion of the anterolateral wall supplied by that vessel. Proximal right coronary artery disease can result in ischemia or infarction of the right ventricular free wall.

Collateral vessels and previous bypass surgery affect the pattern of wall motion as well. If a myocardial segment has a balanced oxygen demand to supply ratio, wall motion will be normal whether blood flow is supplied antegrade by the native vessel, by collateral vessels, or by a bypass graft.

Echocardiographic Views for Evaluation of Left Ventricular Wall Motion

Transthoracic Imaging

Regional systolic function for each segment of the left ventricle can be assessed on transthoracic imaging by combining data from multiple image planes. In the parasternal long-axis view, the basal and midventricular segments of the anterior septum and posterior left ventricular walls are seen. In the parasternal short-axis view, circumferential images of the left ventricle at the base and midventricular levels are obtained. Note that if the transducer is angulated toward the apex from a fixed parasternal position, pro-

gressively more apical segments of the posterior wall are imaged while the *same* segment of the septum is included in the ultrasound image plane. A more parallel alignment between image planes may be obtained by moving the transducer apically to obtain short-axis midventricular and (sometimes) apical views of the left ventricle (Fig. 6–7). In either case, evaluation of wall motion from other windows is helpful for avoiding misdiagnosis related to an oblique image plane. Of note, the apical segments rarely are adequately visualized from the parasternal window.

From the apical window, evaluation of left ventricular wall motion is performed in four-chamber, two-chamber, and long-axis views. Detailed evaluation of the extent of abnormal myocardium is possible by slow rotation of the image plane between the standard views. In the four-chamber view, the inferior septum and lateral wall are seen. Anterior angulation to include the aortic valve allows visualization of portions of the anterior septum. In the two-chamber view, the anterior and inferior free walls are seen. Endocardial and epicardial definition of the anterior wall may be difficult due to attenuation by adjacent overlying lung tissue. This problem can be alleviated by careful patient positioning and imaging during held respiration. In the apical long-axis view, the anterior septum and posterior wall are seen (analogous to the parasternal long-axis view).

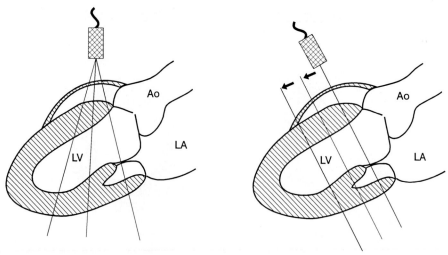

Figure 6–7. Angulation of the transducer from a fixed parasternal position results in short-axis views that intersect similar segments of the septum but progressively more apical segments of the posterior wall. By moving the transducer apically, more parallel image planes can be obtained.

Note that while these three apical image planes are approximately 60° to each other, there is some individual variation in their exact relationship. In addition, variation in coronary anatomy between individuals results in variable patterns of abnormal wall motion. Care is needed in positioning the transducer at the apex, avoiding foreshortening of the ventricle from this approach. Integration of data from parasternal and apical approaches, taking into account image quality in each view, allows assessment of each myocardial segment in at least two views.

Finally, evaluation from a subcostal approach may be helpful. In the subcostal four-chamber view, the inferior septum and lateral wall are imaged. In the subcostal short-axis view, the inferior and posterior walls are nearest the transducer and the anterior and lateral walls most distal (Fig. 6–8).

Transesophageal Imaging

When transthoracic images are inadequate or in certain monitoring situations (e.g., intraoperative monitoring of left ventricular function), regional left ventricular function can be evaluated from a transesophageal approach. From the high left atrial position, a four-chamber view of the left ventricle is obtained (in the transverse plane of the transesophageal echocardiographic probe) showing the inferior septum and lateral wall. Using the probe's longitudinal plane, the anterior and inferior walls are imaged. Note that these views may be foreshortened; that is, the apparent apex represents an oblique plane

through the anterolateral wall, while the true left ventricular apex is not seen.

From the transgastric position the transverse image plane provides short-axis views of the left ventricle at the base (mitral valve) and midventricular (papillary muscle) level. Further advancement of the transducer may allow "apical" four-chamber (in the transverse plane) and long-axis (in the longitudinal plane) views, but again, the ventricle may be foreshortened and the true apex missed if the left ventricular apex does not lie on or near the diaphragm without intervening lung tissue in a position accessible from the transgastric approach.

Transesophageal imaging of left ventricular wall motion is indicated:

1. For intraoperative assessment of global and segmental left ventricular function.
2. In critically ill patients when transthoracic views are inadequate.

Sequence of Events in Ischemia

Irreversible myocardial damage—infarction—results in wall motion abnormalities that are present at rest. With an acute infarction, wall thickness is normal, but systolic wall thickening and endocardial motion are reduced or absent. An old myocardial infarction is characterized by thinning and increased echogenicity of the affected segments due to scarring and fibrosis, in addition to abnormal motion.

In contrast, ischemia is a reversible imbalance in the myocardial oxygen demand/supply ratio.

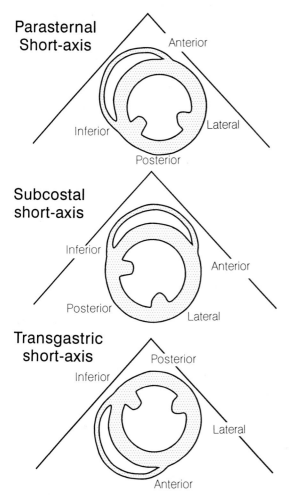

Figure 6–8. The wall segments seen in the short-axis view from a parasternal, subcostal, and transgastric approach are shown. Correct identification of wall segments is facilitated by noting the position of the septum and the papillary muscles.

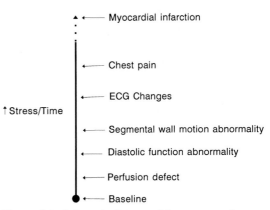

Figure 6–9. Schematic diagram of the sequence of events in myocardial ischemia.

chemical followed by a significant perfusion defect (detectable by radionuclide techniques). Next, regional myocardial dysfunction, characterized by both abnormal diastolic relaxation and compliance and impaired systolic wall thickening and endocardial motion, occurs in rapid succession (within a few cardiac cycles). Ischemic ST-segment depression on electrocardiography and clinical angina are relatively late manifestations of ischemia and are not seen consistently. Echocardiography, by detecting abnormal regional wall motion, provides a useful noninvasive method for evaluating ischemia that should be more sensitive than electrocardiography given this sequence of events. Echocardiography differs from radionuclide techniques in that the functional consequences of ischemia, rather than the pattern of myocardial perfusion, are assessed.

Evaluation of Global and Regional Ventricular Function in Coronary Artery Disease

Global left ventricular systolic function can be evaluated either qualitatively or quantitatively in patients with coronary artery disease using the approaches described in Chapter 4. Since the pattern of left ventricular dysfunction typically is *not* uniform, it is important that qualitative evaluation be based on multiple tomographic views. If quantitative methods are applied, approaches that incorporate endocardial borders from at least two tomographic planes are most appropriate. In patients with coronary artery disease, the left ventricular ejection fraction is essential clinical data because it is a crucial variable in clinical decision making concerning surgical intervention.

Even with substantial coronary artery narrowing, blood flow is adequate for myocardial oxygen demands at rest. However, when the narrowing exceeds 70 percent of the luminal cross-sectional area, blood flow is inadequate to meet increased myocardial oxygen demands with exercise, pharmacologic interventions, or mental stress, resulting in ischemia. When oxygen demand returns to baseline, blood flow again is adequate, ischemia resolves, and wall motion returns to normal. Thus wall motion *at rest* is normal in patients with coronary artery disease if there has been no prior myocardial infarction.

The sequence of changes *as* a region of myocardium becomes ischemic is as follows (Fig. 6–9): The first detectable changes associated with heterogeneity of flow to the left ventricle are bio-

Segmental (or regional) left ventricular systolic function most often is evaluated using a semiquantitative scoring system. The endocardial motion for each defined myocardial segment is described as normal, hypokinetic, akinetic, or dyskinetic, with a score from 1 to 4 corresponding to these descriptive terms. Hyperkinesis also may be noted (Table 6–2). Some clinicians prefer to subclassify the degree of hypokinesis as mild, moderate, or severe, but such a subclassification has significant inter- and intraobserver variability. An overall wall motion score index can be derived by dividing the sum of scores for each segment by the number of segments evaluated:

$$\text{Wall motion score index} = \frac{\text{sum of individual segment scores}}{\text{number of segments visualized}}$$

Several more quantitative approaches to echocardiographic segmental wall motion have been proposed. Most of these represent modifications of angiographic techniques, such as the centerline method for quantitative wall motion analysis. Limitations of the application of these approaches to echocardiographic images include:

1. The need to identify and manually trace the endocardium at end-diastole and end-systole. Accurate automatic edge-detection algorithms will minimize this problem.
2. The need to evaluate wall motion in multiple tomographic views.
3. The need for knowledge of the degree of variability of normal wall motion for each view.
4. The effects of translation, rotation, and torsion of the left ventricle during the cardiac cycle. This potentially could result in imaging different regions of myocardium in systole versus diastole for a given tomographic plane.
5. The question of whether wall thickening or endocardial motion is a more appropriate

method for describing regional ventricular function.

As automated edge-detection programs become faster and are validated for echocardiographic data, quantitative analysis of segmental function will become more feasible in the clinical setting. Approaches that incorporate three-dimensional (3D) reconstruction of the left ventricle also appear promising.

MYOCARDIAL ISCHEMIA

Basic Principles

Since echocardiographic wall motion at rest is normal in a patient with significant coronary artery disease and no prior myocardial infarction, imaging *during ischemia* is needed for diagnosis. Inducing ischemia during echocardiographic imaging is referred to as *stress echocardiography*. Ischemia can be induced by increasing myocardial oxygen demand either with exercise or by pharmacologic interventions (Table 6–3).

Stress Echocardiography

Exercise echocardiography typically is performed using standard exercise-test protocols. Supine or upright bicycle exercise protocols have the advantage that echocardiographic imaging can be performed during exercise at each progressive level of exertion, including maximal exercise. Treadmill exercise protocols have the advantage that a higher total workload can be achieved but the disadvantage that imaging can only be performed after exercise. Wall motion

TABLE 6–2. QUALITATIVE SCALE FOR ASSESSMENT OF SEGMENTAL WALL MOTION ON ECHOCARDIOGRAPHY

SCORE*	WALL MOTION	DEFINITION
1	Normal	Normal endocardial inward motion and wall thickening in systole
2	Hypokinesis	Reduced endocardial motion and wall thickening in systole
3	Akinesis	Absence of inward endocardial motion or wall thickening in systole
4	Dyskinesis	Outward motion or "bulging" of the segment in systole, usually associated with thin, scarred myocardium

*A score of 0 may be used for hyperkinesis, defined as increased endocardial inward motion and wall thickening in systole.

TABLE 6–3. STRESS ECHOCARDIOGRAPHY

TYPE OF STRESS	ADVANTAGES	DISADVANTAGES
Exercise		
Treadmill exercise	Widely available High workload	Imaging post-ETT only
Upright bicycle	Imaging during exercise	Imaging may be technically difficult Lower workload
Supine bicycle	Imaging during exercise	Lower workload Supine position affects exercise physiology
Pharmacologic		
Dobutamine	Continuous imaging Does not require physically active patient	Potential adverse effects of dobutamine Level of stress achieved
Dipyridamole	Continuous imaging Does not require physically active patient	Potential adverse effects of dipyridamole Induction of relative flow inequality rather than ischemia per se

abnormalities that resolve very rapidly after exercise may be missed.

Exercise Echocardiography

Resting images are acquired in digital format for standard views of the left ventricle. Standard exercise protocols are used with monitoring of the 12-lead ECG, blood pressure, and symptoms by a qualified physician during and following the exercise protocol. The risks of exercise echocardiography are the risks of the exercise test itself.

Either during maximal exercise (supine or sitting bicycle) or immediately after exercise (treadmill), image acquisition is repeated. A repetitive cine-loop acquisition cycle is helpful because respiratory motion limits the examiner's ability to select a good-quality beat quickly in real time. Typically, four or more sequential cycles are recorded digitally, and the examiner subsequently chooses the best image for comparison with the baseline views (Fig. 6–10). Next, the rest and exercise cine-loop digital images are displayed side by side so that endocardial motion and wall thickening for each myocardial region can be compared. A systematic approach, comparing each segment in turn, is needed for detection of subtle abnormalities (Fig. 6–11).

Interpretation of an exercise stress echocardiogram includes incorporation of data on the maximum workload achieved (exercise duration), the heart rate and blood pressure response to exercise, the presence of arrhythmias, and clinical symptoms, as well as evaluation of the echocardiographic images.

Dobutamine Stress Echocardiography

Pharmacologic stress testing with intravenous dobutamine is based on the increased heart rate and contractility induced by this potent beta agonist. Typically, infusions are started at a low dose (5 μg/kg/min) and increased incrementally every 3 to 5 minutes with a calibrated infusion pump until the maximum dose (30 to 40 μg/kg/min) or an endpoint has been reached. Atropine is added, if needed, to achieve an appropriate increase in heart rate. In order to minimize the likelihood of significant adverse effects and to optimize the quality of the data obtained, a dobutamine stress echocardiography examination requires a well-defined study protocol performed in the appropriate clinical setting.

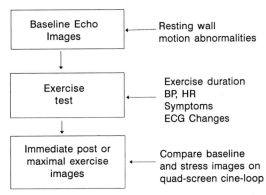

Figure 6–10. Flowchart of an exercise echo protocol.

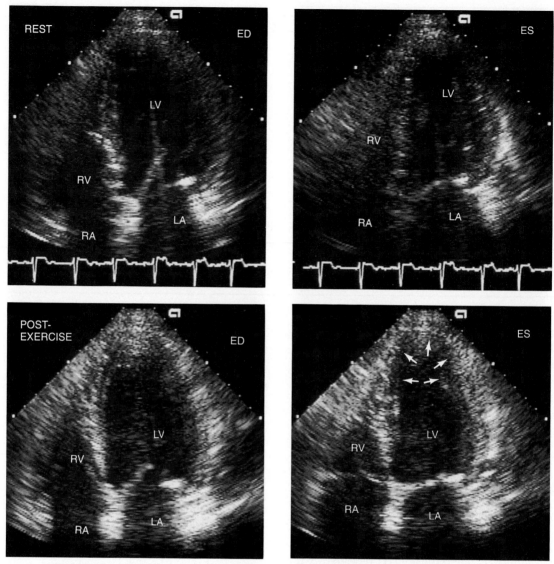

Figure 6–11. Frames from an abnormal exercise echo study showing the development of apical akinesis (*arrows*) with exercise. End-diastolic (ED) images are shown on the left, end-systolic (ES) on the right, with rest images on the top and exercise images on the bottom. The patient was found to have a severe proximal left anterior descending artery stenosis on coronary angiography.

Patient monitoring during dobutamine stress echocardiography includes periodic blood pressure measurement (usually every 2 to 3 minutes), continuous ECG rhythm monitoring, and careful observation for clinical symptoms or signs. Appropriate equipment, medications, and trained personnel should be immediately available in the event of an adverse effect, including a cardiac defibrillator, emergency cardiac medications, intravenous esmolol (a beta blocker that counteracts the effects of dobutamine), and a physician.

After an intravenous line for administration of the dobutamine has been placed, the patient is positioned in a left lateral decubitus position on an echo-stretcher with an apical cutout to allow optimal image acquisition throughout the study protocol. Initially, the intravenous line is filled only with saline while resting data are obtained. At baseline, after 3 minutes at each dosage level, and during recovery, data collection includes recording of heart rate, blood pressure, symptoms, a 12-lead ECG, and echocardiographic images (Fig. 6–12). Standard views include parasternal short-axis images at the base and papillary muscle levels and apical four-chamber, two-

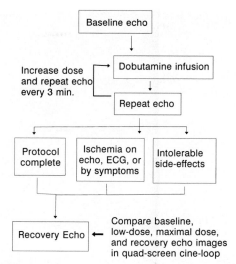

Figure 6–12. Flowchart of dobutamine stress echo protocol.

chamber, and long-axis images. Digital image acquisition in a cine-loop format facilitates interpretation of the study.

Endpoints for stopping the test are (1) reaching the maximum protocol dose, (2) patient discomfort, (3) a definite wall motion abnormality on echocardiography involving two or more adjacent segments, (4) flat or downsloping ST-segment depression >2 mm on ECG, (5) reaching 85 percent of maximum predicted heart rate for age, (6) a systolic blood pressure >200 or <100 mmHg *or* a decline in systolic blood pressure >10 mmHg, and (7) significant ventricular arrhythmias.

Although complications are uncommon when appropriate precautions are observed, reported adverse effects include anxiety, tremulousness, palpitations, arrhythmias, paresthesias, and chest pain. Note that since the purpose of the test is to induce ischemia, a high percentage of patients will have either echocardiographic changes or ECG evidence of ischemia and may experience angina. However, the frequency of angina may be less than with standard ECG stress testing because the protocol can be stopped as soon as wall motion abnormalities are seen (which often is before angina occurs). Hypotension occurs in up to 10 percent of patients but, unlike hypotension with exercise testing, is *not* associated with severe coronary disease or a worse prognosis.

Contraindications to dobutamine stress echocardiography are unstable angina, uncontrolled hypertension, or sensitivity to dobutamine or sulfites.

The echocardiographic images are interpreted after re-formatting the digital images so that each quad screen shows a single view at rest (upper left), low-dose (upper right), maximal dose (lower left), and recovery phase (lower right). For each myocardial segment, wall motion is compared on these images in a systematic fashion. Since wall thickening and endocardial motion normally increase with dobutamine, an abnormal test is defined as the observation of hypo- or akinesis in a region that had normal wall motion at rest (Fig. 6–13).

In addition to detection of ischemic myocardium, dobutamine stress echocardiography has been proposed as a method to evaluate "stunned" or "hibernating" myocardium. For example, in a post–myocardial infarction patient in whom thrombolytic therapy was given, the extent of residual viable myocardium in the area at risk may be unclear early after the event due to myocardial "stunning." Alternatively, a patient with chronic coronary artery disease may have hypokinesis or akinesis at baseline due to "hibernating" myocardium which may recover with revascularization. In both these settings, echocardiographic imaging during low-dose (5 to 10 μg/kg/min) dobutamine infusion has been reported to show improved wall thickening and endocardial motion in viable segments of the myocardium. Of course, at higher dobutamine doses, worsening of regional function may occur due to induction of ischemia.

Other Stress Modalities

Dipyridamole has been proposed for echocardiographic stress testing by some investigators based on the differential pattern of coronary blood flow induced by this agent: increased blood flow in normal coronary arteries with a *relative* decrease in blood flow in diseased vessels. Overall success with this approach has been higher with perfusion imaging (e.g., thallium) because the difference in blood flow between regions supplied by normal versus abnormal coronary arteries can be seen on the radionuclide images. Results with echocardiographic imaging have been less consistent, since actual ischemia (not just a relative difference in blood flow) is needed to discern a wall motion abnormality.

Whichever method of inducing ischemia is used, diagnosis of coronary disease is based on comparison of resting and stress echocardiographic images. Preferably, this is performed using digital image acquisition with cine-loop formatting of a single (good-quality) beat in each tomographic view. Side-by-side display of rest and stress images allows reliable detection of

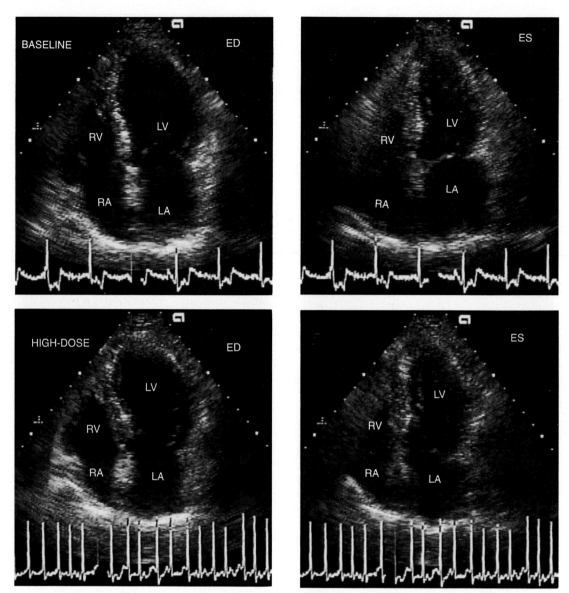

Figure 6–13. Normal dobutamine stress echo. End-diastolic (*left*) and end-systolic (*right*) four-chamber images at baseline (*above*) and at maximal dobutamine dose (*below*) are shown.

new wall motion abnormalities. Typical views for echocardiographic stress testing are a parasternal short-axis view at the papillary muscle level, an apical long-axis view, an apical two-chamber view, and an apical four-chamber view. Other views may be helpful in individual patients depending on image quality and the area of myocardium involved.

Limitations/Technical Aspects

Stress echocardiography has a high sensitivity and specificity for diagnosis of significant coro-

nary artery disease (Tables 6–4 and 6–5). In addition, it allows reliable definition (Tables 6–4 and 6–5) of the anatomic location and extent of ischemic myocardium. However, stress echocardiography does have both technical and physiologic limitations.

The most important potential technical limitation of stress echocardiography is image quality, specifically endocardial definition. Assessment of endocardial wall motion and wall thickening requires adequate delineation of the endocardium for each myocardial segment. Careful attention to patient positioning, transducer orientation, and image-processing param-

TABLE 6–4. SELECTED STUDIES ON THE DIAGNOSTIC ACCURACY OF EXERCISE ECHOCARDIOGRAPHY COMPARED WITH CORONARY ANGIOGRAPHY*

FIRST AUTHOR/YEAR	N	PERCENTAGE WITH DOCUMENTED CAD	SENSITIVITY	SPECIFICITY
Limacher/1984	73	—	91%	88%
Armstrong/1987	123	82%	87	86
Ryan/1988	64	47	78	100
Sawada/1989	57 (women)	49	86	86
Crouse/1991	228	77	97	64
Marwick/1992	179	64	84	86
Quinones/1992	112	77	74	88

*In all studies, significant coronary artery disease was defined as a ≥50 percent stenosis in an epicardial vessel; ETT = exercise treadmill testing.

Data from Limacher et al: Circ 67:1211–18, 1984; Armstrong et al: JACC 10:531–38, 1987; Ryan et al: 11:993–999, 1988; Sawada et al: 14:1440–47, 1989; Crouse et al: AJC 67:1213–18, 1991; Marwick et al: JACC 19:74–81, 1992; Quinones et al: Circ 85:1026–31, 1992.

eters can improve image quality, but definition of certain segments, particularly the anterior wall, may be difficult in some individuals due to adjacent lung tissue.

Exercise and postexercise imaging can be limited by respiratory interference due to a rapid respiratory rate. Digital acquisition in cine-loop format of several cycles, followed by selection of the best images, is necessary for correct interpretation. The possible effects of translation and rotation, both between systole and diastole and between baseline and stress, should be considered in comparisons of wall motion. Given these potential limitations, the interpretation of a stress-echocardiographic study includes a description of image quality as an indicator of the reliability of these results. Suboptimal images should be interpreted with caution.

Potential physiologic limitations are related to the fact that abnormal wall motion occurs only *during* ischemia. First, if the "stress" utilized does *not* induce ischemia, no wall motion abnormality will be seen even if significant coronary disease is present. For example, a patient with limited exercise duration due to hip pain may not achieve a level of exertion that results in ischemia. Similarly, a pharmacologic "stress" that does not induce ischemia will not induce a wall motion abnormality. Second, the duration of ischemia is important. If ischemia has resolved by the time imaging is performed, the wall motion abnormality will not be detected. This is of particular concern with treadmill exercise, since echocardiographic imaging is performed after exertion, although this possible limitation may be offset by the higher maximum workload achieved prior to the recovery period compared with bicycle exercise protocols.

Stress echocardiography in patients with abnormal global or regional function at rest is more difficult to interpret than in subjects with normal resting left ventricular systolic function. The presence of a segmental motion abnormality at rest implies that coronary artery disease, with prior myocardial infarction, is present. With stress imaging, new wall motion abnormalities in regions remote from the site of resting abnormal wall motion indicate additional areas of ischemia. Evaluation of areas adjacent to the resting wall motion abnormality may be problematic due to a potential tethering effect by the abnormal region.

In patients with global systolic dysfunction at rest—which may be due either to end-stage ischemic disease, cardiomyopathy, or chronic valvular disease—stress echocardiography is much less specific for the diagnosis of coronary disease. Differentiation of end-stage ischemic disease from a primary cardiomyopathy is discussed under Myocardial Infarction below. Stress echocardiography also may be helpful in some patients with cardiomyopathy or valvular disease, depending on the specific clinical question.

Alternate Approaches

Exercise Electrocardiography

Exercise ECG remains a standard test for evaluation of patients with suspected or known coronary artery disease. Even though it has a lower sensitivity and specificity for diagnosis of coronary disease compared with imaging techniques, it continues to provide important prognostic data at a low cost in many patients. Imaging techniques most often are needed in subgroups with high false-positive (e.g., women with chest pain) or false-negative rates and in patients with an abnormal resting electrocardiogram which obscures exercise-induced ischemic changes.

Doppler Stress Echocardiography

Doppler stress echocardiography has been proposed as an approach that can be used instead of, or in addition to, evaluation of segmental wall motion. Left ventricular ejection parameters derived from the aortic outflow Doppler velocity curve, including maximum velocity, the velocity-time integral, and the maximum and mean acceleration rates, can be recorded at rest and with stress. The actual changes in an individual patient can be compared with the expected changes for these variables.

Left ventricular diastolic filling is abnormal during ischemia and may be assessed from the Doppler left ventricular inflow curve. Several studies have found that *during* ischemia (e.g., with balloon inflation during percutaneous transluminal angioplasty), the early diastolic filling velocity is reduced, the isovolumic relaxation period is prolonged, and the E/A ratio falls.

These findings are consistent with an acute abnormality in diastolic relaxation. Other studies have found seemingly contradictory results—for example, an increase in the E velocity and E/A ratio with exercise-induced ischemia. Confounding variables that affect the pattern of diastolic filling, most importantly left atrial pressure and heart rate, most likely account for these discrepant results. Another possible explanation is rapid temporal changes in diastolic function during and after ischemia so that the pattern of left ventricular filling varies depending on the time interval between onset of ischemia and the Doppler recording. This possibility is supported by several studies showing that the pattern of left ventricular filling later returns to baseline. Of course, it is simplest to compare changes in an individual patient with his or her own baseline Doppler findings. When comparing patients with each other, other variables that affect diastolic filling, such as age, coexisting mitral regurgitation, PR interval, and ventricular systolic function, further hamper the clinical application of these data. Further studies of the potential utility of this approach are in progress.

Direct Echocardiographic Imaging of the Coronary Arteries

The origins of the right and left coronary arteries often can be identified on transthoracic imaging (Fig. 6–14). On transesophageal imaging, the proximal left coronary can be followed

TABLE 6–5. SELECTED STUDIES ON DIAGNOSTIC ACCURACY OF DOBUTAMINE STRESS ECHOCARDIOGRAPHY COMPARED WITH CORONARY ANGIOGRAPHY

FIRST AUTHOR/ YEAR	SOURCE OF SUBJECTS	N	PERCENTAGE WITH DOCUMENTED CAD	PERCENTAGE STENOSIS CONSIDERED SIGNIFICANT	SENSITIVITY	SPECIFICITY
Berthe/1986	Post-AMI	30	100%	50%	85%	88%
Cohen/1991	Chest pain	70	27	70	86	95
Sawada/1991	Coronary angio	103	44	50	89	85
Mazeika/1992	Coronary angio	50	26	70	78	93
Martin/1992	Coronary angio	40	35	50	76	60
Segar/1992	Coronary angio	85	—	50	95	82
Marcovitz/1992	Coronary angio	141	21	50	96	66
Marwick/1993	Coronary angio	217	65	50	72	83

References: Berthe et al: AJC 58:1167–72, 1986; Cohen et al: AJC 67:1311–18, 1991; Sawada et al: Circ 83:1602–14, 1991; Mazeika et al: JACC 19:1203–11, 1992; Martin et al: AIM 116:190–96, 1992; Segar et al: JACC 19:1197–1202, 1992; Marcovitz et al: AJC 69:1269–73, 1992; Marwick et al: JACC 22:159–167, 1993.

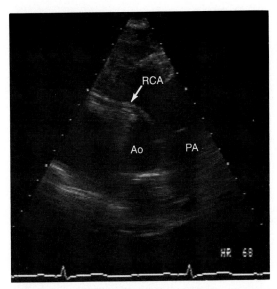

Figure 6–14. Right coronary artery (RCA) seen on a transthoracic parasternal short-axis view.

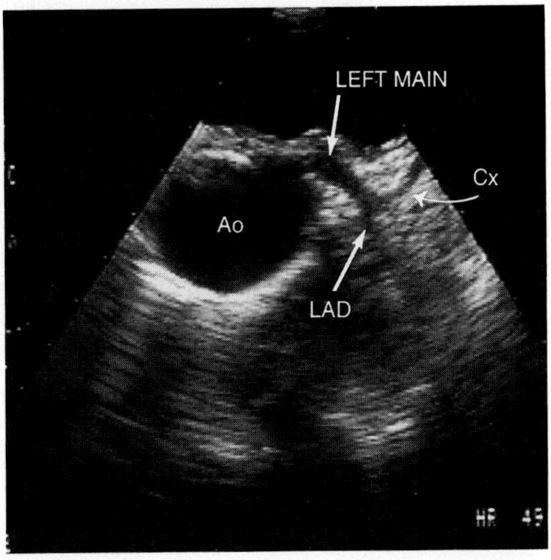

Figure 6–15. Left main coronary artery on transesophageal imaging showing its bifurcation into left anterior descending (LAD) and circumflex (Cx) arteries.

to its bifurcation into left anterior descending and circumflex arteries (Figs. 6–15 and 6–16), and often these branches can be imaged for a portion of their length, as can the right coronary artery. However, clinical decision making usually requires detailed knowledge of the entire extent of the coronary anatomy. Tomographic imaging is a suboptimal method for evaluation of the relatively small coronary vessels which move with the epicardial surface of the heart.

Intravascular ultrasound techniques, in which an imaging transducer is mounted on an intracoronary catheter, provide detailed cross-sectional views of proximal coronary arteries (Fig. 6–17). This application of ultrasound imaging is not covered in this book; suggested readings are indicated at the end of Chapter 3.

Radionuclide Techniques/PET

Radionuclide perfusion imaging techniques with thallium 201 or sestamibi immediately after exercise and at rest after redistribution are well-validated techniques for evaluation of coronary artery disease patients (Fig. 6–18). These techniques also can be performed using dipyridamole to induce heterogeneity in blood flow or with dobutamine to induce ischemia. Compared with stress echocardiography, radionuclide techniques have the advantage that image quality is less dependent on each patient's body habitus, although attenuation due to breast tissue may be a problem in women. Disadvantages of radio-

nuclide techniques include a higher cost, it is less easily performed at the bedside, and it uses ionizing radiation (albeit a low dose). Technical factors are important with both techniques, and data quality at a particular institution depends in part on experience.

Positron emission tomography (PET) combines physiologic and anatomic data and theoretically allows assessment of myocardial metabolism and perfusion. This technique is not widely available clinically, although research applications are considerable.

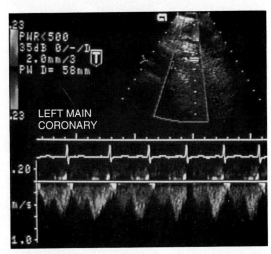

Figure 6–16. Doppler recording of coronary artery blood flow in the left main coronary artery from a transesophageal approach showing predominant diastolic flow.

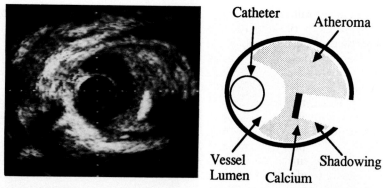

Figure 6–17. Example of typical findings on intravascular ultrasound in a femoral artery with significant disease. Calibrations are 1.0 mm. Note the highly eccentric lumen and the bright echo from calcium with shadowing. (*Reprinted with permission from Linker DT et al: Intra-arterial ultrasound: A potential tool for the vascular surgeon. Eur J Surg 157:373, 1991.*)

Coronary Angiography

Coronary angiography remains the standard of reference for evaluation of coronary artery disease. Cinefluoroscopic films of coronary anatomy in multiple views allow detailed assessment of both proximal and distal coronary anatomy.

Clinical Utility

Diagnosis of Coronary Artery Disease

Stress echocardiography is used for the diagnosis of significant coronary artery disease. The accuracy of stress echocardiography is highly dependent on image quality, specifically endocardial definition, with most investigators reporting success rates for obtaining diagnostic images after treadmill exercise of 85 to 100 percent. The success rate for image acquisition and the quality of the images obtained tend to be greater with supine exercise (in which the patient can be positioned optimally) and with pharmacologic stress (which has the added advantage of little increase in respiratory interference).

Compared with coronary angiography, with significant disease defined as 50 percent narrowing of an epicardial coronary artery, exercise

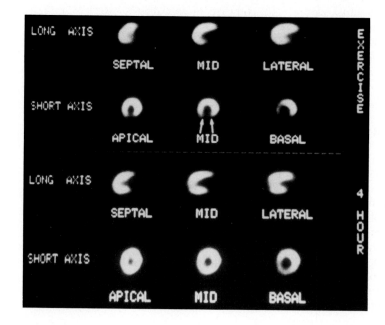

Figure 6–18. Exercise stress thallium study. Three representative vertical long- (septum to lateral wall) and short-axis (apical to basal) tomographic ^{201}Tl images obtained immediately after exercise (*above*) and at 4 hours (*below*). On the exercise images, there is an inferior wall perfusion defect starting in the apical slice on the short-axis view and extending to the midcavity (*arrows*) and basal slice. On the 4-hour images, there is complete redistribution consistent with ischemia without prior infarction in the inferior wall. (*Reprinted with permission from Cerqueira M (ed.): Nuclear Cardiology. Cambridge, Blackwell Scientific, 1994.*)

echocardiography has an overall sensitivity of 74 to 97 percent and a specificity of 64 to 100 percent for diagnosing the presence of coronary artery disease (see Table 6–4). Sensitivity is highest for multivessel disease (>90 percent) and lowest for single-vessel disease (60 to 80 percent) in these studies. In comparison, exercise electrocardiography had a much lower sensitivity at 51 to 63 percent and specificity at 62 to 74 percent, while exercise thallium 201 perfusion imaging tended to have an accuracy similar to echocardiography, with a sensitivity of 61 to 94 percent and a specificity of 81 percent.

Extent and Location of Ischemic Areas

When image quality is adequate, stress echocardiography also allows accurate evaluation of the location and extent of the area of ischemic myocardium. By integrating data from multiple views, a reasonable estimate of the location of significant coronary lesions can be made. Echocardiographic estimates of which and how many coronary arteries are affected correlate well with angiographic findings.

Prognostic Implications

The relationship between stress-echocardiographic results and clinical outcome have been evaluated in several studies. Exercise echocardiography in patients after myocardial infarction predicts subsequent cardiac events with a positive predictive value of 63 to 80 percent and a negative predictive value of 78 to 95 percent. In patients with suspected coronary artery disease, the presence of an inducible wall motion abnormality predicts cardiac events (myocardial infarction, revascularization, death) over the subsequent 12 months with a sensitivity of 45 percent (positive predictive value of only 34 percent) but a specificity of 86 percent (negative predictive value of 91 percent). In patients undergoing noncardiac vascular surgery, dobutamine stress echocardiography is 100 percent sensitive and 69 percent specific for prediction of perioperative unstable angina, myocardial infarction, or death. However, the perioperative cardiac event rate is low, so a positive dobutamine stress echocardiogram has a predictive value of only 19 percent. This test is most helpful when results are *normal*, indicating a low likelihood of a perioperative event (negative predictive value of 100 percent). Further studies on the relationship between stress echocardiography and clinical outcome are needed.

MYOCARDIAL INFARCTION

Basic Principles

Myocardial infarction is irreversible injury to the myocardium due to prolonged ischemia, usually secondary to acute thrombotic occlusion of an epicardial coronary artery at the site of an atherosclerotic plaque. Initially, the affected myocardium becomes akinetic, with normal wall thickness. Over time (4 to 6 weeks), the involved myocardial segments show thinning of the wall and increased echogenicity. A transmural infarction (>50 percent of wall thickness pathologically, Q waves on electrocardiogram clinically) results in a definite area of akinesis and wall thinning. A nontransmural infarction (<50 percent wall thickness pathologically, "non Q wave") may result in a lesser degree of wall thinning and in hypokinesis rather than akinesis.

Since ischemic myocardium also is akinetic in a patient with chest pain, echocardiography cannot distinguish acute infarction from ongoing ischemia. Furthermore, with prolonged ischemia or with successful reperfusion therapy for acute myocardial infarction, a phenomenon called *stunned myocardium* may be seen, where the wall motion abnormality persists for 24 to 72 hours even though irreversible damage has not occurred. Some investigators also propose that prolonged persistence of wall motion abnormalities that can be reversed by reperfusion can occur—termed *hibernating myocardium*. Echocardiographic imaging cannot distinguish between these conditions; it shows the regional myocardial function at the time imaging is performed. The converse of this principle also should be kept in mind. Normal wall motion implies that there is no ischemia *at the time* the images were acquired. Thus normal wall motion *between* episodes of chest pain does not exclude a diagnosis of unstable angina.

Echocardiographic Imaging

The myocardial segments affected and the echocardiographic views for assessment of myocardial infarction are the same as described above for myocardial ischemia.

An occlusion of the left anterior descending artery results in akinesis of the anterior septum, anterior free wall, and apex (Fig. 6–19). Imaging in parasternal long- and short-axis views and in apical views demonstrates these segmental wall motion abnormalities. In the acute setting (Fig. 6–20), the unaffected walls may be hyperkinetic.

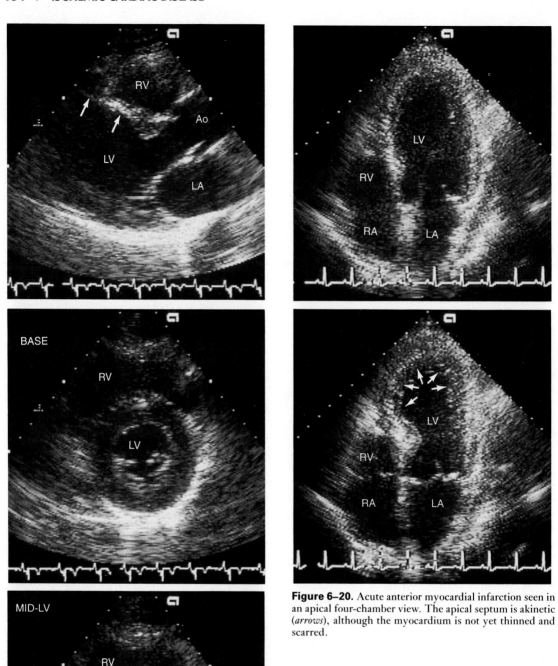

Figure 6–20. Acute anterior myocardial infarction seen in an apical four-chamber view. The apical septum is akinetic (*arrows*), although the myocardium is not yet thinned and scarred.

◄ **Figure 6–19.** Old anterior myocardial infarction with thinning and increased echogenicity of the distal septum (*arrows*) seen in the parasternal long-axis view (*above*) and short-axis views at the mid–left ventricular level (*below*). With this mid-LAD artery occlusion the basal septum (*center*) is normal.

Overall left ventricular systolic function typically is moderately depressed with an average ejection fraction of 41 ± 11 percent after an unreperfused anterior myocardial infarction due to a proximal left anterior descending artery occlusion (Fig. 6–21).

Occlusion of the posterior descending artery results in an inferior myocardial infarction with akinesis of the inferior septum, the inferior free wall, and (to a variable extent) the posterior wall (Figs. 6–22 and 6–23). Parasternal and apical views again are used. The subcostal approach may be particularly helpful in patients with poor image quality from parasternal and apical windows. Typically, overall left ventricular systolic function is only mildly depressed, with an average postinfarction ejection fraction of 53 ± 10 percent after an unreperfused inferior infarction.

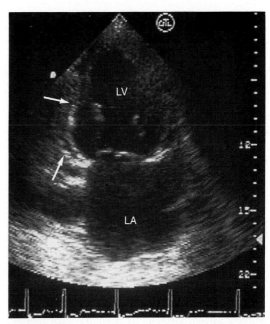

Figure 6–22. Old inferior myocardial infarction with thinning and akinesis of the basal and midventricular segments of the inferior wall (*arrows*) seen in an apical two-chamber view.

With inferior infarction, the echocardiographer should evaluate for possible concurrent right ventricular infarction.

Occlusion of the circumflex artery, resulting in a lateral myocardial infarction, is less common and often is electrocardiographically "silent." Akinesis of the lateral and posterior walls is seen, with a mild to moderately depressed

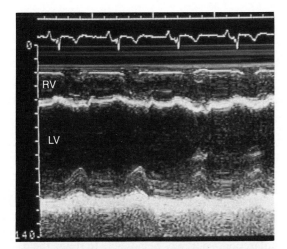

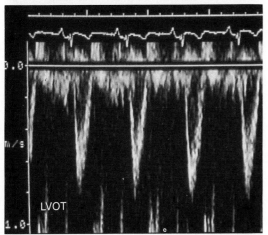

Figure 6–21. M-mode recording of an old anterior myocardial infarction with thinning and increased echogenicity of the septum (*above*). The left ventricular outflow velocity curve shows a reduced antegrade velocity consistent with a reduced stroke volume.

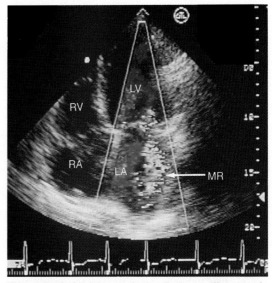

Figure 6–23. Mitral regurgitation due to papillary muscle dysfunction after inferior myocardial infarction.

ejection fraction depending on the extent of myocardium supplied by the circumflex artery in that individual.

Note that these "classic" patterns of wall motion abnormalities will vary with individual variation in coronary anatomy and the location of the occlusion along the length of the coronary artery. Also, these patterns will be altered by the use of reperfusion therapy.

In acute myocardial infarction, diastolic function, as well as systolic function, is abnormal. Acutely, early diastolic relaxation is impaired, with a reduced E velocity on the left ventricular inflow curve. With successful reperfusion, this pattern of diastolic filling tends to normalize over the subsequent 1 to 2 weeks. With large infarctions that are not reperfused, the E velocity also increases postinfarction; however, in this situation, this change in inflow velocity reflects an increased left ventricular end-diastolic pressure rather than "normalization" of the left ventricular filling pattern. In patients with moderate to severely reduced systolic function, the E/A ratio correlates positively with left ventricular end-diastolic and left atrial pressures (i.e., a higher E/A ratio indicates a higher left ventricular end-diastolic pressure) due to the overriding effect of left atrial pressure on the early diastolic filling velocity. It is most helpful to interpret patterns of left ventricular diastolic filling in an individual patient over time with side-by-side comparisons of the echocardiographic findings and integration with other clinical data. Comparisons between patients are limited by the numerous other factors that affect the pattern of left ventricular inflow (see Chap. 5).

Limitations/Alternate Approaches

As for other applications of echocardiography, image quality can be a limiting factor in patients with poor ultrasound tissue penetration. However, with optimal patient positioning, an experienced sonographer, and a state-of-the-art instrument, diagnostic images can be obtained in nearly all patients.

The standard approach to the diagnosis of acute myocardial infarction includes two of the following three findings: (1) a typical clinical presentation, (2) diagnostic electrocardiographic changes, and (3) a consistent pattern of elevation in serum cardiac enzymes. When typical findings of acute myocardial infarction are present, the diagnosis rarely is in doubt. Unfortunately, many patients have an atypical clinical presentation, ECG changes may be nondiagnostic, and cardiac enzymes become elevated only several

hours after the acute event. In these equivocal cases or when a rapid diagnosis is needed for clinical management, prompt echocardiographic imaging may be helpful.

Radionuclide imaging techniques for acute myocardial infarction include thallium perfusion images to detect areas of hypoperfusion. However, an old infarction cannot be distinguished from an acute infarction with this approach.

Coronary angiography, of course, remains the standard of reference for identification of an occluded coronary artery. Concurrent left ventriculography can identify wall motion abnormalities using a right anterior oblique view, showing the anterior wall, apex, and inferior wall in silhouette (Fig. 6–24), and a left anterior oblique view to evaluate the lateral wall (which is superimposed on the ventricular chamber in the right anterior oblique view).

Clinical Utility

Diagnosis of Acute Myocardial Infarction in the Emergency Room

In a patient presenting to the emergency room with chest pain, echocardiographic assessment of global and segmental wall motion can be helpful in clinical decision making. The presence of a segmental wall motion abnormality indicates that coronary artery disease is present—either an acute infarction, ischemia, or an old infarction. Associated hyperkinesis of uninvolved segments suggests an acute event.

Normal wall motion *during pain* is consistent with a very low likelihood of acute myocardial infarction, so it may be possible to triage the patient to a non–coronary-care unit bed depending on the clinical setting. Normal wall motion once pain has resolved is less diagnostic, since unstable angina may be present with wall motion abnormalities seen only *during* episodes of ischemia.

Global left ventricular systolic dysfunction also is an important prognostic sign, indicating significant cardiac disease and the need for further evaluation.

Further studies of the impact of early echocardiographic evaluation of left ventricular wall motion on clinical decision making, clinical outcome, and total costs are needed.

Evaluation of Interventional Therapy for Acute Myocardial Infarction

In a patient with a history suggestive of acute myocardial infarction but a nondiagnostic ECG,

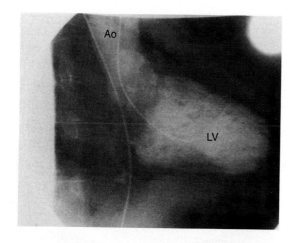

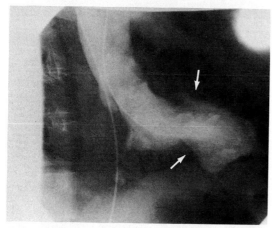

Figure 6–24. Left ventricular angiography showing an akinetic apex (*between arrows*) due to myocardial infarction.

a definite segmental wall motion abnormality on echocardiography may significantly alter decisions regarding reperfusion therapy or may prompt emergent coronary angiography, depending on the specific clinical situation.

In a patient with a definite myocardial infarction by clinical and ECG criteria, echocardiography allows assessment of the location and extent of "myocardium at risk." Once reperfusion therapy has been initiated, echocardiography can be used to assess its effects, although the several-day time lag between successful reperfusion and normalization of wall motion ("stunned" myocardium) makes this evaluation most meaningful before hospital discharge or at outpatient follow-up. However, echocardiography can be helpful in identification of recurrent ischemia in patients with recurrent chest pain by identification of wall motion abnormalities in regions that previously were normal.

At long-term follow-up after myocardial infarction, echocardiography allows assessment of global ventricular function and long-term ventricular dilation due to "infarct expansion."

Complications of Myocardial Infarction

Echocardiography is the procedure of choice for initial evaluation of the post–myocardial infarction patient with a new systolic murmur. Most commonly, the etiology of the murmur is *mitral regurgitation* due to either papillary muscle dysfunction, abnormal wall motion of the segment underlying a papillary muscle, or papillary muscle rupture. The presence and severity of mitral regurgitation are evaluated using Doppler techniques (see Chap. 10), and the etiology is inferred from two-dimensional (2D) imaging. Partial or complete rupture of the papillary muscle is a catastrophic complication that can be recognized as a flail leaflet with an attached mass (the papillary muscle head) that prolapses into the left atrium in systole (Fig. 6–25). Transesophageal imaging is indicated when this diagnosis is suspected and transthoracic images are inadequate.

Another cause of a new systolic murmur after myocardial infarction is a *ventricular septal defect* due to necrosis and rupture of a focal area of the interventricular septum (Fig. 6–26). Identification of the rupture site may be difficult with 2D imaging, especially since this complication tends to occur with *small* infarcts so that the wall motion abnormality may be subtle. Evaluation with Doppler ultrasound establishes the diagnosis, with a high-velocity left-to-right systolic jet recorded with continuous-wave Doppler ultrasound and systolic turbulence on the right ventricular side of the septum recorded with conventional pulsed Doppler or color flow imaging.

When *ventricular rupture* occurs in the free wall of the left ventricle (instead of in the septum), mortality is extremely high due to extravasation of blood into the pericardial space and acute pericardial tamponade. However, some patients have a temporary respite due to containment of the rupture by pericardial adhesions or by thrombosis at the rupture site. In these patients, echocardiography may establish the diagnosis, prompting emergent surgery (Fig. 6–27). Echocardiographic clues of ventricular rupture (in the appropriate clinical setting) include a diffuse or localized pericardial effusion and a discrete segmental wall motion abnormality. Occasionally, the site of rupture can be visualized on 2D imaging, and rarely, flow from the ventricle into the pericardial space can be demonstrated with Doppler techniques.

A chronic, contained ventricular rupture is

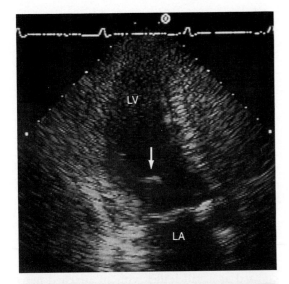

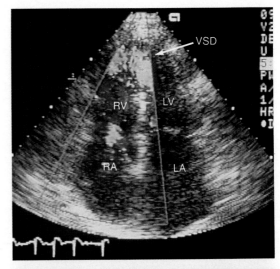

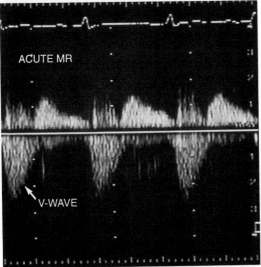

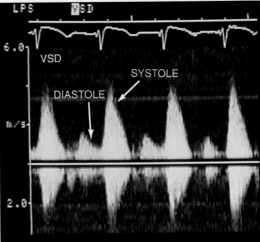

Figure 6–25. Partial rupture of the posteromedial papillary muscle (*arrow*) seen in an apical long-axis view following myocardial infarction (*above*). The continuous-wave Doppler signal (*below*) shows an intense mitral regurgitant jet with a late systolic decline in velocity consistent with a *v* wave.

Figure 6–26. Color flow image showing left-to-right flow across an apical ventricular septal defect (VSD) after myocardial infarction (*above*). Continuous-wave Doppler (*below*) shows high-velocity left-to-right flow in systole with lower-velocity left-to-right flow in diastole across the defect.

called a *pseudoaneurysm*. A left ventricular pseudoaneurysm has a wall composed of pericardium (no myocardial fibers). Characteristic features are a narrow "neck" at the site of rupture with an abrupt transition from normal myocardium to the aneurysm and a ratio of the diameter at the "neck" to the maximum diameter of the aneurysm of <0.5 (Fig. 6–28). Typically, the pseudoaneurysm is partially filled with thrombus. Often, flow in and out of the pseudoaneurysm is seen, and clinically, a corresponding apical murmur may be appreciated on auscultation. While long-term survival has been described oc-

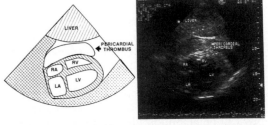

Figure 6–27. Subcostal four-chamber echocardiographic image showing pericardial fluid and a large amount of echodense pericardial thrombus. (*Reprinted with permission from Raitt MH et al: Subacute ventricular free wall rupture complicating myocardial infarction. Am Heart J 126:946–955, 1993.*)

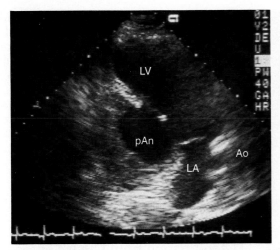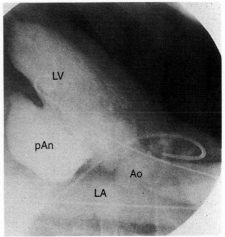

Figure 6–28. Apical long-axis view showing a basal aneurysm filled with thrombus with a narrow neck (*above*) consistent with a pseudoaneurysm (pAn). Angiography (oriented to match the apical long-axis view) shows a similar appearance (*below*).

casionally in patients with a pseudoaneurysm, correct echocardiographic diagnosis is essential. Surgical repair usually is recommended given a high likelihood of spontaneous rupture.

A *pericardial effusion* also can be seen after myocardial infarction as a nonspecific response to transmural infarction. This effusion may be asymptomatic or may be associated with clinical symptoms (chest pain) and signs (ECG changes) of acute pericarditis. While usually benign, tamponade physiology can occur.

Another complication of acute myocardial infarction for which echocardiography is the diagnostic procedure of choice is *right ventricular infarction*. Clinical diagnosis requires a high level of suspicion. Other clinical tests, such as ST-segment elevation in right-sided ECG leads, are not as sensitive or specific as echocardiography. Right ventricular infarction most often is associated with an inferior left ventricular infarct. Echocardiographic findings include right ventricular hypokinesis or akinesis with variable degrees of right ventricular dilation. This diagnosis significantly changes the clinical management of these patients (i.e., low cardiac output is treated with volume infusions rather than with afterload reduction or inotropic agents).

Longer-term complications of acute myocardial infarction include aneurysm formation, left ventricular thrombi, and the sequelae of the irreversible decrease in left ventricular systolic function. A *left ventricular aneurysm* is defined echocardiographically as a dyskinetic region with a diastolic contour abnormality (Fig. 6–29). Apical aneurysms are most common, but inferobasal aneurysms also may be seen. Note that a

"true" left ventricular aneurysm, unlike a "false" or pseudoaneurysm, is lined by (thinned) myocardium. There is a smooth transition from normal myocardium to the thinned area with an obtuse angle between the aneurysm and body of the left ventricle. The ratio of the diameter of the junction between the aneurysm and the remainder of the left ventricle to the maximum aneurysm diameter is >0.5 (see Fig. 8–16).

Left ventricular thrombi form in regions of stasis of blood flow, such as in an apical aneurysm or overlying an area of akinesis in other regions of the left ventricle. Evidence of severely reduced overall ventricular function, an aneurysm, an akinetic area, and the appearance of a spontaneous contrast effect in the left ventricle all increase the likelihood of left ventricular thrombus formation. Only rarely (as in hypereosinophilic syndrome) do ventricular thrombi occur in the absence of an underlying wall motion abnormality.

A thrombus is identified as an area of increased echogenicity within the ventricular chamber, distinct from the endocardium. Often, the thrombus protrudes into the chamber with a convex contour, but laminated thrombus with a concave contour following the endocardial curve also can be seen. Care is needed to distinguish a thrombus from prominent apical trabeculation with a false tendon or "web" traversing the apex of the left ventricular chamber.

Diagnosis of apical thrombi is enhanced by using a 5-MHz transducer (improved near-field resolution), sliding the transducer laterally from the apical window and then angulating medially and superiorly to obtain a short-axis view of the

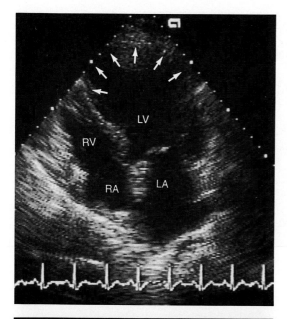

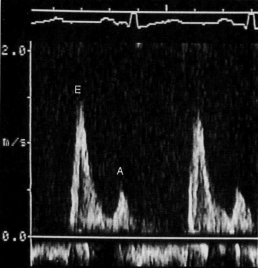

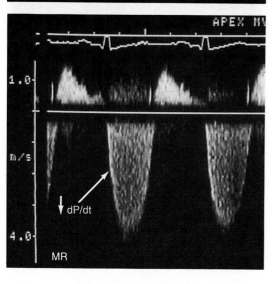

apex. These procedures allow clear definition of the apical endocardium in most individuals. However, if images are suboptimal, appropriate interpretation should indicate that a thrombus "cannot be excluded," especially if the patient is a high risk for left ventricular thrombus formation. Note that transesophageal imaging is rarely helpful for this diagnosis because the apex often cannot be visualized and is in the far field of the image plane (see Figs. 8–16 and 13–18).

END-STAGE ISCHEMIC CARDIAC DISEASE

Differentiation from Other Causes of Left Ventricular Systolic Dysfunction
(Table 6–6)

The diagnosis of coronary artery disease is clear in patients with definite segmental wall motion abnormalities that correspond to the distribution of coronary blood flow. In end-stage ischemic disease, repeated transmural and subendocardial infarctions result in a diffuse pattern of abnormal wall thickening and endocardial motion. Thus, when global systolic dysfunction is present, it may be difficult to differentiate between end-stage ischemic disease and systolic dysfunction due to long-standing valvular disease or a dilated cardiomyopathy (Fig. 6–30).

Echocardiographic Approach

Several features of the echocardiographic examination help in this differentiation. The segmental pattern of left ventricular wall motion is examined carefully in each tomographic plane. While patients with a dilated cardiomyopathy may have a somewhat asymmetrical pattern of wall motion with relative preservation at the ventricular base, definite areas of akinesis or wall thinning suggest ischemic disease. The degree of reduction in overall ventricular function (ejection fraction) is important in patient management but does not assist in determining the etiology of disease.

Right ventricular size and systolic function are normal in patients with ischemic disease un-

◄ **Figure 6–29.** Apical dilation and systolic dyskinesis (*above*) consistent with an apical aneurysm. The pattern of left ventricular inflow (*center*) shows a prominent *E* velocity consistent with an elevated left ventricular end-diastolic pressure. The mitral regurgitant velocity curve in this patient (*below*) shows a reduced *dP/dt*.

TABLE 6–6. DIFFERENTIATION OF LEFT VENTRICULAR SYSTOLIC DYSFUNCTION DUE TO END-STAGE ISCHEMIC DISEASE FROM DILATED CARDIOMYOPATHY OR CHRONIC VALVULAR DISEASE

FINDING	END-STAGE ISCHEMIC DISEASE	DILATED CARDIOMYOPATHY	CHRONIC VALVULAR DISEASE
Left-ventricular ejection fraction	Moderate–severely depressed	Moderate–severely depressed	Moderate–severely depressed
Segmental wall motion abnormalities	May be present	Absent	Absent
Right ventricular systolic function	Normal	Decreased	Variable
Pulmonary artery pressures	Elevated	Elevated	Elevated
Mitral regurgitation	Moderate	Moderate	Moderate–severe
Aortic regurgitation	Not significant	Not significant	Moderate–severe

less there has been a previous right ventricular infarction. Dilated cardiomyopathy occasionally affects the two ventricles in differing degrees but most often results in a symmetrical pattern of right and left ventricular dilation and reduced systolic function.

Mitral valve regurgitation typically accompanies both dilated cardiomyopathy and end-stage ischemic disease due to one of several mechanisms, including mitral annular dilation, reduced papillary muscle systolic function, or malalignment of the papillary muscles. Left ventricular dilation and systolic dysfunction *due to* chronic mitral regurgitation, in contrast to mitral regurgitation due to ventricular dilation and dysfunction, usually are associated with anatomic abnormalities of the mitral leaflets themselves (e.g., myxomatous or rheumatic disease).

Pulmonary artery pressures are elevated to variable degrees in patients with left ventricular dysfunction of any etiology, due to chronic elevation in left ventricular end-diastolic pressure. Pulmonary pressures can be estimated from the tricuspid regurgitant jet velocity or from the pulmonary artery systolic velocity curve as described in Chapter 4.

Mild degrees of tricuspid valve regurgitation are common in ischemic disease, but moderate or severe regurgitation usually is a response to chronic pulmonary hypertension or chronic right ventricular dilation and systolic dysfunction.

Note that aortic regurgitation is *not* a consequence of left ventricular dilation or systolic dysfunction. Left ventricular dilation typically does not result in an increase in the diameter of the aortic annulus or adjacent outflow tract. The

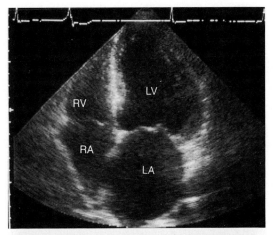

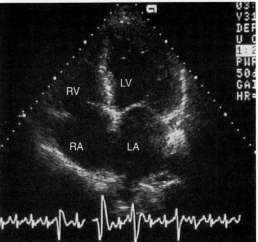

Figure 6–30. End-stage ischemic heart disease (*above*) and a dilated cardiomyopathy (*below*) often appear similar on 2D echocardiography. Note that the ischemic disease patient has normal right ventricular size and systolic function.

finding of moderate or severe aortic regurgitation implies primary valvular disease or aortic root dilation.

Left ventricular thrombi may be present with severe left ventricular dysfunction of any etiology. The observation of reduced systolic function should prompt a search for apical thrombi, but this finding does not help in the differential diagnosis.

Limitations/Alternate Approaches

If a diagnosis of end-stage ischemic disease versus a primary cardiomyopathy would alter patient management, coronary angiography may be needed for a definitive diagnosis, to document the exact site and severity of coronary lesions, and to assess the distal vessel anatomy.

SUGGESTED READING

BASIC PRINCIPLES

1. Kaul S: Echocardiography in coronary artery disease. Curr Prob Cardiol 15:239–298, 1990.
   Concise review of the role of echocardiography in acute myocardial infarction (including complications) and chronic ischemic disease. Brief introduction of concepts of myocardial perfusion imaging, intravascular coronary artery imaging, and tissue characterization. Two hundred and one references.

2. Report of the American Society of Echocardiography Committee on Nomenclature and Standards: Identification of Myocardial Wall Segments. American Society of Echocardiography, Durham, North Carolina, 1982.
   American Society of Echocardiography standards for nomenclature of myocardial wall segments. While several simplifications of this basic 20-segment scheme have been utilized, the concept of dividing the ventricle into thirds from base to apex and the definitions of anterior, lateral, posterior, inferior, and septum are used by all experienced centers.

3. Sheehan FS, Feneley MP, DeBruijn NP, et al: Quantitative analysis of regional wall thickening by transesophageal echocardiography. J Thorac Cardiovasc Surg 103:347–354, 1992.
   Example of the application of quantitative methods for evaluation of regional ventricular function to echocardiographic images. The low variability of the proposed centerline method for normalized wall thickening suggests that this may be a useful standardized approach.

EXERCISE ECHO

4. Armstrong WF: Stress echocardiography for detection of coronary artery disease. Circulation 84(suppl I):43–49, 1991.
   Review of principle of stress echocardiography with a concise review of studies prior to 1991. Fifty references.

5. Quinones MA, Verani MS, Haichin RM, et al: Exercise echocardiography versus ²⁰¹Tl single-photon emission computed tomography in evaluation of cor-

onary artery disease: Analysis of 292 patients. Circulation 85:1026–1031, 1992.
   Direct comparison of simultaneous exercise echocardiography and thallium 201 SPECT perfusion imaging in 292 patients (112 underwent coronary angiography). Echo and SPECT agreed in 88 percent of cases (normal versus abnormal) and had an agreement rate of 82 percent by ventricular region. Of note, about a third of regions with fixed defects on SPECT showed wall thickening on echocardiography. Conversely, fixed wall motion abnormalities on echo often showed some degree of perfusion on SPECT.

6. Marwick TH, Nemec JJ, Pashkow FJ, et al: Accuracy and limitations of exercise echocardiography in a routine clinical setting. J Am Coll Cardiol 19:74–81, 1992.
   In 179 post-treadmill stress echocardiograms, factors that limited accuracy were a submaximal exercise test (<85 percent of age-predicted maximal heart rate), less severe coronary narrowing, and single-vessel disease. Accuracy was maintained over a wide range of image quality.

7. Sheikh KH, Bengtson JR, Helmy S, et al: Relation of quantitative coronary lesion measurements to the development of exercise-induced ischemia assessed by exercise echocardiography. J Am Coll Cardiol 15:1043–1051, 1990.
   In 34 patients with single-vessel coronary artery disease, the development of wall motion abnormalities on exercise echocardiography correlated with the degree of coronary narrowing measured quantitatively. This suggests that exercise echo may be a useful modality for assessing the physiologic significance of a coronary artery lesion.

DOBUTAMINE STRESS ECHO

8. Mertes H, Sawada SG, Ryan T, et al: Symptoms, adverse effects, and complications associated with dobutamine stress echocardiography: Experience in 1118 patients. Circulation 88:15–19, 1993.
   Complications of dobutamine stress echocardiography that required termination of the test protocol included noncardiac symptoms (nausea, anxiety, headache, tremor, urgency) in 3 percent, and angina pectoris in 19.3 percent (which was relieved by sublingual nitroglycerin or a short-acting beta blocker in all cases). Arrhythmias included premature ventricular contractions in 15 percent, premature atrial contractions in 8 percent, and nonsustained ventricular tachycardia in 40 (3.5 percent) patients. There were no deaths, myocardial infarctions, or episodes of sustained ventricular tachycardia.

9. Segar DS, Brown SE, Sawada SG, et al: Dobutamine stress echocardiography: Correlation with coronary lesion severity as deter mined by quantitative angiography. J Am Coll Cardiol 19:1197–1202, 1992.
   In 85 patients, the sensitivity of dobutamine stress echocardiography (DSE) for detection of ≥50 percent stenosis was similar for the three major coronary arteries. Abnormal wall motion on DSE correlated best with a minimum lumen diameter <1 mm on quantitative coronary angiography. Abnormal wall motion at a heart rate ≤125 beats per minute was predictive of multivessel disease.

10. Marcovitz PA, Armstrong WF: Accuracy of dobutamine stress echocardiography in detecting coronary artery disease. Am J Cardiol 69:1269–1273, 1992.
   In 141 patients with suspected coronary artery disease, dobutamine stress echocardiography had a sensitivity of 96 percent for detecting coronary artery disease but a specificity of only 66 percent. Specificity increased to 91 percent (and sensitivity decreased to 87 percent) when only subjects with normal resting wall motion were considered. Resting abnormal-

ities leading to false-positive results most often were due to cardiomyopathy or valvular heart disease.

11. Mazeika PK, Nadazdin A, Oakley CM: Dobutamine stress echocardiography for detection and assessment of coronary artery disease. J Am Coll Cardiol 19: 1203–1211, 1992.
Sensitivity of dobutamine stress echocardiography for diagnosis of coronary artery disease (≥ 70 percent stenosis) was dependent on the number of vessels involved: one-vessel (50 percent), two-vessel (60 percent), and three-vessel disease (sensitivity 86 percent). It was observed that in addition to wall motion, the presence of inducible mitral regurgitation improves sensitivity and maintains specificity for diagnosis of coronary artery disease.

12. Marwick T, Willemart B, D'Hondt AM, et al: Selection of the optimal nonexercise stress for the evaluation of ischemic regional myocardial dysfunction and malperfusion. Circulation 87:345–354, 1993.
In 97 patients without previous infarction, dobutamine stress echocardiography had a sensitivity of 85 percent with a specificity of 82 percent for significant coronary artery disease, defined as >50 percent stenosis. In the same patients, dobutamine sestamibi had a sensitivity and specificity of 80 percent and 74 percent, adenosine echocardiography had a sensitivity of 58 percent and a specificity of 87 percent, and adenosine sestamibi had a sensitivity of 86 percent and specificity of 71 percent.

13. Poldermans D, Fioretti PM, Forster T, et al: Dobutamine stress echocardiography for assessment of perioperative cardiac risk in patients undergoing major vascular surgery. Circulation 87:1506–1512, 1993.
In 136 patients undergoing vascular surgery, dobutamine stress echocardiography showed a new or worsened wall motion abnormality in 35 of 131 completed studies. All 15 patients with a cardiac complication (unstable angina, pulmonary edema, or death due to myocardial infarction) had an abnormal dobutamine stress echocardiographic test.

14. Eichelberger JP, Schwarz KQ, Black ER, et al: Predictive value of dobutamine echocardiography just before noncardiac vascular surgery. Am J Cardiol 72:602–607, 1993.
In 75 patients undergoing noncardiac vascular surgery there were 5 (7 percent) perioperative cardiac events (unstable angina, myocardial infarction, or death). Dobutamine stress echocardiography had a positive predictive value of 19 percent and a negative predictive value of 100 percent for perioperative cardiac events.

DOPPLER STRESS ECHO

15. Mehdirad AA, Williams GA, Labovita AJ, et al: Evaluation of left ventricular function during upright exercise: Correlation of exercise Doppler with postexercise two-dimensional echocardiographic results. Circulation 75:413–419, 1987.
See comment with Suggested Reading 14.

16. Harrison MR, Smith MD, Friedman BJ, DeMaria AN: Uses and limitations of exercise Doppler echocardiography in the diagnosis of ischemic heart disease. J Am Coll Cardiol 10:809–817, 1987.
See comment with Suggested Reading 14.

17. Christie J, Sheldahl LM, Tristani FE, et al: Determination of stroke volume and cardiac output during exercise: Comparison of two-dimensional and Doppler echocardiography, Fick oximetry, and thermodilution. Circulation 76:539–547, 1987.
These three studies present the use of Doppler measures of ventricular function in conjunction with exercise testing in small series of subjects. Aortic flow velocity, acceleration,

and percentage change in peak ejection velocity are proposed as useful measures of overall left ventricular systolic function.

MYOCARDIAL INFARCTION

18. Kloner RA, Parisi AF: Acute myocardial infarction: Diagnostic and prognostic applications of two-dimensional echocardiography. Circulation 75:521–524, 1987.
Editorial outlining the potential role of echocardiography in optimizing the use of thrombolytic therapy for patients with acute myocardial infarction.

19. Fleishmann KE, Goldman L, Robiolio PA, et al: Echocardiographic correlates of survival in patients with chest pain. J Am Coll Cardiol 23:1390–1396, 1994.
In 513 presenting to the emergency room with chest pain, 92 percent were admitted to the hospital, 48 percent had ischemic changes on ECG, 46 percent had a history of corollary artery disease, and 21 percent suffered an acute myocardial infarction. At 28.5 month follow-up 20 percent had died (57 percent cardiovascular) with echocardiographic predictors of overall mortality and death from, cardiovascular causes being severe left ventricular systolic dysfunction and moderate or severe mitral regurgitation (even when adjusted for clinical and ECG variables).

20. Bourdillon PDV, Broderick TM, Williams ES, et al: Early recovery of regional left ventricular function after reperfusion in acute myocardial infarction assessed by serial two-dimensional echocardiography. Am J Cardiol 63:641–646, 1989.
Wall motion assessed by echocardiography showed improvement over the first 3 days after reperfusion for acute myocardial infarction, with no further improvement at 7 days.

21. Otto CM, Stratton JR, Maynard C, et al: Echocardiographic evaluation of segmental wall motion early and late after thrombolytic therapy in acute myocardial infarction: The Western Washington Tissue Plasminogen Activator Emergency Room Trial. Am J Cardiol 65:132–138, 1990.
Concordance between infarct location by echocardiography and angiography was 81 percent (versus 76 percent for ECG) in 92 acute myocardial infarction patients. Improvement in wall motion between the acute presentation and 3-month follow-up was seen only in subjects with reperfusion within 2 hours of symptom onset.

22. Picard MH, Wilkins GT, Ray PA, Weyman AE: Natural history of left ventricular size and function after acute myocardial infarction. Assessment and prediction by echocardiographic endocardial surface mapping. Circulation 82:484–494, 1990.
Left ventricular endocardial "maps" were used to quantitate the area of abnormal wall motion in 57 patients with acute myocardial infarction studied at entry and at 3 months. Infarct expansion at the apex was seen in subjects with anterior infarctions and an increased endocardial surface area index at entry.

MYOCARDIAL VIABILITY

23. Cigarroa CG, deFilippi CR, Brickner E, et al: Dobutamine stress echocardiography identifies hibernating myocardium and predicts recovery of left ventricular function after coronary revascularization. Circulation 88:430–436, 1993.
In 25 patients with multivessel coronary artery disease and depressed ventricular function, dobutamine stress echocardiography was performed preoperatively and after revascularization. After revascularization, ventricular function im-

proved in 9/11 patients with contractile reserve (defined as improvement in wall thickening in 2 adjacent segments or greater than a 20 percent improvement in the regional wall thickening score) but in only 2/14 patients without contractile reserve.

24. Smart SC, Sawada S, Ryan T, et al: Low-dose dobutamine echocardiography detects reversible dysfunction after thrombolytic therapy of acute myocardial infarction. Circulation 88:405–415, 1993.
In 51 patients with dobutamine echocardiographic studies performed within 7 days and again 4 weeks post–myocardial infarction, dobutamine-responsive wall motion had a specificity of 90 percent and a sensitivity of 86 percent for reversible myocardial dysfunction.

COMPLICATIONS OF ACUTE MYOCARDIAL INFARCTION

25. Panidis IP, Mintz GS, Goel I, et al: Acquired ventricular septal defect after myocardial infarction: Detection by combined two-dimensional and Doppler echocardiography. Am Heart J 111:427–429, 1986.
Classic article describing the echocardiographic diagnosis of ventricular septal defect after myocardial infarction.

26. Come PC, Riley MF, Weintraub R, et al: Echocardiographic detection of complete and partial papillary muscle rupture during acute myocardial infarction. Am J Cardiol 56:787–789, 1985.
Mechanism and echocardiographic diagnosis of post–myocardial infarction mitral regurgitation are discussed.

27. Raitt MH, Kraft CD, Gardner CJ, et al: Subacute ventricular free wall rupture complicating myocardial infarction. Am Heart J 126:946–955, 1993.
Review of the literature and four case reports of left ventricular rupture after myocardial infarction emphasizing that this diagnosis may be made by echocardiography and can be successfully treated surgically. 73 references.

28. Visser CA, Kan G, Meltzer RS, et al: Incidence, timing, and prognostic value of left ventricular aneurysm formation after myocardial infarction: A prospective, serial echocardiographic study in 158 patients. Am J Cardiol 57:729–732, 1986.
Left ventricular aneurysm formation was seen within 3 months in 22 percent of patients with nonreperfused myocardial infarctions—29/90 (32 percent) anterior and 6/68 (9 percent) posterior infarctions.

29. Asinger RW, Mikell FL, Elsperger J, Hodges M: Incidence of left ventricular thrombosis after acute transmural myocardial infarction. N Engl J Med 305:297–302, 1981.
In the prethrombolytic era, the incidence of apical thrombus detectable by two-dimensional echocardiography was 0/35 inferior infarctions and 12/35 (34 percent) anterior infarctions. Thrombi occurred only in areas of akinesis or dyskinesis.

30. Kinch JW, Ryan TJ: Right ventricular infarction. N Engl J Med 330:1211–1217, 1994.
A concise and well-written review of the clinical presentation, diagnosis, and management of right ventricular infarction. The echocardiographic approach is emphasized and compared with ECG and hemodynamic and radionuclide findings. 78 references.

CLINICAL OUTCOME AFTER MYOCARDIAL INFARCTION

31. Voller H, von Ameln H, Spielberg C, et al: Hemodynamic response to exercise-induced myocardial ischemia detected by transmitral filling patterns derived from Doppler echocardiography. J Am Soc Echocardiogr 6:255–264, 1993.
Diastolic left ventricular filling during exercise-induced ischemia in 13 patients was compared with exercise changes in 15 patients with old myocardial infarction (but no ischemia) and 11 normal controls. With ischemia, A velocity was lower and the E/A ratio was higher than in the normal individuals or old myocardial infarction patients. The mechanism is postulated to be a greater increase in left atrial pressure with exercise.

32. Lewis BS, Emmott SN, Smyllie J, et al: Left ventricular systolic and diastolic function, and exercise capacity six to eight weeks after acute myocardial infarction. The DEFIANT Study Group. Am J Cardiol 72:149–153, 1993.
In 115 patients with a median left ventricular ejection fraction of 43 percent, the left ventricular inflow Doppler A velocity was related inversely and the E/A ratio was related directly to exercise capacity. In contrast, measures of left ventricular systolic dysfunction did not predict exercise workload.

33. Pozzoli M, Capomolla S, Opasich C, et al: Left ventricular filling pattern and pulmonary wedge pressure are closely related in patients with recent anterior myocardial infarction and left ventricular dysfunction. Eur Heart J 13:1067–1073, 1992.
The E/A ratio and early diastolic deceleration time correlated with pulmonary wedge pressure in 50 patients after anterior myocardial infarction with an ejection fraction <40 percent. An E/A ratio ≥1 predicted a pulmonary wedge pressure >20 mmHg with a sensitivity of 100 percent and specificity of 86 percent.

34. Crawford MH: Risk stratification after myocardial infarction with exercise and Doppler echocardiography. Circulation 84(suppl 3):I163–166, 1991.
Summary of the utility of exercise echocardiography for predicting prognosis after myocardial infarction.

35. Krivokapich J, Child JS, Gerber RS, et al: Prognostic usefulness of positive or negative exercise stress echocardiography for predicting coronary events in ensuing twelve months. Am J Cardiol 71:646–651, 1993.
In 360 patients with suspected coronary artery disease (60 percent of whom had resting wall motion abnormalities on echocardiography), an inducible wall motion abnormality on exercise echocardiography predicted cardiac events (myocardial infarction, revascularization, or death) over 12 months follow-up with a sensitivity of 45 percent and a specificity of 86 percent. Patients unable to reach an appropriate stress level had a high rate of cardiac events even when the echocardiogram was nondiagnostic (17 of 27 patients).

36. St. John Sutton M, Pfeffer MA, Plappert T, et al: Quantitative two-dimensional echocardiographic measurements are major predictors of adverse cardiovascular events after acute myocardial infarction. Circulation 89:68–75, 1994.
In 512 patients with echocardiograms 11 days and 1 year post–myocardial infarction, baseline left ventricular (LV) end-systolic area and percent change in area were strong predictors of cardiac death and cardiac events. Patients treated with captopril had smaller LV areas at 1 year with a greater percent change in cavity area in the captopril group and a lower rate of adverse outcomes (risk reduction 35 percent). These data suggest that LV enlargement and function after myocardial infarction are predictors of outcome and that prevention of LV enlargement, as assessed by echocardiography, improves clinical outcome.

ECHOCARDIOGRAPHIC APPROACH TO THE CARDIOMYOPATHIES, HYPERTENSIVE HEART DISEASE, POST-CARDIAC TRANSPLANT PATIENT, AND PULMONARY HEART DISEASE

Right Ventricular Pressure
Overload
Secondary Tricuspid Regurgitation
Limitations/Technical Considerations

Clinical Utility
Alternate Approaches
SUGGESTED READING

INTRODUCTION

Cardiomyopathy is defined as a primary disease of the myocardium, excluding myocardial dysfunction due to ischemia or chronic valvular disease. There are several possible approaches to classification of cardiomyopathies, such as etiology or anatomy, but a physiologic classification is most useful clinically. The three basic physiologic categories of cardiomyopathy are dilated, hypertrophic, and restrictive. The disease process in an individual patient may correspond closely with one of these physiologic categories; however, overlap between these categories (particularly between dilated and restrictive) can occur. Echocardiographic evaluation focuses on confirming the diagnosis and type of cardiomyopathy present and on defining the physiologic consequences of the disease process in that individual (Table 7–1).

While hypertensive and pulmonary heart disease, strictly speaking, are not cardiomyopathies, they are included in this chapter because

their clinical and echocardiographic presentation may mimic a cardiomyopathy. In addition, evaluation of the post-cardiac transplant patient is included here.

DILATED CARDIOMYOPATHY

Basic Principles

Dilated cardiomyopathy is characterized by four-chamber enlargement with impaired systolic function of both ventricles. The list of possible etiologies is long and includes postviral, toxins (e.g., alcohol), parasitic diseases (e.g., Chagas' disease), peripartum, and idiopathic (Table 7–2). The physiology is characterized predominantly by impaired contractility with a reduced cardiac output and elevated left ventricular end-diastolic pressure. Patients most often present with heart failure symptoms. Coexisting mitral regurgitation frequently is present sec-

TABLE 7–1. TYPICAL FEATURES OF THE THREE PHYSIOLOGIC TYPES OF CARDIOMYOPATHY

	DILATED	HYPERTROPHIC	RESTRICTIVE
Left ventricular systolic function	Moderately–severely ↓	Normal	Normal
Left ventricular diastolic function	May be abnormal	Abnormal	Abnormal
Left ventricular hypertrophy	↑ Left ventricular mass due to left ventricular dilation with normal wall thickness	Asymmetrical left ventricular hypertrophy	Concentric left ventricular hypertrophy
Chamber dilation	All four chambers	Left atrial dilation if mitral regurgitation is present	Left and right atrial dilation
Outflow tract obstruction	Absent	Dynamic left ventricular outflow tract obstruction may be present	Absent
Left ventricular end-diastolic pressure	Elevated	Elevated	Elevated
Pulmonary artery pressures	Elevated	Elevated	Elevated

TABLE 7–2. EXAMPLES OF POTENTIAL CAUSES OF DILATED CARDIOMYOPATHY

Idiopathic

Toxins (alcohol, medications, cobalt, snake bites)

Metabolic (thiamine deficiency, acromegaly)

Peripartum

Infections (Chagas' disease, postviral)

Systemic diseases (e.g., immune-mediated injury)

Inherited disorders (Duchenne's muscular dystrophy, sickle cell anemia)

---

ondary to left ventricular and mitral annular dilation. Pulmonary hypertension may develop in response to the chronic elevation in left atrial pressure. Left ventricular diastolic dysfunction may be present but typically is not the predominant feature of this disease.

Echocardiographic Approach
(Table 7–3)

Two-dimensional (2D) imaging from standard windows allows evaluation of the size and function of all four cardiac chambers (Figs. 7–1 and 7–2). Qualitative evaluation of right ventricular size and systolic function and quantitative evaluation of left ventricular size and systolic function provide important clinical data. In addition to 2D imaging, other signs of poor left ventricular systolic function include the M-mode findings of an increased mitral E-point to septal separation due to ventricular dilation, and reduced anteroposterior aortic root motion reflecting reduced left atrial filling and emptying (Fig. 7–3). Doppler findings may include a reduced aortic ejection velocity and velocity-time integral, indicating a reduced stroke volume, but compensatory mechanisms (including left ventricular dilation) result in a normal stroke volume at rest in many individuals. A slow rate of rise in velocity of the mitral regurgitant jet indicates a reduced rate of rise in left ventricular pressure in early systole (dP/dt).

Associated atrioventricular valve regurgitation can be assessed with Doppler techniques (see Chap. 10) and often is moderate in severity (Fig. 7–4). Pulmonary pressures usually are elevated and can be estimated from the velocity in the tricuspid regurgitant jet, as described in Chapter 4.

The pattern of left ventricular diastolic filling

TABLE 7–3. ECHOCARDIOGRAPHIC APPROACH TO THE PATIENT WITH A SUSPECTED CARDIOMYOPATHY

QUALITATIVE	QUANTITATIVE
2D/M-mode Imaging	
Chamber dimensions	LV-EDV, LV-ESV
Degree and pattern of LV hypertrophy	LV-mass
Evidence for dynamic outflow tract obstruction	
SAM of the mitral valve	
Aortic valve midsystolic closure	
LV systolic function	EF
Doppler Echo	
Associated valvular regurgitation	
Estimates of PA pressure	TR jet, TPV in PA
Pattern of LV diastolic filling	
Pattern of LA filling (pulmonary venous inflow)	
Evidence for dynamic outflow tract obstruction	
High-velocity, late-peaking jet in systole	ΔP (max and mean)
Color flow demonstration of turbulence in the LV outflow tract	
HPRF localization of the level of obstruction	
Provocative maneuvers (Valsalva, amyl nitrate inhalation) may be needed	

Notes: 2D = two-dimensional; LA = left atrial; LV = left ventricular; EDV = end-diastolic volume; ESV = end-systolic volume; TR = tricuspid regurgitation; TPV = time to peak velocity; ΔP = pressure gradient; PA = pulmonary artery; EF = ejection fraction; HPRF = high pulse repetition frequency.

can be evaluated with Doppler recordings of left ventricular inflow. A high E velocity with a small A velocity indicates "pseudonormalization" with a high left atrial pressure (increased gradient from left atrium to left ventricle at mitral valve opening) and a high end-diastolic pressure (reduced A velocity) (Fig. 7–5). The M-mode finding of a delayed rate of mitral valve closure—a "B-bump" or "AC-shoulder" (see Fig. 7–3)—correlates with an elevated end-diastolic pressure. Earlier in the disease course, a reduced E velocity and increased A velocity consistent with impaired early diastolic relaxation may be observed.

When significant left ventricular systolic dysfunction is present (ejection fraction ≤35 percent), a careful search for apical left ventricular thrombus is indicated (Fig. 7–6). Details on the

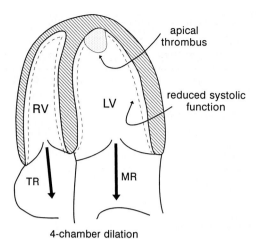

Figure 7–1. Schematic diagram of the key features of dilated cardiomyopathy in an apical four-chamber view. All four chambers are enlarged with reduced left and right ventricular (LV and RV) systolic function. Dashed lines indicate the limited extent of endocardial motion between end-diastole and end-systole. An apical thrombus is present. Secondary mitral and tricuspid regurgitation are indicated by the arrows (LA = left atrium; RA = right atrium).

technical aspects of identifying a left ventricular thrombus are given in Chapter 6.

Limitations/Technical Considerations

Echocardiography rarely can establish the *etiology* of a dilated cardiomyopathy, even though it is instrumental both in confirming the diagnosis and in providing prognostic data. The

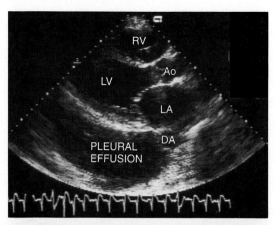

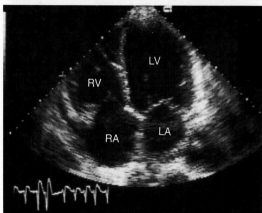

Figure 7–2. 2D images in a patient with dilated cardiomyopathy. In the parasternal long-axis view (*above*), left ventricular and atrial enlargement is seen. A pleural effusion is present posteriorly. A Swan-Ganz catheter is seen in the enlarged right ventricular outflow tract. In the apical four-chamber view (*below*), dilation of all four chambers is seen. In real time, right and left ventricular systolic function is severely reduced (DA = descending aorta).

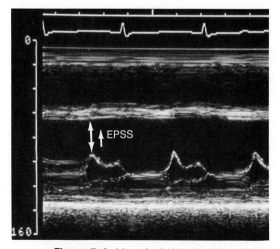

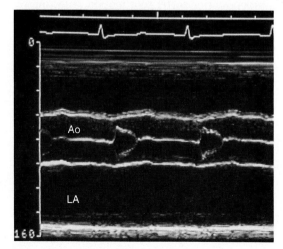

Figure 7–3. M-mode findings in dilated cardiomyopathy. There is increased mitral *E*-point septal separation (EPSS) and a "B-bump" (*left*) and decreased aortic root motion with early closure of the aortic valve (*right*).

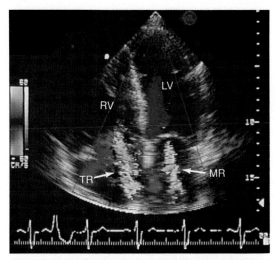

Figure 7–4. Color Doppler of mitral and tricuspid regurgitation due to ventricular dilation and systolic dysfunction in a patient with a dilated cardiomyopathy.

echocardiographic appearance of a dilated cardiomyopathy is fairly uniform despite a wide range of disease processes. One exception is Chagas' heart disease; these patients typically have a left ventricular apical aneurysm with minimal involvement of the ventricular septum. In patients with endomyocardial fibrosis due to Chagas' disease, there is apical obliteration of a small ventricle with atrial enlargement and atrioventricular valve regurgitation. While Chagas' disease is rare in North America, it is endemic in South and Central America and may be diagnosed in immigrants from those areas. Recognition of the echocardiographic features of this disease may prompt the correct diagnosis in a nonendemic area.

In most patients with dilated cardiomyopathy, an exact etiology cannot be identified, even when all diagnostic modalities are utilized. The most useful additional data are a careful patient history to uncover possible precipitating factors. An endomyocardial biopsy is rarely diagnostic except when an infiltrative process (e.g., amyloid, sarcoid, hemochromatosis) is present. Findings of "myocarditis" are nonspecific and usually do not change the therapeutic approach.

Clinical Utility

Echocardiographic evaluation is indicated at the initial presentation of a patient with symptoms consistent with dilated cardiomyopathy. If an echocardiogram performed in a patient with a suspected dilated cardiomyopathy shows no significant impairment of left ventricular systolic dysfunction, a careful search is needed for other causes of heart failure symptoms, such as pericardial constriction, restrictive or hypertrophic cardiomyopathy, ischemic disease, or valvular disease (Table 7–4).

If the echocardiogram is consistent with the clinical diagnosis of dilated cardiomyopathy, detailed information on ventricular function, chamber sizes, associated valvular disease, and pulmonary artery pressures is obtained.

While "routine" follow-up studies are not indicated, repeat echocardiograms may be needed if a significant change in clinical status occurs suggesting an interval change in ventricular

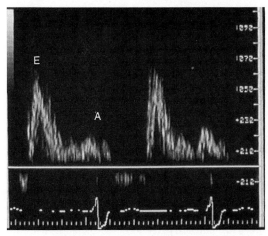

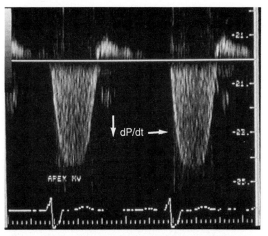

Figure 7–5. Doppler findings in dilated cardiomyopathy. Left ventricular diastolic inflow shows a high *E* velocity and low *A* velocity suggestive of "pseudonormalization" due to an elevated end-diastolic pressure (*left*). The mitral regurgitant jet shows a slow rate of rise in velocity consistent with a reduced *dP/dt* (*right*).

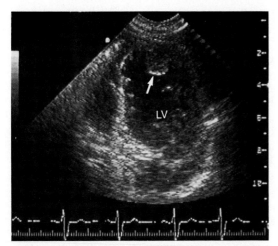

Figure 7–6. Left ventricular apical thrombus (*arrow*) in a posteriorly angulated apical four-chamber view in a patient with dilated cardiomyopathy.

function. Since ventricular function is a strong predictor of outcome, assessment of the patient's current status allows appropriate tailoring of medical therapy. A severe decrease in ventricular systolic function may prompt consideration of cardiac transplantation.

In the intensive-care unit, echocardiographic evaluation can be helpful in patients with dilated cardiomyopathy to assess left ventricular function, pulmonary artery pressures, and the degree of coexisting mitral regurgitation, and to estimate left ventricular filling pressures. Evaluation of an individual patient's response to afterload reduction therapy can be performed by repeat 2D echo ejection fraction measurements or by sequential measurements of stroke volume

TABLE 7–4. ECHOCARDIOGRAPHIC DIFFERENTIAL DIAGNOSIS OF "HEART FAILURE"

Ischemic disease

Valvular disease

Hypertensive heart disease

Cardiomyopathy
 Dilated
 Hypertrophic
 Restrictive

Pericardial disease
 Constriction
 Tamponade

Pulmonary heart disease

and cardiac output using Doppler and 2D echo techniques (see Chap. 3 and Fig. 7–7).

Alternate Approaches

If measurement of pulmonary vascular resistance is needed (e.g., in a heart transplant candidate), cardiac catheterization is indicated. Although echocardiographic measures of pulmonary pressure are accurate, calculation of pulmonary vascular resistance currently is not reliable enough for clinical decision making.

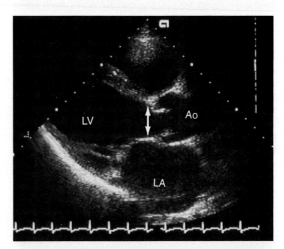

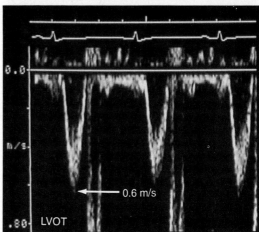

Figure 7–7. Calculation of stroke volume in a patient with dilated cardiomyopathy. Outflow tract diameter is measured from a parasternal long-axis view for calculation of a circular cross-sectional area (CSA_{LVOT}). The left ventricular outflow tract velocity-time integral (VTI_{LVOT}) is recorded just proximal to the aortic valve from an apical approach using a pulsed Doppler sample volume length of 5 to 10 mm. Stroke volume (SV) is calculated as $VTI \times CSA$. Cardiac output is stroke volume times heart rate.

HYPERTROPHIC CARDIOMYOPATHY

Basic Principles

Hypertrophic cardiomyopathy is an autosomal dominant inherited disease of the myocardium (with variable penetrance) related to abnormalities in the beta-myosin heavy-chain gene. Predominant anatomic features of this disease are (1) asymmetrical hypertrophy of the left ventricle, (2) normal ventricular systolic function, and (3) impaired diastolic left ventricular function (Fig. 7–8). Subaortic dynamic obstruction to left ventricular outflow is present in some individuals. Other important clinical features of this disease are a high risk of sudden death (especially during exertion); symptoms of angina, exercise intolerance, and syncope; and a systolic murmur on cardiac auscultation.

The pattern of left ventricular hypertrophy can be quite variable, ranging from "classic" septal hypertrophy to isolated apical hypertrophy. In addition, the degree of myocardial thickening is quite variable, even within a family. The common feature of all these hypertrophy patterns is normal thickness (or "sparing") of the basal posterior left ventricular wall. In the parasternal long- and short-axis views, this region is seen at the base (between the papillary muscle and mitral annulus) posterior to the mitral valve leaflets. Hypertrophy may be confined to the anterior segment of the ventricular septum (type I) or may involve the anterior and posterior segments of the septum (type II) with sparing of the lateral, posterior, and inferior walls. Some pa-

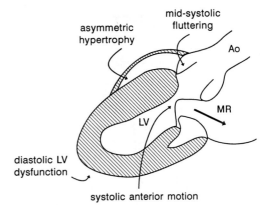

Figure 7–8. Schematic diagram of the typical features of hypertrophic cardiomyopathy in a parasternal long-axis view. There is midsystolic closure and coarse fluttering of the aortic valve leaflets, asymmetrical septal hypertrophy with sparing of the basal posterior wall, normal left ventricular systolic function with impaired diastolic function, dynamic outflow tract obstruction with systolic anterior motion of the mitral valve leaflets, and mitral regurgitation.

tients have extensive ventricular hypertrophy with normal wall thickness seen only in the basal segment of the posterior wall (type III). An unusual pattern of hypertrophy is *apical hypertrophic cardiomyopathy* (type IV), which is of particular note to the echocardiographer because it can be missed if the marked displacement of the apical endocardium is not recognized. Clinically, the clue to this pattern of hypertrophy is inverted precordial T waves on the electrocardiogram (Fig. 7–9).

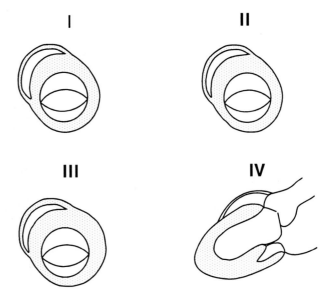

Figure 7–9. Schematic diagram of patterns of ventricular hypertrophy in hypertrophic cardiomyopathy in a parasternal basal short-axis view. Type I = hypertrophy confined to anterior septum; type II = anterior and posterior septum involved; type III = extensive hypertrophy sparing only the basal posterior wall; type IV = apical hypertrophy (in a long-axis schematic view).

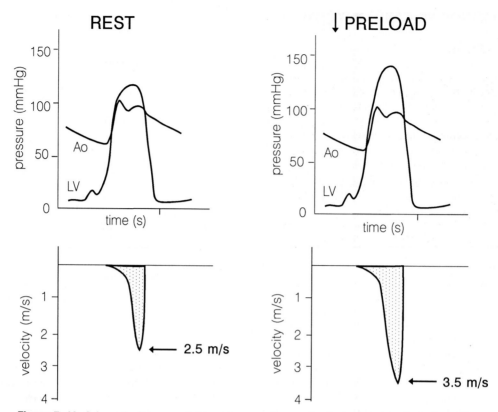

Figure 7–10. Schematic diagrams of the pressure gradient and velocity curve in dynamic outflow obstruction due to hypertrophic cardiomyopathy. At rest, a small gradient is present only in late systole between the left ventricle (LV) and aorta (Ao). The continuous-wave Doppler curve shows a late-peaking velocity of 2.5 m/s, with the origin of this velocity being the subaortic region. With alterations in loading conditions (decreased preload), the degree of obstruction increases dramatically. A late-peaking, high-velocity (3.5 m/s) Doppler curve now is obtained.

In patients with subaortic obstruction, apposition of the anterior leaflet of the mitral valve against the hypertrophied ventricular septum is seen in systole. This obstruction is *dynamic* rather than fixed, both in the sense that it occurs only in mid to late systole and in the sense that the presence and severity of obstruction can be altered by loading conditions. These features contrast with the fixed obstruction of aortic valve stenosis, which persists from onset to end-ejection and in which the severity of the stenosis is relatively insensitive to changes in loading conditions. Dynamic outflow obstruction in hypertrophic cardiomyopathy typically has a pattern of onset in midsystole, with the maximum left ventricular to aortic pressure gradient occurring in late systole (Figs. 7–10 and 7–11). Controversy persists regarding (1) the mechanism of dynamic obstruction and (2) the lack of a clear relationship between clinical status and hemodynamic findings. Of note, late systolic obstruction occurs after the majority of the stroke volume has been ejected, thus minimally affecting forward stroke volume in most patients.

Obstruction can be diminished by maneuvers that increase ventricular volume—an increase in preload or a decrease in contractility—or by maneuvers that increase afterload. Conversely, the degree of obstruction is increased by a reduction

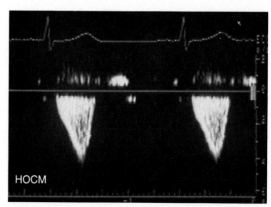

Figure 7–11. Continuous-wave Doppler in a patient with hypertrophic cardiomyopathy shows the characteristic late-peaking high-velocity curve due to dynamic outflow tract obstruction.

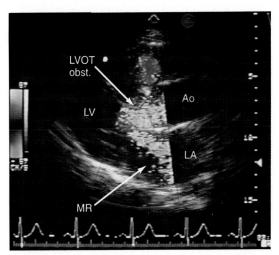

Figure 7–12. Color flow image of mitral regurgitation in a patient with hypertrophic cardiomyopathy showing a posteriorly directed jet originating from the malcoapted segment of the mitral leaflets in association with systolic anterior motion. Turbulence in the outflow tract is seen due to subaortic dynamic obstruction.

in preload, an increase in contractility, or a decrease in afterload. All these conditions are similar in that they reduce left ventricular volume. Some patients with no or minimal evidence of outflow obstruction at rest develop obstruction with maneuvers performed during the physical examination or with echocardiography. Clinically useful maneuvers include examination during a post-premature contraction beat (increased contractility), with Valsalva maneuver (decreased preload), or after inhalation of amyl nitrate (decreased afterload and preload).

Dynamic outflow obstruction usually is associated with mitral regurgitation, since the systolic anterior motion of the leaflets in systole disrupts normal coaptation. A posteriorly directed mitral regurgitant jet of mild to moderate severity originates at the malcoapted segment of the leaflets (Fig. 7–12).

Left ventricular systolic function typically is normal. However, left ventricular diastolic function is abnormal, accounting for many of the heart failure symptoms in patients with hypertrophic cardiomyopathy. The thickened myocardium exhibits impaired relaxation and decreased compliance.

Echocardiographic Approach

Left Ventricular Asymmetric Hypertrophy

Evaluation of the pattern and extent of left ventricular hypertrophy is made from multiple tomographic views. In the parasternal long-axis view, particular attention is focused on the posterobasal wall between the papillary muscle and the mitral annulus. While the wall in this region is not thickened in patients with hypertrophic cardiomyopathy, it is thickened in patients with concentric hypertrophy due to other etiologies (e.g., hypertension, restrictive cardiomyopathy). 2D guided M-mode tracings provide the best endocardial definition for measurement of septal and posterior wall thickness, although 2D measurements can be used when image quality is adequate. 2D imaging in both long- and short-axis views is used to ensure that the M-mode beam is perpendicular to the left ventricular walls and to avoid inclusion of right ventricular trabeculation in the septal wall thickness.

The parasternal long-axis view also offers the best opportunity to define the exact relationship between the pattern of septal hypertrophy and the outflow tract (Fig. 7–13). This is important when a surgical approach, such as myotomy-myectomy, is being considered, since surgical visualization usually is retrograde across the aortic valve, allowing only limited direct inspection of the septal endocardium and little information on the extent of septal thickening or the degree of septal curvature. Parasternal short-axis views from base to apex allow assessment of the lateromedial extent of the hypertrophic process.

Apical views again allow visualization of the pattern and extent of hypertrophy. Diagnosis of apical hypertrophy can be difficult, since endocardial definition may be poor and the endocardial surface (which may be located up to one-third the distance from the apical epicardium to the base) may be missed if image quality is suboptimal. In some cases, the epicardium may be mistaken for the apical endocardium. A careful examination, when the referring physician has alerted the echocardiographer to this possible diagnosis, avoids this potential pitfall. Color or pulsed Doppler examination is helpful in demonstrating the absence of blood flow in the "apical" region which is occupied by the hypertrophied myocardium.

Qualitative and quantitative evaluation of left ventricular systolic function is performed using standard approaches (see Chap. 4).

Left Ventricular Diastolic Function

Left ventricular diastolic function is evaluated from the Doppler inflow velocity curve recorded at the mitral valve leaflet tips. The E velocity, the A velocity, the E/A ratio, and the early diastolic deceleration slope can be measured. Se-

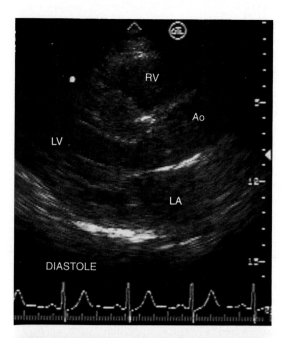

DIASTOLE

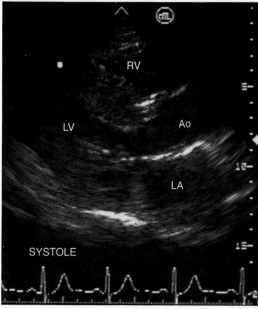

SYSTOLE

Figure 7–13. 2D images of hypertrophic cardiomyopathy in a parasternal long-axis view at end-diastole (*above*) and end-systole (*below*).

quential studies, in conjunction with clinical data, allow inferences about left ventricular diastolic function (see Chap. 5). Typical changes include a prolonged isovolumic relaxation time, reduced E velocity, and enhanced A velocity; however, there is marked patient variability. Changes in the filling pattern after medical or surgical therapy may be seen consistent with improved diastolic filling.

Dynamic Outflow Tract Obstruction

2D/M-Mode Imaging. In a patient with dynamic left ventricular outflow tract obstruction, the parasternal long-axis view shows systolic anterior motion of the mitral valve leaflets. This can be appreciated better on M-mode recordings showing the systolic anterior motion and leaflet-septal apposition in mid to late systole. Note that the rate of anterior leaflet motion is more rapid than the anterior motion of the posterior wall in systole (Fig. 7–14). A "contact lesion" on the ventricular septum at the site of mitral leaflet impingement may be seen on 2D long- and short-axis imaging in some patients.

Short-axis parasternal views also show the systolic anterior motion of the mitral valve leaflets. Frame-by-frame analysis shows the cross-sectional area of the outflow tract throughout systole.

Apical 2D views are helpful for demonstrating the abnormal mitral leaflet motion, especially the apical long-axis and the anteriorly angulated four-chamber views. Note that the degree of systolic anterior motion may not be uniform from medial to lateral across the mitral leaflets, so imaging in multiple planes with slight adjustments in transducer angulation may be needed to demonstrate the presence and extent of dynamic outflow obstruction.

The aortic valve shows normal leaflet opening in early systole, followed by midsystolic abrupt partial closure with coarse fluttering of the aortic valve leaflets in late systole due to the late systolic dynamic outflow obstruction. Again, these rapid leaflet movements are best documented on M-mode recordings (Fig. 7–15). The aortic leaflets themselves may be sclerotic due to chronic

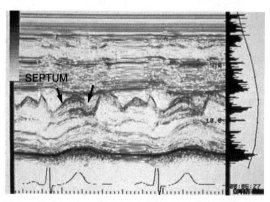

Figure 7–14. M-mode at the mitral valve level (*left*) in a patient with dynamic outflow obstruction due to hypertrophic cardiomyopathy showing the classic septal hypertrophy and systolic anterior motion (SAM) of the mitral leaflets (*arrows*).

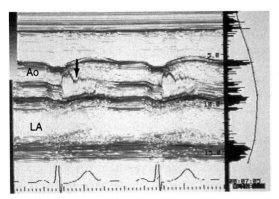

Figure 7–15. An M-mode at the aortic valve level (in the same patient as in Fig. 7–14) shows midsystolic closure of the aortic valve (*arrow*) followed by coarse fluttering of the leaflets.

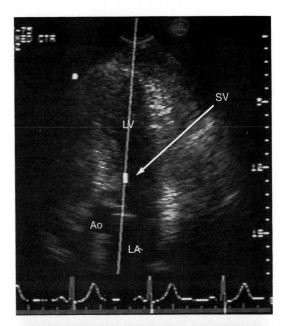

impact of a turbulent jet as a result of subaortic obstruction, and some degree of coexisting aortic regurgitation may be noted.

Doppler Evaluation. Doppler studies provide a more direct evaluation of the presence, location, and degree of dynamic subaortic obstruction than do 2D or M-mode techniques. With conventional pulsed or color flow imaging, the site of obstruction is identified based on the location of the poststenotic turbulence. Both parasternal and apical long-axis views are useful for this examination.

Using pulsed Doppler from an apical approach, the sample volume is slowly moved from the apex progressively toward the base, recording the velocity curve at each step. Proximal to the outflow obstruction, velocities are normal. At the site of obstruction, the velocity increases abruptly to a velocity reflecting the degree of obstruction (as stated in the Bernoulli equation). This approach, using stepwise evaluation with pulsed Doppler ultrasound, is advantageous in that intracavity gradients due to apical hypertrophy or apposition of the papillary muscle with the septum will be recognized and not mistaken for *subaortic* dynamic obstruction (Fig. 7–16).

Continuous-wave Doppler from an apical approach typically shows a late-peaking high-ve-

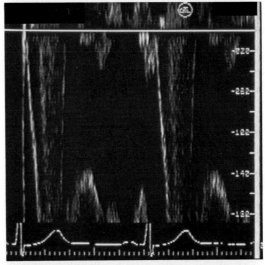

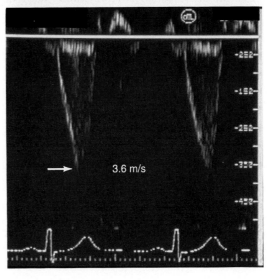

Figure 7–16. Example of the use of a stepwise pulsed-Doppler examination to localize the level of outflow tract obstruction. With the sample volume at the mitral valve level in the outflow tract (*top*), pulsed Doppler shows a marked increase in velocity with signal aliasing (*middle*). This velocity can be resolved with high pulse repetition frequency Doppler (*bottom*) or with continuous-wave Doppler ultrasound (as shown in Fig. 7–11).

locity systolic jet in patients with dynamic left ventricular outflow tract obstruction. The shape of this curve is distinctive, corresponding to the temporal course of the left ventricular to aortic pressure gradient (see Fig. 7–10). Again, since continuous-wave Doppler measures velocities along the entire length of the ultrasound beam, other techniques are needed to confirm the depth of origin of the signal along the ultrasound beam. Occasionally, hypertensive heart disease or hypovolemia will result in a late-peaking high-velocity waveform, but the site of obstruction is *not* subaortic; it is closer to the apex, at the midventricular level.

When features suggestive of hypertrophic cardiomyopathy are present and there is no evidence for outflow obstruction at rest, maneuvers to "provoke" outflow obstruction may be performed in order to make a definite diagnosis or to relate the patient's symptoms to the echocardiographic findings. When only a modest degree of obstruction is seen at rest, interventions to increase the degree of obstruction may be performed for similar reasons.

A spontaneous premature ventricular contraction (PVC) results in an increased degree of obstruction on the post-PVC beat due to increased left ventricular contractility. The strain phase of the Valsalva maneuver increases obstruction by decreasing preload (smaller left ventricular cavity size) but is difficult to perform simultaneously with echocardiography due to changes in cardiac position and lung interference as the patient performs the maneuver. A simple and reasonably safe method to provoke dynamic outflow obstruction in the echocardiography laboratory is amyl nitrate inhalation with direct physician supervision. This medication results in a brief decrease in preload (venodilation) and decrease in afterload (arterial dilation), both of which increase the degree of obstruction. A moderate degree of tachycardia may occur, but the duration of action of this inhaled medication is brief. The sonographer records the continuous-wave Doppler signal in the left ventricular outflow tract before, during, and following administration of amyl nitrate by the physician to document the effects of the medication on the degree of outflow obstruction. Attention is needed to maintain a parallel intercept angle between the ultrasound beam and the high-velocity jet, particularly with respect to the phase of the respiratory cycle. The physician monitors heart rate, rhythm, symptoms, and blood pressure. Care is needed to ensure that only the patient (and not the other individuals in the room) are exposed to the medication.

Mitral Valve Abnormalities

The mitral valve is anatomically and functionally abnormal in the majority of patients with hypertrophic cardiomyopathy. Functionally, mitral regurgitation results from systolic anterior motion of the leaflets into the outflow tract leading to late systolic failure of coaptation and a consequent posteriorly directed regurgitant jet. However, anatomic abnormalities are present as well. Both autopsy and echocardiographic studies have demonstrated that the mitral leaflets have an increased surface area and a longer length (particularly the anterior leaflet) than in normal subjects. In addition, the degree of coaptation is excessive, and the coaptation plane is displaced posteriorly. About 10 percent of patients have anomalous papillary muscle anatomy with direct insertion of the papillary muscle into the leaflet.

Limitations/Technical Considerations

As discussed earlier, it is important to distinguish hypertrophic cardiomyopathy with dynamic subaortic obstruction associated with systolic anterior motion of the mitral leaflet from a concentrically hypertrophied ventricle due to other disease processes (such as hypertension). In some situations, the hypertrophied ventricle may be hyperdynamic, with midcavity obliteration resulting in an intracavity gradient. The distinction between hypertrophic cardiomyopathy and a hyperdynamic concentrically hypertrophied ventricle can be made by careful attention to the 2D images (sparing of the basal posterior wall in hypertrophic cardiomyopathy) and M-mode findings (characteristic aortic and mitral valve motion) and evaluation of the depth of origin of the high-velocity jet using conventional pulsed, high-pulse-repetition-frequency, and color Doppler techniques (Fig. 7–17).

Another difficult problem is separating the degree of outflow obstruction due to dynamic subaortic obstruction from that due to valvular aortic stenosis in the rare patient with both conditions. In the presence of serial stenoses, an accurate measure of the pressure drop across each narrowing may not be possible, since the simplified Bernoulli equation applies to a single stenosis. However, high-pulse-repetition-frequency Doppler may allow examination of velocities at each site, indicating the relative contribution of each site to the total degree of

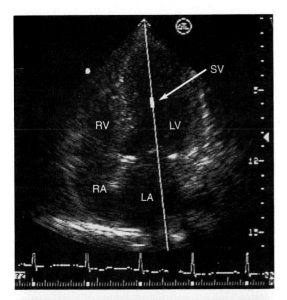

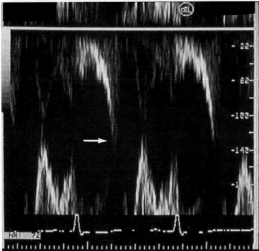

Figure 7–17. Example of a concentrically hypertrophied hyperdynamic left ventricle with midcavity obliteration at end-systole (*above*) resulting in a late-peaking high-velocity outflow tract Doppler curve (*below*). This condition must be distinguished from the dynamic subaortic obstruction seen in hypertrophic cardiomyopathy. SV = sample volume.

obstruction to ventricular outflow. Occasionally, a patient with valvular aortic stenosis and a hypertrophied ventricle will demonstrate dynamic subaortic obstruction only *after* aortic valve replacement. Some of these patients have hypertrophic cardiomyopathy that is "unmasked" by the afterload reduction of valve replacement. Others have a hyperdynamic ventricle with a midcavity pressure gradient that may resolve as the degree of left ventricular hypertrophy decreases postoperatively.

Clinical Utility

Diagnosis and Screening

Echocardiography is the procedure of choice for accurate diagnosis of hypertrophic cardiomyopathy. Since this is an inherited disorder, screening with echocardiography is indicated for all first-degree relatives of the affected individual. This diagnosis significantly changes clinical management even in asymptomatic individuals, given the high risk of sudden death with exertion, and has important implications for genetic counseling.

Evaluation of Medical Therapy

In patients with a definite diagnosis of hypertrophic cardiomyopathy, Doppler findings can be used to assess the impact of medical therapy. Specifically, the pattern of left ventricular diastolic filling after institution of therapy to improve diastolic function (such as beta blockers or calcium channel blockers) may show an improvement in early diastolic filling. The degree of dynamic outflow obstruction also may show improvement on medical therapy.

Surgical Therapy

Pre- and intraoperative echocardiographic evaluation of the patient undergoing surgical treatment for hypertrophic cardiomyopathy is essential. Preoperative knowledge of the extent, distribution, and curvature of septal hypertrophy guides the surgeon in terms of the location and size of the muscle segment to be removed. Intraoperative monitoring allows evaluation of the adequacy of the procedure in relieving outflow tract obstruction, using both 2D imaging and Doppler techniques. Images are obtained at baseline and immediately following the procedure (after cardiopulmonary bypass is discontinued). Note that while transesophageal imaging provides adequate images of the myectomy site in some cases, epicardial imaging often is preferable, since the septum is located anteriorly relative to the esophagus. Color flow imaging from a transesophageal or transepicardial approach allows evaluation of the flow pattern in the left ventricular outflow tract as an indicator of residual obstruction. Since the degree of obstruction is influenced dramatically by loading conditions, the postbypass study should be performed under hemodynamic conditions as similar as possible to the baseline state. It may be difficult to obtain an accurate continuous-wave Doppler recording of the degree of outflow obstruction in the operating room because the transesophageal approach rarely provides a transgastric apical view from which the beam can be aligned parallel to the jet. An epicardial apical position may not be obtainable with a median sternotomy because the transducer often is too large to fit under the ribs at the apex. Placement of a sterile transducer on the ascending aorta with inferior angulation toward the outflow tract may allow a parallel intercept angle in some patients.

Postmyectomy complications that are detectable by intraoperative echocardiography include a ventricular septal defect at the site of the myectomy as well as residual outflow tract obstruction.

Alternate Approaches

Usually, echocardiography provides all the data needed for clinical management of a patient with suspected or diagnosed hypertrophic cardiomyopathy. Alternate tomographic imaging techniques can provide data on the anatomic pattern of hypertrophy but do not allow evaluation of abnormal diastolic filling or the presence and degree of dynamic outflow tract obstruction.

In cases where the echocardiographic findings and clinical presentation are discrepant, cardiac catheterization may be helpful. First, evaluation of coronary anatomy may be indicated, since coexisting epicardial coronary artery disease may explain some symptoms in a patient with hypertrophic cardiomyopathy. Second, recordings of left ventricular and aortic pressures at rest and after provocative maneuvers to increase or decrease dynamic outflow obstruction and with slow "pullback" across the outflow tract and aortic valve allow more detailed hemodynamic evaluation. This is particularly helpful in the patient with sequential stenoses in the subaortic region and at the aortic valve level.

In the operating room, direct left ventricular and aortic pressure measurements after myectomy may be helpful if residual obstruction is suspected.

RESTRICTIVE CARDIOMYOPATHY

Basic Principles

Restrictive cardiomyopathy is characterized by normal left ventricular systolic function with impaired diastolic function due to a stiff, hypertrophied left ventricle. Heart failure symptoms are due to the resultant elevation in left ventricular end-diastolic pressure and the inability to increase cardiac output with exercise due to impaired diastolic filling. Note that *heart failure*—defined as the inability to maintain a normal cardiac output or maintenance of a normal cardiac output *only* with an elevated left ventricular end-diastolic pressure—can occur with normal systolic function. In many patients with restrictive cardiomyopathy, *right-sided* failure predominates initially with symptoms of peripheral edema and ascites.

As the disease process progresses, an individual patient may progress from an anatomic/hemodynamic pattern consistent with restrictive cardiomyopathy to a pattern showing some features of dilated cardiomyopathy, ending with a picture indistinguishable from dilated cardiomyopathy.

The etiology of restrictive cardiomyopathy includes infiltrative processes such as amyloidosis and hemochromatosis and inflammatory diseases such as sarcoidosis (Table 7–5). Compared with dilated cardiomyopathy, restrictive cardiomyopathy is a rare diagnosis. An unusual cause of restrictive cardiomyopathy is the hypereosinophilic syndrome. This systemic disease is characterized by hypereosinophilia with involvement of the lungs, bone marrow, brain, and heart. Cardiac involvement is typical and exhibits unique echocardiographic features. In this syndrome, left ventricular thrombus formation occurs *in the absence of an underlying wall motion abnormality* (particularly in the apex), resulting in gradual apical "obliteration" (as seen on angiography) or filling in of the apex with an echogenic mass (on echocardiography). Thrombus formation also occurs under the posterior mitral valve leaflet, leading to adherence of the posterior leaflet to the endocardium and significant mitral regurgitation.

TABLE 7–5. ETIOLOGY OF RESTRICTIVE CARDIOMYOPATHY (EXAMPLES)

Amyloidosis

Hemochromatosis

Sarcoidosis

Hypereosinophilic syndrome (Löffler's endocarditis)

Glycogen storage diseases

Echocardiographic Approach

2D echocardiographic imaging in patients with restrictive cardiomyopathy typically shows a nondilated, thick-walled left ventricle with normal systolic function and abnormal diastolic function. The right ventricular free wall often is thickened as well, and biatrial enlargement is seen. Secondary signs of moderate pulmonary hypertension may be present, including paradoxic septal motion and tricuspid regurgitation (Figs. 7–18 and 7–19).

Doppler evaluation confirms moderate pulmonary hypertension based on (1) time to peak velocity in the pulmonary artery and (2) tricuspid regurgitant jet velocity plus an estimate of right atrial pressure (see Chap. 3). Note that in the untreated patient, right atrial pressure usually is high, so the inferior vena cava is dilated with reduced respiratory variation (Fig. 7–20).

The pattern of left ventricular diastolic filling parallels the abnormalities in left ventricular diastolic function in this disease. However, interpretation is complicated both by the numerous confounding factors that affect left ventricular diastolic filling (see Chap. 5) and by temporal changes in diastolic filling as the disease progresses in an individual patient. Early in the disease course, impaired diastolic relaxation of the left ventricle results in impaired *early* diastolic filling. The Doppler left ventricular inflow curve shows a reduced *E* velocity, increased *A* velocity, prolonged isovolumic relaxation time, and decreased early diastolic deceleration slope (Fig. 7–21).

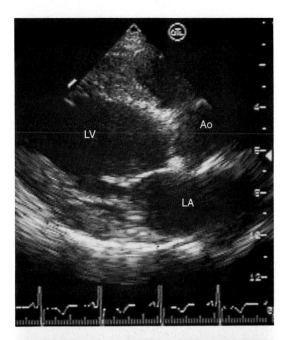

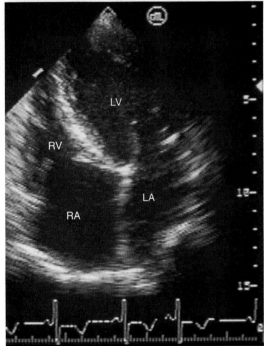

Figure 7–19. Parasternal long-axis (*above*) and apical four-chamber (*below*) 2D echocardiographic images in a patient with a restrictive cardiomyopathy due to amyloidosis. There is biventricular hypertrophy, biatrial enlargement, and both systolic and diastolic dysfunction of the left ventricle.

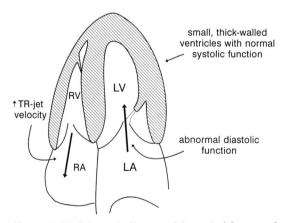

Figure 7–18. Schematic diagram of the typical features of restrictive cardiomyopathy, which include a thick-walled, small left ventricle (LV) with impaired diastolic function, left and right atrial enlargement (LA, RA), and signs of secondary pulmonary hypertension, including paradoxical septal motion and a high-velocity tricuspid regurgitant (TR) jet.

As the disease progresses, left atrial pressure rises, resulting in an increased pressure gradient from the left atrium to left ventricle at mitral valve opening. Along with reduced diastolic

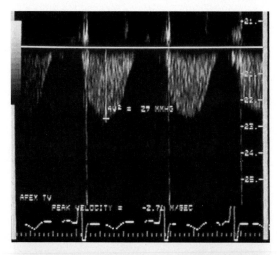

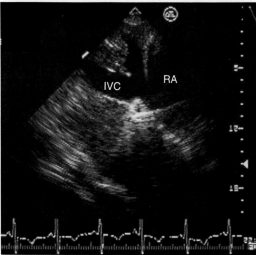

Figure 7–20. Tricuspid regurgitant jet velocity of 2.7 m/s in the same patient with restrictive cardiomyopathy as shown in Figure 7–19. Right atrial pressure estimated from the size and respiratory motion of the inferior vena cava was 20 mmHg. Estimated pulmonary artery systolic pressure then is 49 mmHg.

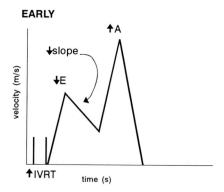

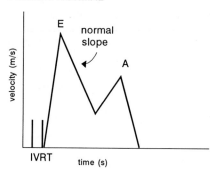

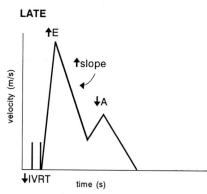

Figure 7–21. Schematic diagrams of left ventricular diastolic filling in restrictive cardiomyopathy. Early in the disease course ventricular relaxation abnormalities predominate, and the E velocity and early deceleration slope are reduced while the isovolumic relaxation time and A velocity are increased. Pseudonormalization occurs as left ventricular end-diastolic pressure rises, resulting in relatively normal E and A velocities. With advanced (late) disease, ventricular compliance decreases, resulting in a high E velocity, steep deceleration slope, short isovolumic relaxation time, and reduced A velocity.

compliance of the left ventricle, this increased mitral opening pressure leads to an increased E velocity and a rapid deceleration slope. The A velocity is reduced due to a combination of increased left ventricular end-diastolic pressure and reduced atrial contractile function (Fig. 7–22). Thus the pattern of diastolic filling in advanced restrictive cardiomyopathy (which may coincide with the initial clinical presentation) is similar to the "big E, little A" pattern seen in normal young individuals. This "pseudonormal" pattern can be distinguished from normal by (1) the rapid early diastolic deceleration slope, (2) the patient's age, clinical presentation, and associated echocardiographic findings, and (3) the pattern of pulmonary venous inflow into the left

atrium. With a pseudonormal left ventricular inflow pattern, pulmonary venous flow shows either blunting or reversal of the normal diastolic phase of atrial inflow. When atrial contraction occurs, the increased resistance to left ventricular filling results in flow reversal in the lower resistance pulmonary veins. Thus pul-

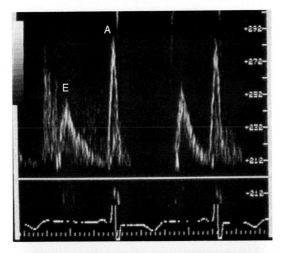

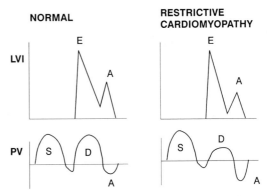

Figure 7–23. Schematic diagrams of left ventricular inflow (LVI) and pulmonary vein (PV) Doppler flow patterns with normal diastolic function and in restrictive cardiomyopathy. Although the inflow patterns are similar superficially, the "pseudonormal" pattern has a steeper deceleration slope and lower *A* velocity. The pulmonary vein flow shows reduced diastolic filling and prominent *A* reversal compared with the normal pattern.

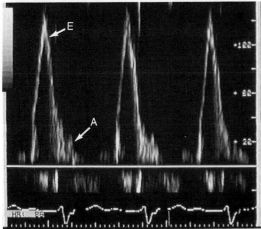

Figure 7–22. Left ventricular diastolic filling in a patient with an early restrictive cardiomyopathy shows impaired early diastolic relaxation (*above*). In contrast, an elderly patient with advanced amyloid heart disease (*below*) shows "pseudonormalization" with a prominent *E* velocity and low *A* velocity consistent with reduced diastolic compliance.

monary venous flow shows a reduced diastolic phase, normal systolic phase, and prominent *a*-wave flow reversal. This is in contrast to the normal pattern of nearly equal systolic and diastolic pulmonary venous inflow curves (Fig. 7–23) and a small *a* wave.

Examination of right atrial filling by recording hepatic vein (or superior vena cava) flow patterns also can be helpful. These patterns correspond to the physical findings of the neck vein pulsations seen in patients with restrictive cardiomyopathy. Using this analogy, the hepatic vein flow pattern typically shows a prominent reverse flow phase with atrial contraction (*a* wave) followed by a rapid filling curve in systole (*x* descent). The diastolic phase of right atrial filling is blunted corresponding to a diminished

v wave and *y* descent. These findings correspond to the pattern of right atrial pressure recordings at catheterization; the *x* descent represents the "dip," and the blunted systolic filling phase represents the "plateau" of the dip-and-plateau pattern.

Limitations/Technical Considerations

Differentiation of restrictive cardiomyopathy from constrictive pericarditis is problematic. Both have a similar clinical presentation, and both are characterized by preserved left ventricular systolic function with impaired diastolic filling. Features that distinguish these two conditions include the patterns of atrial and ventricular diastolic filling, the presence or absence of pericardial thickening, and the degree of associated pulmonary hypertension. However, no single feature is diagnostic of either condition (see Table 8–5).

Attention to technical details is necessary in recording Doppler atrial and ventricular filling patterns, particularly their relationship to the phase of respiration. Respiratory variation is assessed most reliably using a respirometer to mark the onsets of inspiration and expiration. Prior to recording Doppler signals, 2D and color flow imaging is utilized to convince the sonographer that there is no significant respiratory variation in the angle between the ultrasound beam and the direction of blood flow. Respiratory changes in intercept angle could result in apparent changes in velocity even under constant-flow conditions due to the erroneous assumption that cos θ remains 1 in the Doppler equation. Once a constant intercept angle is ascertained, recordings of left ventricular diastolic inflow are made with the sample volume positioned first at the mitral annulus level and then at the mitral leaflet tips.

Recording right atrial filling patterns is straightforward using a subcostal approach with the pulsed Doppler sample volume positioned in the central hepatic vein. This vein connects directly to the inferior vena cava and right atrium, with no intervening venous valve, and conveniently lies parallel to the direction of the ultrasound beam from the subcostal window.

Left atrial filling is more technically challenging to record due to signal attenuation at the depth of the pulmonary veins from an apical approach. Other transthoracic acoustic windows rarely allow interrogation of pulmonary vein flow at a near-parallel intercept angle. A transesophageal approach is helpful if recordings of pulmonary vein flow are inadequate on transthoracic interrogation and are needed for patient management.

Clinical Utility

In a patient with heart failure symptoms, a diagnosis of restrictive cardiomyopathy may not have been suspected on clinical grounds. In some cases, echocardiographic findings may provide the first clues pointing toward this diagnostic possibility. In a patient with known restrictive cardiomyopathy, echocardiography can be used to follow disease progression. A meticulous examination with careful attention to technical details and with integration of 2D, Doppler, and clinical data may allow differentiation of restrictive cardiomyopathy from constrictive pericarditis.

Alternate Approaches

Diagnostic evaluation of the patient with probable restrictive cardiomyopathy may include cardiac catheterization with measurement of intracardiac pressures at rest and with volume loading, endomyocardial biopsy, and chest computed tomographic imaging (to detect pericardial calcification or thickening). In some cases, constrictive pericarditis may remain a diagnostic possibility despite the results of these tests. The diagnosis of constrictive pericarditis is critical, since it can be treated by removal of the adher-

ent pericardial layers. In patients in whom there is a high level of suspicion but nondiagnostic test results, thoracotomy may be indicated to confirm (and treat) or exclude a diagnosis of pericardial constriction.

In the future, tissue characterization based on analysis of the back-scattered acoustic signal may prove helpful in evaluation of infiltrative cardiomyopathies.

HYPERTENSIVE HEART DISEASE

Basic Principles

Hypertensive heart disease is an end-organ consequence of systemic hypertension. Chronic systemic pressure overload results in left ventricular hypertrophy to maintain normal wall stress. Initially, diastolic function is impaired, while systolic function remains normal. With long-standing hypertension, systolic dysfunction and ventricular dilation can occur. Other cardiac abnormalities associated with chronic hypertension include aortic root dilation, aortic valve sclerosis, mitral annular calcification, left atrial enlargement and atrial fibrillation.

Echocardiographic Approach

Ventricular Hypertrophy (Table 7–6)

Standard 2D views demonstrate concentric left ventricular hypertrophy with increased wall thickness and a nondilated chamber (Fig. 7–24). In contrast to hypertrophic cardiomyopathy, the pattern of hypertrophy is symmetrical, including involvement of the basal posterior wall. M-mode recordings confirm an increased end-diastolic wall thickness (>11 mm). Left ventricular mass can be calculated from the M-mode data, assuming hypertrophy is symmetrical, but preferably is calculated from 2D data (Fig. 7–25; also see Chap. 4).

Diastolic Function

Left ventricular diastolic function is characterized by impaired early diastolic relaxation. This results in a reduced E velocity, reduced E/A ratio, and prolonged deceleration slope. Interestingly, in individuals with physiologic hypertrophy (due to physical conditioning), diastolic dysfunction is not seen even when increased wall thickness is present. In pathologic hypertrophy (due to hypertension), diastolic

TABLE 7–6. CONDITIONS WITH INCREASED LEFT VENTRICULAR WALL THICKNESS

	HYPERTENSIVE HEART DISEASE	HYPERTROPHIC CARDIOMYOPATHY	RESTRICTIVE CARDIOMYOPATHY
Left ventricular hypertrophy	+	+	+
Pattern of hypertrophy	Concentric	Asymmetrical	Concentric
Clinical history of hypertension	+	Absent	Absent
Outflow obstruction	Midventricular cavity obliteration	Dynamic subaortic obstruction	Absent
Right ventricular hypertrophy	Absent	May be present	+
Pulmonary hypertension	Mild	Mild	Moderate
Left ventricular systolic function	Normal initially but may be reduced late in disease course	Normal	Normal initially but may be reduced late in disease course
Left ventricular diastolic function	Abnormal	Abnormal	Abnormal

+ = present.

dysfunction often is the first evidence of end-organ damage, usually antedating clear evidence of anatomic hypertrophy.

Systolic Function

Typically, systolic function is preserved early in the disease course. Segmental wall motion abnormalities are not seen unless coexisting coronary artery disease is present. With a small, hypertrophied, normally functioning left ventricular chamber, midcavity obliteration at end-systole may be seen with an associated Doppler velocity curve showing a brief, late-systolic high-velocity signal (see Fig. 7–17). The duration of this intracavity gradient is briefer than that seen with hypertrophic cardiomyopathy, the level of obstruction is midventricular rather than subaortic, and systolic anterior motion of the mitral leaflets is not seen. Midcavity obliteration is exacerbated by hypovolemia or increased contractility.

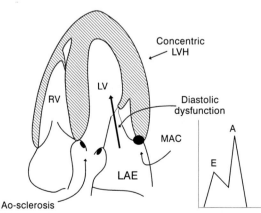

Figure 7–24. Schematic diagram of hypertensive heart disease in an anteriorly angulated apical four-chamber view. Note concentric left ventricular hypertrophy (LVH), mitral annular calcification (MAC), left atrial enlargement (LAE), aortic (Ao) valve sclerosis, aortic root dilation, and impaired early diastolic relaxation ($E < A$).

Other Echocardiographic Findings

Aortic root dilation often is present in hypertensive patients and is associated with increased tortuosity of the ascending aorta, arch, and descending aorta. Increased irregular echogenicity of the aortic walls, representing atherosclerosis, also may be noted. In uncomplicated hypertension, the aortic annulus itself is not dilated. The aortic valve leaflets usually show fibrocalcific changes and associated mild aortic regurgitation. Mitral annular calcification often is present in patients with chronic hypertension and is one cause of mild to moderate mitral regurgitation in

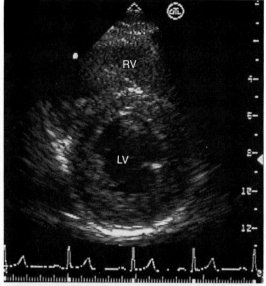

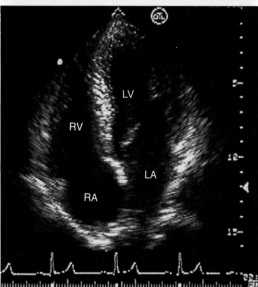

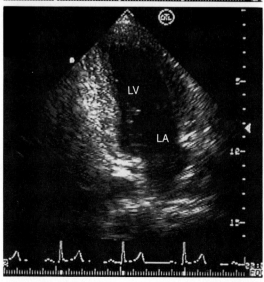

these patients. Left atrial enlargement is due to a combination of a chronically elevated left ventricular end-diastolic pressure and mitral regurgitation.

Limitations/Technical Considerations

Left ventricular mass determinations are dependent on optimal image quality with clear definition of endocardial and epicardial surfaces and on correct endocardial border tracing at end-diastole and end-systole. Differentiation of hypertensive heart disease from hypertrophic or restrictive heart disease is based on the pattern of hypertrophy, associated echocardiographic findings, and integration of the echocardiographic and clinical data.

Clinical Utility

Diagnosis and Prognosis

Left ventricular mass, measured by echocardiography, is a strong predictor of clinical outcome in patients with hypertension. In subjects with borderline hypertension, increased left ventricular mass identifies a subgroup of patients with a poor prognosis without medical therapy. In patients with definite hypertension, the degree of left ventricular hypertrophy reflects the chronic elevation of systemic pressure, in theory serving as an index of the temporally averaged blood pressure over long periods of time. Thus left ventricular mass may be a more accurate method for assessing the severity of hypertension than occasional blood pressure recordings in the physician's office or even 24-hour recordings of blood pressure.

Choices of Medical Therapy

Some hypertension clinics tailor medical therapy in individual patients based on noninvasive Doppler echo evaluation of hemodynamics. Since blood pressure equals cardiac output times systemic vascular resistance, hypertension can

◀ **Figure 7–25.** 2D echo views needed for left ventricular mass determination in a hypertensive patient. Parasternal short-axis (*above*), apical four-chamber (*center*) and two-chamber (*below*) views at end-diastole are shown. Epicardial and endocardial borders in the short-axis view and an apical length measurement are needed to calculate left ventricular mass using Eq. (4.22).

be due to elevation of either one or both of the components of this equation. To assess hemodynamics noninvasively in hypertensive patients, cardiac output is measured using Doppler recordings of ascending aortic flow and 2D aortic diameter measurements (see Chap. 4). Systemic vascular resistance then is calculated from the cuff blood pressure and Doppler cardiac output. Appropriate medications are chosen based on the specific hemodynamics in each patient.

Efficacy of Medical Therapy

Determination of left ventricular mass also is useful in assessing the long-term effect of medical therapy. Again, rather than measuring blood pressure at rare intervals in the disease course, the chronic end-organ effects of hypertension on the left ventricle are measured. It seems plausible that effective antihypertensive therapy should reverse end-organ changes; specifically, it should result in regression of left ventricular hypertrophy.

Evaluation of Heart Failure Symptoms in a Patient with Hypertension

In a patient with chronic hypertension, heart failure symptoms may be due to diastolic or systolic left ventricular dysfunction, superimposed coronary artery disease, or superimposed valvular disease. Early in the disease course, pathologic hypertrophy is associated with impaired early diastolic filling. Impaired ventricular filling leads to elevated left atrial pressures and pulmonary venous hypertension, resulting in dyspnea. Diagnosis of diastolic dysfunction with preserved systolic function can be made by echocardiography and has important clinical implications, since the therapy for heart failure symptoms is quite different for diastolic versus systolic dysfunction.

An extreme form of preserved systolic function with left ventricular hypertrophy and heart failure symptoms has been observed in hypertensive patients and has been termed *hypertensive hypertrophic cardiomyopathy of the elderly*. This condition is characterized by normal to hyperdynamic systolic function, concentric hypertrophy, diastolic dysfunction, and a midventricular late systolic gradient due to cavity obliteration. Strictly speaking, this combination of findings is not a "cardiomyopathy" but simply represents severe end-organ damage due to hypertension. However, awareness of this specific clinical picture results in consideration of this diagnosis in patients whom otherwise might be suspected of having a restrictive cardiomyopathy.

With long-standing hypertension, impairment of left ventricular contractility can occur, even in the absence of coexisting coronary artery disease. Physiologically, elevated afterload (as in valvular aortic stenosis) is the proximate cause of systolic dysfunction. However, systolic function may not improve even with aggressive antihypertensive therapy when systolic dysfunction is long-standing, suggesting that irreversible changes in ventricular contractility have occurred. End-stage hypertensive heart disease has an echocardiographic appearance similar to end-stage dilated cardiomyopathy.

Alternate Approaches

The need for routine echocardiographic evaluation of patients with hypertension is controversial. Medical management based on intermittent office blood pressure measurements remains standard practice at many medical centers. Estimates of the chronicity of blood pressure elevation can be obtained by 24-hour blood pressure monitors or evaluation of other end-organ damage (e.g., renal function, retinal examination). While electrocardiographic estimates of left ventricular hypertrophy are less accurate and precise than echocardiographic measurements, there is a substantial cost differential between these diagnostic tests.

EVALUATION OF THE POST-CARDIAC TRANSPLANT PATIENT

Basic Principles

Echocardiographic evaluation of the post-cardiac transplant patient typically is directed toward one of two goals: (1) assessment of cardiac anatomy and physiology prompted by a specific clinical problem or (2) the elusive goal of noninvasive diagnosis of early rejection of the transplanted heart.

Clinical problems encountered in the post-cardiac transplant patient include:

1. Pericardial effusion, particularly early postoperatively.

2. Right ventricular systolic dysfunction due to inadequate myocardial preservation at the time of transplantation, persistently elevated pulmonary vascular resistance, or transplant rejection.

3. Left ventricular systolic dysfunction due to inadequate myocardial preservation, acute re-

jection early posttransplantation, or superimposed coronary artery disease at a longer interval posttransplantation.

Primary valvular disease, of course, is uncommon due to screening of donor hearts before transplantation. However, mitral or tricuspid regurgitation secondary to ventricular dysfunction and annular dilation may be seen. Diastolic dysfunction clearly occurs and may be a marker of early rejection. Unfortunately, evaluation of diastolic function after cardiac transplantation is fraught with difficulty due to the confounding effects of loading conditions, heart rate, patient age, coexisting mitral regurgitation, and other factors, as detailed in Chapter 5.

Echocardiographic Approach

Normal Findings after Cardiac Transplantation

A normal echocardiogram after cardiac transplantation shows biatrial enlargement due to the conjunction of donor and recipient atria at the time of transplantation (Fig. 7–26). The suture lines between the donor and recipient portions of the atrium, for both right and left atria, may be prominent and should not be mistaken for an abnormal atrial mass (Fig. 7–27). Typically, right and left ventricular size, wall thickness, and systolic function are normal in the absence of perioperative complications or rejection. Valvular anatomy and function are normal, with small amounts of mitral, tricuspid, and pulmonic regurgitation present at a prevalence similar to that in normal individuals. The suture lines in the aorta and pulmonary artery may be difficult to appreciate, depending on the dis-

tance of the suture lines from the valve planes. A small pericardial effusion is seen early postoperatively but rarely persists beyond a few weeks. Paradoxical (postoperative) septal motion may be present. Pulmonary artery pressures may show some degree of persistent elevation as calculated from the velocity in the tricuspid regurgitant jet and estimates of right atrial pressure.

Evaluation of Abnormal Findings

The echocardiographic approach to the posttransplant patient with suspected cardiac dysfunction is similar to that in any patient, with the proviso that the expected findings after transplantation (such as the atrial suture line) are recognized.

Pericardial effusions often are loculated due to postoperative pericardial adhesions, so careful examination in multiple tomographic planes from parasternal, apical, and subcostal windows is essential when this diagnosis is suspected.

Echocardiographic Diagnosis of Transplant Rejection

With severe rejection, right and left ventricular systolic dysfunction occurs and can be recognized by echocardiography. With mild or early rejection, 2D echocardiographic changes are subtle and are not accurate or reproducible

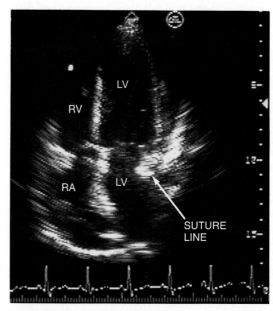

Figure 7–27. Apical four-chamber view in a posttransplant patient showing biatrial enlargement with a prominent suture line (*arrow*).

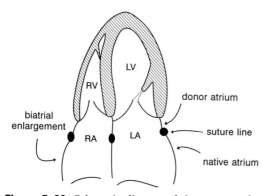

Figure 7–26. Schematic diagram of the posttransplant heart. Note the suture line between the donor and native atria resulting in an appearance of biatrial enlargement. Right and left ventricular size and systolic function are normal.

enough to allow adjustment of immunosuppressive medications in individual patients. Instead, proposed echocardiographic approaches to diagnosis of early rejection have focused on measures of diastolic function, specifically measures of early diastolic relaxation. Approaches have included assessment of diastolic filling based on digitized M-mode posterior wall motion, Doppler recording of right and left ventricular diastolic inflow, Doppler recordings of superior vena cava flow and M-mode or Doppler recordings of the interval between aortic valve closure and mitral valve opening (isovolumic relaxation time, or IVRT). In general, transplant rejection is associated with a "restrictive" filling pattern with a prolonged IVRT, an increased early diastolic filling velocity, a shortened pressure half-time (more rapid early diastolic deceleration), and a loss of forward systolic flow in the superior vena cava. Although some centers have found these measures clinically useful, they have not yet gained wide acceptance for patient management. More refined approaches to ultrasonic tissue characterization also appear promising, since they may detect interstitial edema early in the course of rejection.

Limitations/Technical Considerations/Alternate Approaches

The standard method for evaluation of transplant rejection remains transvenous endomyocardial biopsy. Some centers use echocardiographic (rather than fluoroscopic) guidance for this procedure. Since echocardiographic images are tomographic, any segment of the biotome shaft going through the image plane will appear to be the "tip." Thus it is crucial to identify the open forceps of the biotome for correct identification of the biopsy site. A subcostal window often is most practical, since, with the patient supine, clear views of the right ventricle and septum are obtained, and the sonographer is clear of the sterile field (usually the right internal jugular vein approach is used). In some cases, the apical view also may be helpful.

PULMONARY HEART DISEASE

Chronic versus Acute Pulmonary Disease

Chronic pulmonary hypertension, whether due to intrinsic lung disease, recurrent pulmo-

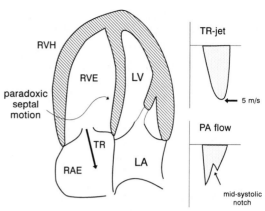

Figure 7–28. Schematic diagram of the key features of pulmonary heart disease. Right ventricular hypertrophy (RVH) and enlargement (RVE) are seen with paradoxic septal motion. Secondary tricuspid regurgitation (TR) and right atrial enlargement (RAE) are common. Elevated pulmonary artery pressures will be reflected in the high-velocity tricuspid regurgitant jet velocity and midsystolic notching in the pulmonary artery velocity curve.

nary emboli, or primary pulmonary hypertension, results in a group of clinical signs and symptoms termed *cor pulmonale*. The underlying pathophysiology of this clinical syndrome is chronic pressure overload of the right ventricle as it ejects into a high-resistance pulmonary vascular bed. Initially, compensatory hypertrophy of the right ventricle occurs with preserved systolic function. Over time, right ventricular contractility deteriorates, and right ventricular dilation, moderate to severe tricuspid regurgitation, and consequent right atrial enlargement are seen (Fig. 7–28).

Acute pulmonary embolism also can affect right-sided heart function due to sudden onset of elevated pulmonary vascular resistance. Echocardiographic evaluation may be helpful in assessing pulmonary artery pressures and right ventricular function both in patients with chronic and in those with acute pulmonary hypertension.

Echocardiographic Approach

Pulmonary Pressures

Standard approaches for noninvasive evaluation of pulmonary pressures, as described in Chapter 4, are applicable to the patient with suspected or known pulmonary hypertension. The most reliable approach is to record the maximum tricuspid regurgitant jet velocity for calculation of the right ventricular to right atrial systolic pressure difference (Fig. 7–29). Care is needed

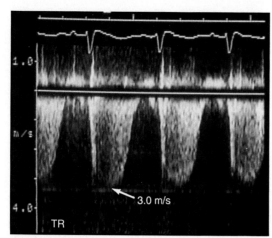

Figure 7–29. Tricuspid regurgitant jet in a patient with pulmonary heart disease. The maximum velocity of 3 m/s indicates a right ventricular to right atrial pressure difference of 36 mmHg. Right atrial pressure was elevated at 20 mmHg, so estimated pulmonary artery systolic pressure is 56 mmHg.

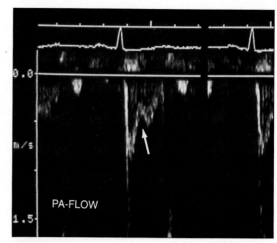

Figure 7–30. Pulmonary artery velocity curve showing midsystolic notching (*arrow*) due to severe pulmonary hypertension.

to interrogate the tricuspid regurgitant jet from multiple acoustic windows (apical, parasternal) with careful transducer angulation to obtain a parallel intercept angle between the ultrasound beam and jet. Right atrial pressure is estimated from the size and respiratory variation in the inferior vena cava. Then pulmonary artery systolic pressure (in the absence of pulmonic stenosis) is calculated as

$$PAP = 4V_{TR}^2 + RAP$$

Pulmonary mean pressure can be estimated from the time to peak velocity of the pulmonary artery or right ventricular outflow tract velocity curve. Diastolic pulmonary artery pressure can be estimated from the velocities in the pulmonic regurgitant Doppler curve.

Indirect signs of pulmonary hypertension often are seen on echocardiography which indicate the presence, but not the exact severity, of pulmonary hypertension. An M-mode recording through the pulmonic valve shows a reduced *a* dip and midsystolic closure of the valve. This pattern has a reasonably high specificity (>90 percent) for detecting pulmonary hypertension but a low sensitivity (30 to 60 percent). This motion pattern is paralleled by the Doppler velocity curve, which shows an abrupt midsystolic deceleration of flow (Fig. 7–30). Signs of right ventricular pressure overload, including abnormal ventricular septal motion, may be valuable clues suggesting the presence of pulmonary hypertension, as detailed below.

Right Ventricular Pressure Overload

The response of the right ventricle to chronic pressure overload is concentric hypertrophy. This increase in thickness of the right ventricular free wall is best seen on the subcostal view. Ventricular septal motion is abnormal or "paradoxical" with anterior motion of the septum during systole both on M-mode and 2D imaging. A rational explanation for this pattern of septal motion is based on the concept that the septum moves toward the center of mass of the heart during systole. With right ventricular hypertrophy, the center of mass is shifted anteriorly, so the septum moves toward the center of the right ventricle instead of the normal pattern of motion toward the center of the left ventricle. On 2D imaging, the curvature of the septum is reversed.

With long-standing or acute pulmonary hypertension, right ventricular systolic dysfunction can occur, with secondary dilation serving as a compensatory mechanism to maintain forward stroke volume. However, right ventricular dilation leads to tricuspid regurgitation due to annular dilation and malalignment of the papillary muscles. This superimposed volume overload results in further right ventricular dilation and more tricuspid regurgitation. Right atrial dilation is due to both pressure (*v* wave) and volume (tricuspid regurgitation) overload of the right atrium. When right ventricular volume and pressure overload coexist, septal motion shows abnormal diastolic flattening as well as systolic anterior motion. This pattern is due to increased volume flow into the right ventricle

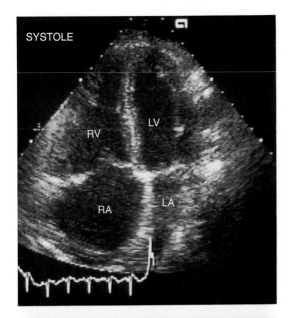

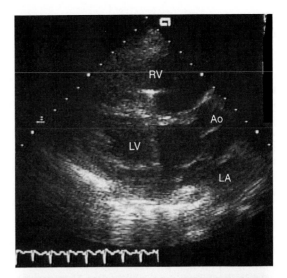

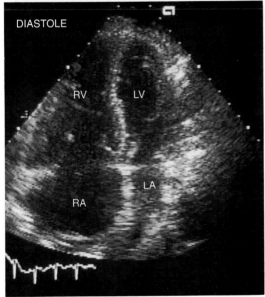

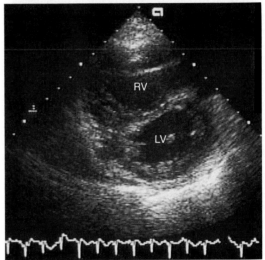

Figure 7-32. Parasternal views in the same patient as in Figure 7-30 shows flattening of the ventricular septum in diastole and right ventricular enlargement. A Swan-Ganz catheter (with reverberation artifact) is seen in the right ventricular outflow tract.

Figure 7-31. Apical four-chamber view at end-diastole (*above*) and end-systole (*below*) in a patient with cor pulmonale. There is right ventricular enlargement, right ventricular hypertrophy, paradoxical septal motion, and reduced systolic function of the right ventricle.

(compared with the left ventricle) in diastole (Figs. 7-31 and 7-32).

Secondary Tricuspid Regurgitation

Tricuspid regurgitation secondary to pulmonary hypertension and/or right ventricular systolic dysfunction can be evaluated with color Doppler flow imaging from parasternal, apical, and subcostal views. Severe regurgitation results in systolic flow reversal in the inferior vena cava and hepatic veins. Careful attention to tricuspid valve anatomy is needed to ensure that other etiologies of tricuspid regurgitation (e.g., vegetation, rheumatic, Ebstein's) are not present.

The intensity of the continuous-wave Doppler tricuspid regurgitant jet relates to the severity of regurgitation, but the *velocity* relates to the right ventricular to right atrial pressure difference. With acute tricuspid regurgitation, a rapid fall-off in velocity in late systole may be seen consistent with a right atrial *v* wave.

Limitations/Technical Considerations

The major limitation of echocardiography in evaluation of cor pulmonale is poor ultrasound tissue penetration resulting in poor image quality and low Doppler signal strength. Hyperexpanded lungs obscure the standard acoustic windows in many patients with chronic lung disease. However, adequate image quality may be obtained by careful patient positioning. Subcostal views provide diagnostic data in most cases.

Assessment of the severity of pulmonary hypertension depends on obtaining a parallel intercept angle between the ultrasound beam and tricuspid regurgitant jet. Underestimation of pulmonary artery pressures should be considered in all patients, especially when Doppler signal strength is suboptimal or when the Doppler data and clinical setting are discrepant. The absence of a recordable tricuspid regurgitant jet does *not* indicate normal pulmonary pressures. In this situation, the echocardiographer should indicate that the data are inadequate and alternate diagnostic approaches should be considered.

Clinical Utility

Echocardiography allows confirmation of a clinical diagnosis of cor pulmonale, assessment of the degree of pulmonary hypertension, and evaluation of right ventricular size and systolic dysfunction. In addition, it offers at least the potential for evaluating changes in pulmonary pressures with therapeutic interventions.

In the patient with an acute pulmonary embolus, imaging may show a residual thrombus originating from or in transit through (from a deep vein thrombosis) the right side of the heart. Transesophageal imaging can demonstrate thrombus in the main, right, or left pulmonary artery. However, the sensitivity of echocardiography for *diagnosis* of pulmonary embolism based on demonstrating a thrombus is *low* because the thrombus is lodged more distally in the pulmonary vasculature in most cases.

Indirect signs of pulmonary embolism include evidence of acute right ventricular pressure overload with elevated pulmonary artery pressures, right ventricular dilation and dysfunction, and tricuspid regurgitation. Similar findings may be seen in patients with chronic recurrent pulmonary emboli. The possibility of pulmonary embolism should be strongly considered in patients with these findings even when a different working clinical diagnosis or "reason for echo" was entertained. Often patients who are subsequently diagnosed with pulmonary embolism are initially referred for nonspecific indications including "chest pain," "dyspnea," or "heart failure."

Alternate Approaches

Cardiac catheterization allows direct measurement of right ventricular and pulmonary artery pressures and calculation of pulmonary vascular resistance. Right ventricular size and systolic function can be evaluated by angiography.

Clinically, the standard approach for diagnosis of pulmonary embolism is a radionuclide lung ventilation-perfusion scan. These data often are combined with a radionuclide or vascular diagnostic evaluation for deep venous thrombus. In some cases, pulmonary angiography is needed with injection of contrast material directly into the main pulmonary artery. The risk of pulmonary angiography is relatively high, especially in patients with pulmonary hypertension, so noninvasive approaches are preferable whenever possible.

SUGGESTED READING

1. Waller BF: Pathology of the cardiomyopathies. J Am Soc Echocardiogr 1:4–19, 1988.
   Review of the pathology and pathophysiology of cardiomyopathies. Excellent illustrations.

2. Acquatella H, Schiller NB: Echocardiographic recognition of Chagas' disease and endomyocardial fibrosis. J Am Soc Echocardiogr 1:60–68, 1988.
   Review of the echocardiographic findings in Chagas' disease.

3. Vanoverschelde J-LJ, Raphael DA, Robert AR, Cosyns JR: Left ventricular filling in dilated cardiomyopathy: Relation to functional class and hemodynamics. J Am Coll Cardiol 15:1288–1295, 1990.
   In patients with dilated cardiomyopathy (n = 34), more severe symptoms were associated with a higher E velocity, lower atrial filling fraction, higher E/A ratio, shorter IVRT, and shorter time to peak filling rate. Severely symptomatic patients also had a higher pulmonary artery wedge pressure, lower cardiac output, and more severe mitral regurgitation. Diastolic parameters of left ventricular function correlated better than systolic parameters with functional class.

4. Shen W-F, Tribouilloy C, Rey JL, et al: Prognostic significance of Doppler-derived left ventricular diastolic filling variables in dilated cardiomyopathy. Am Heart J 124:1524–1533, 1992.
   In 62 consecutive patients with dilated cardiomyopathy, the E/A ratio was the only significant Doppler predictor of clinical outcome at 31 ± 14 month follow-ups (27 cardiac events, 23 deaths, and 4 cardiac transplants). The cardiac

event rate was 77 percent with an E/A ratio >2 versus 19 percent for E/A ≤2 (p < 0.001). Clinical functional improvement was associated with normalization of left ventricular filling parameters.

5. Simonson JS, Schiller NB: Descent of the base of the left ventricle: An echocardiographic index of left ventricular function. J Am Soc Echocardiogr 2:25–35, 1989.
   The extent of apical motion of the mitral annulus in systole is a simple measure of left ventricular systolic function. A "descent of the base" (annular apical motion) of <8 mm in the apical four-chamber view corresponded to an EF < 50 percent with a sensitivity of 98 percent and specificity of 82 percent.

6. Douglas PS, Morrow R, Ioli A, Reichek N: Left ventricular shape, afterload and survival in idiopathic dilated cardiomyopathy. J Am Coll Cardiol 13:311–315, 1989.
   In 36 patients with dilated cardiomyopathy, poorer survival was related to a more spherical left ventricle (overall cavity shape or ratio of short- to long-axis dimensions), but not to systolic cavity dimensions, wall thickness, or fractional shortening.

7. Lewis JF, Webber JD, Sutton LL, et al: Discordance in degree of right and left ventricular dilation in patients with dilated cardiomyopathy: Recognition and clinical implications. J Am Coll Cardiol 21:649–654, 1993.
   In 67 patients with dilated cardiomyopathy, patients with greater involvement of the left than the right ventricle had a better outcome than those with equal degrees of dilation and systolic dysfunction of right and left ventricles.

8. Isaaz K, Pasipoularides A: Noninvasive assessment of intrinsic ventricular load dynamics in dilated cardiomyopathy. J Am Coll Cardiol 17:112–121, 1990.
   A new method to evaluate the net force of ejection using noninvasive Doppler data is proposed. Net force F of ejection is

   $$F = A \cdot dv/dt + B \cdot v^2$$

   where v is ejection velocity and A and B are variables related to left ventricular chamber and outflow tract geometry. In patients with dilated cardiomyopathy, maximal ejection force, peak local acceleration, and outflow velocity were depressed compared with normal.

9. Kusumoto FM, Muhiudeen IA, Kuecherer HF, et al: Response of the interatrial septum to transatrial pressure gradients and its potential for predicting pulmonary capillary wedge pressure: An intraoperative study using transesophageal echocardiography in patients during mechanical ventilation. J Am Coll Cardiol 21:721–728, 1993.
   The curvature of the interatrial septum depends on the relative right and left atrial pressures. Midsystolic brief reversal is seen in normal individuals due to a transient right to left atrial pressure increase. The presence/absence of midsystolic atrial septum curvature reversal had a sensitivity of 89 percent and specificity of 95 percent for prediction of a pulmonary capillary wedge pressure ≤15 mmHg.

10. Rakowski H, Sasson Z, Wigle ED: Echocardiographic and Doppler assessment of hypertrophic cardiomyopathy. J Am Soc Echocardiogr 1:31–47, 1988.
    Excellent review of the echocardiographic approach in patients with hypertrophic cardiomyopathy. Forty-four references.

11. Wong M, Johnson G, Shabetai R, et al. for the V-HeFT VA Cooperative Studies Group: Echocardiographic variables as prognostic indicators and thera- peutic monitors in chronic congestive heart failure: Veterans Affairs Cooperative Studies V-HeFT I and II. Circulation 87(suppl VI):65–70, 1993.
    Echocardiographic variables including EPSS, systolic left ventricular interval dimension, and the ratio of ventricular radius to wall thickness were shown to be predictors of mortality in patients with congestive heart failure in a large randomized trial (V-HeFT).

12. Maron BJ: Hypertrophic cardiomyopathy. Curr Probl Cardiol 18:637–704, 1993.
    Review of hypertrophic cardiomyopathy including morphologic features, clinical presentation, natural history, and echocardiographic findings. 177 references.

13. Solomon SD, Wolff S, Watkins H, et al: Left ventricular hypertrophy and morphology in familial hypertrophic cardiomyopathy associated with mutations of the beta-myosin heavy chain gene. J Am Coll Cardiol 22:498–505, 1993.
    Two-dimensional echocardiograms were compared in 39 genetically affected and 30 unaffected family members. The spectrum of abnormal findings in genetically affected individuals was broad, with a maximal LV wall thickness ranging from 11 to 40 (mean 24) mm. In the affected group, 62 percent had systolic anterior motion of the mitral leaflet, 79 percent had reversed septal curvature, and 77 percent had a septal/free wall ratio >1.3.

14. Webb JG, Sasson Z, Rakowski H, et al: Apical hypertrophic cardiomyopathy: Clinical follow-up and diagnostic correlates. J Am Coll Cardiol 15:83–90, 1990.
    Description of findings and clinical course of 26 patients with apical hypertrophic cardiomyopathy. None had dynamic outflow obstruction.

15. Karam R, Lever HM, Healy BP: Hypertensive hypertrophic cardiomyopathy or hypertrophic cardiomyopathy with hypertension? A study of 78 patients. J Am Coll Cardiol 13:580–584, 1989.
    These authors emphasize that the clinical and echocardiographic features of elderly hypertensive patients with "hypertensive hypertrophic cardiomyopathy" are similar to those of normotensive patients with hypertrophic cardiomyopathy alone.

16. Panza JA, Petrone RK, Fananapazir L, Maron BJ: Utility of continuous wave Doppler echocardiography in the noninvasive assessment of left ventricular outflow tract pressure gradient in patients with hypertrophic cardiomyopathy. J Am Coll Cardiol 19:91–99, 1992.
    Validation of Doppler measurement of the subaortic gradient in patients with hypertrophic cardiomyopathy compared with cardiac catheterization in 28 patients. Correlations were excellent at baseline (r = 0.93), after provocative maneuvers (r = 0.89), and on a beat-to-beat basis in a single patient (r = 0.98) for maximum gradient by Doppler versus catheterization. Interobserver variability for Doppler data was low (r = 0.99). Several examples of the characteristic late-peaking velocity signal of dynamic outflow obstruction are shown.

17. Klues HG, Maron BJ, Dollar AL, Roberts WC: Diversity of structural mitral valve alterations in hypertrophic cardiomyopathy. Circulation 85:1651–1660, 1992.
    Detailed anatomic study of mitral valve abnormalities seen in hypertrophic cardiomyopathy. Abnormalities were present in 66 percent of 94 valves and included increased leaflet area, elongation of the leaflets, and anomalous direct insertion of the anterior mitral leaflet into the papillary muscle.

18. Stewart WJ, Schiavone WA, Salcedo EE, et al: Intraoperative Doppler echocardiography in hypertrophic cardiomyopathy: Correlations with the obstructive gradient. J Am Coll Cardiol 10:327–335, 1987.
Evaluation of the accuracy of intraoperative assessment of the degree of dynamic outflow obstruction before and after myectomy. Of note, a parallel intercept angle between the jet and Doppler beam was obtained by placing a sterile continuous-wave transducer directly on the ascending aorta with angulation toward the outflow tract. Careful positioning was required to obtain the highest-velocity signal.

19. Grigg LE, Wigle ED, Williams WG, et al: Transesophageal Doppler echocardiography in obstructive hypertrophic cardiomyopathy: Clarification of pathophysiology and importance in intraoperative decision making. J Am Coll Cardiol 20:42–52, 1992.
Discussion of the utility of intraoperative transesophageal echocardiography in planning the extent of myotomy/myectomy, assessing the immediate results of the procedure, and evaluating for any potential complications. Abnormalities of the mitral valve also are described. Note that accurate assessment of the subaortic pressure gradient may be difficult from a transesophageal approach due to a nonparallel intercept angle between the jet and the ultrasound beam.

20. Marwick TH, Stewart WJ, Lever HM, et al: Benefits of intraoperative echocardiography in the surgical management of hypertrophic cardiomyopathy. J Am Coll Cardiol 20:1066–1072, 1992.
In 50 patients, the impact of the combined use of preoperative transthoracic and intraoperative transesophageal echocardiography on patient management are discussed. In 10 patients (20 percent), a persistent outflow gradient >50 mmHg or increased moderate mitral regurgitation prompted reinstitution of cardiopulmonary bypass for further myectomy or mitral valve repair.

21. Gottdiener JS, Maron BJ, Schooley RT, et al: Two-dimensional echocardiographic assessment of the idiopathic hypereosinophilic syndrome. Anatomic basis of mitral regurgitation and peripheral embolization. Circulation 67:572–578, 1983.
Cardiac manifestations of the hypereosinophilic syndrome include (1) mitral regurgitation due to posterior leaflet thickening and adherence to the posterior left ventricular wall and (2) apical left ventricular thrombi in the absence of abnormal wall motion.

22. Klein AL, Hatle LK, Taliercio CP, et al: Prognostic significance of Doppler measures of diastolic function in cardiac amyloidosis. A Doppler echocardiography study. Circulation 83:808–816, 1991.
Left ventricular diastolic filling in cardiac amyloidosis is characterized by reduced early diastolic filling and an enhanced atrial contribution to filling early in the disease course; with progression to rapid early filling and a reduced atrial contribution late in the disease course ("pseudonormalization"). The Doppler pattern of left ventricular diastolic filling was predictive of clinical outcome in 63 consecutive patients. Those with a deceleration time ≤150 ms had a 1-year probability of survival of 49 percent compared with 76 percent in those with a deceleration time >150 ms (p < 0.001).

23. Devereux RB, de Simone G, Ganau A, et al: Left ventricular hypertrophy and hypertension. Clin Exp Hypertens 15(6):1025–32, 1993.
Review of the left ventricular response to chronic hypertension emphasizing the value of ventricular mass in predicting outcome in patients with hypertension, the role of echocardiography in assessing the degree of end-organ damage, and the potential role of echocardiographic data in clinical decision making in hypertensive patients.

24. De Simone G, Devereux, RB, Roman MJ, et al: Assessment of left ventricular function by the mid-wall fractional shortening/end-systolic stress relation in human hypertension. J Am Coll Cardiol 23:1444–1451, 1994.
The ratio of observed to predicted midwall shortening in 474 hypertensive patients was found to be above the 95th percentile of normal in only 4 percent of hypertensive subjects. In 16 percent, midwall shortening was below the 5th percentile of normal. These patients also were older, and had concentric left ventricular hypertrophy, a pattern associated with higher cardiovascular risk.

25. Ren JF, Pancholy SB, Iskandrian AS, et al: Doppler echocardiographic evaluation of the spectrum of left ventricular diastolic dysfunction in essential hypertension. Am Heart J 127:906–913, 1994.
In 41 patients with essential hypertension, left ventricular mass was inversely correlated with the normalized peak filling rate (r = −0.89). In patients with concentric hypertrophy, the normalized peak filling rate was decreased despite normal end-diastolic and end-systolic volumes, sugesting that diastolic dysfunction occurs early in the clinical course of hypertensive heart disease and may precede evidence of systolic dysfunction.

26. Gibbons RS: Doppler echocardiography for rejection surveillance in the cardiac allograft recipient. J Am Soc Echocardiogr 4:97–104, 1991.
Detailed description of the technical factors affecting echocardiographic evaluation of transplant rejection and review of posttransplant echocardiographic findings.

27. Miller LW, Labovitz AJ, McBride LA, et al: Echocardiographically guided endomyocardial biopsy. A 5-year experience. Circulation 78:99–102, 1988.
Description of utility of echocardiography for guiding endomyocardial biopsy in 4700 individual biopsies in 58 patients. Only two complications occurred.

28. Desruennes M, Corcos T, Cabrol A, et al: Doppler echocardiography for the diagnosis of acute cardiac allograft rejection. J Am Coll Cardiol 12:63–70, 1988.
On serial studies in 55 consecutive patients, a 20 percent decrease in pressure half-time had a sensitivity of 88 percent and a specificity of 87 percent for diagnosis of acute rejection using endomyocardial biopsy as the standard of reference.

29. Simmonds MB, Lythall DA, Slorach C, et al: Doppler examination of superior vena caval flow for the detection of acute cardiac rejection. Circulation 86(suppl II):259–266, 1992.
In 30 patients, a forward systolic flow velocity ≤ 17 cm/s had a sensitivity of 100 percent and a specificity of 80 percent for diagnosis of acute rejection. The postulated mechanism of this observation was diminished long-axis shortening of the right ventricle.

30. Come PC: Echocardiographic evaluation of pulmonary embolism and its response to therapeutic interventions. Chest 101(suppl 4):151S–162S, 1992.
Review of echocardiographic findings in pulmonary embolism emphasizing that with an acute event, pressures are only moderately elevated (about 40 mmHg mean pulmonary artery pressure). Thus higher right-sided pressures suggest chronic or recurrent disease.

31. Hunter JJ, Johnson KR, Karagianes TG, Dittrich HC: Detection of massive pulmonary embolus-in-transit by transesophageal echocardiography. Chest 100:1210–1214, 1991.
Description of the visualization of pulmonary emboli "in transit" through the right side of the heart using transesophageal echocardiography.

CHAPTER 8

PERICARDIAL DISEASE: TWO-DIMENSIONAL ECHOCARDIOGRAPHIC AND DOPPLER FINDINGS

NORMAL PERICARDIAL ANATOMY AND PHYSIOLOGY

The pericardium consists of two serous surfaces surrounding a closed, complex, saclike potential space. The visceral pericardium is continuous with the epicardial surface of the heart. The parietal pericardium is a dense but thin, fibrous structure which is closely apposed to the pleural surfaces laterally and blends with the central tendon of the diaphragm inferiorly. Around the right and left ventricles and the ventricular apex, the pericardial space is a simple ellipsoid structure conforming to the shape of the ventricles. Around the systemic and pulmonary venous inflows and around the great vessels, the parietal and visceral pericardia meet to close the "ends" of the sac—these areas often are referred to as *pericardial reflections*. The pericardial space encloses the right atrium and right atrial appendage anteriorly and laterally, with pericardial reflections around the superior and inferior vena cava near their junction with the right atrium. Superiorly, the pericardium extends a short distance along the great vessels, with a small "pocket" of pericardium surrounding the great arteries posteriorly—the *transverse sinus*. The pericardial space extends lateral to the left atrium, and a blind pocket of the pericardium extends posterior to the left atrium, between the four pulmonary veins—the *oblique sinus* (Fig. 8–1). The pericardial space normally contains a small amount (5 to 10 ml) of fluid which may be detectable by echocardiography.

Anatomically, the pericardium isolates the heart from the rest of the mediastinum and from the lungs and pleural spaces. In addition, it may serve a lubricating function to allow normal rotation and translation of the heart during the cardiac cycle. However, the normal physiologic function of the pericardium is unclear. Some investigators suggest that the pericardium exerts a "restraining" effect on normal cardiac filling, while others argue that the pericardium has no significant hemodynamic function. In either case, the importance of the pericardium becomes clear with disease processes such as inflammation, infection, or malignancy.

PERICARDITIS

Basic Principles

Pericarditis is inflammation of the pericardium, and it can be due to a wide variety of causes, including infection, postviral, trauma, uremia, and transmural myocardial infarction (Table 8–1). Clinically, the diagnosis is based on the characteristic triad of chest pain, electrocardiographic changes, and the presence of a pericardial rub on auscultation. While it is probable that most patients with pericarditis have a pericardial effusion at some point in the disease course, a pericardial effusion is not a necessary criterion for diagnosis of pericarditis, nor does the presence of an effusion indicate a diagnosis of pericarditis. Interestingly, there is no correlation between the size of the pericardial effusion and the presence or absence of a pericardial "rub" on physical examination.

Echocardiographic Approach

In a patient with suspected pericarditis, the echocardiogram may show a pericardial effusion of any size or pericardial thickening with or without an effusion, or it may be entirely normal. A pericardial effusion is recognized as an echolucent space around the heart, as described in detail below (Fig. 8–2).

Pericardial thickening is evidenced by increased echogenicity of the pericardial reflection on two-dimensional (2D) imaging and as multiple parallel reflections posterior to the left ventricle on M-mode recordings (Fig. 8–3). However, since the pericardium typically is the most echogenic structure in the image, it can be difficult to distinguish normal from thickened pericardium.

A careful echocardiographic examination from several windows is needed when pericarditis is

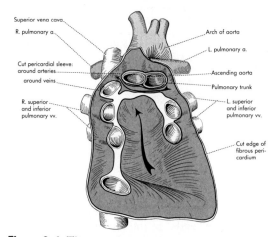

Figure 8–1. The posterior wall of the pericardial sac after the heart has been removed by severing its continuity with the great arteries and veins and by cutting the two pericardial sleeves that surround the arteries and veins. The parietal serous pericardium is pink; the fibrous pericardium is white; the horizontal arrow is in the transverse sinus; the vertical arrow is in the oblique sinus of the pericardium. *(Reprinted with permission from Hollingshead WH, Rosse C: Textbook of Anatomy. Philadelphia, Harper and Row, 1985.)*

TABLE 8–1. DIFFERENTIAL DIAGNOSIS OF PERICARDIAL EFFUSION/PERICARDITIS

I. Infections
    A. Postviral pericarditis
    B. Bacterial
    C. Tuberculosis
II. Malignant
    A. Metastatic disease (e.g., lymphoma, melanoma)
    B. Direct extension (lung carcinoma, breast carcinoma)
    C. Primary cardiac malignancy
III. "Inflammatory"
    A. Post-myocardial infarction (Dressler's syndrome)
    B. Uremia
    C. Collagen-vascular disease
    D. Post-cardiac surgery
IV. Intracardiac-pericardial communications
    A. Blunt or penetrating chest trauma
    B. Post-catheter procedures (electrophysiology studies, coronary angioplasty or atherectomy, valvuloplasty)
    C. Left ventricular rupture post-myocardial infarction

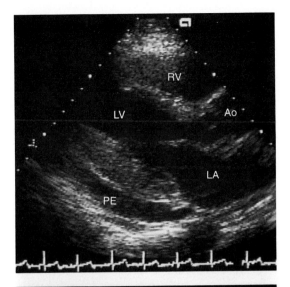

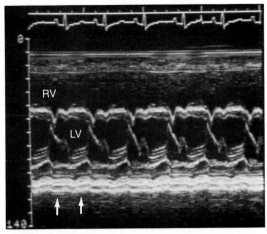

Figure 8–3. Pericardial thickening on M-mode echocardiography appears as multiple parallel dense echoes posterior to the left ventricular epicardium (*arrows*).

PERICARDIAL EFFUSION

Basic Principles and Tamponade Physiology

A wide variety of disease processes can result in a pericardial effusion with a differential diagnosis similar to that for pericarditis (see Table 8–1). The physiologic consequences of fluid in the pericardial space depend both on the volume and rate of fluid accumulation. A slowly expanding pericardial effusion can become quite large (>1000 ml) with little rise in pericardial pressure, whereas rapid accumulation of even a small volume of fluid (50 to 100 ml) can lead to a marked rise in pericardial pressure (Fig. 8–4).

Tamponade physiology occurs when the pressure in the pericardium exceeds the pressure in

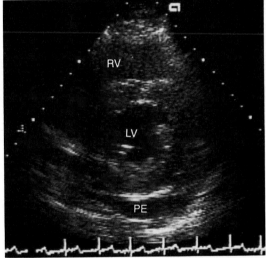

Figure 8–2. Parasternal long- and short-axis views of a small to moderate posterior pericardial effusion (PE).

suspected, since effusion or thickening can be localized and may be seen in only certain tomographic views. If a pericardial effusion is present, the possibility of tamponade physiology should be considered (see below). If pericardial thickening is present, examination for evidence of constrictive physiology (see below) should be considered.

Clinical Utility

Pericarditis is a clinical diagnosis that cannot be made independently by echocardiography. The goal of the echo examination is to evaluate for pericardial effusion or thickening.

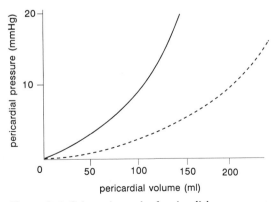

Figure 8–4. Schematic graph of pericardial pressure versus pericardial volume for an acute effusion (*solid line*, with a steep pressure-volume relationship) and for a chronic effusion (*dashed line*, where large volumes may lead to only mild pressure elevation).

the cardiac chambers, resulting in impaired cardiac filling. As pericardial pressure rises, filling of each cardiac chamber is sequentially impaired, with lower-pressure chambers (atria) being affected before higher-pressure chambers (ventricles). The compressive effect of the pericardial fluid is seen most clearly in the phase of the cardiac cycle when pressure is lowest in that chamber—systole for the atrium, diastole for the ventricles. Filling pressures become elevated as a compensatory mechanism to maintain cardiac output. In fully developed tamponade, diastolic pressures in all four cardiac chambers are equal (and elevated) due to exposure of the entire heart to the elevated pericardial pressure.

Clinically, tamponade physiology is manifested as low-cardiac-output symptoms, hypotension, and tachycardia. Jugular venous pressure is elevated and pulsus paradoxus (an inspiratory decline >10 mmHg in systemic blood pressure) is present on physical examination. The clinical finding of pulsus paradoxus is closely related to the echo findings of reciprocal respiratory changes in right and left ventricular filling and emptying (Fig. 8–5).

Echocardiographic Approach to Diagnosis of Pericardial Effusion

Diffuse Effusion

A pericardial effusion is recognized on 2D echocardiography as an echolucent space adjacent to the cardiac structures. In the absence of prior pericardial disease or surgery, pericardial effusions usually are diffuse and symmetrical

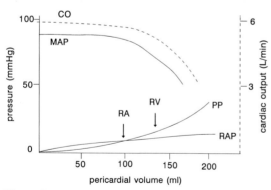

Figure 8–5. Schematic graph showing the relationship between pericardial pressure (PP), right atrial pressure (RAP), mean arterial pressure (MAP), and cardiac output (CO). Note that when pericardial pressure exceeds right atrial (RA) pressure, blood pressure and cardiac output fall. When right ventricular (RV) pressure is exceeded (at the arrow), cardiac output and mean arterial pressure fall further.

with clear separation between the parietal and visceral pericardium (Fig. 8–6). A relatively echogenic area anteriorly, in the absence of a posterior effusion, most likely represents a pericardial fat pad. M-mode recordings are helpful, especially with a small effusion, showing the flat posterior pericardial echo reflection and the moving epicardial echo with separation between the two in both systole and diastole.

In patients with recurrent or long-standing pericardial disease, fibrinous stranding within the fluid and on the epicardial surface of the heart may be seen (Fig. 8–7). When a malignant

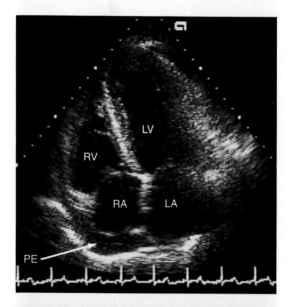

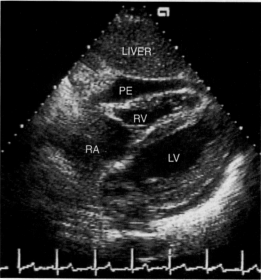

Figure 8–6. Pericardial effusion seen from an apical four-chamber view (*above*) and from a subcostal view (*below*).

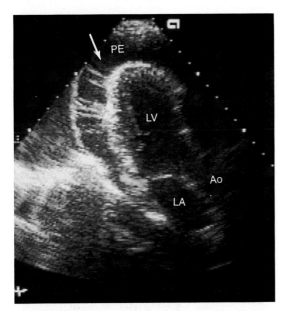

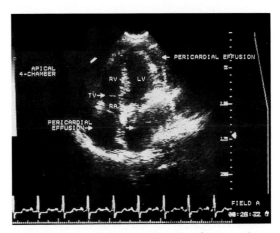

Figure 8–8. Apical four-chamber view demonstrating a loculated pericardial effusion (PE) after cardiac surgery with severe compression of both the left and right atria by loculated fluid collections. Note the relative absence of fluid around the right and left ventricles. *(Reprinted with permission from Otto CM et al: A case of delayed postoperative cardiac tamponade with unusual echocardiographic findings. Chest 97:1003, 1990.)*

Figure 8–7. Fibrinous stranding with adhesions between the visceral and parietal pericardia in a chronic effusion seen on an apical long-axis view.

effusion is suspected, it is difficult to distinguish this nonspecific finding from metastatic disease. Features suggesting the latter include a nodular appearance, evidence of extension into the myocardium, and the appropriate clinical setting.

The size of the pericardial effusion is considered to be small when the separation between parietal and visceral pericardium is <0.5 cm, moderate when it is 0.5 to 2 cm, and large when it is >2 cm. More quantitative measures of the size of the pericardial effusion rarely are needed in the clinical setting.

Loculated Effusion

In the postoperative patient or the patient with recurrent pericardial disease, a *loculated* pericardial effusion can occur. In this situation, the effusion may be localized by adhesions to a small area of the pericardial space or may consist of several separate areas of pericardial effusion. Recognition of a loculated effusion is especially important because hemodynamic compromise can occur with even a small, strategically located fluid collection and because drainage may not be possible from a percutaneous approach (Fig. 8–8).

Distinguishing from Pleural Fluid

Echocardiographic evaluation for a pericardial effusion thus requires a careful examination from multiple acoustic windows. The parasternal approach demonstrates the extent of the fluid collection at the base of the heart in both long- and short-axis views. Note that pericardial fluid may be seen posterior to the left atrium (in the oblique sinus) as well as posterior to the left ventricle. Care should be taken that the coronary sinus or descending thoracic aorta are not mistaken for pericardial fluid. In fact, these structures can help in distinguishing pericardial from pleural fluid, since a left pleural effusion will extend posterolateral to the descending aorta, while a pericardial effusion will track anterior to the descending aorta (Figs. 7–2 and 8–9).

In the apical views, the lateral, medial, and apical extent of the effusion can be appreciated. In the apical four-chamber view, an isolated echo-free space superior to the right atrium most likely represents pleural fluid. The subcostal view demonstrates fluid between the diaphragm and right ventricle and is particularly helpful in echo-guided pericardiocentesis. The sensitivity and specificity of echocardiography for detection of a pericardial effusion are very high.

Echocardiographic Approach to Pericardial Tamponade (Fig. 8–10)

When cardiac tamponade occurs with a diffuse moderate to large pericardial effusion, the associated physiologic changes are evident on

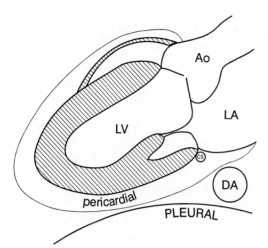

Figure 8–9. Schematic diagram of the relationship between a pericardial effusion and the descending aorta (DA) compared with a left pleural effusion. Pericardial fluid tracks posterior to the left atrium (LA) in the oblique sinus and anterior to the descending aorta.

echocardiographic and Doppler examination (Table 8–2).

Right Atrial Systolic Collapse

When intrapericardial pressure exceeds right atrial systolic pressure (lowest point of pressure curve), inversion or collapse of the right atrial free wall occurs. Since the right atrial free wall is a thin, flexible structure, *brief* right atrial wall inversion can occur in the absence of tamponade

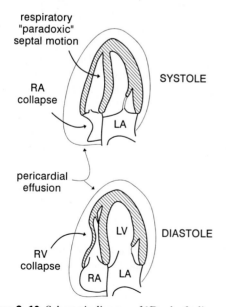

Figure 8–10. Schematic diagram of 2D echo findings with tamponade physiology.

TABLE 8–2. PERICARDIAL TAMPONADE

Clinical Findings

Low cardiac output

Elevated venous pressures

Pulsus paradoxus

Hypotension

2D-Echo

Moderate–large pericardial effusion

Right atrial systolic collapse (duration greater than a third of systole)

Right ventricular diastolic collapse

Reciprocal changes in right and left ventricular volumes (varying pattern of septal motion) with respiration

Doppler

Respiratory variation in right and left ventricular diastolic filling

Increased right ventricular filling on first beat after inspiration

Decreased left ventricular filling on first beat after inspiration

Inferior vena cava plethora (indicator of elevated right atrial pressure)

physiology. However, the longer the duration of right atrial inversion relative to the cycle length, the greater is the likelihood of cardiac tamponade. Inversion for greater than a third of systole has a sensitivity of 94 percent and a specificity of 100 percent for the diagnosis of tamponade. Careful frame-by-frame 2D image analysis is needed for this evaluation (Fig. 8–11).

Right Ventricular Diastolic Collapse

Right ventricular diastolic collapse occurs when intrapericardial pressure exceeds right ventricular diastolic pressure *and* when the right ventricular free wall is normal in thickness and compliance. The presence of right ventricular hypertrophy or infiltrative diseases of the myocardium may allow development of a pressure gradient between the pericardial space and right ventricular chamber without inversion of the normal contour of the free wall. Right ventricular diastolic collapse is best appreciated in the parasternal long-axis view or from a subcostal window. If the timing of right ventricular wall motion is not clear on 2D imaging, an M-mode

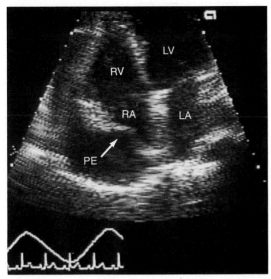

Figure 8–11. Apical four-chamber view showing systolic collapse on the right atrial free wall in a patient with clinical tamponade. PE = pericardial effusion.

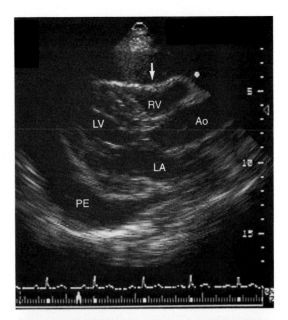

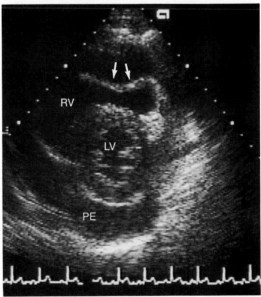

Figure 8–12. Parasternal long- (*above*) and short-axis (*below*) views showing right ventricular diastolic collapse (*arrows*).

through the right ventricular free wall is helpful. The presence of right ventricular diastolic collapse is somewhat less sensitive (60 to 90 percent) but more specific (85 to 100 percent) than brief right atrial systolic collapse for diagnosing tamponade physiology (Fig. 8–12).

Reciprocal Changes in Ventricular Volumes

Reciprocal respiratory variation in right and left ventricular volumes may be seen on 2D imaging when tamponade is present. In the apical four-chamber view, an increase in right ventricular volume with inspiration (shift in septal motion toward the left ventricle in diastole and toward the right ventricle in systole) and a decrease during expiration (normalization of septal motion) can be appreciated. This pattern of motion corresponds to the physical finding of pulsus paradoxus. The proposed explanation for this observation is that total pericardial volume (heart chambers plus pericardial fluid) is fixed in tamponade so that as intrathoracic pressure becomes more negative during inspiration, enhanced right ventricular filling limits left ventricular diastolic filling. This pattern reverses during expiration (Fig. 8–13).

Respiratory Variation in Diastolic Filling

Doppler recordings of right and left ventricular diastolic filling in patients with tamponade physiology show a similar pattern. With inspiration, the right ventricular early diastolic filling velocity is augmented, while left ventricular diastolic filling diminishes (Figs. 8–14 and 8–15). In addition, the flow velocity integral in the pulmonary artery increases with inspiration, while the aortic flow velocity integral decreases. In the acutely ill patient, these changes can be difficult to demonstrate in part due to respiratory changes in the intercept angle between the Dop-

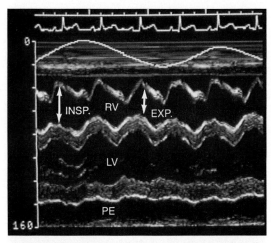

Figure 8–13. M-mode tracing showing reciprocal changes in right and left ventricular volumes with respiration when tamponade is present.

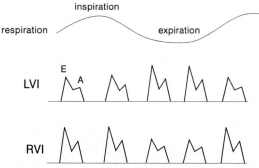

Figure 8–14. Schematic diagram of left and right ventricular diastolic inflow (RVI and LVI). Doppler curves with tamponade physiology showing enhanced right ventricular (and reduced left ventricular) diastolic filling with inspiration and a reversal of this pattern during expiration.

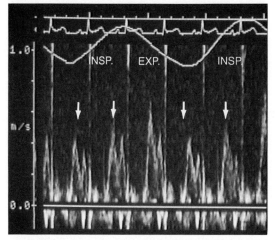

Figure 8–15. Doppler recording of left ventricular inflow in a patient with tamponade showing reduced filling during inspiration.

pler beam and the flow of interest causing artifactual apparent velocity changes. Differentiating the normal respiratory variation in diastolic filling from the excessive variation (>25 percent) seen in tamponade may be subtle in borderline cases. Tamponade physiology is not an all-or-none phenomenon; a patient may exhibit varying degrees of hemodynamic impairment as the degree of pericardial compression (pericardial pressure) increases.

Plethora of the Inferior Vena Cava

Inferior vena cava plethora, a dilated inferior vena cava with <50 percent inspiratory reduction in diameter near the inferior vena cava–right atrium junction, also has been proposed as a sensitive (97 percent), albeit nonspecific (40 percent), indicator of tamponade physiology. This simple finding reflects the elevated right atrial pressure seen in tamponade.

Limitations/Alternate Approaches

Echocardiography is very sensitive for the diagnosis of pericardial effusion, even when loculated, if care is taken to examine the heart in multiple tomographic planes from multiple acoustic windows. Loculated effusions can be difficult to assess in certain locations, particularly if localized to the atrial region, since the effusion itself may be mistaken for a normal cardiac chamber.

The etiology of the pericardial effusion is not always evident on echocardiographic examination. Irregular pericardial or epicardial masses in a patient with a known malignancy certainly raise the possibility of a malignant effusion, but this appearance can be mimicked by fibrinous organization of a long-standing pericardial effusion. Masses adjacent to the cardiac structures (in the mediastinum) resulting in pericardial effusion can be missed by echocardiography. Wide-view tomographic imaging procedures, such as computed tomography or magnetic resonance imaging, are helpful in these cases.

Obviously, whether a pericardial effusion is infected or inflammatory in etiology cannot be determined by echocardiography. Depending on the associated clinical findings in each case, diagnostic pericardiocentesis may be indicated to establish the correct diagnosis.

With cardiac rupture, either after myocardial infarction, after cardiac procedures, or with chest trauma, the site of rupture itself rarely can be detected, so a high level of suspicion is needed when this diagnosis is a possibility. In some cases, the site of left ventricular rupture is "contained" by pericardial adhesions, resulting in formation of a pseudoaneurysm. A *pseudoaneurysm* is defined as a saccular structure communicating with the ventricle with walls composed of pericardium (Fig. 8–16). In contrast, the walls of a "true" aneurysm are composed of thinned, scarred myocardium. A pseudoaneurysm (see Fig. 8–16) can be distinguished from a true aneurysm by echocardiography based on (1) an abrupt transition from normal thickness of myocardium to the thin walled sac, (2) an acute angle between the contour of the aneurysm and the left ventricle, and (3) a narrow opening between the ventricular chamber and the aneurysm ("neck") with a ratio of the neck diameter to maximum diameter of <0.5. This distinction is important because pseudoaneurysms are prone to rupture and require surgical correction, whereas a diagnosis of a true aneurysm does not mandate surgical intervention.

Clinical Utility

Diagnosis of Pericardial Effusion

Echocardiography is the procedure of choice for diagnosis of pericardial effusion. When transthoracic images are inadequate, as occa-

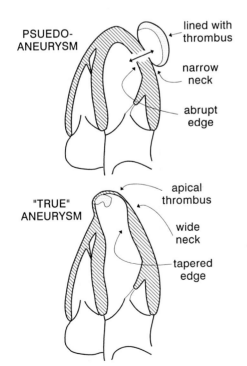

PSUEDO-ANEURYSM

lined with thrombus

narrow neck

abrupt edge

"TRUE" ANEURYSM

apical thrombus

wide neck

tapered edge

Figure 8–16. Schematic diagram of a pseudoaneurysm versus a true aneurysm.

sionally occurs (especially in postoperative patients), transesophageal imaging or an alternate tomographic imaging procedure (MRI, CT) may be needed. Echocardiography can be helpful in establishing a diagnosis of pericardial tamponade but requires integration with other clinical data.

In evaluating a patient for cardiac tamponade, it is essential to remember that tamponade is a clinical and hemodynamic diagnosis. Furthermore, varying degrees of tamponade physiology may be seen. The most important finding on echocardiography in a patient with suspected pericardial tamponade is whether or not a pericardial effusion is present. The absence of a pericardial effusion *excludes* the diagnosis, again taking care that a loculated effusion is not missed. Only rarely does tamponade physiology result from other mediastinal contents under pressure (i.e., air due to barotrauma or a compressive mass). Conversely, in a patient with convincing clinical evidence for tamponade, the presence of a moderate to large pericardial effusion on echocardiography *confirms* the diagnosis.

In intermediate cases, either when the clinical diagnosis has not been considered or when the clinical evidence is equivocal, 2D findings of chamber collapse and inferior vena cava plethora and Doppler findings showing marked respiratory variation in right and left ventricular filling may be helpful. Since none of these findings has a positive predictive value of 100 percent, each needs to be considered in conjunction with the clinical data. Other diagnostic tests that are helpful in making this diagnosis include right-sided heart catheterization showing a depressed cardiac output and equalization of right atrial, right ventricular diastolic, and pulmonary artery wedge pressures.

Echo-Guided Pericardiocentesis

The success rate without complications of percutaneous needle pericardiocentesis can be enhanced by using echocardiographic guidance. With the patient in the position planned for the procedure, the optimal transcutaneous approach is identified based on the location of the effusion, the distance from the chest wall to the pericardium, and the absence of intervening structures. The transducer angle and pericardial depth are noted, and the transducer position is marked prior to prepping the site for the procedure. After the procedure, the residual amount of pericardial fluid is assessed using standard tomographic views. If monitoring during the procedure is needed, an acoustic window that allows visualization of the effusion but does not

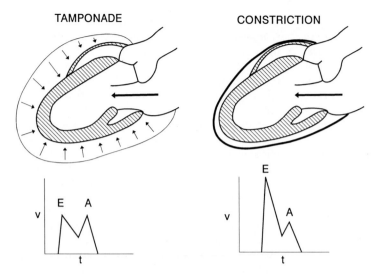

Figure 8–17. Schematic diagram of pericardial tamponade compared with pericardial constriction. With tamponade, diastolic filling is impaired in both early and late diastole due to the elevated pericardial pressures "compressing" the heart. With constriction, early diastolic filling is rapid but ends abruptly when the volume limits of the rigid pericardial space are reached.

compromise the sterile field is identified. (Alternatively, a sterile sleeve is used for the transducer.) Note that with *tomographic* imaging it is difficult to identify the *tip* of the needle, since any segment of the needle passing through the image plane may appear to be the tip. Scanning in both superoinferior and lateromedial directions during imaging helps minimize this source of error. Confirmation that the needle tip is in the pericardial space can be made by injecting a *small* amount of agitated sterile saline through the needle to achieve an echo-contrast effect.

PERICARDIAL CONSTRICTION

Basic Principles

In constrictive pericarditis, the visceral and parietal layers of the pericardium are adherent, thickened, and fibrotic, resulting in impairment of diastolic ventricular filling. Pericardial constriction can occur after repeated episodes of pericarditis, after cardiac surgery, after radiation therapy, and from a variety of other causes. The diagnosis often is delayed because clinical symptoms are nonspecific—fatigue and malaise due to low cardiac output—and physical findings either are subtle (elevated jugular venous pressure, distant heart sounds) or occur only late in the disease course (ascites and peripheral edema).

The physiology of constrictive pericarditis is characterized by impaired diastolic cardiac filling due to the abnormal pericardium surrounding the cardiac structures, acting like a rigid "box" (Fig. 8–17). Early diastolic filling is rapid,

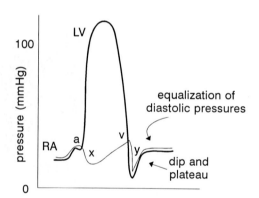

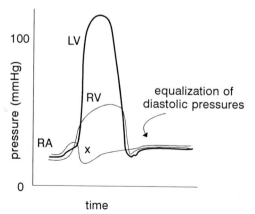

Figure 8–18. Typical pressure tracings in tamponade and constriction.

with an abrupt cessation of ventricular filling as diastolic pressure rises—when the "box" is "full." Pressure tracings typically show (1) a brief, rapid fall of ventricular pressure in early diastole followed by a high early diastolic pressure plateau (*dip-plateau* or *square-root sign*), (2) a rapid descent of right atrial pressure with the onset of ventricular filling (*y* descent), (3) only modest elevation of right ventricular and pulmonary artery systolic pressures, (4) a right ventricular diastolic pressure plateau that is a third or more of systolic pressure, and (5) equalization of diastolic pressures in the right ventricle and left ventricle even after volume loading (Fig. 8–18).

Echocardiographic Approach
(Table 8–3)

2D/M-Mode Imaging

Typically, left ventricular wall thickness, internal dimensions, and systolic function are normal in the patient with constrictive pericarditis. Left atrial enlargement is seen due to chronic left

---

TABLE 8–3. ECHO DOPPLER FINDINGS IN CONSTRICTIVE PERICARDITIS

M-mode/2D

Pericardial thickening

Normal left ventricular size and systolic function

Left atrial enlargement

Flattened diastolic wall motion

Abrupt posterior motion of the ventricular septum in early diastole

Dilated inferior vena cava and hepatic veins

Doppler

Prominent *y* descent on hepatic vein or superior vena cava flow pattern

Left ventricular inflow shows prominent *E* velocity with a rapid early diastolic deceleration slope and a small or absent *A* velocity

Increase in LV-IVRT by >20 percent on first beat after inspiration

Respiratory variations in right ventricular/left ventricular diastolic filling (difference >25 percent) with increase in right ventricular filling and decrease in left ventricular filling with inspiration

Pulmonary venous flow shows prominent *a* wave and blunting of systolic phase of left atrial filling

---

atrial pressure elevation. Pericardial thickening may be evident on 2D imaging as increased echogenicity in the region of the pericardium (Fig. 8–19). Careful examination from several acoustic windows is needed because the spatial distribution of pericardial thickening may be asymmetrical. From the parasternal approach, an M-mode recording shows multiple dense echos, posterior to the left ventricular epicardium, moving parallel with each other. These echos persist even at a low-gain setting. M-mode recordings also may demonstrate an abrupt pos-

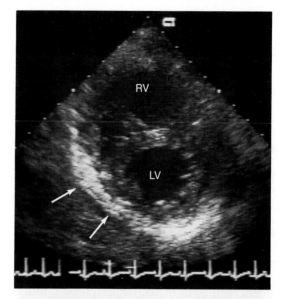

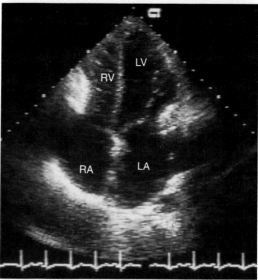

Figure 8–19. Constrictive pericarditis from a parasternal short-axis and apical four-chamber view. Note the thickened pericardium (*arrow*), biatrial enlargement, and small ventricles.

terior motion of the ventricular septum in early diastole, with flat motion in middle to late diastole (Fig. 8–20). This pattern of motion appears to be due to initial rapid right ventricular diastolic filling, followed by equalization of filling of right and left ventricles as the "plateau" phase of the pressure curve is reached. The left ventricular posterior wall endocardium shows little posterior motion during diastole (<2 mm from early to late diastole) due to the impairment of diastolic filling resulting in a "flat" pattern of diastolic posterior wall motion. On subcostal views, the inferior vena cava and hepatic veins are dilated, reflecting the elevated right atrial pressure.

Doppler Examination

The Doppler findings in constrictive pericarditis reflect the abnormal hemodynamics in this condition (Fig. 8–21). Pulsed Doppler recordings of hepatic vein flow (from a subcostal approach) measure right atrial filling and show a prominent a wave and a deep y descent (Fig. 8–22). Similarly, pulsed Doppler recordings of pulmonary vein flow (transthoracic apical four-chamber view or transesophageal approach) indicate left atrial filling and again show a prominent a wave, prominent y descent, and blunting of the systolic phase of atrial filling.

Both right and left ventricular diastolic filling show a high E velocity due to rapid early diastolic filling occurring simultaneously with the initial high atrial to ventricular pressure difference during the brief early diastolic "dip" in ventricular pressure. As left ventricular pressure rises, filling abruptly ceases, reflected in a short deceleration time of the E-velocity curve. Little

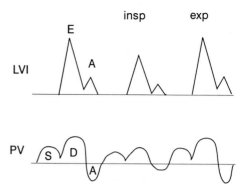

Figure 8–21. Schematic diagram of the Doppler flow patterns in constrictive pericarditis. Left ventricular inflow shows reduced early diastolic filling with inspiration, while the pulmonary vein shows a prominent a wave and blunting of the systolic filling phase.

ventricular filling occurs in late diastole due to the elevated left ventricular diastolic pressure (the "plateau") and the constrictive effect of the thickened pericardium. Doppler recordings of ventricular inflow thus show a very small A velocity following atrial contraction.

Marked reciprocal respiratory variations in right and left ventricular diastolic inflow velocities are seen due to the differing effects of changes in intrapleural pressure on filling of the two ventricles. With inspiration, intrapleural pressure becomes more negative, resulting in

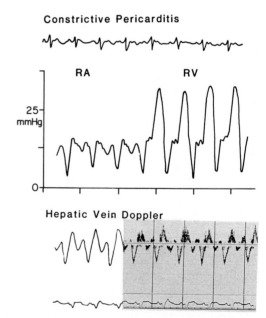

Figure 8–22. Pressure tracing and hepatic vein flow in a patient with constrictive pericarditis. Note the prominent a wave, flat diastolic segment, and prominent y descent, all consistent with the "square-root sign" or dip and plateau in the pressure tracings.

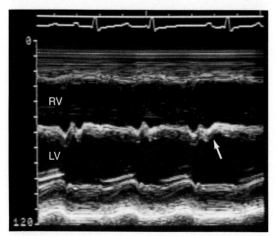

Figure 8–20. M-mode in constrictive pericarditis showing rapid anterior motion of the septum in early systole.

augmentation of right ventricular diastolic filling and inflow velocity. Left ventricular filling velocities *decrease* with inspiration and *increase* with expiration. Similar directional changes occur in normal individuals, with the respiratory changes being more marked (variation >25 percent) with constrictive pericarditis. The left ventricular isovolumic relaxation time—measured from the aortic closure to the mitral opening click on Doppler recordings—increases by a mean of 20 percent with inspiration in patients with constrictive pericarditis.

Comparison of Pericardial Tamponade, Constrictive Pericarditis, and Restrictive Cardiomyopathy (Table 8–4)

Although the hemodynamics of pericardial tamponade and pericardial constriction have some similarities, differentiating between these two diagnoses usually is straightforward based on the presence or absence of a pericardial effusion. Differentiating constrictive pericarditis from a restrictive cardiomyopathy is more difficult. Both are characterized by clinical signs and symptoms of elevated venous pressure and low cardiac output, and both show a normal-sized left ventricular chamber with normal systolic function on 2D echocardiography. Pericardial thickening may be difficult to appreciate, and other 2D and M-mode findings may not reliably differentiate between these two diagnoses. A difference (>25 percent) in maximum E velocity from expiration to inspiration has been suggested as a useful method for distinguishing constrictive pericarditis from restrictive cardiomyopathy. These characteristic Doppler findings may favor one clinical diagnosis over another and, in conjunction with other clinical data, may be definitive in some cases. However, Doppler

TABLE 8–4. COMPARISON OF PERICARDIAL TAMPONADE, PERICARDIAL CONSTRICTION, AND RESTRICTIVE CARDIOMYOPATHY

	PERICARDIAL TAMPONADE	CONSTRICTIVE PERICARDITIS	RESTRICTIVE CARDIOMYOPATHY
Hemodynamics			
Right atrial pressure	↑	↑	↑
Right/left ventricular filling pressures	↑, RV = LV	↑, RV = LV	↑, LV > RV
Pulmonary artery pressures	Normal	Mild elevation (35–40 mmHg systolic)	Moderate-severe elevation (≥60 mmHg systolic)
Right ventricular diastolic pressure plateau		>1/3 peak RV pressure	<1/3 peak RV pressure
Radionuclide Diastolic Filling		Rapid early filling, impaired late filling	Impaired early filling
2D Echo	Moderate-large PE	Pericardial thickening without effusion	Left ventricular hypertrophy Normal systolic function
Doppler Echo	Reciprocal respiratory changes in right and left ventricular filling Inferior vena cava plethora	$E > a$ on LV inflow Prominent y descent in hepatic vein Pulmonary venous flow = prominent a wave, reduced systolic phase Respiratory variation in IVRT and in E velocity	(1) Early in disease $e < A$ on LV inflow (2) Late in disease $E > a$ (3) Constant IVRT (4) Absence of significant respiratory variation
Other Diagnostic Tests	Therapeutic/diagnostic pericardiocentesis	CT or MRI for pericardial thickening	Endomyocardial biopsy

CT = computed tomography, IVRT = isovolumic relaxation time, LV = left ventricle, MRI = magnetic resonance imaging, PE = pericardial effusion, RV = right ventricular.

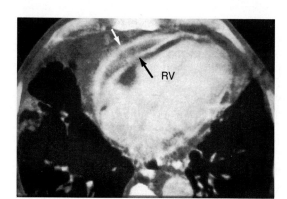 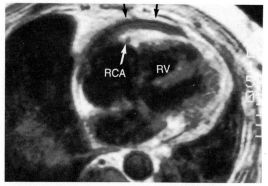

Figure 8–23. In a patient with tuberculous constrictive pericarditis, chest CT (*left*) shows thickening of visceral and parietal pericardial layers surrounding consolidated caseous material as alternating bands of light and dark anterior to the right ventricle (*arrows*). In a second patient with constrictive pericarditis, the chest MRI (*right*) shows pericardial thickening as a low signal band (*dark area*) anterior to the right ventricle (*arrow*). Epicardial fat is high signal (*white*) with the right coronary artery (RCA) indicated.

data are far from absolutely accurate due to overlap between groups in the Doppler findings and due to differing hemodynamics in patients with restrictive cardiomyopathy depending on disease stage (see Chap. 7). One of the most helpful findings on Doppler examination is estimation of pulmonary artery systolic pressure from the tricuspid regurgitant jet. Patients with restrictive cardiomyopathy typically have moderate to severe pulmonary hypertension, while those with constrictive pericarditis have only mild elevations in pulmonary pressures.

Limitations/Alternate Approaches

When the diagnosis of constrictive pericarditis is in question, several alternate approaches may be helpful. Chest fluoroscopy shows calcification of the pericardium in about 50 percent of cases of constrictive pericarditis. Both chest CT or MRI scanning are more definitive for detection of pericardial thickening, especially when it is asymmetrical (Fig. 8–23). Evaluation of early diastolic ventricular filling on frame-by-frame angiography or by radionuclide techniques also has been proposed as a method to distinguish constrictive pericarditis from restrictive cardiomyopathy. Endomyocardial biopsy occasionally will confirm a diagnosis of restrictive cardiomyopathy due to an infiltrative process.

Right- and left-sided heart catheterization with recording of intracardiac pressures and waveforms, including simultaneous recording of right ventricular and left ventricular diastolic pressures after volume loading, remains the standard of reference for diagnosis of constric-

tive pericarditis. However, even with this technique some cases will be missed, so exploratory thoracotomy may be needed to make a definitive diagnosis. If present, pericardial constriction then can be relieved by surgical removal of the pericardium.

Clinical Utility

The diagnosis of pericardial constriction remains problematic, with no single diagnostic feature on echocardiographic or Doppler examination. However, the conjunction of several findings in a patient in whom the level of clinical suspicion is high increases the likelihood of this diagnosis and may be definitive in some cases. Conversely, the echo and Doppler findings may provide the first clues for this diagnosis in a patient in whom it was not previously considered—for example, a patient presenting with ascites and no prior cardiac history.

SUGGESTED READING

1. Markiewicz W, Brik A, Brook G, et al: Pericardial rub in pericardial effusion: Lack of correlation with amount of fluid. Chest 77:643–646, 1980.
   In 76 patients with a pericardial effusion, a rub was noted on auscultation in 4 of 13 (30 percent) with a small, 23 of 40 (58 percent) with a moderate, and 10 of 23 (43 percent) patients with a large effusion. These findings suggest that the size of the effusion cannot be predicted from the presence or absence of a rub.

2. Markiewicz W, Monakier I, Brik A, et al: Clinical-echocardiographic correlations in pericardial effusion. Eur Heart J 3:260–266, 1982.
   Of 100 patients with an effusion on echocardiography, 49 had a clinical course consistent with acute pericarditis (id-

iopathic in 23 of 49, after radiation in 7, Dressler's syndrome in 7, purulent in 4, and other in 7), while the remainder had a less acute presentation. In the latter group, the etiology was carcinoma in 20 of 51, heart disease in 12, uremia in 7, rheumatoid arthritis in 5, and chronic idiopathic pericarditis in 4 patients (3 other).

3. Permanyer-Miralda G, Sagrista-Sauleda J, Soler-Soler J: Primary acute pericardial disease: A prospective series of 231 consecutive patients. Am J Cardiol 56: 623–630, 1985.
Of 231 patients with primary acute pericarditis, "therapeutic pericardiocentesis" was performed in 44 for tamponade physiology, while 32 had a "diagnostic" pericardiocentesis for suspected purulent pericarditis. The diagnostic yield was 29 percent for therapeutic and 6 percent for diagnostic pericardiocentesis. The overall diagnostic yield of pericardial biopsy was 22 percent.

4. Gillam LD, Guyer DE, Gibson TC, et al: Hydrodynamic compression of the right atrium: A new echocardiographic sign of cardiac tamponade. Circulation 68:294–301, 1983.
Right atrial free wall systolic inversion which persists for a third or more of the cycle length had a sensitivity of 94 percent and specificity of 100 percent for the diagnosis of tamponade physiology in 127 patients (19 with tamponade).

5. Leimgruber P, Klopfenstein HS, Wann LS, Brooks HL: The hemodynamic derangement associated with right ventricular diastolic collapse in cardiac tamponade: An experimental echocardiographic study. Circulation 68:612–620, 1983.
In an experimental model, right ventricular diastolic collapse occurred when intrapericardial pressure exceeded right ventricular diastolic pressure and was associated with a 21 percent reduction in cardiac output (but no change in mean aortic pressure). Of note, right ventricular diastolic collapse did not occur in the presence of right ventricular hypertrophy.

6. Reddy PS, Curtiss EI, Uretsky BF: Spectrum of hemodynamic changes in cardiac tamponade. Am J Cardiol 55:1487–1491, 1990.
The range of hemodynamic compromise that can be seen with tamponade physiology is emphasized in this study of 77 consecutive patients with >150 ml of pericardial fluid. In group I, intrapericardial pressures were less than right atrial and pulmonary artery wedge pressures. In group II, intrapericardial and right atrial pressures had equaled. In group III, intrapericardial, right atrial, and pulmonary artery wedge pressures were equal. All subjects improved after pericardiocentesis, with the greatest improvement seen in group III.

7. Gonzalez MS, Basnight MA, Appleton CP: Experimental cardiac tamponade: A hemodynamic and Doppler echocardiographic reexamination of the relation of right and left heart ejection dynamics to the phase of respiration. J Am Coll Cardiol 18:243–252, 1991.
In this model, there was an inverse relationship between peak left and right ventricular systolic pressures and ejection times, and between pulmonary and aortic flow velocities, when tamponade physiology was present. This suggests that the mechanism of pulsus paradoxus is the reciprocal changes in right and left ventricular filling due to a "fixed" total cardiac volume in tamponade.

8. Gonzalez MS, Basnight MA, Appleton CP: Experimental pericardial effusion: Relation of abnormal respiratory variation in mitral flow velocity to hemodynamics and diastolic right heart collapse. J Am Coll Cardiol 17:239–248, 1991.

Respiratory changes in left ventricular diastolic filling are exaggerated in tamponade, with this variation occurring before equalization of intracardiac pressures and definite right-sided heart collapse. The presence of excessive respiratory variation, but not its magnitude, is predictive of tamponade physiology.

9. Leeman DE, Levine MJ, Come PC: Doppler echocardiography in cardiac tamponade: Exaggerated respiratory variation in transvalvular blood flow velocity integrals. J Am Coll Cardiol 11:572–578, 1988.
Exaggerated respiratory variation in left ventricular filling on Doppler examination was noted in 13 patients with tamponade physiology, with resolution of these changes after pericardiocentesis.

10. Picard MH, Sanfilippo AJ, Newell JB, et al: Quantitative relation between increased intrapericardial pressure and Doppler flow velocities during experimental cardiac tamponade. J Am Coll Cardiol 18:234–242, 1991.
In contrast to Suggested Reading 8 above, these authors did note a quantitative relationship between the degree of increase in intrapericardial pressure and the percentage change in inflow/outflow patterns with respiration.

11. Chuttani K, Pandian NG, Mohanty PK, et al: Left ventricular diastolic collapse: An echocardiographic sign of regional cardiac tamponade. Circulation 83: 1999–2006, 1991.
Loculated effusions, especially after cardiac surgery, can cause compression of individual cardiac chambers leading to tamponade physiology. Conventional signs of tamponade may be absent on echocardiography in these cases.

12. Himelman RB, Kircher B, Rockey DC, Schiller NB: Inferior vena cava plethora with blunted respiratory response: A sensitive echocardiographic sign of cardiac tamponade. J Am Coll Cardiol 12:1470–1477, 1988.
Dilation of the inferior vena cava reflects an elevated right atrial pressure. Plethora of the inferior vena cava had a sensitivity of 97 percent but a specificity of only 40 percent for the diagnosis of pericardial tamponade. False-positive results occurred in patients with right ventricular failure, tricuspid regurgitation, and pulmonary hypertension.

13. Eisenberg MJ, Schiller NB: Bayes' theorem and the echocardiographic diagnosis of cardiac tamponade. Am J Cardiol 68:1242–1244, 1991.
Using Bayes' theorem, the predictive values of right ventricular collapse, right atrial collapse, and inferior vena cava plethora for the diagnosis of tamponade were calculated (using published sensitivities and specificities for these variables). When the pretest probability of tamponade is high (50 percent), both right atrial and right ventricular collapse have high positive and negative predictive values. With a medium (10 percent) or low (1 percent) pretest likelihood, all three variables have a high (≥97 percent) negative predictive value (i.e., tamponade can be excluded if absent) but a low positive predictive value.

14. Levine MJ, Lorell BH, Diver DJ, Come PC: Implications of echocardiographically assisted diagnosis of pericardial tamponade in contemporary medical patients: Detection before hemodynamic embarrassment. J Am Coll Cardiol 17:59–65, 1991.
Echocardiography identified right heart chamber collapse in the presence of an effusion (i.e., tamponade) in patients with minimal evidence of hemodynamic compromise. Symptoms persisted even with hemodynamic improvement after pericardiocentesis in many patients. When malignancy was the cause of tamponade, 1-year survival was only 17 percent.

15. Schnittger I, Bowden RE, Abrams J, Popp RL: Echocardiography: Pericardial thickening and constrictive pericarditis. Am J Cardiol 42:388–395, 1978.
Description of echocardiographic diagnosis of pericardial thickening and correlation with surgical, autopsy, and catheterization findings.

16. Agatston AS, Rao A, Price RJ, Kinney EL: Diagnosis of constrictive pericarditis by pulsed Doppler echocardiography. Am J Cardiol 54:929–930, 1984.
Brief early report describing the pattern of left ventricular filling in patients with constrictive pericarditis.

17. von Bibra H, Schober K, Jenni R, et al: Diagnosis of constrictive pericarditis by pulsed Doppler echocardiography of the hepatic vein. Am J Cardiol 63:483–488, 1989.
In patients with constrictive pericarditis, hepatic vein flow showed abrupt reversal in late systole and in mid-diastole, similar to the "W pattern" seen on physical examination of the neck veins. This hepatic vein flow pattern had a sensitivity of 68 percent and a specificity of 100 percent for the diagnosis of constrictive pericarditis in 51 patients (13 with constrictive pericarditis, 13 controls, 12 with right ventricular pressure overload, and 12 with right ventricular pressure and volume overload).

18. Hatle LK, Appleton CP, Popp RL: Differentiation of constrictive pericarditis and restrictive cardiomyopathy by Doppler echocardiography. Circulation 79:357–370, 1989.
Patients with constrictive pericarditis showed marked respiratory variation in left and right ventricular inflow velocities and isovolumic relaxation times, while patients with restrictive cardiomyopathy did not have respiratory variation. With constrictive pericarditis, the first beat after inspiration showed a decrease in left ventricular inflow velocity, an increase in right ventricular inflow velocity, and an increase in left ventricular isovolumic relaxation time. These changes resolve after pericardiectomy.

19. Aroney CN, Ruddy RD, Dighero H, et al: Differentiation of restrictive cardiomyopathy from pericardial constriction: Assessment of diastolic function by radionuclide angiography. J Am Coll Cardiol 13:1007–1014, 1989.
Diastolic filling curves were evaluated using radionuclide techniques. In patients with constrictive pericarditis, the rate of early diastolic filling and the time to peak filling rate were increased, while the atrial contribution to left ventricular filling was decreased compared with patients with restrictive cardiomyopathy and normal individuals.

20. Catherwood E, Mintz GS, Kotler MN, et al: Two-dimensional echocardiographic recognition of left ventricular pseudoaneurysm. Circulation 62:294–303, 1980.
Characteristic echocardiographic findings in left ventricular pseudoaneurysm are presented.

21. Gatewood RP Jr, Nanda NC: Differentiation of left ventricular pseudoaneurysm with two-dimensional echocardiography. Am J Cardiol 46:869–878, 1980.
Characteristic echocardiographic findings in left ventricular pseudoaneurysm are presented.

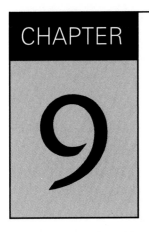

CHAPTER 9

VALVULAR STENOSIS: DIAGNOSIS, QUANTITATION, AND CLINICAL APPROACH

BASIC PRINCIPLES

Approach to Evaluation of Valvular Stenosis

Narrowing, or stenosis, of a cardiac valve can be due to a congenitally abnormal valve, a post-inflammatory process (e.g., rheumatic), or degenerative calcification. As the degree of valve opening decreases, the increasing obstruction to blood flow results in an increased flow velocity and pressure gradient across the valve. In isolated valve stenosis, clinical symptoms typically occur when the valve orifice is reduced to one-quarter its normal size. In mixed stenosis and regurgitation, symptoms can occur when each lesion, if isolated, would be considered only moderate in severity.

Secondary changes in patients with valvular stenosis include the response of the specific cardiac chambers affected by pressure overload. The ventricular response to pressure overload is hypertrophy; the atrial response is dilation. Chronic pressure overload also can lead to irreversible changes in other upstream cardiac chambers and in the pulmonary vascular bed (e.g., in mitral stenosis).

Complete echocardiographic evaluation of the patient with valvular stenosis includes (1) diagnostic imaging of the valve to define the etiology of stenosis, (2) quantitation of stenosis severity, (3) evaluation of coexisting valvular lesions, (4) assessment of left ventricular systolic function, and (5) the response to chronic pressure overload of other upstream cardiac chambers and the pulmonary vascular bed. This echocardiographic evaluation then is integrated with pertinent clinical data for a complete evaluation of the patient.

Fluid Dynamics of Valvular Stenosis

High-Velocity Jet

The fluid dynamics of a stenotic valve are characterized by the formation of a laminar, high-velocity jet in the narrowed orifice. The flow profile in cross section at the origin of the jet is relatively blunt (or flat) and remains blunt as the jet reaches its narrowest cross-sectional area in the vena contracta, slightly downstream from the anatomic orifice (Fig. 9–1). Thus the narrowest cross-sectional area of flow (physiologic orifice area) is smaller than the anatomic orifice area. The magnitude of this difference between physiologic and anatomic area depends on orifice geometry and the Reynold's number (a descriptor of the inertial and shear stress properties of the fluid). The ratio of the physiologic to anatomic orifice area is known as the *discharge coefficient*.

The length of the high-velocity jet is dependent on orifice geometry as well and can be variable in the clinical setting with, for example, a very short jet across a deformed, irregular, calcified aortic valve and a longer jet across a smoothly tapering, symmetrical, rheumatic mitral valve or a congenitally stenotic semilunar valve (Fig. 9–2).

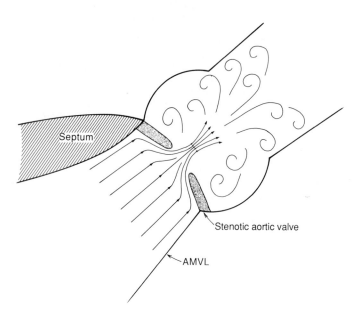

Septum

Stenotic aortic valve

AMVL

Figure 9–1. Schematic illustration of the fluid dynamics of the stenotic aortic valve in systole. The left ventricular outflow tract (LVOT) is bounded by the septum and anterior mitral valve leaflet (AMVL). As LVOT flow accelerates and converges, a relatively flat velocity profile occurs proximal to the stenotic valve, as indicated by the arrows. Flow accelerates in a spatially small zone adjacent to the valve as blood enters the narrowed orifice. In the stenotic orifice, a high-velocity laminar jet is formed with the narrowest flowstream (vena contracta, indicated by the dots) occurring downstream from the orifice. Beyond the jet, flow is disturbed, with blood cells moving in multiple directions and velocities. *(Reprinted with permission from Judge KW, Otto CM: Cardiol Clin 8:203, 1990.)*

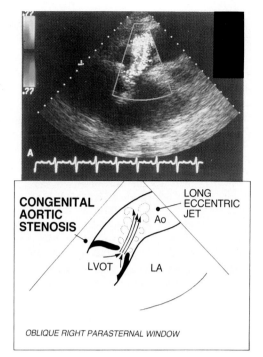

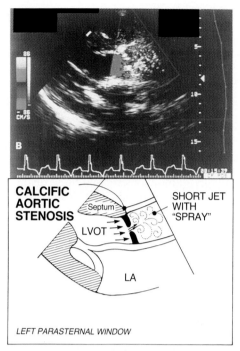

Figure 9–2. Color flow imaging in congenital valvular aortic stenosis (*left*) from an oblique high right parasternal window and in calcific aortic stenosis (*right*) from a left parasternal window, with corresponding line drawings below. In the congenital case, note the domed valve with a long, eccentric jet; in the calcific case, note the short jet with a diffuse "spray" (LV = left ventricle; Ao = aorta, LA = left atrium). (*Reprinted with permission from Judge KW, Otto CM: Cardiol Clin 8:203, 1990.*)

Relationship Between Pressure Gradient and Velocity

The pressure gradient across the stenotic valve is related to the velocity in the jet, according to the unsteady Bernoulli equation:

Bernoulli equation (9.1)

$$\Delta P = 1/2\rho(V_2^2 - V_1^2) + \rho\left(\frac{dv}{dt}\right)dx + R(v)$$

Convective   Local   Viscous
acceleration   acceleration   resistance

where ΔP is the pressure gradient across the stenosis (mmHg), ρ is the mass density of blood (1.06×10^3 kg/m³), V_2 is velocity in the stenotic jet, V_1 is velocity proximal to the stenosis, $(dv/dt)dx$ is the time-varying velocity at each distance along the flow stream, and R is a constant describing the viscous losses for that fluid and orifice. Historically, the first description of this equation was proposed about 1738 by Daniel Bernoulli from studies of steady water flow in rigid tubes. The concepts were later expanded and refined by Euler. Of note, these equations may not be strictly applicable to pulsatile blood flow in compliant chambers and vessels, although clinical studies have shown that remarkably accurate pressure-gradient predictions can

be made with this approach. This equation was first applied to Doppler data from stenotic cardiac valves by Dr. Holen (1976) and Dr. Hatle (1979).

Eliminating the terms for viscous losses and acceleration, substituting known values for the mass density of blood, and adding a conversion factor for measuring velocity in units of meters per second (m/s) and pressure gradient in millimeters of mercury (mmHg), the Bernoulli equation can be reduced to

$$\Delta P = 4(V_2^2 - V_1^2) \qquad (9.2)$$

If the proximal velocity is ≤ 1.0 m/s, as is commonly the case for stenotic valves, it becomes even smaller when squared [for example, $(0.8)^2 = 0.64$]. Thus the proximal velocity often can be ignored in the clinical setting so that:

Simplified Bernoulli equation (9.3)
$$\Delta P = 4v^2$$

This equation allows highly accurate and reproducible calculation of maximum pressure gradients (from maximum velocity) and mean pressure gradients (by integrating the instantaneous pressure difference over the flow period).

Distal Flow Disturbance

Distal to the stenotic jet, the flowstream becomes disorganized with multiple blood flow velocities and directions, although fully developed turbulence, as strictly defined in fluid dynamic terms, may not occur. The distance that this flow disturbance propagates downstream is related to stenosis severity. In addition, the *presence* of a downstream flow disturbance can be extremely useful in defining the exact anatomic site of obstruction, e.g., allowing differentiation of subvalvular outflow obstruction (flow disturbance on the ventricular side of the valve) from valvular obstruction (flow disturbance only distal to the valve).

Proximal Flow Patterns

Proximal to a stenotic valve, flow is smooth and organized (laminar) with a normal flow velocity. The spatial flow velocity profile proximal to a stenotic valve depends on valve anatomy, inlet geometry, and the degree of flow acceleration. For example, in calcific aortic stenosis, the acceleration of blood flow by ventricular systole coupled with a tapering outflow tract geometry results in a relatively uniform flow velocity (a "flat" flow profile) across the outflow tract just proximal to the stenotic valve. Immediately adjacent to the valve orifice there is acceleration as

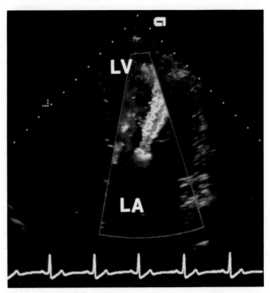

Figure 9–4. Color flow of a mitral stenosis jet (*left*). A well-defined proximal isovelocity surface area is seen.

flow converges to form the high-velocity jet, but this region of proximal acceleration is spatially small. The flow profile differs slightly for congenital aortic stenosis in that the proximal acceleration region under the domed leaflets in systole is larger but is similar in that a relatively flat velocity profile is present at the aortic annulus.

In contrast, the flow pattern proximal to the stenotic mitral valve is quite different (Figs. 9–3 and 9–4). Here, the left atrial to left ventricular pressure gradient drives flow passively from the large inlet chamber (the left atrium) abruptly across the stenotic orifice. Proximal flow acceleration is prominent over a large region of the left atrium. The three-dimensional (3D) velocity profile is curved; that is, flow velocities are faster adjacent to and in the center of a line continuous with the jet direction through the narrowed orifice and slower at increasing radial distances from the valve orifice. The proximal velocity profile of an atrioventricular valve thus is hemispherical (or possibly hemielliptical), unlike the more flattened velocity profile proximal to a stenotic semilunar valve. Any 3D surface area proximal to a narrowed orifice at which all the blood velocities are equal can be referred to as a *proximal isovelocity surface area* (PISA).

The clinical importance of these flow patterns is that stroke volume can be calculated proximal to a stenotic valve based on knowledge of the cross-sectional area of flow and the spatial mean flow velocity over the period of flow, as de-

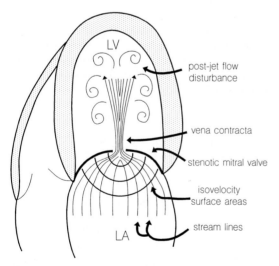

Figure 9–3. Schematic diagram of the fluid dynamics of rheumatic mitral stenosis. The stream lines of flow accelerate as they approach the stenotic orifice, with several curved proximal isovelocity surface areas indicated. The mitral stenosis jet is long, with the postjet flow disturbance occurring adjacent and distal to the laminar jet.

post-jet flow disturbance

vena contracta

stenotic mitral valve

isovelocity surface areas

stream lines

scribed in Chapter 4. This concept applies to the flat flow profile proximal to a stenotic aortic valve (used in the continuity equation), to the proximal flow patterns seen in mitral stenosis, and to the proximal isovelocity surface areas seen with regurgitant lesions (see Chap. 10).

AORTIC STENOSIS

Diagnostic Imaging of the Aortic Valve (Fig. 9–5)

Calcific Aortic Stenosis

The most common etiology of valvular aortic stenosis in adults is degenerative calcification of an apparently normal trileaflet valve. Calcification occurs slowly over many years and may be seen on two-dimensional (2D) echo as aortic valve "sclerosis"—areas of increased echogenicity, typically at the base of or on the valve leaflets, without significant obstruction to left ventricular outflow. Clinically significant obstruction tends to occur at the ages of 70 to 85 years. When obstruction is present, 2D imaging shows a marked increase in echogenicity of the leaflets consistent with fibrocalcific disease and reduced systolic opening. When aortic stenosis

is suspected, a systolic leaflet separation of 15 mm or more by 2D or 2D-guided M-mode echocardiography reliably excludes severe obstruction. When the leaflets are abnormal and systolic separation is less than 15 mm, the degree of obstruction may be mild, moderate, or severe and cannot be reliably quantitated by imaging techniques. Direct measurement of valve area on short-axis 2D imaging is possible only occasionally either from a transthoracic or from a transesophageal approach because of the complex 3D anatomy of the orifice in calcific degenerative stenosis.

Bicuspid Aortic Valve

Secondary calcification of a bicuspid aortic valve can be difficult to distinguish from calcification of a trileaflet valve once stenosis becomes severe. Average age at symptom onset is younger for adults with bicuspid valve stenosis, with presentation typically at the ages of 45 to 65 years.

Earlier in the disease course a bicuspid valve can be identified on 2D parasternal short-axis views by demonstrating that there are only two open leaflets in systole (Fig. 9–6). Long-axis views show systolic bowing of the leaflets into the aorta, resulting in a "domelike" appearance.

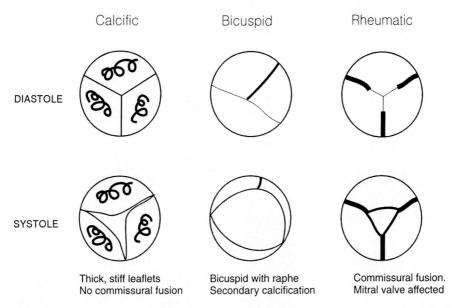

| Calcific | Bicuspid | Rheumatic |

DIASTOLE

SYSTOLE

Thick, stiff leaflets
No commissural fusion

Bicuspid with raphe
Secondary calcification

Commissural fusion.
Mitral valve affected

Figure 9–5. Schematic diagram of the three most common causes of valvular aortic stenosis. *Calcific* aortic stenosis is characterized by fibrocalcific masses on the aortic side of the leaflet that result in increased leaflet stiffness without commissural fusion. A *congenital* bicuspid valve undergoes secondary degenerative changes. The diagnostic features of *rheumatic stenosis* are commissural fusion and mitral valve involvement.

M-mode recordings may help in identifying a bicuspid valve if an eccentric closure line is present but can be misleading in terms of the degree of leaflet separation if the M-mode is taken through the base, rather than the tips, of the bowed leaflets. Typically, the two leaflets are unequal in size, with the anterior (if the leaflet opening is anteroposterior) or rightward (if the leaflet opening is lateromedial) leaflet being larger. Many bicuspid valves have a raphe in the larger leaflet so that the closed valve in diastole appears trileaflet; accurate identification of the number of aortic valve leaflets can be made only in systole. Doppler interrogation of the aortic

valve should be performed whenever a bicuspid valve is suspected to evaluate for stenosis and/or regurgitation.

Rheumatic Aortic Stenosis

Rheumatic valvular disease preferentially involves the mitral valve, so rheumatic aortic stenosis is diagnosed when aortic disease occurs concurrently with rheumatic mitral valve disease. The rheumatic disease process results in commissural fusion of the aortic leaflets, similar to the pathology seen in rheumatic mitral ste-

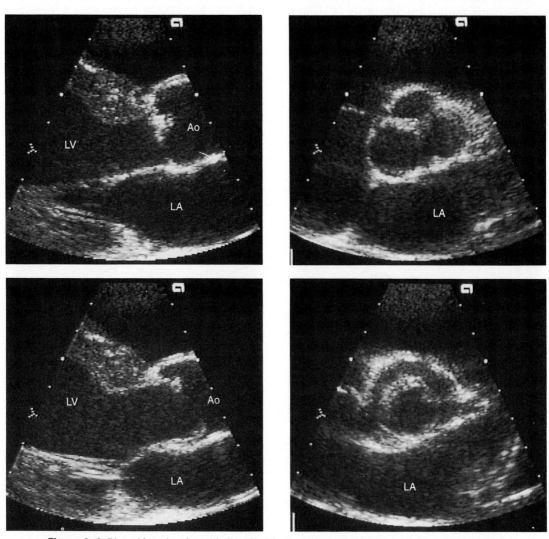

Figure 9–6. Bicuspid aortic valve with diastolic (*above*) and systolic (*below*) frames shown in parasternal long-axis (*left*) and short-axis (*right*) views. Note the diastolic sagging and systolic doming of the leaflets in the long-axis view. In short axis, only two leaflets are seen to open in systole with the commissures at 4 and 10 o'clock.

nosis. Two-dimensional imaging may show increased echogenicity along the leaflet edges, commissural fusion, and systolic doming of the aortic leaflets. Often, however, the echocardiographic images appear similar to those of calcific aortic stenosis (other than the presence of rheumatic mitral valve disease).

Congenital Aortic Stenosis

Congenital aortic stenosis usually is diagnosed in childhood, but some patients may not become symptomatic until young adulthood or may present with restenosis after surgical valvotomy performed in childhood or adolescence. These patients most often have a unicuspid valve with a single eccentric orifice and prominent systolic doming.

Differential Diagnosis (Table 9–1)

The differential diagnosis of left ventricular outflow obstruction includes fixed subvalvular obstruction (a subaortic membrane or a muscular subaortic stenosis), dynamic subaortic obstruction (hypertrophic cardiomyopathy), and supravalvular stenosis. In a patient with a clinical diagnosis of valvular aortic stenosis, the echocardiographic study should demonstrate whether the obstruction is, in fact, valvular or if one of these other diagnoses accounts for the clinical presentation (Fig. 9–7).

A subaortic membrane should be suspected in young adults when the valve anatomy is not clearly stenotic, yet Doppler examination reveals a high transaortic pressure gradient. The membrane may be poorly visualized in a transthoracic study; biplane transesophageal imaging can be helpful. The spatial orientation of the jet and the shape of the continuous-wave Doppler velocity curve are similar for fixed obstructions, whether sub-, supra-, or valvular, but careful pulsed Doppler or color flow imaging allows localization of the level of obstruction by detection of the poststenotic flow disturbance.

In dynamic outflow obstruction, the timing and shape of the late-peaking continuous-wave Doppler velocity curve are distinctive. In addition, the degree of obstruction changes dramatically with provocative maneuvers, as detailed in Chapter 7. In the occasional patient with both subvalvular *and* valvular obstruction, high-pulse-repetition-frequency Doppler ultrasound can be helpful in defining the maximum velocities at each site of obstruction.

Quantitation of Stenosis Severity

The severity of valvular aortic stenosis can be determined accurately using equations derived from our understanding of the fluid dynamics of a stenotic valve.

Pressure Gradients

Maximum transaortic pressure gradient (ΔP_{max}) can be calculated from the maximum aortic jet velocity (V_{max}) using the simplified Bernoulli equation (Fig. 9–8):

$$\Delta P_{max} = 4V_{max}{}^2 \qquad \text{maximum gradient} \quad (9.4)$$

Mean pressure gradient (ΔP_{mean}) can be calculated by digitizing the aortic jet velocity curve (where $V_1, \ldots, V_n$ are instantaneous velocities) and averaging the instantaneous gradients over the systolic ejection period:

$$\text{Mean gradient} \quad (9.5)$$
$$\Delta P_{mean} = \frac{4v_1^2 + 4v_2^2 + 4v_3^2 + \cdots + 4v_n^2}{n}$$

Interestingly, in native aortic valve stenosis, transaortic pressure gradient correlates closely and linearly with maximum transaortic gradient so that mean gradient can be approximated from published regression equations as

$$\text{Mean gradient} \quad (9.6)$$
$$\text{regression equation}$$
$$\Delta P_{mean} = \frac{(\Delta P_{max})}{1.45} + 2 \text{ mmHg}$$

TABLE 9–1. ECHOCARDIOGRAPHIC DIFFERENTIAL DIAGNOSIS OF LEFT VENTRICULAR OUTFLOW TRACT OBSTRUCTION

Valvular aortic stenosis
  Calcific aortic stenosis
  Bicuspid valve with secondary calcification
  Rheumatic aortic stenosis
  Congenital aortic stenosis (e.g., unicuspid or fused trileaflet valve)

Subaortic stenosis
  Membranous
  Muscular
  Dynamic (e.g., hypertrophic cardiomyopathy)

Supravalvular stenosis

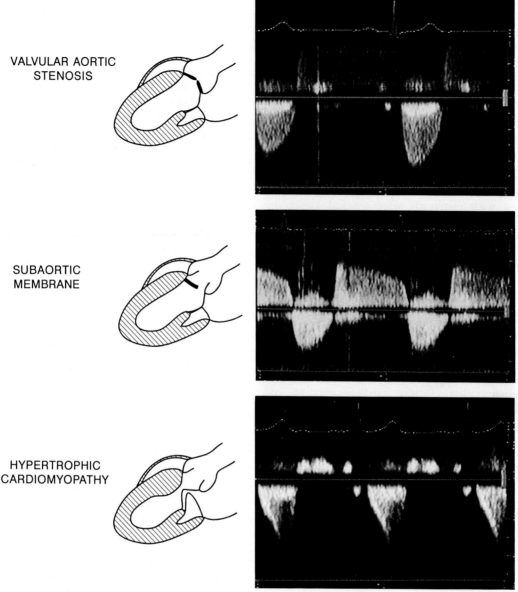

VALVULAR AORTIC
STENOSIS

SUBAORTIC
MEMBRANE

HYPERTROPHIC
CARDIOMYOPATHY

Figure 9–7. Examples of the shape of the continuous-wave Doppler velocity curve in valvular aortic stenosis, fixed subvalvular obstruction due to a subaortic membrane, and dynamic obstruction due to hypertrophic cardiomyopathy. Note that the continuous-wave curves for subvalvular and valvular aortic stenosis are similar, although coarse fluttering of the valve with subvalvular obstruction results in a "rough" appearance of the systolic velocity curve. These can be distinguished by 2D and color flow imaging. The shape of the curve with dynamic obstruction is distinctly different with velocity peaking in late systole.

or (from a different study):

$$\Delta P_{\mathrm{mean}} = 2.4(V_{\mathrm{max}})^2 \qquad (9.7)$$

Note that these two equations give similar results.

With careful attention to technical details, Doppler-determined pressure gradients are accurate, as has been demonstrated in numerous in vitro and animal models and in clinical studies

(Table 9–2). Note that while Doppler maximum gradients correspond to maximum instantaneous gradients by catheter measurement and that Doppler mean gradients correspond to catheter-measured mean gradients, neither Doppler gradient correlates with the peak-to-peak gradient reported at catheterization. In fact, peak aortic and peak left ventricular pressures do not occur simultaneously, so none of the instantaneous ve-

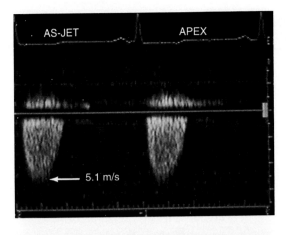

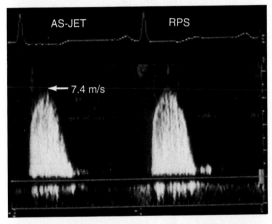

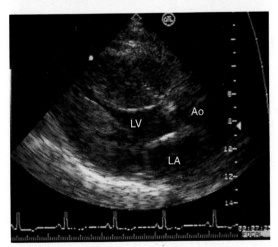

Figure 9–8. Continuous-wave Doppler recording of an aortic stenosis jet recorded from an apical (*above*) and a high right parasternal (*center*) approach in a 56-year-old man with a systolic murmur. The highest-velocity jet (right parasternal in this case) is used because it represents the most parallel intercept angle between the direction of blood flow and the stenotic jet. Maximum pressure gradient is calculated as $\Delta P = 4v^2$, with mean pressure gradient determined by integrating the instantaneous gradients over the systolic ejection period. Severe concentric left ventricular hypertrophy also was present (*below*).

locities recorded with Doppler ultrasound are strictly comparable with this clinical measurement. Potential confusion about Doppler pressure gradient data in an individual patient can be avoided by clearly identifying the specific type of gradient measured—"maximum instantaneous" or "mean systolic" (Fig. 9–9).

Physiologic changes in pressure gradient should be taken into consideration when comparing nonsimultaneous data recordings and in patient management decisions. Pressure gradients depend on volume flow rate, as well as the degree of valve narrowing, so in an individual patient the pressure gradient will rise when transaortic stroke volume increases (e.g., anxiety, exercise) and will fall when stroke volume decreases (e.g., sedation, hypovolemia).

The dependence of pressure gradients on volume flow rate can lead to erroneous conclusions about stenosis severity in adult patients with either a chronically elevated or depressed transaortic stroke volume. For example, a patient with coexisting aortic regurgitation will have a high transaortic pressure gradient with only a moderate degree of valve narrowing. Conversely, a patient with left ventricular systolic dysfunction or coexisting mitral regurgitation may have a low transaortic pressure gradient despite severe aortic stenosis. These coexisting conditions are common in adults with valvular aortic stenosis, so determination of the stenotic orifice area is essential for complete evaluation of disease severity (Figs. 9–10 and 9–11).

Continuity Equation Valve Area

Aortic valve area can be calculated based on the principle of continuity of flow (Table 9–3). Specifically, the stroke volume (SV) just proximal to the aortic valve (SV_{LVOT}) and that in the stenotic valve orifice (SV_{Ao}) are equal:

$$SV_{LVOT} = SV_{Ao} \qquad (9.8)$$

If flow is laminar with a spatially flat velocity profile,

$$SV = CSA \times VTI \qquad (9.9)$$

where CSA is the cross-sectional area of flow (cm^2), SV is stroke volume (cm^3), and VTI is the velocity-time integral (cm). Since flow both proximal to and in the aortic jet itself is laminar with a reasonably flat velocity profile,

$$CSA_{LVOT} \times VTI_{LVOT} = CSA_{Ao} \times VTI_{Ao} \qquad (9.10)$$

All the variables in this equation can be measured with 2D or Doppler echo except CSA_{Ao}, which is the stenotic aortic valve area (AVA) itself. Rearranging the equation,

TABLE 9–2. SELECTED STUDIES VALIDATING DOPPLER PRESSURE GRADIENTS IN VALVULAR STENOSIS (IN VIVO SIMULTANEOUS DATA)

FIRST AUTHOR, YEAR	N	STUDY GROUP/MODEL	R	RANGE (mmHg)	SEE (mmHg)
Callahan, 1985	120	Supravalvular constriction (canines)	$0.99\ (\Delta P_{max})$ $0.98\ (\Delta P_{mean})$	7–179 N/A	5.2 4.3
Smith, 1985	88	Supravalvular constriction (canines)	$0.98\ (\Delta P_{max})$ $0.98\ (\Delta P_{mean})$	5–166 5–116	5.3 3.3
Currie, 1985	100	Adults with valvular aortic stenosis	$0.92\ (\Delta P_{max})$ $0.92\ (\Delta P_{mean})$	2–180 0–112	15 10
Smith, 1986	33	Adults with valvular aortic stenosis	$0.85\ (\Delta P_{max})$	27–138	N/A
Simpson, 1985	24	Adults with valvular aortic stenosis	$0.98\ (\Delta P_{max})$	0–120	N/A
Burwash, 1993	98	Chronic valvular aortic stenosis (canines)	$0.95\ (\Delta P_{max})$ $0.91\ (\Delta P_{mean})$	10–128 5–77	8.4 5.3

Data from Callahan et al: Am J Cardiol 56:989–993, 1985; Smith et al: JACC 6:1306–1314, 1985; Currie et al: Circ 71:1162–1169, 1985; Smith et al: Am Heart J 111:245–252, 1986; Simpson et al: Br Heart J 53:636–639, 1985; Burwash et al: Am J Physiol, 265 (Heart Circ. Physiol 34): HI734–HI743, 1993.

Continuity equation (9.11)

$$AVA = CSA_{LVOT} \times \frac{VTI_{LVOT}}{VTI_{Ao}}$$

Thus the measurements needed to calculate valve area with the continuity equation are (Fig. 9–12):

1. The circular outflow tract cross-sectional area (CSA), calculated from outflow tract diameter measured on a 2D parasternal long-axis systolic image;

2. The velocity-time integral in the outflow tract, recorded with pulsed Doppler-echocardiography from an apical approach;

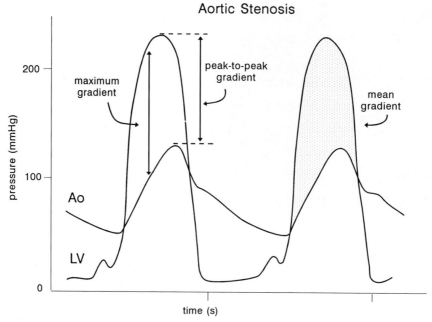

Figure 9–9. Example of left ventricular (LV) and aortic (Ao) pressures measured with fluid-filled catheters in a patient with severe valvular aortic stenosis. Note that the maximum instantaneous gradient is greater than the peak-to-peak gradient. Mean gradient is indicated by the shaded area.

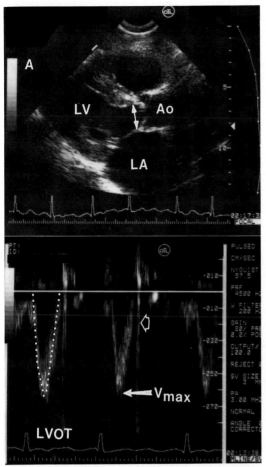

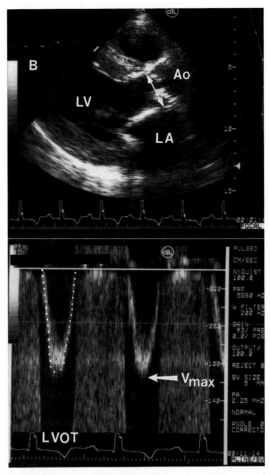

Figure 9–10. Left ventricular outflow tract diameter and velocity in a patient with low transaortic volume flow. Pressure gradients alone will underestimate stenosis severity in this setting. *(Reprinted with permission from Judge KW, Otto CM: Cardiol Clin 8:203, 1990.)*

Figure 9–11. Left ventricular outflow tract diameter and velocity in a patient with mixed moderate aortic stenosis and moderate aortic regurgitation. Both the outflow tract velocity and aortic jet velocity are elevated due to the elevated transaortic volume flow rate. Calculation of valve area remains accurate in this setting. *(Reprinted with permission from Judge KW, Otto CM: Cardiol Clin 8:203, 1990.)*

3. The velocity-time integral in the aortic stenosis jet, recorded with continuous-wave Doppler ultrasound.

For clinical use, the continuity equation can be simplified by substituting maximum velocities (V) for velocity-time integrals. The shape and timing of outflow tract and aortic jet velocity curves are similar, so their ratios are nearly identical:

$$\frac{\text{VTI}_{\text{LVOT}}}{\text{VTI}_{\text{Ao}}} \approx \frac{V_{\text{LVOT}}}{V_{\text{Ao}}} \quad \begin{array}{c}\text{Velocity} \\ \text{ratio}\end{array} \quad (9.12)$$

The simplified continuity equation then is:

$$\text{Simplified continuity equation} \quad (9.13)$$
$$\text{AVA} = \text{CSA}_{\text{LVOT}} \times \frac{V_{\text{LVOT}}}{V_{\text{Ao}}}$$

Attempts to further simplify the continuity equation by eliminating the need to measure outflow tract diameter have been unsuccessful. While the group mean outflow tract diameter is smaller in women than in men, there is substantial overlap in the range of diameters in men and women. Although outflow tract diameter correlates with body size when people of all ages from infancy to adulthood are considered, in the adult population, the relationship between body size (either body surface area, height, or weight) and outflow tract diameter is weak. Thus outflow tract diameter must be measured in each patient for accurate valve area calculations. On the other hand, outflow tract diameter tends to remain constant in a given adult patient over time. Apparent differences in diameter at follow-up visits are more likely to represent measurement error

TABLE 9–3. SELECTED STUDIES OF AORTIC VALVE AREA DETERMINATION

FIRST AUTHOR, YEAR	COMPARISON	N	STUDY GROUP	R*	RANGE (cm²)	SEE* (cm²)
Hakki, 1981	Simplified vs original Gorlin formula	60	Aortic stenosis	0.96	0.2–2.0	0.10
Skjaerpe, 1985	Cont eq vs Gorlin	30	Aortic stenosis	0.89	0.4–2.4	0.12
Zoghbi, 1986	Cont eq vs Gorlin	39	Aortic stenosis	0.95	0.4–2.0	0.15
Otto, 1988	Cont eq vs Gorlin	103	Aortic stenosis	0.87	0.2–3.7	0.34
Teirstein, 1986	Cont eq vs Gorlin	30	Aortic stenosis	0.88	0.3–1.6	0.17
Oh, 1988	Cont eq vs Gorlin	100	Aortic stenosis	0.83	0.2–1.8	0.19
Danielson, 1989	Cont eq vs Gorlin	100	Aortic stenosis	0.96	0.4–2.0	—
Cannon, 1985	Gorlin vs videotape of valve opening	42	Porcine valves in pulsatile flow model	0.87	0.6–2.5	0.28
	New formula vs actual orifice area	42	Porcine valves in pulsatile flow model	0.98	0.6–2.5	0.11
Segal, 1987	Cont eq vs actual valve area		In vitro pulsatile flow with orifice plates	0.99	0.05–0.5	0.016
	Gorlin formula vs actual valve area			0.87		0.047
Cannon, 1988	Gorlin vs known valve area	135	Prosthetic aortic valves	0.39	0.6–2.3	—
Come, 1987	Gorlin vs Gorlin	28	AS	0.42	0.3–1.1	—
	Cont eq vs Gorlin	40	Pre-BAV	0.71	0.2–1.1	—
			Post-BAV	0.85	0.5–2.6	—
Nishimura, 1988	Cont eq vs Gorlin	55	Pre-BAV	0.72	0.2–0.9	0.10
			Post-BAV	0.61	0.5–1.3	0.17
Desnoyers, 1988	Cont eq vs Gorlin	42	Pre-BAV	0.74	0.3–1.3	—
Stoddard, 1989	Cont eq vs Gorlin	41	Pre-BAV	0.84	0.2–0.8	0.08
			Post-BAV	0.87	0.3–1.2	0.10

*If not stated in the publication, statistics were calculated from the raw data provided in tables. A blank indicates that data for this calculation were not available.

Note: AS = aortic stenosis; BAV = balloon aortic valvuloplasty; Cont eq = continuity equation; Gorlin = Gorlin formula valve area.

Data from Hakki et al: Circ 63:1050–1055, 1981; Skjaerpe et al: Circ 72:810–818, 1985; Zoghbi et al: Circ 73:452–459, 1986; Otto et al: Arch Intern Med 148:2553–2560, 1988; Teirstein et al: JACC 8:1059–1065, 1986; Oh et al: JACC 11:1227–1234, 1988; Danielson et al: Am J Cardiol 63:1107–1111, 1989; Cannon et al: Circ 71:1170–1178, 1985; Segal et al: JACC 9:1294–1305, 1987; Cannon et al: Am J Cardiol 62:113–116, 1988; Come et al: JACC 10:115–124, 1987; Nishimura et al: Circ 78:791–799, 1988; Desnoyers et al: Am J Cardiol 62:1078–1084, 1988; Stoddard et al: JACC 14:1218–1228, 1989.

Reprinted with permission from Otto CM et al: Am J Cardiol 69:1607, 1992.

than an actual interval anatomic change. Thus the ratio of outflow tract velocity to aortic jet velocity can be used to follow disease progression in individual patients.

Velocity Ratio

Although not strictly comparable to valve area, the velocity ratio also may be a useful measure of stenosis severity that, in effect, is "indexed" for body size. Obviously, normal valve area is dependent on body size—infants and children have smaller valve areas than adults and large adults are expected to have larger valve areas than small adults. One way to take the effect of body size into account is to "index" valve area by dividing it by body surface area (BSA):

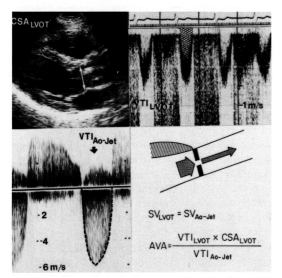

Figure 9–12. Continuity equation aortic valve area (AVA) calculations require measurement of left ventricular outflow tract diameter on a parasternal long-axis view for circular cross-sectional area (CSA) calculation (*above, left*), pulsed Doppler recording of the left ventricular outflow tract velocity-time integral (VTI) from an apical approach (*above, right*), and continuous-wave Doppler recording of the aortic stenosis velocity-time integral (VTI AS-jet) from whichever window gives the highest-velocity signal. (*Reprinted with permission from Otto CM, Pearlman AS: Arch Intern Med 148:2553–2560, 1988.*)

TABLE 9–4. PITFALLS IN ECHOCARDIOGRAPHIC EVALUATION OF AORTIC STENOSIS

Technical

Acoustic access

Intercept angle between aortic stenosis jet and ultrasound beam

Outflow tract diameter imaging

Respiratory motion

Learning-curve effect

Interpretation

Identification of flow signal origin (AS vs. MR)

Beat-to-beat variability (AF, PVCs)

Intra- and interobserver measurement variability

Calculation errors

Physiology

Interim changes in heart rate or stroke volume

Dependence of velocity and ΔP on volume flow rate

Progression of AS severity

Standards of reference
    Maximum vs. peak-to-peak ΔP
    Continuity vs. Gorlin formula valve areas

$$\text{Aortic valve index} = \frac{\text{AVA}}{\text{BSA}} \quad (9.14)$$

An alternate approach is to define the "normal" valve area for that individual as the cross-sectional area of the outflow tract. Then, the increase in velocity from outflow tract to aortic jet reflects stenosis severity regardless of body size. If

$$\text{"Normal" AVA} = \text{CSA}_{\text{LVOT}} \quad \text{and} \quad (9.15)$$
$$\text{Actual AVA} \cong \text{"normal" AVA} \times \frac{V_{\text{LVOT}}}{V_{\text{Ao}}}$$

then

$$\frac{\text{Actual AVA}}{\text{"Normal" AVA}} \cong \frac{V_{\text{LVOT}}}{V_{\text{Ao}}}$$

A velocity ratio near 1 indicates little obstruction, a velocity ratio of 0.5 indicates a valve area that is one-half normal, and a velocity ratio of 0.25 indicates a valve area reduced to one-quarter its normal value.

Technical Considerations and Potential Pitfalls (Table 9–4)

Continuity equation valve areas have been well validated in comparison with Gorlin formula valve areas calculated from invasive measurements of pressure gradient and cardiac output. Some of the discrepancies between Doppler echo and invasive measurements of valve area are due to measurement variability for the invasive data and to limitations of the Gorlin formula itself. However, technical considerations in recording the Doppler and 2D echo data and the measurement variability of the noninvasive technique also are important.

With careful attention to technical details, an experienced laboratory can obtain accurate noninvasive data for calculation of transaortic pressure gradients and valve areas in nearly all adults with valvular aortic stenosis. However, accurate noninvasive quantitation of aortic stenosis severity is a technically demanding procedure, and a significant learning-curve effect is seen in each laboratory for this clinical application. There are several potential pitfalls in the Doppler approach, as detailed below. Each laboratory should confirm the accuracy of its data by comparison with those of an experienced echocardiography laboratory or with other diagnostic tests.

The Aortic Jet. Owing to the high velocities seen in aortic stenosis (usually 3 to 7 m/s), continuous-wave Doppler ultrasound is needed for accurate measurement of the aortic jet signal. High-pulse-repetition-frequency Doppler echo also can be used but is more time-consuming and technically demanding, since sample volume depth as well as beam direction must be optimized.

In recording the aortic jet velocity signal, a search is made for the highest-frequency shift. This signal then is assumed to represent a near-parallel intercept angle (θ) between the ultrasound beam and the direction of the jet. In this situation, cos θ equals 1 and thus can be ignored in the Doppler equation (see Chap. 1). Any deviation from a nonparallel intercept will result in underestimation of the jet velocity. For example, an intercept angle of 30° will result in a measured velocity of 4.3 m/s when the actual velocity is 5.0 m/s. Underestimation of velocity, which is squared in the Bernoulli equation, results in a large error in calculated pressure gradient. Intercept angles within 15° of parallel will result in an error in velocity measurement of 5 percent or less.

The direction of the aortic jet often is eccentric relative to either the plane of the aortic valve or the long axis of the aorta and rarely can be predicted from the 2D images. Occasionally, jet direction can be visualized with color flow imaging, but, more often, the direction of the short jet of calcific stenosis cannot be identified. Even when jet direction is seen in a single tomographic plane, the orientation of the jet in the elevational plane remains unknown.

Pragmatically, the solution to the problem of aligning the ultrasound beam parallel to an aortic jet of unknown direction is to perform a careful search from several acoustic windows with optimal patient positioning and multiple transducer angulations. The highest-velocity signal obtained then is assumed to represent the most parallel intercept angle. At a minimum, the aortic jet should be interrogated from an apical approach with the patient in a steep left lateral decubitus position on an examination bed with an apical cutout, from a high right parasternal position with the patient in a right lateral decubitus position, and from the suprasternal notch with the patient supine and the neck extended. Even then, the possibility of underestimation of jet velocity due to a nonparallel intercept angle cannot be excluded. In some cases, the highest-velocity signal may be recorded from a subcostal or left parasternal window.

When the continuous-wave beam is aligned with the aortic jet, a smooth velocity curve is seen with a well-defined peak velocity and spectral darkening along the outer edge of the velocity curve. Audibly, the signal is high frequency and tonal. The spectral recording should be made with an appropriate velocity scale (at least 1 m/s higher than the observed maximum jet velocity), with wall filters set at a high level, and with gain adjustment to provide clear definition of the maximum velocity. Maximum velocity is measured at the edge of the dark velocity envelope. The velocity-time integral is measured by digitizing the velocity curve over systole.

Care is needed that the high-velocity jet is correctly identified. Other high-velocity systolic jets (Table 9–5 and Fig. 9–13) may be mistaken for aortic stenosis if inadequate attention is paid to timing, shape, and associated diastolic flow curves. In some cases, 2D "guided" continuous-wave Doppler may be helpful in correct identification of the jet.

Outflow Tract Diameter. Left ventricular outflow tract diameter is measured in midsystole, just proximal to and parallel with the plane of the stenotic aortic valve, from the inner edge of the septal endocardial echo to the leading edge of the base of the anterior mitral leaflet. A parasternal long-axis view provides the most accurate measurement because it depends on the axial (rather than lateral) resolution of the ultrasound beam. Outflow tract cross-sectional area (CSA) is assumed to be circular:

$$CSA_{LVOT} = \pi(D/2)^2 \quad \text{Outflow tract CSA} \quad (9.16)$$

Note that small errors in outflow tract diameter measurement may lead to large errors in calculated cross-sectional area. Furthermore, of the measurements made for evaluating aortic stenosis severity, outflow tract diameter shows the greatest intra- and interobserver variability. Several measurements should be averaged to minimize this potential source of error.

Outflow Tract Velocity. The outflow tract systolic velocity signal is recorded from an apical

---

TABLE 9–5. OTHER HIGH-VELOCITY SYSTOLIC JETS THAT MAY BE MISTAKEN FOR AORTIC STENOSIS

Subaortic obstruction (fixed or dynamic)

Mitral regurgitation

Tricuspid regurgitation

Ventricular septal defect

Pulmonic or branch pulmonary artery stenosis

Peripheral vascular stenosis (e.g., subclavian artery)

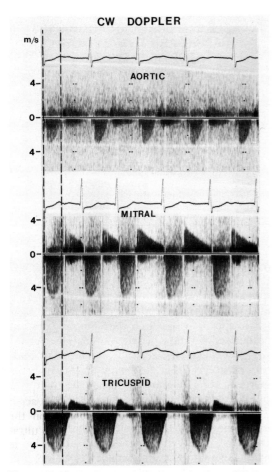

CW DOPPLER

AORTIC

MITRAL

TRICUSPID

Figure 9–13. From an apical approach, three different high-velocity systolic jets directed away from the transducer were recorded in this patient with mild to moderate aortic stenosis, severe mitral stenosis with mild mitral regurgitation, and severe pulmonary hypertension. These three flow signals can be differentiated on the basis of timing, shape, and associated diastolic flow signals.

approach using pulsed Doppler echo. Either an anteriorly angulated four-chamber view or an apical long-axis view can be used. A sample volume 5 to 10 mm in length is positioned just proximal to the region of acceleration into the stenotic jet. Correct positioning is ensured by starting with the sample volume *in* the jet and slowly repositioning it apically until a smooth velocity curve with a well-defined peak velocity and little spectral broadening is seen. The presence of an aortic valve closing (but not opening) click indicates that the sample volume is immediately adjacent to the valve. A transducer position is chosen initially that indicates a parallel alignment between the ultrasound beam and the long axis of the outflow tract on 2D imaging. Then, transducer position and angulation are adjusted, based on the audible Doppler signal

and the velocity curve, to record the highest-velocity signal proximal to the flow acceleration region. In addition, the sample volume is moved laterally across the outflow tract in each apical view to document a flat flow velocity profile.

The rationale for this protocol for sample volume positioning is that the outflow tract diameter and velocity signals need to be recorded *at the same* anatomic site for accurate transaortic stroke volume calculations. Necessarily, these two recordings are made nonsimultaneously from different acoustic windows because of the need for a parallel orientation between the Doppler beam and the direction of blood flow for accurate velocity measurement and for a perpendicular orientation between the 2D echo beam and the outflow tract for accurate diameter measurement. Measuring both immediately adjacent to the stenotic valve provides a reference point that ensures that both measurements are made at the same spatial location.

The maximum outflow tract velocity is measured at the edge of the darkest spectral signal. The time-velocity integral is measured by digitizing the systolic velocity curve. Wall filters are set low enough that the systolic ejection period is clearly defined.

Coexisting Valvular Disease

A high percentage (about 80 percent) of patients with predominant aortic stenosis also have aortic regurgitation, most often mild or moderate in severity. The degree of regurgitation can be evaluated as described in Chapter 10. Although coexisting aortic regurgitation will result in an increase in the transaortic pressure gradient (due to increased transaortic volume flow), valve area calculations will be accurate because the stroke volume in the continuity equation represents transaortic stroke volume.

Coexisting mitral regurgitation also is common due to mitral annular calcification in adults with calcific aortic stenosis. Again, mitral regurgitant severity can be evaluated as described in Chapter 10. Particular attention should be directed toward aortic valve area calculations when mitral regurgitation is present. Otherwise, severe aortic stenosis may be missed if the transaortic pressure gradient is low due to low transaortic volume flow.

Patients with rheumatic aortic stenosis may have significant mitral stenosis, mitral regurgitation, or mixed mitral disease. Evaluation of aortic stenosis severity is unaffected by these coexisting lesions other than the aforementioned potential for a low transaortic pressure gradient if the transaortic volume flow rate is depressed.

Response of the Left Ventricle to Valvular Aortic Stenosis

The left ventricular response to the chronic pressure overload of valvular aortic stenosis is concentric hypertrophy—an increase in left ventricular mass due to increased wall thickness without chamber dilation. Hypertrophy tends to normalize left ventricular wall stress, since:

$$\text{Wall stress} \cong \frac{r}{t} \cdot P \quad \begin{array}{l} \text{Left ventricular} \\ \text{wall stress} \end{array} \quad (9.17)$$

where r is ventricular radius, t is wall thickness, and P is left ventricular pressure. The relative wall thickness (the ratio of wall thickness to radius) is a useful and simple measure of the degree of hypertrophy. Left ventricular mass (which can be indexed for body size) can be calculated from tracings of endocardium and epicardium at end-diastole, as described in Chapter 4.

In aortic stenosis, left ventricular systolic function tends to be preserved until late in the disease course. When left ventricular systolic dysfunction does occur, it may be due to the increased afterload of outflow obstruction and thus is reversible after valve replacement. Ventricular systolic function can be evaluated qualitatively or quantitatively, as described in Chapter 4. Even a qualitative evaluation has significant prognostic implications in unoperated adults with aortic stenosis.

Interestingly, there appear to be gender differences in the response of the left ventricle to aortic stenosis. Women tend to have more hypertrophied, smaller ventricles with preserved systolic function, while men tend to show less increase in wall thickness, more left ventricular dilation, and a higher prevalence of systolic dysfunction.

Clinical Applications in Specific Patient Populations (Table 9–6)

Symptomatic Adults with Valvular Aortic Stenosis Being Considered for Surgical Intervention

Doppler echocardiography now is the diagnostic test of choice for symptomatic adults being considered for valve replacement. A complete echocardiographic examination includes evaluation of stenosis severity, assessment of left ventricular systolic function, and evaluation of

TABLE 9–6. ECHOCARDIOGRAPHIC APPROACH TO VALVULAR AORTIC STENOSIS

1. Valve anatomy, etiology of stenosis

2. Exclude other causes of left ventricular outflow obstruction

3. Stenosis severity
   a. Jet velocity
   b. Mean pressure gradient
   c. Continuity equation valve area

4. Degree of coexisting aortic regurgitation

5. Left ventricular hypertrophy and systolic function

coexisting valvular lesions, as described above. While all the clinical and Doppler echo data should be considered in clinical decision making for each individual patient, a generalized diagnostic approach based on the Doppler data can be derived for this patient population. As for any generalization, exceptions do occur in clinical practice, so this diagnostic approach serves more as a useful frame of reference than as a rigid patient management scheme (Fig. 9–14).

For initial evaluation of aortic stenosis severity, aortic jet maximum velocity is the simplest and most useful quantitative measure. This is not surprising, since maximum velocity is predictably related to maximum pressure gradient

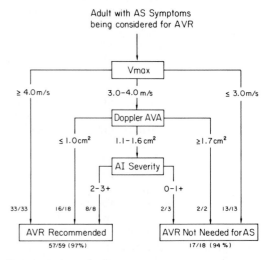

Figure 9–14. Diagnostic approach for evaluation of adults with aortic stenosis symptoms being considered for valve replacement. The number of subjects in each group (denominator) and the number in whom this echo approach was correct (numerator) are shown. Overall diagnostic accuracy of this approach is 96 percent. (*Reprinted with permission from Otto CM, Pearlman AS: Arch Intern Med 148:2553–2560, 1988.*)

(via the simplified Bernoulli equation), which, in turn, is linearly related to mean pressure gradient in native valvular aortic stenosis. Thus maximum velocities, maximum gradients, and mean gradient measurements are redundant, simply describing the same data in different ways.

When the aortic jet velocity is >4.0 m/s, the presence of severe aortic valve disease is confirmed, and valve replacement is needed. Note that some subjects with a jet velocity >4.0 m/s may have only moderate stenosis with coexisting moderate regurgitation. However, if symptoms consistent with aortic valve disease are present, the high jet velocity confirms the clinical diagnosis, and valve replacement for mixed stenosis and regurgitation is needed. In these subjects, findings at cardiac catheterization are similar, with a high pressure gradient despite only a moderate reduction in valve area.

When the aortic jet velocity is <3.0 m/s, significant aortic valve disease is not present, and valve replacement is not needed. Caution is needed in this situation to ensure that the jet velocity measurement is accurate—a nonparallel intercept angle between the aortic jet and the Doppler beam can result in underestimation of jet velocity and the erroneous conclusion that severe stenosis is not present. If severe left ventricular systolic dysfunction is present, severe aortic stenosis may be present despite a low velocity (and low gradient). In these patients, calculation of valve area is needed.

In symptomatic adults with an aortic jet velocity between 3.0 and 4.0 m/s, further evaluation of stenosis severity is needed. These patients may have only moderate stenosis with normal transaortic volume flow, mild stenosis with coexisting aortic regurgitation, or severe stenosis with low transaortic volume flow. In aortic stenosis, low transaortic volume flow is not necessarily identifiable by 2D imaging. For example, a hypertrophied left ventricle with normal systolic function but a small ventricular chamber will have a small stroke volume. Thus calculation of aortic valve area with the continuity equation is especially important in patients with only a moderate increase in jet velocity (3 to 4 m/s) and a corresponding modest mean pressure gradient (20 to 40 mmHg). In addition, evaluation of the degree of coexisting aortic regurgitation is needed because valve replacement may be warranted in the symptomatic patient with only mild to moderate aortic stenosis and significant aortic regurgitation.

This diagnostic approach has been shown to be accurate and cost-effective in evaluating symptomatic adults with valvular aortic stenosis. Again, it must be emphasized that this approach is only as accurate as the Doppler echo data upon which it is based. Careful attention to technical details is needed during the Doppler examination. In cases where the clinical situation is discrepant with the echo findings, other diagnostic tests such as cardiac catheterization may be helpful. Coronary angiography is needed in most patients if valve replacement is planned (for possible coronary artery bypass grafting) and often is needed if valve replacement is *not* planned to evaluate alternate etiologies for the patient's symptoms.

Disease Progression in Asymptomatic Aortic Stenosis

In following individual patients over time, the reproducibility of a technique, as well as its accuracy, is important. Reproducibility of Doppler echo data includes both recording variability (e.g., intercept angle, wall filters, signal strength, acoustic window), measurement variability (e.g., identification of the maximum velocity, outflow tract diameter), and physiologic variability (e.g., interim changes in heart rate, stroke volume, or pressure gradient). Aortic jet maximum velocity measurement is reproducible as described by the mean coefficient of variation with an intraobserver variability of 3.2 percent and an interobserver variability of 3.1 percent. Outflow tract velocity, recorded by two experienced sonographers, also is reproducible with intra- and interobserver variability of 3.0 and 3.9 percent. Measurement of outflow tract diameter shows the greatest variability, with intra- and interobserver mean coefficients of variation of 5.1 and 7.9 percent. These variabilities indicate that for values at the middle of the range, a change greater than measurement variability is >0.2 m/s for maximum jet velocity, >0.1 m/s for outflow tract velocity, >0.2 cm for outflow tract diameter, and >0.15 cm^2 for aortic valve area.

Doppler echo has been used to follow disease progression in asymptomatic adults with valvular aortic stenosis. Several observations from these studies are noteworthy. First, prognosis depends on the presence or absence of clinical symptoms and not on hemodynamic severity per se. There is significant overlap in all measures of hemodynamic severity between symptomatic and asymptomatic adults, and it is not unusual to see asymptomatic individuals with a jet velocity >4.0 m/s. Second, the rate of hemodynamic progression is extremely variable from patient to patient. The increase in jet velocity ranges from −0.3 to +1.0 (mean +0.36) m/s per year, mean pressure gradient increases by −7 to +23 (mean +8) mmHg per year, and valve area decreases by 0 to 0.5 (mean 0.1) cm² per year. To date, no baseline characteristics have been identified that predict the rate of progression in individual patients. Third, while hemodynamic progression may present as an increase in aortic jet velocity (and transaortic pressure gradient), disease progression can occur with no change in jet velocity if there is a concurrent decrease in transaortic volume flow rate (Fig. 9–15).

The optimal timing of follow-up Doppler echo examination for asymptomatic aortic stenosis has not been defined. It could be argued that once the baseline examination has established the diagnosis, the patient can be followed only clinically, since the timing of valve replacement is determined by symptom onset. On the other hand, adults with aortic stenosis often have significant comorbid disease, and knowledge of hemodynamic severity can be important in patient management. In the clinically stable patient, annual examinations are appropriate

because significant hemodynamic progression rarely occurs at a more rapid rate.

Assessment of a Systolic Murmur

Echocardiography for evaluation of a systolic murmur allows a correct anatomic diagnosis, determination of the etiology of disease, and evaluation of hemodynamic severity. Evaluation is particularly useful in certain clinical situations.

In the pregnant woman with valvular aortic stenosis, echocardiography can be used to optimize management during pregnancy and to plan the optimal approach to labor and delivery in terms of hemodynamic monitoring, anesthesia, induction of labor, and mode of delivery.

In the patient with a systolic murmur undergoing noncardiac surgery, echocardiographic evaluation can be used to determine the potential need for aortic valve replacement prior to other surgery or may allow a more conservative approach with careful perioperative hemodynamic monitoring given an accurate assessment of aortic stenosis severity.

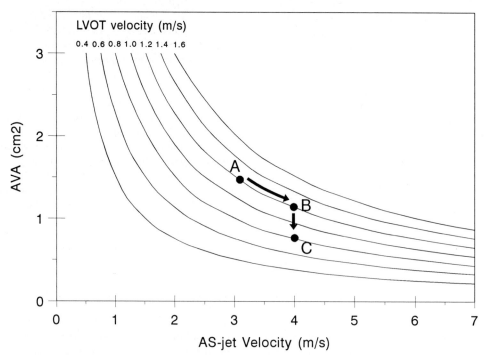

Figure 9–15. Graph of the relationship between aortic valve area (AVA) and aortic stenosis jet velocity for left ventricular outflow tract (LVOT) velocities ranging from 0.4 to 1.6 m/s. In the example shown, a patient initially has a jet velocity of 3.0 m/s and a valve area of 1.5 cm² (A). As stenosis severity increases, jet velocity increases to 4.0 m/s and valve area decreases to 1.2 cm² (B). However, with further disease progression (C), jet velocity was unchanged at 4 m/s, but valve area decreased to 0.8 cm² in the setting of decreased transaortic volume flow (LVOT velocity 1.2 to 0.8 m/s).

Case Examples

Case 1

A 39-year-old woman presented with syncope and was successfully resuscitated. She had a history of aortic valve disease but had refused surgical treatment in the past. Physical examination showed a IV/VI aortic stenosis murmur, a I/VI aortic regurgitation murmur, and bibasilar rales. Echocardiography showed:

2D echo: Aortic valve thickened with systolic doming and reduced systolic opening

Left ventricular hypertrophy with normal systolic function

Left ventricular outflow tract diameter = 2.0 cm

Doppler: Aortic stenotic jet = 5.9 m/s (Figs. 9–16 and 9–17)

Left ventricular outflow tract velocity = 0.9 m/s

AR: 1+, MR: 2+

From these data, outflow tract cross-sectional area is:

$$CSA_{LVOT} = \pi\left(\frac{2.0}{2}\right)^2 = 3.14 \text{ cm}^2$$

Aortic valve area, calculated with the simplified continuity equation, is:

$$AVA = \frac{3.14 \text{ cm}^2 \times 0.9 \text{ m/s}}{5.9 \text{ m/s}} = 0.5 \text{ cm}^2$$

and the velocity ratio is:

$$Velocity \ ratio = \frac{0.9}{5.9} = 0.15$$

At surgery, the patient had a severely stenotic and thickened unicuspid aortic valve. Aortic valve replacement was performed, and the patient has done well.

Case 2

A 56-year-old man presented with nephrolithiasis, a III/VI systolic murmur on auscultation, and no cardiac symptoms. Echocardiography showed:

2D echo: Abnormal aortic valve (probably bicuspid) with severe fibrocalcific changes

Severe left ventricular hypertrophy

Doppler: Left ventricular outflow tract diameter = 2.4 cm

Aortic stenotic jet = 7.4 m/s (see Fig. 9–8)

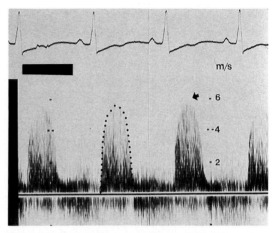

Figure 9–16. Aortic stenosis jet recorded with continuous-wave Doppler from a suprasternal notch approach in a 39-year-old woman with syncope. These data provide a definitive diagnosis in this clinical setting.

Left ventricular outflow tract velocity = 1.2 m/s

AR: 2+

From these data,

$\Delta P_{max} = 4(7.4)^2 = 219$ mmHg

$\Delta P_{mean} = 2.4(7.4)^2 = 131$ mmHg

Velocity ratio = 1.2/7.4 = 0.16

$CSA_{LVOT} = \pi(2.4/2)^2 = 4.5$ cm^2

$AVA = 4.5$ cm$^2 \times (1.2/7.4) = 0.7$ cm^2

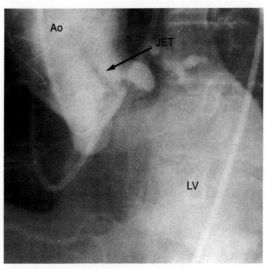

Figure 9–17. Supravalvular aortogram in the same patient as in Figure 9–16 with a jet of unopacified blood from the left ventricle highlighted against the background of contrast material in the aortic root.

Case 3

A 69-year-old man presented with severe congestive heart failure. Examination showed a soft systolic murmur but a single S_2. Echocardiography showed:

2D echo: Calcified trileaflet aortic valve with reduced systolic opening

Moderate left ventricular dilation with moderately reduced systolic function and global left ventricular hypokinesis

Doppler: Aortic stenotic jet = 3.2 m/s (Fig. 9–18)

Left ventricular outflow tract diameter = 2.0 cm

VTI_{Ao} = 70 cm

Left ventricular outflow tract velocity = 0.9 m/s

VTI_{LVOT} = 20.1 cm

From these data,

$$\Delta P_{max} = 4(3.2)^2 = 41 \text{ mmHg}$$
$$\Delta P_{mean} = 2.4(3.2)^2 = 25 \text{ mmHg}$$
$$\text{Stroke volume} = CSA_{LVOT} \times VTI_{LVOT}$$
$$= \pi(2.0/2)^2 \times 20.1 = 63 \text{ ml}$$
$$\text{Cardiac output} = SV \times HR = 63 \times 80 \text{ bpm}$$
$$= 5.0 \text{ L/min}$$
$$\text{AVA (using VTIs)} = CSA_{LVOT} \times (20.1/70)$$
$$= 0.9 \text{ cm}^2$$
$$\text{AVA (using velocities)} = CSA_{LVOT} \times (0.9/3.2)$$
$$= 0.9 \text{ cm}^2$$

MITRAL STENOSIS

Diagnostic Imaging of the Mitral Valve

Rheumatic Disease

Rheumatic disease predominantly affects the mitral valve and is the most common cause of mitral stenosis. Rheumatic valvular disease is characterized by commissural fusion which results in bowing or doming of the valve leaflets in diastole (Fig. 9–19). The base and midsections

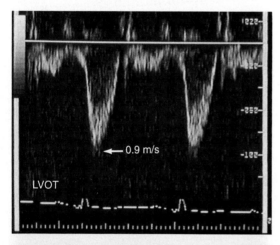

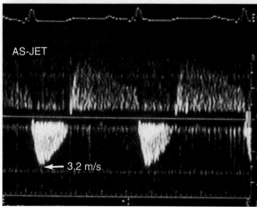

Figure 9–18. Left ventricular outflow tract (LVOT) velocity (*above*) and aortic stenosis jet (*below*) in an elderly patient with severe aortic stenosis with a low V_{max} of 3.2 m/s and coexisting left ventricular systolic dysfunction with a low stroke volume.

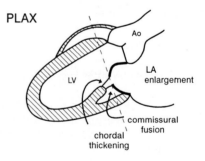

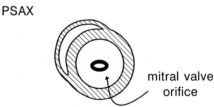

Figure 9–19. Schematic diagram of the 2D echo findings in mitral stenosis. In the parasternal long-axis view (PLAX), commissural fusion with diastolic doming of the mitral leaflets is seen, as well as chordal thickening and fusion. In a parasternal short-axis view (PSAX), at the mitral valve orifice, the area of opening can be planimetered. The plane of the short-axis view is indicated by a dashed line on the long-axis image.

of the leaflets move toward the ventricular apex, while the motion of the leaflet tips is restricted due to fusion of the anterior and posterior leaflets along the medial and lateral commissures. Thickening at the leaflet tips occurs frequently, but the remainder of the leaflets can show variable degrees of thickening and/or calcification. If the base and midportions of the leaflets are relatively thin, leaflet mobility is normal other than the fused commissures. The rheumatic process also typically affects the subvalvular region with fusion, shortening, fibrosis, and calcification of the mitral chordae.

In rheumatic mitral stenosis, 2D echo allows detailed evaluation of mitral valve morphology, including assessment of leaflet thickness, leaflet mobility, the degree of calcification, and the extent of subvalvular involvement on transthoracic parasternal and apical views (Fig. 9–20). Occasionally, if transthoracic images are suboptimal, transesophageal imaging may be needed for evaluation of mitral valve anatomy, although definition of subvalvular disease may be limited due to shadows and reverberations from calcification of the mitral valve and annulus.

Mitral Annular Calcification and Calcific Mitral Stenosis

Mitral annular calcification is a common incidental finding on echocardiography in elderly subjects. Mild annular calcification appears as an isolated area of calcification on the left ventricular side of the posterior annulus, near the base of the posterior mitral leaflet. In more severe mitral annular calcification, increased echogenicity is seen in a hemielliptical pattern involving the entire posterior annulus. The area of fibrous continuity between the anterior mitral leaflet and the aortic root rarely is involved. The etiology of mitral annular calcification is considered to be a "degenerative" age-related process. It can result in mild to moderate mitral regurgitation due to increased rigidity of the mitral annulus. Occasionally, the calcification extends into the base of the mitral leaflets themselves, resulting in functional mitral stenosis due to narrowing of the diastolic flow area. Calcific mitral stenosis can be distinguished from rheumatic disease by careful imaging techniques to demonstrate thin and mobile mitral leaflet tips without commissural fusion.

Differential Diagnosis (Table 9–7)

In patients referred for echocardiography with suspected mitral stenosis, the initial differ-

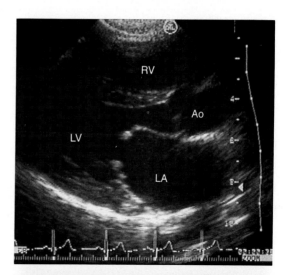

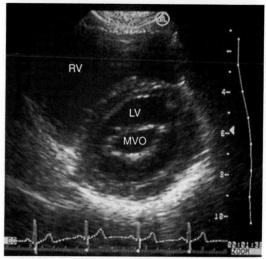

Figure 9–20. Parasternal long-axis view (*above*) of a patient with mild rheumatic mitral stenosis showing the typical doming of the anterior mitral leaflet due to commissural fusion. Left atrial enlargement is present. The short-axis view (*below*) allows accurate planimetry of the mitral orifice (MVO) area if care is taken to identify the smallest opening by scanning slowly from apex toward the base.

ential diagnosis includes other causes of pulmonary congestion. Standard echo Doppler evaluation will reveal whether left ventricular systolic dysfunction, aortic valve disease, or mitral regurgitation is present. The possibility of diastolic left ventricular dysfunction also should be considered. The rare case of an atrial myxoma or other atrial tumor obstructing left ventricular inflow, thus mimicking the clinical presentation of mitral stenosis, can easily be diagnosed by 2D imaging (see Chap. 13). Rarely, a patient with mild obstruction due to cor triatriatum may present as an adult.

TABLE 9–7. ECHOCARDIOGRAPHIC DIFFERENTIAL DIAGNOSIS OF LEFT VENTRICULAR INFLOW OBSTRUCTION

Mitral valve stenosis
  Rheumatic mitral stenosis
  Calcific mitral stenosis (rare)
  Congenital mitral stenosis

Left atrial tumor (myxoma)

Left atrial thrombus

Left ventricular diastolic dysfunction

Congenital disease
  Congenital mitral stenosis
  Cor triatriatum

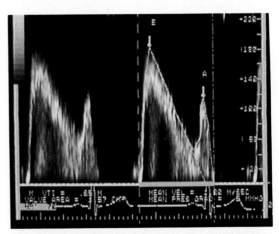

Figure 9–21. Transmitral flow curve in the same patient as in Figure 9–20. Using this velocity curve, pressure gradients can be calculated with the Bernoulli equation and valve area by the pressure half-time method. Note the well-defined maximal velocity and the clearly defined, linear deceleration slope. An *A* velocity is seen because sinus rhythm is present.

Quantitation of Mitral Stenosis Severity

Pressure Gradients (Fig. 9–21)

The mean diastolic transmitral pressure gradient can be determined from the transmitral velocity curve using the simplified Bernoulli equation:

$$\text{Mean mitral } \Delta P = \frac{4(V_1^2 + V_2^2 + V_3^2 + \cdots V_n^2)}{n} \quad (9.17)$$

With severe stenosis, the mean pressure gradient may be as high as 20 to 30 mmHg, but it may be as low as 5 to 15 mmHg. The variability in pressure gradients in severe mitral stenosis is due to the dependence of pressure gradients on volume flow rate as well as valve area. Severe mitral stenosis may be associated with a low stroke volume (due to the limitation of left ventricular diastolic filling), resulting in a relatively low mean gradient. If volume flow rate increases, for example with exercise, an increase in transmitral gradient is seen. As for other types of valvular stenosis, calculation of valve area, taking both pressure gradient and volume flow rate into account, is helpful in quantitating mitral stenosis severity.

Mitral Valve Area

2D Echo Valve Area (Fig. 9–22). Compared with valvular aortic stenosis, the 3D anatomy of rheumatic mitral stenosis is simpler with a planar elliptical orifice that is relatively constant in position in middiastole. Thus 2D short-axis imaging of the diastolic orifice allows direct planimetry of valve area. This approach has

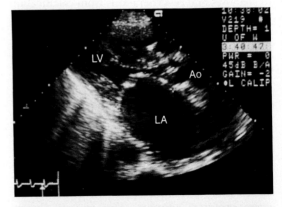

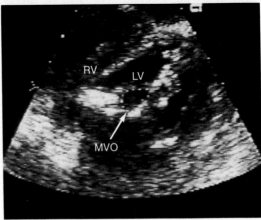

Figure 9–22. Long-axis (*above*) and short-axis (*below*) views of severe mitral stenosis. Note the commissural fusion, diastolic doming, and marked thickening and calcification of the valve leaflets. Aortic valve involvement and severe left atrial enlargement are present.

been well validated compared with measurement of valve area at surgery and in comparison with catheterization-determined valve areas. Since the shape of the mitral valve inflow region is similar to a funnel, with the narrowest cross-sectional area at the leaflet tips, it is important to begin the 2D scan at the apex, slowly moving the image plane toward the mitral valve to identify the smallest orifice. With a low overall 2D gain setting, the inner edge of the black-white interface is traced. Given the accuracy of this technique, 2D echo mitral valve area should be measured in patients with mitral stenosis whenever image quality is adequate.

Pressure Half-Time Valve Area (Fig. 9–23). Calculation of mitral valve area by the pressure half-time method is based on the concept that the *rate* of pressure decline across the stenotic mitral orifice is determined by the cross-sectional area of the orifice: the smaller the orifice, the slower is the rate of pressure decline. The influence of left atrial and left ventricular compliance on the rate of pressure decline is assumed to be negligible—an assumption that is

not always warranted, especially immediately after balloon commissurotomy.

The pressure half-time is defined as the time interval (in milliseconds) between the maximum early diastolic transmitral pressure gradient and the time point where the pressure gradient is half the maximum value. Initially, the pressure half-time concept was evaluated using invasive measurements of left atrial and left ventricular pressure. Pressure half-time was found to be constant for a given individual, even with exercise-induced changes in volume flow rate, suggesting that this measurement is a constant measure of stenosis severity for a given valve area.

This concept then was adapted to transmitral Doppler flow velocity curves. Given the quadratic relationship between velocity and pressure gradients, the half-time is determined from a Doppler spectral velocity curve as the time interval from the maximum mitral velocity (V_{max}) to the point where the velocity has fallen to $V_{max}/\sqrt{2}$ (Fig. 9–24). Initial studies comparing Doppler half-time data with invasively determined Gorlin valve areas found a linear relationship, with a half-time of about 220 ms corresponding to a valve area of 1.0 cm². The empirical formula

$$\mathrm{MVA} = \frac{220}{T_{1/2}} \qquad \begin{array}{l}\text{Pressure half-time}\\\text{MVA}\end{array} \qquad (9.18)$$

was proposed and has been shown to correlate well with invasive valve areas in several clinical studies (Table 9–8).

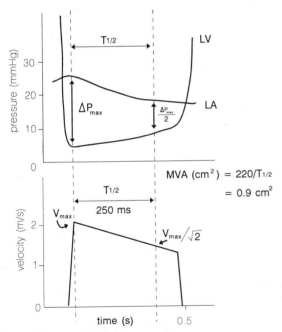

Figure 9–23. Schematic diagram showing the relationship between left ventricular (LV) and left atrial (LA) pressures (*above*) and the transmitral velocity curve (*below*) recorded with Doppler ultrasound. The shape of the pressure gradient is reflected in the Doppler velocity curve. The pressure half-time ($T_{1/2}$) is the same whether measured from the pressure data or from the velocity data. Mitral valve area (MVA) is calculated using an empirical constant as 220/$T_{1/2}$, where valve area is in square centimeters (cm²) and $T_{1/2}$ is in milliseconds (ms).

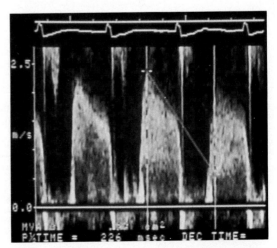

Figure 9–24. Pressure half-time measurement in a patient with severe mitral stenosis. Maximum velocity and the diastolic slope are identified as shown, yielding a pressure half-time of 226 ms corresponding to a mitral valve area of 1.0 cm². There is no *a* wave because atrial fibrillation is present.

TABLE 9–8. SELECTED STUDIES OF MITRAL VALVE AREA DETERMINATION

FIRST AUTHOR, YEAR	COMPARISON	N	STUDY GROUP	R	RANGE (cm²)	SEE (cm²)
Gorlin, 1951	MVA by Gorlin formula vs direct autopsy or surgery	11	Mitral stenosis	0.89	0.5–1.5	0.15
Hakki, 1981	MVA by original vs simplified Gorlin formula	40	Mitral stenosis	0.94	0.4–2.6	0.19
Libanoff, 1968	$T_{1/2}$ at rest vs exercise	20	Mitral valve disease	0.98	20–340 ms	21 ms
Henry, 1975	2D echo vs direct measurement at surgery	20	MS pts undergoing surgery	0.92	0.5–3.5	—
Holen, 1977	MVA by Doppler vs Gorlin	10	Mitral stenosis	0.98	0.6–3.4	0.18
Hatle, 1979	$T_{1/2}$ vs Gorlin MVA	32	Mitral stenosis	−0.74	0.4–3.5	—
Smith, 1986	2D echo vs Gorlin	37	MS alone	0.83	0.4–2.3	0.26
		35	Prior commissurotomy	0.58		0.28
	$T_{1/2}$ MVA vs Gorlin	(37)	MS alone	0.85		0.22
		(35)	Prior commissurotomy	0.90		0.14
Reid, 1987	$T_{1/2}$ MVA vs Gorlin	12	Pre-CBV	0.80	0.6–3.6	0.4
			Post-CBV	0.30		0.3
	2D echo vs Gorlin		Pre- and post-CBV	0.80		
Come, 1988	$T_{1/2}$ MVA vs Gorlin	37	Pre-CBV	0.51	0.6–1.3	—
			Post-CBV	0.47	1.2–3.8	—
	Gorlin vs Gorlin	23	Repeat-cath	0.74	0.4–1.4	—
Thomas, 1988	Predicted vs actual $T_{1/2}$	18	Pre-CBV	0.93–0.96		
			Post-CBV	0.52–0.66		
Abascal, 1988	2D echo vs Gorlin	17	Pre-CBV	0.81		
			Post-CBV	0.75		
			Pre- and post-CBV	0.88	0.5–3.0	
	$T_{1/2}$ MVA vs Gorlin	17	Pre-CBV	0.75		
			Immediately post-CBV	0.46		
			Follow-up	0.78	0.8–3.0	
Chen, 1989	$T_{1/2}$ MVA vs Gorlin	18	Pre-CBV	0.81	0.4–1.2	0.11
			Immediately post-CBV	0.84	1.3–2.6	0.20
			24–48 h post-CBV	0.72	1.3–2.6	0.49

Note: CBV = catheter balloon valvuloplasty; Gorlin = Gorlin formula valve area; MS = mitral stenosis; MVA = mitral valve area; 2D = two-dimensional; $T_{1/2}$ = pressure half-time.

Data from Gorlin et al: Am Heart J 41:1–29, 1951; Hakki et al: Circ 63:1050–1055, 1981; Libanoff et al: Circ 38:144–150, 1968; Henry et al: Circ 51:827–831, 1975; Holen et al: Acta Med Scand 201:83–88, 1977; Hatle et al: Circ 60:1096–1104, 1979; Smith et al: Circ 73:100–107, 1986; Reid et al: Circ 76:628–636, 1987; Come et al: Am J Cardiol 61:817–825, 1988; Thomas et al: Circ 78:980–993, 1988; Abascal et al: JACC 12:606–615, 1988; Chen et al: JACC 13:1309–1313, 1989.

Reprinted with permission from Otto CM et al: Am J Cardiol 69:1607, 1992.

Continuity Equation Mitral Valve Area.

The continuity principle for calculation of valve area also can be applied to the mitral orifice:

$$MVA = \frac{\text{transmitral SV}}{\text{VTI}_{\text{MS-jet}}} \quad \substack{\text{Continuity} \\ \text{equation MVA}} \quad (9.19)$$

where SV is stroke volume (cm³/s), VTI is the velocity-time integral in the mitral stenosis jet, and MVA is the mitral valve area. Stroke volume can be determined from the left ventricular outflow tract cross-sectional area and velocity-time integral (in the absence of aortic regurgitation) or from the pulmonary artery diameter and velocity-time integral. Note that stroke volume measured at either of these sites will represent transmitral volume flow accurately only if there is no significant mitral regurgitation.

Proximal Isovelocity Surface Area Method.

In theory, transmitral volume flow rate can be calculated accurately in mitral stenosis even when mitral regurgitation is present using the proximal isovelocity surface area method. The color Doppler flow parameters are adjusted to demonstrate a well-defined hemispherical aliasing surface area on the left atrial side of the mitral orifice. The velocity at this location equals the Nyquist limit (the "aliasing" velocity). The cross-sectional area of the aliased boundary can be calculated as the surface area of a hemisphere with diameter measured from the color flow image. Multiplying cross-sectional area times the known velocity yields the volume flow rate, which then can be used in conjunction with the transmitral velocity time interval in the continuity equation. One difficulty with this approach is that the volume flow rate must be integrated over the diastolic filling period; a single color image yields only the volume flow rate at one time point in diastole. Because of this problem, the proximal isovelocity method has not been widely applied for evaluation of mitral valve area.

Technical Considerations and Potential Pitfalls (Table 9–9)

Currently, assessment of the severity of mitral stenosis in an individual patient typically includes calculation of the mean transmitral pressure gradient, planimetry of the 2D echo valve area, and calculation of the pressure half-time valve area. Besides the physiologic limitations of pressure gradient and valve area measurements in mitral stenosis, potential technical problems deserve attention and in specific instances, other approaches to evaluating stenosis severity may be utilized. Evaluation of coexisting lesions also is important.

TABLE 9–9. PITFALLS IN EVALUATION OF MITRAL STENOSIS SEVERITY

Pressure Gradient

Intercept angle between mitral stenosis jet and ultrasound beam

Beat-to-beat variability in atrial fibrillation

Dependence on transvalvular volume flow rate (e.g., exercise, coexisting mitral regurgitation)

2D Valve Area

Image orientation

Tomographic plane

2D gain settings

Intra- and interobserver variability in planimetry of orifice

Poor acoustic access

Deformed valve anatomy post-commissurotomy

T$_{1/2}$ Valve Area

Definition of V_{max} and early diastolic slope

Nonlinear early diastolic velocity slope

Sinus rhythm with a wave superimposed on early diastolic slope

Influence of coexisting aortic regurgitation

Changing left ventricular and left atrial compliances immediately after commissurotomy

Continuity Equation Mitral Valve Area

Accurate measurement of transmitral stroke volume

As for any intracardiac blood flow, accurate pressure gradient calculations depend on accurate velocity measurements, which require a near-parallel intercept angle between the direction of blood flow and the Doppler beam. The mitral stenosis jet nearly always can be recorded from an apical approach, but careful transducer positioning and angulation are needed to record an optimal signal. Color flow imaging may be helpful in defining the jet direction in a given tomographic plane. Depending on the maximum jet velocity, the velocity curve can be recorded with conventional pulsed, high-pulse-repetition-frequency, or continuous-wave Doppler ultrasound. Pulsed Doppler recordings may show better definition of the maximum velocity and early diastolic slope than continuous-wave Doppler recordings because of a better signal-to-noise ratio.

Direct planimetry of mitral valve area on 2D short-axis images has proven to be a valid technique in most clinical situations. However, definition of valve area may be difficult if image quality is poor or if there is extensive distortion of the valve anatomy. Valve area can be underestimated if gain settings are too high and can be overestimated if the smallest area at the leaflet tips is not recorded. Low gain settings and careful scanning in a short-axis plane from the apex toward the base helps avoid these potential problems.

Pressure half-time valve area calculations have significant limitations in certain clinical settings. When coexisting aortic regurgitation is present, left ventricular filling occurs both antegrade across the mitral valve and retrograde across the aortic valve. This may result in a more rapid rise in left ventricular diastolic pressure than if there were no aortic regurgitation, resulting in a shorter half-time measurement. Conversely, if severe aortic regurgitation impairs mitral leaflet opening, functional mitral stenosis may be superimposed on anatomic mitral stenosis, with lengthening of the half-time measurement. In clinical practice, if the 2D echo shows rheumatic mitral stenosis and only mild to moderate aortic regurgitation is present, the half-time method remains a useful approach for evaluation of stenosis severity. If aortic regurgitation is severe, or if the mitral valve anatomy is atypical, the potential influence of coexisting lesions should be considered.

A major assumption of the half-time method is that left atrial and left ventricular compliances do not significantly affect the rate of pressure gradient decline across the stenotic orifice. While this assumption appears to be warranted in clinically stable patients with mitral stenosis, it is *not* justified in the period immediately after catheter mitral valvuloplasty. After relief of mitral stenosis, the fall in left atrial pressure and the increase in left ventricular filling are accompanied by directionally opposite changes in left atrial and left ventricular compliance. During the 24 to 72 hours after the procedure, equilibrium has not been reached, and the pressure half-time may not be an accurate reflection of orifice area. After this adjustment period, compliances stabilize, and the pressure half-time method again provides useful information.

Even under physiologically stable conditions, accurate pressure half-time measurements require careful recording of the mitral stenosis velocity curve. While a parallel intercept angle is somewhat less important than for pressure gradient calculations (since the *shape* of the curve is the same even at a nonparallel angle), it is im-portant that the intercept angle be *constant* throughout diastole to avoid artifactual distortion in the shape of the curve. The maximum early diastolic velocity and the early diastolic deceleration slope should be well defined. Pressure half-times are most easily and reproducibly measured if the deceleration slope is linear. If a linear slope cannot be obtained even after careful adjustment of transducer position and angulation, the half-time measurement should be made using the middiastolic slope of the curve, extrapolating back to the initial maximum velocity (Fig. 9–25).

In atrial fibrillation, several beats are averaged, since mean gradient will vary with the R-R interval. While the half-time will be relatively constant despite variation in the length of diastole, only beats where the diastolic filling period is long enough to show the early diastolic slope clearly are appropriate for measurement. In sinus rhythm, the increase in velocity due to atrial contraction may obscure the early diastolic slope, particularly at high heart rates, so that half-time measurements may not be possible.

Continuity equation mitral valve area determinations are most accurate in patients without significant coexisting mitral regurgitation. In this subgroup, continuity equation mitral valve area calculations provide a useful alternate to the pressure half-time method, especially in situations of altered chamber compliances. The accuracy of the continuity equation method, as in aortic stenosis, depends on a parallel intercept angle between the mitral stenotic jet and the ultrasound beam and a careful stroke volume calculation from diameter and velocity recordings. Accurate pulmonary artery diameter measurement for stroke volume calculations can be dif-

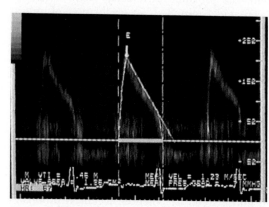

Figure 9–25. In this patient with mitral stenosis, the diastolic deceleration slope is nonlinear on some beats (*left*) with a steeper early than middiastolic slope. If attempts to record a more linear slope (*center*) are unsuccessful, the middiastolic slope should be measured.

ficult in adult patients due to poor acoustic access. Left ventricular outflow tract diameter nearly always can be imaged reliably. However, many patients with mitral stenosis have some degree of coexisting aortic or mitral regurgitation so that transaortic stroke volume does not equal transmitral stroke volume.

The proximal isovelocity surface area method avoids the problem of measuring transmitral stroke volume when coexisting regurgitant lesions are present because it measures transmitral volume flow directly. However, there are significant methodologic problems with this approach, specifically accurate calculation of the surface area of the aliasing signal and temporal averaging of the volume flow calculation. Although this method is not widely used because of these problems, it remains a theoretically sound approach to valve area determination.

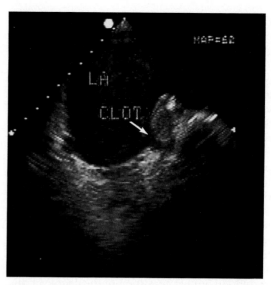

Figure 9–26. Clot in the atrial appendage of a patient with mitral stenosis, seen on transesophageal imaging.

Coexisting Lesions in Mitral Stenosis

Left Atrial Enlargement and Thrombus

Chronic pressure overload of mitral stenosis leads to gradual enlargement of the left atrium. Left atrial size can become extremely large in long-standing severe mitral stenosis. In conjunction with a low volume flow rate due to the stenotic valve, left atrial enlargement results in stasis of blood flow and thrombus formation. Thrombi are located preferentially in the left atrial appendage but also can occur in the body of the atrium as protruding or as laminated thrombus along the atrial wall or interatrial septum (Fig. 9–26).

Transthoracic echo has a high specificity for detection of left atrial thrombus (i.e., if it is visualized, it most likely is a real finding), but the sensitivity is less than 50 percent. In part, this relates to the difficulty of imaging the left atrial appendage in adults. Sometimes the left atrial appendage can be visualized in laterally angulated parasternal short-axis views at the aortic valve level or from apical two-chamber views angulated slightly superiorly. More often it cannot be visualized at all, or image quality is too poor at the depth of the left atrium to allow reliable exclusion of atrial thrombus. Ultrasound penetration is poor, and beam width artifact can be substantial at the depth of the left atrium from surface imaging.

Transesophageal echo has a high sensitivity (>99 percent) and specificity (>99 percent) for detection of left atrial thrombus. The left atrial appendage can be well visualized, and the higher transducer frequencies (5 MHz) and lower imaging depths result in high-resolution images. By careful tomographic imaging, the entire body of the left atrium can be examined. Laminated thrombus may be difficult to identify, especially along the interatrial septum, and should be suspected if the septum appears excessively thickened.

Pulmonary Hypertension

In mitral stenosis, increased left atrial pressure results in pulmonary venous hypertension and consequent pulmonary artery hypertension. Initially, the increase in pulmonary artery pressure is "passive"—the pressure difference across the pulmonary bed (pulmonary artery minus left atrial pressure) is normal. In this situation, although pulmonary pressures are elevated, pulmonary vascular resistance is normal, and pulmonary pressures will fall toward normal after relief of mitral stenosis. With long-standing pulmonary venous hypertension, irreversible changes in the pulmonary vascular bed occur, leading to elevated pulmonary vascular resistance and persistent pulmonary hypertension after relief of mitral stenosis.

The presence of pulmonary hypertension can be suspected in mitral stenosis when there is midsystolic partial closure (or "notching") of the pulmonic valve M-mode, a short interval between the onset of flow and maximum velocity, or midsystolic abrupt deceleration in the right ventricular outflow velocity curve. With severe pulmonary hypertension, 2D echo may show right ventricular hypertrophy and enlargement, paradoxical septal motion, and tricuspid regurgitation secondary to annular dilation.

The degree of pulmonary hypertension can be quantitated from the velocity in the tricuspid regurgitant jet and the appearance of the inferior vena cava. The simplified Bernoulli equation is used to calculate the right ventricular to right atrial maximum systolic pressure difference (Fig. 9–27) from the continuous-wave Doppler tricuspid regurgitant jet recording. This difference is added to an estimate of right atrial pressure based on the size and respiratory variation of the inferior vena cava as it enters the right atrium. While pulmonary vascular resistance cannot be determined with Doppler echo techniques (since an absolute measure of left atrial pressure is not available), pulmonary hypertension out of proportion to the degree of mitral stenosis raises the possibility of a coexisting pulmonary disease process.

Mitral Regurgitation

Some degree of coexisting mitral regurgitation is common in patients with mitral stenosis. Mitral regurgitant severity can be evaluated using standard techniques (see Chap. 10) and is an important factor in deciding on appropriate therapy. For example, significant mitral regurgitation is a contraindication to surgical or balloon commissurotomy. Coexisting mitral regurgitation elevates the transmitral pressure gradient (due to increased transmitral volume flow rate), but both 2D echo and pressure half-time valve area measurements remain accurate.

Other Coexisting Valvular Disease

The rheumatic disease process also can affect the aortic valve (second in frequency to the mitral valve) and, less commonly, the tricuspid valve. Aortic valve involvement may result in stenosis and/or regurgitation which can be evaluated with appropriate 2D and Doppler echo techniques. Evaluation of aortic regurgitation by color flow imaging may be complicated in the presence of mitral stenosis due to merging of the two diastolic flow disturbances in the left ventricle. Imaging the aortic regurgitant jet in short axis just proximal to the aortic valve and using other Doppler methods for evaluation of regurgitant severity will avoid this potential problem.

Rheumatic tricuspid stenosis may be difficult to appreciate on 2D imaging. Doppler flow patterns are similar to mitral stenosis, and the same quantitative methods for evaluation of stenosis severity can be applied. Even in the absence of rheumatic involvement of the tricuspid valve, significant tricuspid regurgitation is common (due to pulmonary hypertension and annular dilation) in patients with mitral stenosis. Careful evaluation of tricuspid regurgitation severity is especially important preoperatively in case tricuspid annuloplasty is needed at the time of mitral valve surgery.

Left Ventricular Response

The left ventricle in mitral stenosis is small and nonhypertrophied, with normal systolic function. The presence of left ventricular dilation suggests that significant coexisting mitral or aortic regurgitation or primary myocardial dysfunction (cardiomyopathy or ischemic disease) is present.

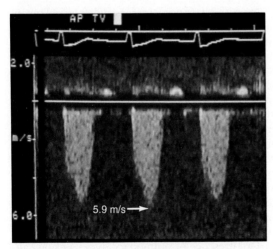

Figure 9–27. Tricuspid regurgitant jet of 5.2 m/s in a patient with severe mitral stenosis indicating a right ventricular to right atrial pressure difference of 108 mmHg. Given a normal right atrial pressure, this corresponds to a pulmonary systolic pressure of about 115 to 120 mmHg. This patient also had right ventricular enlargement and paradoxical septal motion, as seen in Figure 9–22. Pulmonary hypertension of this severity represents irreversible pulmonary vascular disease.

Clinical Applications in Specific Patient Populations (Table 9–10)

Diagnosis, Hemodynamic Progression, and Timing of Intervention

Echo Doppler is the standard clinical method for evaluation of the presence and severity of valvular mitral stenosis. Disease progression can be followed and the timing of intervention can be determined using Doppler echo and clinical

TABLE 9–10. ECHOCARDIOGRAPHIC APPROACH TO MITRAL STENOSIS

1. Valve morphology

2. Exclude other causes of clinical presentation

3. Mitral stenosis severity
   a. Mean transmitral pressure gradient
   b. 2D valve area
   c. $T_{1/2}$ valve area

4. Coexisting mitral regurgitation

5. Left atrial enlargement

6. Pulmonary artery pressure (from TR jet and IVC)

7. TEE for evaluation of left atrial clot if CBV is planned

8. Coexisting tricuspid regurgitation severity

CBV = catheter balloon valvuloplasty; IVC = inferior vena cava; TR = tricuspid regurgitation; TEE = transesophageal echocardiography.

TABLE 9–11. MITRAL VALVE MORPHOLOGY BY TWO-DIMENSIONAL ECHOCARDIOGRAPHY

MORPHOLOGY	SCORE
Mobility	
Highly mobile valve with only leaflet tips restricted	1
Leaflet middle and base portions have normal mobility	2
Valve continues to move forward in diastole, mainly from the base	3
No or minimal forward movement of the leaflets in diastole	4
Leaflet Thickening	
Leaflets near normal in thickness (4–5 mm)	1
Midleaflets normal, marked thickening of margins (5–8 mm)	2
Thickening extending through the entire leaflet (5–8 mm)	3
Marked thickening of all leaflet tissue (>8–10 mm)	4
Subvalvular Thickening	
Minimal thickening just below the mitral leaflets	1
Thickening of chordal structures extending up to one-third of the chordal length	2
Thickening extending to the distal third of the chordal length	3
Extensive thickening and shortening of all chordal structures extending down to the papillary muscles	4
Calcification	
A single area of increased echo brightness	1
Scattered areas of brightness confined to leaflet margins	2
Brightness extending into the mid-portion of the leaflets	3
Extensive brightness throughout much of the leaflet tissue	4
Total score is obtained by adding the scores for each of the four features	

Reprinted with permission from Reid CL et al: Influence of mitral valve morphology on mitral balloon commissurotomy: Immediate and 6-month results from the NHLBI Balloon Valvuloplasty Registry. Am Heart J 124:657, 1992.

data alone. Evaluation by cardiac catheterization rarely is needed.

Pre- and Post-Catheter Balloon Commissurotomy

In the potential candidate for catheter balloon mitral commissurotomy, echo Doppler evaluation of mitral valve morphology is important in patient selection both in terms of predicted hemodynamic results and in terms of the risk of procedural complications. Mitral valve morphology may be described by a qualitative assessment, an additive scoring system (Table 9–11), or quantitative measurements of leaflet mobility. Whatever approach is used, the important features to consider are leaflet mobility, leaflet thickness, leaflet and commissural calcification, and subvalvular involvement. In general, the best hemodynamic results are seen with thin, mobile leaflets that have commissural fusion but little calcification or subchordal thickening. However, some patients with a relatively unfavorable morphology do have relief of mitral stenosis with balloon commissurotomy. It is noteworthy that patients with the most heavily calcified and deformed valves (and the most severe stenosis) are more likely to suffer procedure-related morbidity and mortality.

Another factor to consider in this patient population is the degree of coexisting mitral regurgitation, since commissurotomy is contradicted if moderate or severe regurgitation is present. In addition, since any left atrial thrombi may be dislodged by the catheters during the procedure,

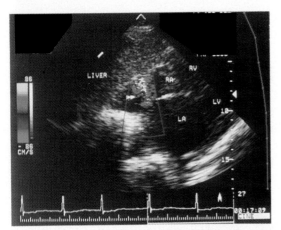

Figure 9–28. Small atrial septal defect with left-to-right flow seen on a subcostal view using color flow imaging in a patient after catheter mitral balloon commissurotomy.

transesophageal echocardiography is needed to evaluate for left atrial thrombus.

After catheter balloon valvuloplasty, echo Doppler allows identification of complications, permits assessment of hemodynamic results, and provides a baseline for future disease progression. Potential complications include (1) an increase in the severity of mitral regurgitation and (2) the presence of an atrial septal defect (usually small) at the transseptal catheter puncture site (Fig. 9–28). Hemodynamic results can be evaluated with standard echo Doppler techniques, again with an awareness of the potential inaccuracies in the half-time method in the immediate postcommissurotomy period. Doppler evaluation of postprocedure pulmonary artery systolic pressure also can be helpful.

Pre-, Intra-, and Postoperative Valvotomy

Considerations for pre- and postoperative evaluation of the patient undergoing surgical valvotomy are similar to those for catheter valvuloplasty. In addition, intraoperative monitoring with transesophageal echocardiography may be performed to evaluate the hemodynamic results and degree of mitral regurgitation immediately after repair. If significant mitral regurgitation or residual stenosis is present, valve replacement then can be performed at the same operative procedure.

Evaluation of the Pregnant Patient with Pulmonary Congestion

When echocardiography is requested in a pregnant patient with pulmonary congestion,

the possibility of valvular mitral stenosis should be considered. Symptoms due to mitral stenosis often occur initially during pregnancy due to increased metabolic demands and volume flow rate, and the murmur may not be appreciated on auscultation. Careful imaging of the valve and recording of the transmitral flow velocity curve allow exclusion or confirmation of this possibility.

Case Examples

Case 1 (Fig. 9–29)

A 56-year-old woman presented with increasing dyspnea on exertion. Echocardiography showed rheumatic mitral stenosis with:

Mitral valve morphology score = 4
Mitral valve area: 2D 1.2 cm^2
  $T_{1/2}$ 1.2 cm^2

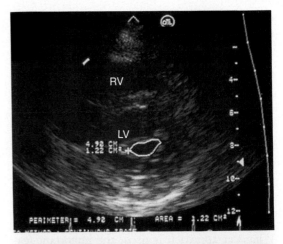

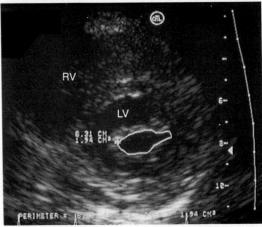

Figure 9–29. 2D short-axis mitral valve area before (1.2 cm^2) and 2 years after (1.9 cm^2) balloon mitral commissurotomy.

Mitral regurgitation = 2+
Moderate left atrial enlargement

The patient underwent balloon commissurotomy. At 2-year follow-up she remains asymptomatic with a 2D mitral valve area of 1.9 cm².

Case 2 (Fig. 9–30)

A 61-year-old woman was referred for possible balloon mitral commissurotomy. Echocardiography showed rheumatic mitral valve disease.

$T_{1/2}$ = 110 ms
MVA = $220/T_{1/2}$ = 2.0 cm²
Mitral regurgitation = 4+
Tricuspid regurgitant jet = 3.8 m/s
Estimated right atrial pressure = 10 mmHg
Estimated pulmonary artery systolic pressure = 68 mmHg

Based on these data, it was concluded that valvuloplasty was not appropriate. The patient underwent mitral valve replacement without complications.

TRICUSPID STENOSIS

Tricuspid stenosis is uncommon in adult patients. Rheumatic disease can occur and is associated with rheumatic mitral disease in nearly all cases. Carcinoid heart disease affects both tricuspid and pulmonic valves and can lead either to stenosis or to regurgitation. Right atrial tumors, large vegetations, or a large atrial thrombus (which may have embolized from the venous bed) can obstruct right ventricular inflow and mimic tricuspid stenosis.

2D echo images show thickening and shortening of the tricuspid valve leaflets (Fig. 9–31). Commissural fusion and diastolic bowing indicate rheumatic disease. Doppler recordings of the transvalvular flow velocity allow calculation

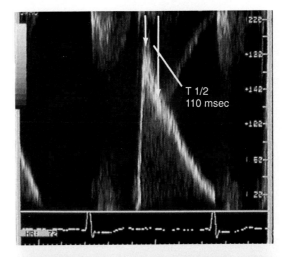

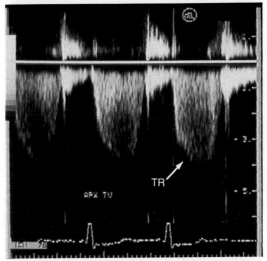

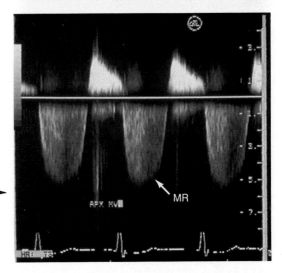

Figure 9–30. Left ventricular inflow curve (*above*) across the rheumatic mitral valve recorded with pulsed Doppler. The maximum velocity is elevated due to increased transmitral volume flow secondary to mitral regurgitation, but the deceleration slope is only moderately prolonged. The pressure half-time is 110 ms, corresponding to a mitral valve area of 2.0 cm². The tricuspid regurgitant jet (*center*) shows a maximum velocity of 3.8 m/s. Note that the tricuspid regurgitant jet has a longer duration, different shape, lower maximum velocity, and different associated diastolic flow curve than the mitral regurgitant jet (*below*) in this patient.

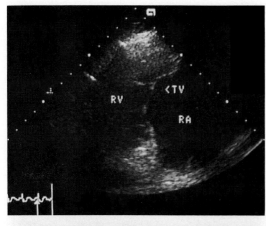

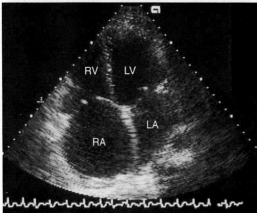

Figure 9–31. 2D right ventricular inflow (*above*) and apical four-chamber (*below*) views in a patient with rheumatic tricuspid valve disease. The leaflets are thickened, shortened, and immobile, resulting in a fixed orifice in systole and diastole. Right ventricular and right atrial enlargement secondary to volume overload are evident.

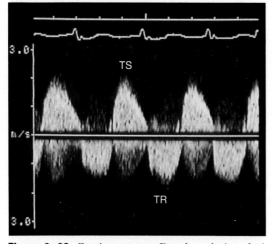

Figure 9–32. Continuous-wave Doppler velocity of tricuspid valve flow in the same patient as in Figure 9–31 showing the increased antegrade velocity in diastole. Severe tricuspid regurgitation is present with a high-intensity signal but low maximum velocity because pulmonary pressures are not elevated.

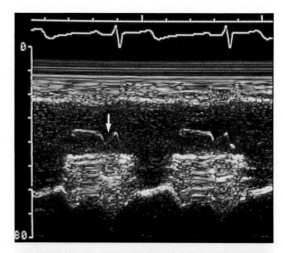

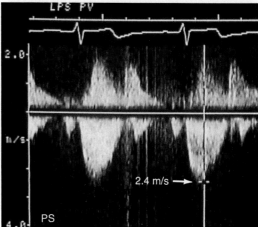

Figure 9–33. M-mode recording (*above*) of the pulmonic valve in a patient with mild pulmonic stenosis showing an increased *a* wave (note timing relative to the QRS complex and P wave). Continuous-wave Doppler from a left parasternal approach shows a pulmonary artery systolic velocity curve with a maximum velocity of 2.4 m/s corresponding to a maximum pressure gradient of 24 mmHg (*below*).

of mean gradient and pressure half-time valve area as described for the mitral valve (Fig. 9–32).

PULMONIC STENOSIS

Pulmonic stenosis in adults is most often due to congenital disease, either clinically insignificant or residual stenosis after reparative surgery in childhood. Pulmonic stenosis may occur in conjunction with other congenital lesions such as ventricular inversion (C-TGA) or tetralogy of Fallot.

2D echo imaging of the pulmonic valve shows thickened leaflets with systolic bowing. On Doppler interrogation, the antegrade velocity is increased with corresponding maximum and mean pressure gradients via the Bernoulli equation. Pulmonic valve area is not usually calculated, but the continuity equation principle can be applied in this situation, using an appropriate intracardiac location for stroke volume determination. Poststenotic pulmonary artery dilation may be present. Differentiation of valvular pulmonic stenosis from sub- or supravalvular obstruction can be difficult by 2D echo. Careful examinations with color flow and conventional pulsed Doppler can be very helpful in defining the site of the poststenotic flow disturbance (and thus the site of obstruction) (Fig. 9–33).

SUGGESTED READING

BASIC PRINCIPLES OF THE FLUID DYNAMICS OF VALVULAR STENOSIS

1. Yoganathan AP, Cape EG, Sung H-W, et al: Review of hydrodynamic principles for the cardiologist: Applications to the study of blood flow and jets by imaging techniques. J Am Coll Cardiol 12:1344–1353, 1988.
   Review of basic principles of blood flow, including Bernoulli relationships, volume flow calculation, and the fluid dynamics of jets.

2. Pasipoularides A: Clinical assessment of ventricular ejection dynamics with and without outflow obstruction. J Am Coll Cardiol 15:859–882, 1990.
   Detailed review of the physiology of left ventricular ejection emphasizing pressure-flow relationships.

3. Thomas JD, Weyman AE: Fluid dynamics model of mitral valve flow: Description with in vitro validation. J Am Coll Cardiol 13:221–233, 1989.
   Fluid dynamic model of the mitral valve with emphasis on the implications for Doppler and invasive pressure gradient and valve area calculations.

4. Flachskampf FA, Weyman AE, Guerrero JL, Thomas JD: Influence of orifice geometry and flow rate on effective valve area: An in vitro study. J Am Coll Cardiol 15:1173–1180, 1990.
   Further details on transmitral flow dynamics emphasizing variations in the discharge coefficient.

5. Segal J, Lerner DJ, Miller DC, et al: When should Doppler-determined valve area be better than the Gorlin formula? Variation in hydraulic constants in low flow states. J Am Coll Cardiol 9:1294–1305, 1987.
   Evaluation of the effects of variations in the discharge coefficient on calculated valve areas, especially at low cardiac outputs.

AORTIC STENOSIS

6. Hatle L, Angelsen BA, Tromsdal A: Non-invasive assessment of aortic stenosis by Doppler ultrasound. Br Heart J 43:284–292, 1980.
   Original description of noninvasive calculation of transaortic pressure gradients from continuous-wave Doppler using the Bernoulli equation in patients with aortic stenosis.

7. Currie PJ, Seward JB, Reeder GS, et al: Continuous-wave Doppler echocardiographic assessment of severity of calcific aortic stenosis: A simultaneous Doppler-catheter correlative study in 100 adult patients. Circulation 71:1162–1169, 1985.
   Simultaneous Doppler and catheter measurements of transaortic pressure gradients in adults with aortic stenosis.

8. Smith MD, Dawson PL, Elion JL, et al: Correlation of continuous-wave Doppler velocities with cardiac catheterization gradients: An experimental model of aortic stenosis. J Am Coll Cardiol 6:1306–1314, 1985.
   Detailed evaluation of the instantaneous pressure gradients in experimental aortic stenosis.

9. Otto CM, Pearlman AS: Doppler echocardiography in adults with symptomatic aortic stenosis: Diagnostic utility and cost-effectiveness. Arch Intern Med 148:2553–2560, 1988.
   Use of Doppler measures of jet velocity and valve area in the management of patients with symptomatic aortic stenosis.

10. Galan A, Zoghbi WA, Quinones MA: Determination of severity of valvular aortic stenosis by Doppler echocardiography and relation of findings to clinical outcome and agreement with hemodynamic measurements determined at cardiac catheterization. Am J Cardiol 67:1007–1012, 1991.
    Clinical outcome in relation to noninvasive Doppler findings in a large series of patients with aortic stenosis emphasizing the high degree of accuracy (97 percent) of this noninvasive approach.

11. Otto CM, Pearlman AS, Gardner CL: Hemodynamic progression of aortic stenosis in adults assessed by Doppler echocardiography. J Am Coll Cardiol 13:545–550, 1989.
    Reproducibility of Doppler echo data. In 42 asymptomatic adults followed for a mean of 20 months, 21 patients developed symptoms of aortic stenosis. The rate of increase in mean pressure gradient was higher in the symptomatic patients (15 versus 7 mmHg per year). No baseline variables that predict rate of progression were identified.

12. Roger VL, Tajik AJ, Bailey KR, et al: Progression of aortic stenosis in adults: New appraisal using Doppler echocardiography. Am Heart J 119:331–338, 1990.
    Of 112 adults with valvular aortic stenosis, an increase in jet velocity of 0.33 ± 0.50 m/s per year was seen in the 38 patients who became symptomatic during a mean 25-month follow-up period. In those who remained asymptomatic, jet velocity increased by 0.18 ± 0.26 m/s per year. Baseline variables did not predict outcome.

13. Burwash IG, Thomas DD, Sadahiro M: Dependence of Gorlin formula and continuity equation valve areas on transvalvular volume flow rate in valvular aortic stenosis. Circulation 89:827–835, 1994.
    In a model of chronic valvular aortic stenosis, with anatomy and hemodynamics similar to degenerative aortic valve disease, both invasively derived Gorlin formula and Doppler-echo continuity equation valve areas varied linearly with volume flow rate. The magnitude of the change in valve area was a 28 percent change in Gorlin formula valve area and a 22 percent change in continuity equation valve area for a doubling in mean flow rate. The authors propose that the mechanism of this observation is an actual increase in the degree of valve opening with increases in volume flow rate.

MITRAL STENOSIS

14. Henry WL, Griffith JM, Michaelis LL, et al: Measurement of mitral orifice area in patients with mitral valve disease by real-time, two-dimensional echocardiography. Circulation 51:827–831, 1975.
    Validation of 2D echo planimetry of mitral valve area compared with measurements at operation. 2D echo valve area

was within 0.3 cm² of surgical area in 12 of 14 (86 percent) patients.

15. Smith MD, Handshoe R, Handshoe S, et al: Comparative accuracy of two-dimensional echocardiography and Doppler pressure half-time methods in assessing severity of mitral stenosis in patients with and without prior commissurotomy. Circulation 73:100–107, 1986.
    In 74 patients with mitral stenosis, correlations were good for Doppler or 2D echo valve areas versus catheterization (r = 0.80 and 0.83), but Doppler correlated better (r = 0.90) than 2D echo (r = 0.58) in the 35 patients with prior commissurotomy. Reproducibility was 0.14 cm² for 2D echo and 0.15 cm² for Doppler data.

16. Holen J, Aaslid R, Landmark K, Simonsen S: Determination of pressure gradient in mitral stenosis with a non-invasive ultrasound Doppler technique. Acta Med Scand 199:455–460, 1976.
    Original description of Doppler measurement of transmitral pressure gradients.

17. David D, Lang RM, Marcus RH, et al: Doppler echocardiographic estimation of transmitral pressure gradients and correlations with micromanometer gradients in mitral stenosis. Am J Cardiol 67:1161–1164, 1991.
    Detailed study of pressure-velocity relations across the stenotic mitral valve.

18. Libanoff AJ, Rodbard S: Evaluation of the severity of mitral stenosis and regurgitation. Circulation 33:218–226, 1966.
    Original description of pressure half-time with catheterization data.

19. Hatle L, Angelsen B, Tromsdal A: Noninvasive assessment of atrioventricular pressure half-time by Doppler ultrasound. Circulation 60:1096–1104, 1979.
    Application of pressure half-time concept to Doppler data.

20. Thomas JD, Weyman AE: Doppler mitral pressure half-time: A clinical tool in search of theoretical justification. J Am Coll Cardiol 10:923–929, 1987.
    Review of theoretical background of pressure half-time concept emphasizing potential effects of left atrial and left ventricular compliance as well as the influence of mitral valve area.

21. Thomas JD, Wilkins GT, Choong CYP, et al: Inaccuracy of mitral pressure half-time immediately after percutaneous mitral valvotomy: Dependence on transmitral gradient and left atrial and ventricular compliance. Circulation 78:980–993, 1988.
    Evaluation of pressure half-time before and after mitral balloon commissurotomy illustrating reciprocal changes in left atrial and left ventricular compliance after valvuloplasty.

22. Abascal VM, Wilkins GT, Choong CYP, et al: Echocardiographic evaluation of mitral valve structure and function in patients followed for at least 6 months after percutaneous balloon mitral valvuloplasty. J Am Coll Cardiol 12:606–615, 1988.
    In patients under mitral balloon commissurotomy, the 16-point mitral valve morphology score was higher in patients with a decrease in valve area >25 percent at follow-up (mean mitral morphology score = 11 ± 2 versus 7 ± 2, p < 0.002).

23. Reid CL, McKay CR, Chandraratna PAN, et al: Mechanisms of increase in mitral valve area and influence of anatomic features in double-balloon, catheter balloon valvuloplasty in adults with rheumatic mitral stenosis: A Doppler and two-dimensional echocardiographic study. Circulation 76:628–636, 1987.
    Mitral valve leaflet mobility was predictive of postvalvuloplasty mitral valve area. Calcification of the commissures is associated with a small increase in valve area after valvuloplasty.

24. Reid CL, Otto CM, David KB, et al. and the NHLBI-BVR investigators: Influence of mitral valve morphology on mitral balloon commissurotomy: Immediate and six-month results from the NHLBI Balloon Valvuloplasty Registry. Am Heart J 124:657–665, 1992.
    In 555 patients undergoing balloon mitral commissurotomy, total leaflet morphology score was only weakly related to valve area after the procedure. On multivariate analysis, the strongest predictors of postprocedure valve area were preprocedure valve area (p < 0.001), left atrial size (p = 0.01), balloon diameter (p = 0.02), cardiac output (p = 0.004), and leaflet mobility (p = 0.01).

25. Complications and mortality of percutaneous balloon mitral commissurotomy. A report from the National Heart, Lung, and Blood Institute Balloon Valvuloplasty Registry. Circulation 85:2014–2024, 1992.
    Overall 30-day mortality was 0.6 percent with a serious complication rate of 12 percent. On multivariate analysis, predictors of early death were a higher echo score and smaller preprocedure valve area (p < 0.001).

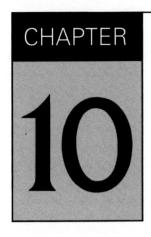

CHAPTER 10

VALVULAR REGURGITATION: DIAGNOSIS, QUANTITATION, AND CLINICAL APPROACH

INTRODUCTION

Echocardiographic evaluation of the patient with valvular regurgitation includes assessment of valve anatomy, the severity of regurgitation, chamber dilation due to the imposed volume overload, ventricular function, and the degree of pulmonary hypertension. In some clinical situations, the clinical significance of valvular regurgitation is related to the *presence* of abnormal regurgitation, regardless of severity. For example, detection of aortic regurgitation in a patient with chest pain and an enlarged aortic root heightens the suspicion of aortic dissection. Detection of regurgitation also may be important in terms of endocarditis risk and the need for prophylactic antibiotics in patients with a cardiac murmur. In other situations, e.g., endocarditis with acute mitral regurgitation, the *severity* of regurgitation is a key factor in clinical decision making regarding surgical intervention. In contrast, in chronic mitral regurgitation due to myxomatous valve disease, the *response of the left ventricle to chronic volume overload*, not regurgitant severity per se, is the most important factor in deciding on the timing of valve surgery.

BASIC PRINCIPLES

Etiology of Valvular Regurgitation

Valvular regurgitation may be due to congenital or acquired abnormalities of the valve leaflets or to abnormalities of the associated supporting structures. For example, aortic root dilation can result in aortic regurgitation even with anatomically normal valve leaflets. Similarly, left ventricular dilation can result in mitral regurgitation even with an otherwise normal valve apparatus. Echocardiographic examinations allow defini-

tion of the etiology of valvular regurgitation in most cases. Even when a single definite etiology is not evident, the differential diagnosis of the etiology of regurgitation often can be narrowed to the few most likely possibilities. The examination also may provide clues as to whether regurgitation is acute or chronic in duration.

Fluid Dynamics of Valvular Regurgitation (Table 10–1)

The fluid dynamics of a regurgitant valve are, in many ways, similar to the fluid dynamics of a stenotic valve, as described in Chapter 9 (Fig. 10–1). The regurgitant valve can be thought of as having a regurgitant orifice, which is characterized physiologically, in simple terms, by a high-velocity laminar jet even though the anatomy of the regurgitant orifice may be quite complex. The instantaneous velocity in this jet (v) is related to the instantaneous pressure difference (ΔP) across the valve, as stated in the simplified Bernoulli equation: $\Delta P = 4v^2$. Recording this high-velocity jet with continuous-wave Doppler allows assessment of the time course of the pressure difference between the two chambers on either side of the valve.

On the upstream side of the regurgitant valve, flow acceleration proximal to the regurgitant orifice is present, and a proximal isovelocity surface area (PISA) can be defined similar to that seen on the left atrial side of the stenotic mitral valve. This observation provides an alternate method for quantitative evaluation of regurgitant stroke volume.

As the high-velocity jet enters the chamber receiving the regurgitant flow, the flow pattern becomes disturbed with nonlaminar flow, multiple blood flow velocities, and multiple blood flow directions. Evaluation of the spatial extent of the flow disturbance (often called the *jet*) in the

TABLE 10–1. RELATIONSHIP BETWEEN FLUID DYNAMICS OF VALVULAR REGURGITATION AND DIAGNOSTIC APPROACH

FLUID DYNAMIC CHARACTERISTIC	DIAGNOSTIC APPROACH
High-velocity jet in regurgitant orifice	Pressure/velocity relationship of continuous-wave Doppler curve
Proximal acceleration	Proximal isovelocity surface area
Flow disturbance in chamber receiving regurgitant flow	Flow mapping
Increased volume flow across valve	Increased antegrade velocity, volume flow at two sites
Conservation of momentum	Regurgitant orifice area, momentum calculations

Valvular Regurgitation

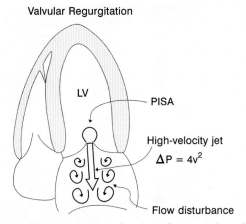

Figure 10–1. Schematic drawing of a regurgitant jet showing the proximal isovelocity surface area (PISA), the jet through the regurgitant orifice, and the flow disturbance in the receiving chamber.

receiving chamber provides a semiquantitative measure of regurgitant severity (see below).

The fluid dynamics of the regurgitant flow disturbance are complex and not fully understood. However, several generalizations are possible (Table 10–2). The shape and direction of the regurgitant jet depend on multiple factors, including the anatomy and orientation of the regurgitation orifice, the driving force across the valve, and the size and compliance of the receiving chamber. Jets are "pulled" toward adjacent walls (e.g., mitral regurgitation in the left atrium) if within a critical distance from the wall at the entry site and also are "pulled" toward

---

TABLE 10–2. FACTORS THAT AFFECT REGURGITANT JET SIZE AND SHAPE

Physiologic

Regurgitant volume

Driving pressure

Size and shape of regurgitant orifice

Receiving chamber constraint

Wall impingement

Timing relative to the cardiac cycle

Influence of coexisting jets or flowstreams

Technical

Ultrasound system gain, pulse repetition frequency, transducer frequency, frame rate

Image plane, depth, signal strength

---

other flowstreams (e.g., aortic regurgitation and mitral stenosis). Jets that adhere to the wall of the chamber will have a smaller cross-sectional area on tomographic color flow imaging (and a smaller three-dimensional volume) since entrainment of additional fluid elements into the jet occurs on only one side, instead of on all sides, as with a central jet.

Another approach to quantitation of valvular regurgitation is calculation of the total momentum in the regurgitant jet. *Momentum*, defined as volume flow times velocity, remains constant in any closed fluid system. Thus the total momentum of the regurgitant jet must equal the initial momentum across the narrowed orifice based on the law of conservation of momentum. This observation may prove to be useful in developing new methods for quantitation of regurgitant severity (see below).

Volume Overload

Chronic valvular regurgitation results in progressive volume overload of the ventricle. Volume overload of the left ventricle results in chamber dilation with normal wall thickness so that total left ventricular mass is increased (eccentric hypertrophy). An important clinical feature of chronic left ventricular volume overload is that an irreversible decrease in systolic function can occur in the absence of symptoms. In fact, an irreversible decrease in contractility can occur despite a normal ejection fraction due to the altered loading conditions of the ventricle when regurgitation is present.

In patients with regurgitant valves, the term *total stroke volume* refers to the total volume of blood pumped by the ventricle on each beat. *Forward stroke volume* is the amount of blood delivered to the peripheral circulation, and *regurgitant volume* is the amount of backflow across the abnormal valve (Fig. 10–2).

Detection of Valvular Regurgitation

Valvular regurgitation can be detected with either conventional pulsed Doppler, color flow imaging, or continuous-wave Doppler ultrasound. While two-dimensional (2D) imaging provides detailed information about valve anatomy and chamber dilation and function, it provides only indirect evidence for the presence or absence of valvular incompetence. The finding of an anatomically abnormal mitral valve in the presence of left atrial and left ventricular dilation

Mitral Regurgitation

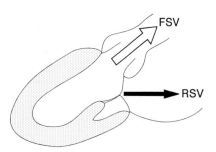

Total SV = Forward SV + Regurgitant SV

Figure 10–2. When mitral regurgitation is present, total stroke volume is the sum of the regurgitant (RSV) and forward stroke volumes (FSV).

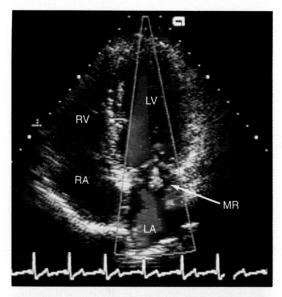

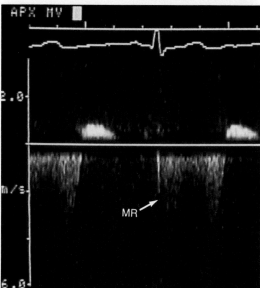

Figure 10–3. Example of "physiologic" mitral regurgitation recorded with pulsed (*above*) and continuous-wave (*below*) Doppler in a normal individual. Note the low signal strength compared with antegrade flow and the incomplete systolic signal.

suggests that mitral regurgitation may be present, but Doppler examination is necessary for direct confirmation or exclusion of the diagnosis. Although a few M-mode findings have been shown to be specific for diagnosing valvular regurgitation (e.g., high-frequency fluttering of the anterior mitral leaflet in aortic regurgitation), these findings are not sensitive enough to reliably exclude regurgitation when suspected on clinical grounds.

With conventional pulsed Doppler ultrasound, detection of regurgitation is based on identification of the flow disturbance on the upstream side of the valve. A small sample volume is placed on the immediate upstream side of the closed valve; the flow disturbance is identified both audibly and on the spectral display. Care is needed to ensure that the sample volume is correctly positioned (e.g., on the left ventricular side of the aortic valve in *diastole* and on the left atrial side of the mitral valve in *systole*), since considerable motion of the valve planes occurs during the cardiac cycle. Mild regurgitation may not extend throughout systole (for atrioventricular valve regurgitation) or diastole (for semilunar valve regurgitation) (Fig. 10–3).

When the examination is performed correctly, pulsed Doppler ultrasound is extremely sensitive (nearly 100 percent) and specific (nearly 100 percent) for diagnosing valvular regurgitation as compared with angiography. In fact, Doppler ultrasound is so sensitive that regurgitation often is detected that is not audible by auscultation. These cases most often are true positives, as evidenced by angiographic confirmation. False-positive results can occur with pulsed Doppler when the origin of the flow signal is mistaken. For example, if the sample volume inadvertently is on the left ventricular side of the mitral valve

in systole, normal left ventricular outflow may be mistaken for mitral regurgitation. False-negative results occur when signal strength is poor due to poor acoustic access or attenuation due to the depth of interrogation. False-negative results also occur if the examiner fails to interrogate the valve in multiple tomographic views, thereby missing a localized or eccentric regurgitant signal.

Color flow imaging similarly has a high sensitivity (88 percent) and specificity (100 percent) for detection of valvular regurgitation when instrument settings and examination technique are optimal. False-negative results again occur if signal strength is poor, if multiple image planes are not utilized, or if color flow processing parameters are set incorrectly.

Continuous-wave Doppler detection of valvular regurgitation is based on identification of the high-velocity jet through the regurgitant orifice. An advantage of continuous-wave Doppler is that beam width is broad at the level of the valves when interrogated from an apical approach. Identification of the regurgitant signal utilizes the velocity, shape, timing, and associated antegrade flow signal to correctly identify the origin of the signal.

Valvular Regurgitation in Normal Individuals

Given the high sensitivity of Doppler ultrasound for detection of regurgitation, it has become apparent that a small degree of regurgitation is present in a high percentage of otherwise normal individuals. Typically, regurgitation detected in otherwise normal individuals is spatially restricted to the area immediately adjacent to valve closure, may be short in duration, and represents only a small regurgitant volume (see Fig. 10–3). When meticulously searched for, mitral regurgitation can be detected in 70 to 80 percent, tricuspid regurgitation in 80 to 90 percent, and pulmonic regurgitation in 70 to 80 percent of normal individuals. Thus a small degree of regurgitation of these three valves is normal and appears to have no adverse clinical implications. Aortic regurgitation is found in only a small percentage (5 percent) of individuals with an otherwise normal echocardiographic study and may be important in terms of endocarditis risk.

Approaches to Evaluation of the Severity of Regurgitation
(Table 10–3)

Doppler Flow Mapping

Semiquantitative evaluation of regurgitant severity is extremely useful in patient management. Often the clinical question is whether only mild regurgitation or hemodynamically significant regurgitation is present. In these settings, precise quantitation of the severity of regurgitation is unnecessary.

TABLE 10–3. APPROACHES TO EVALUATION OF REGURGITATION SEVERITY

Semiquantitative

Flow mapping (pulsed or color)

Continuous-wave Doppler signal intensity

Distal flow reversals

Quantitative

Volume flow at two sites

Descending aortic flow reversal

Proximal isovelocity surface area

Jet momentum

Flow *mapping* is evaluation of the extent of the flow disturbance in the chamber receiving the regurgitant jet either with conventional pulsed Doppler or color flow imaging. With conventional pulsed Doppler, a small sample volume is sequentially moved across the chamber, beginning at the valve plane and moving progressively more distally. At each site, it is noted whether an abnormal flow signal with appropriate timing (i.e., systole for mitral regurgitation, diastole for aortic regurgitation) is present or absent. The examiner then builds a mental 2D image of the extent of the flow disturbance in that tomographic plane. By integrating data from multiple tomographic planes, the three-dimensional (3D) size and shape of the regurgitant jet can be estimated. Multiple image planes allow detection and correct interpretation of the extent of eccentric jets which may not be recorded in each image plane.

The overall 3D extent of the regurgitant jet then is described on a 0 to 4+ scale, where 1+ is mild regurgitation (a small jet), 2 to 3+ is moderate regurgitation, and 4+ is severe regurgitation (a jet that nearly fills the receiving chamber) (Figs. 10–4 and 10–5).

Flow mapping depends on the timing and location of the Doppler signals and *not* absolute blood flow velocity. Thus flow mapping can be performed from windows where the intercept angle between the ultrasound beam and the direction of regurgitant flow is nonparallel. In fact, these windows may allow a shorter distance from the transducer to the flow region of interest, resulting in a better signal-to-noise ratio. For example, aortic regurgitation often is evaluated from parasternal long- and short-axis views.

Flow Mapping for AR

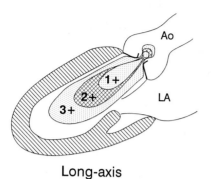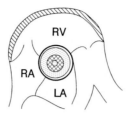

Long-axis

Short-axis just below aortic valve

Figure 10–4. Semiquantitation of aortic regurgitant severity using color flow mapping in parasternal long- and short-axis views. The depicted jet areas are only rough guides. In the clinical setting, multiple views are utilized, and jets often are eccentric in direction and asymmetrical in shape.

Although the long-axis view of the aortic regurgitant jet is nearly perpendicular to the ultrasound beam, multiple flow directions within the jet allow detection of the diastolic flow disturbance with this Doppler technique. It is the location and timing of the velocity signal and not the absolute velocity that are of interest in this application of Doppler ultrasound. Of course, an accurate blood velocity determination cannot be made both because of the nonparallel intercept angle and because the velocity exceeds the Nyquist limit of the pulsed Doppler mode.

Color flow imaging can be utilized for flow mapping, based on the same approach described for conventional pulsed Doppler, with the advantages that Doppler velocity signals across a tomographic plane can be sampled simultaneously and the visual format is easily understood by referring physicians. Since color flow imaging basically is pulsed Doppler ultrasound with somewhat different signal processing and display formats, it is important to remember that signal aliasing still occurs. Again, the use of

multiple tomographic image planes and acoustic windows is essential for appropriate evaluation of regurgitant jets. The appearance of a regurgitant jet with color flow imaging will vary depending on the ultrasound system, transducer frequency, and specific instrument settings. Correct visual interpretation depends on experience with a particular instrument and knowledge of the influence of instrument settings on the visual display. On most systems, a "variance" color scale results in a green regurgitant signal superimposed on the normal red-blue flow patterns. A "velocity" scale results in a mosaic of red, blue, and white pixels in the regurgitant jet. Since the goal of this application is to identify the location and timing of abnormal flow signals in a tomographic format, the exact color scale used is not particularly important so long as it displays the boundaries of the flow disturbance accurately.

With either a variance or a velocity color flow scale, it is obvious that an abnormal color pattern is not synonymous with abnormal flow

Flow Mapping for MR

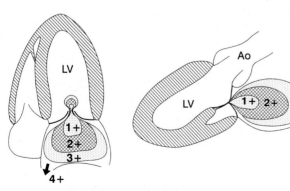

Apical 4-chamber   **Parasternal long-axis**

Figure 10–5. Mitral regurgitation semiquantitative flow mapping. Again, multiple views are used during the examination, and jet geometry is considered in conjunction with jet area in grading the degree of regurgitation. Severe (4+) mitral regurgitation is associated with systolic flow reversal in the pulmonary veins.

given the physics of pulsed Doppler color flow imaging. An abnormal color pattern can be seen even with normal intracardiac flow patterns. For example, the normal antegrade flow velocity of laminar flow across the aortic valve exceeds the Nyquist limit, resulting in aliasing and an "abnormal" color pattern. Conversely, abnormal flow signals may not demonstrate variance or a mosaic pattern if the flow velocities are within the Nyquist limit for that interrogation depth. For example, the low velocities seen in pulmonic regurgitation result in a uniform color display even though the flow pattern is abnormal. Most physicians choose a color scale that highlights the potential abnormalities most clearly. Caution in interpretation of the color flow display is needed whichever display mode is chosen.

Evaluation of the exact timing of a flow signal in relation both to valve closing and to the QRS complex can be helpful in correct identification of the signal. With conventional pulsed Doppler, the spectral output of velocity versus time provides high temporal resolution. The mitral regurgitant signal, for example, can be distinguished from the immediately adjacent aortic outflow signal based on its timing: Mitral regurgitation starts with mitral valve closure, while aortic outflow starts slightly later, after isovolumic contraction (Fig. 10–6). Even if the aortic outflow signal appears to originate spatially from a sample volume positioned in the left atrium due to beam width artifact, the timing of the signal allows correct identification. With 2D color flow imaging, temporal resolution is sacrificed for spatial resolution so that a Doppler sampling

rate of only 15 to 30 frames per second is achieved. If the signal origin is unclear, use of 2D guided color "M-mode" may be helpful by providing higher time resolution. The color Doppler signal is displayed at each depth along a single line of interrogation (y axis) versus time (x axis) at a higher sampling rate (Fig. 10–7).

Continuous-Wave Doppler Approach

Several types of information regarding the severity of valvular regurgitation can be derived from the spectral display of the continuous-wave Doppler signal. First, signal intensity is proportional to the number of blood cells contributing to the regurgitant signal. Since the ultrasound beam is relatively broad and signals from the entire length of the beam are recorded, much of the regurgitant jet can be encompassed in the beam with appropriate adjustment of beam direction. It is particularly helpful to compare the intensity

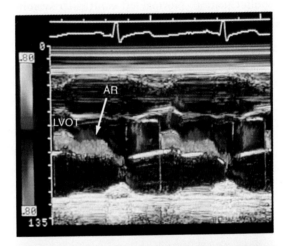

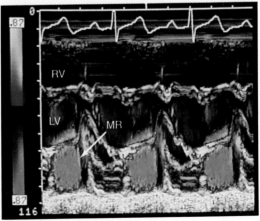

Figure 10–7. Color M-mode of aortic (*above*) and mitral (*below*) regurgitation shows the high time resolution of this approach.

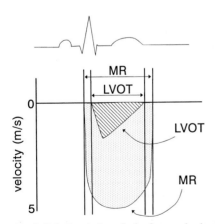

Figure 10–6. Relative timing of mitral regurgitation (MR) and left ventricular outflow tract (LVOT) flow signal. Mitral regurgitation extends from the onset of isovolumic contraction to the end of isovolumic relaxation. Left ventricular outflow is shorter in duration, occurring only during ejection.

of the regurgitant signal to antegrade flow across the same valve as a qualitative estimate of regurgitant severity. A weak signal reflects mild regurgitation, whereas a signal nearly equal in intensity to antegrade flow reflects severe regurgitation. Moderate regurgitation has an intermediate signal strength.

Second, the associated antegrade velocity across the regurgitant valve provides useful information. Regurgitation results in an increase in the antegrade volume flow rate across the valve which is reflected in an increase in the antegrade velocity across the valve. The greater the severity of regurgitation, the higher is the antegrade velocity. Of course, the possibility of coexisting valvular stenosis also must be considered.

Third, the shape of the velocity curve depends on the time-varying pressure gradient across the regurgitant valve. Each instantaneous velocity is related to the instantaneous pressure gradient across the valve, as stated in the Bernoulli equation. Normal left ventricular systolic pressure is 100 to 150 mmHg and normal left atrial pressure is 5 to 15 mmHg, so the left ventricular to left atrial pressure difference in systole is 85 to 145 mmHg. Thus the mitral regurgitant velocity curve typically shows a maximum velocity of 5 to 6 m/s. When ventricular function is normal, there is rapid acceleration to peak velocity, with a maintained high-velocity in systole and with rapid deceleration prior to diastolic opening of the mitral valve. An increase in end-systolic left atrial pressure (a *v* wave) results in a decline in the instantaneous pressure gradient and in the instantaneous velocity (Fig. 10–8). Similarly, the shape of the aortic regurgitant velocity curve depends on the time course of the diastolic pressure difference across the aortic valve. When left ventricular end-diastolic pressure is low and aortic end-diastolic pressure is normal or mildly reduced, a large pressure difference (and high velocity) across the valve is present throughout diastole with a slow rate of pressure decline (Fig. 10–9). Acute regurgitation results in more rapid equalization of left ventricular and aortic pressures with a more rapid velocity decline in diastole.

Upstream Flow Reversal

When atrioventricular valve regurgitation is severe enough that a significant volume of blood

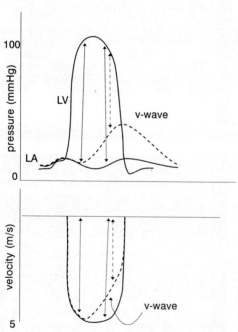

Figure 10–8. Left ventricular (LV) and left atrial (LA) pressures and the Doppler velocity curve in chronic (*solid lines*) and acute (*dashed lines*) mitral regurgitation are shown. Note that the shape of the velocity curve reflects the shape of the pressure difference between the left ventricle and the left atrium so that a late-systolic rise in left atrial pressure (*v* wave) is seen as a more rapid decrease in velocity in late systole on the Doppler curve.

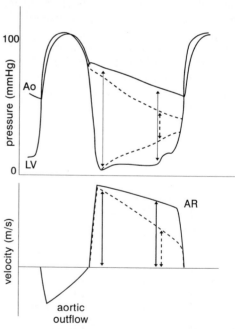

Figure 10–9. Left ventricular (LV) and central aortic (Ao) pressures and the corresponding Doppler velocity curve are shown for chronic (*solid lines*) and acute (*dashed lines*) aortic regurgitation. Again, the shape of the velocity curve is related to the instantaneous pressure differences across the valve, as stated in the Bernoulli equation. With acute aortic regurgitation, aortic pressure falls more rapidly and ventricular diastolic pressure rises more rapidly, resulting in a steeper deceleration slope on the Doppler curve.

is displaced by the regurgitant jet, flow reversal is seen in the veins entering the atrium. With severe tricuspid regurgitation, the normal pattern of systolic inflow into the right atrium from the superior and inferior vena cava is reversed. This can be demonstrated with a pulsed Doppler sample volume positioned in the central hepatic vein (Fig. 10–10). Severe mitral regurgita-

tion results in reversal of the normal patterns of systolic inflow into the left atrium from the pulmonary veins. This may be difficult to demonstrate on a transthoracic study due to signal attenuation at the depth of the pulmonary vein but is easily recorded from a transesophageal approach (Fig. 10–11).

Regurgitation of a semilunar valve results in reversal of flow in the associated great vessel as blood flows from the great vessel, across the incompetent valve, and into the ventricle. The distance from the valve plane that this flow reversal extends in the great vessel is proportional to regurgitant volume.

Volume Flow at Two Intracardiac Sites

Regurgitant stroke volume can be calculated from the difference between total and forward stroke volume. Total stroke volume is calculated from antegrade flow across the regurgitant valve as the cross-sectional area of flow times the velocity-time integral of transvalvular flow (see discussion of stroke volume calculation in Chap. 4). Forward stroke volume is calculated as antegrade flow across a different (and nonregurgitant) valve (Fig. 10–12).

For example, with aortic regurgitation, transaortic stroke volume (SV) represents total left

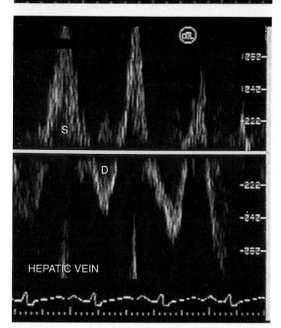

Figure 10–10. With the sample volume (SV) positioned in the central hepatic vein from a subcostal approach, systolic (S) flow reversal in the hepatic vein Doppler velocity curve is seen when severe tricuspid regurgitation is present. Forward flow into the right atrium in diastole (D) also is seen.

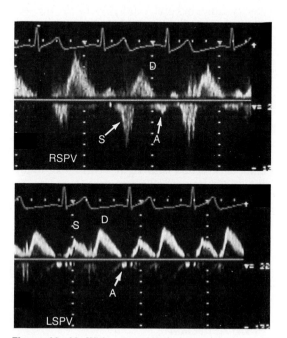

Figure 10–11. With severe mitral regurgitation, systolic flow reversal in the right superior pulmonary vein Doppler velocity curve (*above*) and blunting of systolic flow in the left superior pulmonary vein (*below*) are seen on transesophageal imaging in a patient with an eccentric, anteromedially directed regurgitant jet. D = diastolic flow, A = atrial reversal.

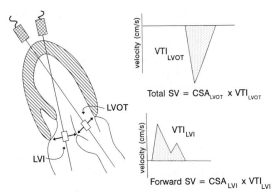

Total SV = CSA$_{LVOT}$ × VTI$_{LVOT}$

Forward SV = CSA$_{LVI}$ × VTI$_{LVI}$

Regurg. SV = Total SV - Forward SV

Figure 10–12. Calculation of aortic regurgitant stroke volume (SV) by measurement of transvalvular volume flow rate at two intracardiac sites is illustrated. Transaortic flow, representing total stroke volume, is calculated from the cross-sectional area (CSA) and velocity-time integral (VTI) of the left ventricular outflow tract (LVOT). Transmitral flow, representing forward stroke volume, is calculated from the cross-sectional area and velocity-time integral of left ventricular inflow (LVI) across the mitral annulus. Regurgitant stroke volume is the difference between total and forward stroke volume.

ventricular stroke volume and can be calculated as:

$$SV_{total} = CSA_{LVOT} \times VTI_{LVOT} \quad (10.1)$$

where CSA is cross-sectional area, VTI is the velocity-time integral, and LVOT is the left ventricular outflow tract. Forward stroke volume is represented by left ventricular inflow across the mitral valve, since the amount of blood filling the ventricle equals the amount of blood delivered to the body on each beat, and can be calculated as:

$$SV_{forward} = CSA_{LVI} \times VTI_{LVI} \quad (10.2)$$

With aortic regurgitation, alternate sites for measurement of forward stroke volume are the pulmonary artery and right ventricular inflow region. Then, regurgitant stroke volume is:

$$SV_{regurgitant} = SV_{total} - SV_{forward} \quad \begin{array}{l} \text{Regurgitant stroke volume} \quad (10.3) \end{array}$$

and regurgitant fraction (RF) is:

$$RF = \frac{SV_{regurgitant}}{SV_{total}} \quad \begin{array}{l} \text{Regurgitant} \\ \text{fraction} \end{array} \quad (10.4)$$

Proximal Isovelocity Surface Area (PISA) Approach

Another approach for determining regurgitant stroke volume is to examine the flow pattern on the upstream side of the valve (proximal to the regurgitant orifice). Acceleration of flow occurs

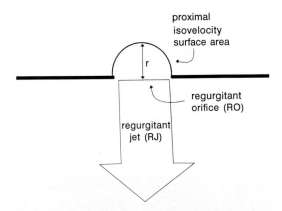

regurg. volume = PISA × velocity

RO area= regurg. volume/VTI$_{RJ}$

Figure 10–13. Proximal to a regurgitant orifice, flow accelerates resulting in concentric proximal isovelocity surface areas (PISAs). The color Doppler aliasing velocity allows identification of one of these PISAs, which then can be used to calculate the regurgitant volume based on the aliasing velocity. The radius (r) is used to calculate the PISA. In combination with the velocity-time integral (VTI) of the continuous-wave Doppler recording of the regurgitant jet (RJ), regurgitant orifice area (RO) can be calculated.

proximal to the valve plane with, conceptually, a series of isovelocity "surfaces" leading to the high-velocity jet in the regurgitant orifice. Immediately adjacent to the orifice, these surfaces are small with high-velocity flow; at increasing distances from the orifice, areas are larger and velocities are lower. Based on the principle of volume flow calculation by Doppler techniques, the volume flow rate (in this case, regurgitant flow) for any of these surfaces, when averaged over the temporal flow period, is (Fig. 10–13):

$$Regurgitant\ volume = PISA \times velocity \quad (10.5)$$

The velocity for a PISA can be determined from the color flow image as the aliasing velocity—where a distinct red-blue interface is seen (Fig. 10–14). At this interface, the velocity is known, being equivalent to the Nyquist limit on the velocity color scale. The size of the PISA can be maximized to allow more accurate regurgitant flow rate calculations by decreasing the velocity range and shifting the velocity baseline.

The shape of the isovelocity surface proximal to a regurgitant valve tends to be hemispherical with a tendency toward a hemielliptical shape closer to the orifice (Fig. 10–14). Assuming a hemispherical shape, the PISA is calculated from measurements of the distance from the aliasing velocity to the regurgitant orifice as:

$$PISA = 2\pi r^2 \quad (10.6)$$

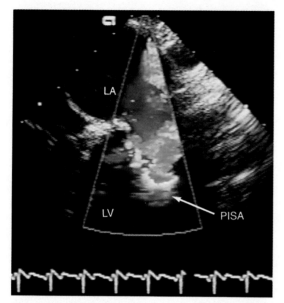

Figure 10–14. Color flow image of a proximal isovelocity surface area in mitral regurgitation seen on transesophageal imaging. The aliasing velocity is 61 cm/s.

Note that the PISA method for calculating regurgitant volume is analogous to calculation of stroke volume proximal to a stenotic valve. The differences between these approaches are (1) the differing shapes of the proximal velocity stream lines, (2) the use of color flow, rather than pulsed Doppler, to measure velocity at a given location, and (3) the need for temporal averaging when color data from single images are used.

The PISA method can be combined with the velocity-time integral of continuous-wave Doppler recording through the regurgitant orifice VTI_{RO} to calculate regurgitant orifice area based on the principle of conservation of mass (the continuity equation). Since the regurgitant volume (RV) proximal to and *in* the regurgitant orifice are equal,

$$RV = ROA \times VTI_{RO} \qquad (10.8)$$

or

$$ROA = \frac{RV}{VTI_{RO}} \qquad (10.9)$$

Of course, other methods for measuring regurgitant stroke volume can be substituted in this equation.

Jet Momentum

Yet another approach to quantification of the severity of valvular regurgitation is based on the principle of conservation of momentum. Momentum is defined as the product of volume flow rate (Q) and velocity (v):

$$Momentum = Q \times v \qquad (10.10)$$

At any cross-sectional plane perpendicular to a regurgitant jet, momentum is equal to any other plane perpendicular to the jet (including at the orifice). In simple terms, this means that as the volume of the jet increases distal to the regurgitant valve, velocity decreases accordingly.

Since volume flow rate equals cross-sectional area times velocity,

$$Q = area \times v \qquad (10.11)$$

substituting Eq. (10.11) for Q in Eq. (10.10) yields:

$$Momentum = area \times v^2 \qquad (10.12)$$

Thus momentum can be calculated in the regurgitant orifice from regurgitant orifice area (using Eq. 10.9) and the continuous-wave (CW) Doppler signal of jet velocity. Alternatively, momentum can be calculated from measurement of the color flow jet cross-sectional area and velocity measured with pulsed Doppler (PD) at any plane perpendicular to the long axis of the jet.

If regurgitant orifice area is unknown, it can be calculated from determinations of momentum in the jet distal to the orifice plus the continuous-wave Doppler signal, since:

$$Momentum_{orifice} = momentum_{jet} \qquad (10.13)$$

Using Eq. (10.12),

$$ROA \times V^2_{CW} = area\ of\ jet \times V^2_{PD} \qquad (10.14)$$

so

$$ROA = (area\ of\ jet \times V^2_{PD})/V^2_{CW} \qquad (10.15)$$

Several investigators have hypothesized that jet momentum and regurgitant orifice area may be useful descriptors of regurgitant severity and have shown that color regurgitant jet areas correlate well with momentum or regurgitant orifice area. While promising research tools, these methods are tedious and prone to error in the clinical setting and as yet have not gained wide acceptance.

Alternate Approaches/ Technical Considerations

Etiology of Valve Disease

If transthoracic images are suboptimal or nondiagnostic for evaluation of aortic or mitral valve anatomy and the etiology of regurgitation, transesophageal imaging may be helpful. With aortic root disease, visualization of the ascending aorta may be suboptimal on transthoracic imaging, so transesophageal echocardiography, gated computed tomographic scanning, magnetic resonance imaging, or aortography may be needed to fully define the extent and severity of disease.

Left Ventricular Size and Systolic Function

While serial echocardiographic evaluation of left ventricular size in chronic aortic or mitral regurgitation has become a standard method of clinical evaluation, two factors potentially limit the reliability of this approach. First, suboptimal image quality or recording techniques may result in erroneous measurements. Care is needed to ensure that the dimensions are measured perpendicular to the long and short axes of the left ventricle, and instrument settings must be adjusted for optimal endocardial definition.

Second, the reproducibility of left ventricular measurements must be considered. Overall reproducibility includes variation in *recording* the data, variation in *measuring* the data, and *physiologic* variation (such as heart rate and loading conditions) that may affect the measurement. Reproducibility of 2D guided M-mode measurements of the left ventricle suggests that an interval change of >8 mm in end-systolic or end-diastolic dimensions represents a definite clinical change.

Similar concerns apply to serial qualitative or quantitative evaluations of left ventricular systolic function. While accurate when carefully performed, image orientation and endocardial definition must be carefully optimized, and endocardial border tracing must be performed by an experienced individual. Alternate methods for evaluation of left ventricular size and systolic function include radionuclide or angiographic ventriculography.

Regurgitant Severity

Doppler evaluation of valvular regurgitant severity has become a standard clinical tool; however, there are numerous potential pitfalls and limitations of this method. Doppler flow mapping provides only a semiquantitative estimate of regurgitant severity. Attempts to refine this approach by measurement of jet area or even 3D jet volume are fraught with difficulty due to the complex fluid dynamics of valvular regurgitation. First, the size and shape of the regurgitant jet depend not only on regurgitant volume but also on regurgitant orifice shape and orientation, the shape and compliance of the receiving chamber, entrainment into the jet of static blood within the receiving chamber, deflection of the jet toward adjacent walls, and confluence with other flowstreams within the chamber (e.g., left ventricular inflow and aortic regurgitation). Second, the size and shape of the jet vary temporally during the cardiac cycle. Third, transducer frequency, depth of interrogation, instrument settings, and recording parameters all affect the appearance of the regurgitant jet on color flow images.

The utility of the continuous-wave Doppler curve depends, in large part, on technical factors in data recording as well as on correct data interpretation. The high-velocity regurgitant signal is optimized when the high-pass ("wall") filter is set at the maximum level, and the gain and velocity scale are adjusted to show the peak velocities clearly. Accurate pressure gradient calculations assume a near-parallel intercept angle between the direction of the ultrasound beam and the regurgitant jet, thus requiring examination from multiple acoustic windows with careful transducer angulation to obtain this parallel alignment. Use of a dedicated, small, continuous-wave transducer often facilitates the examination and provides a better signal-to-noise ratio than 2D guided continuous-wave Doppler. In addition, the 2D image may distract the examiner from searching for the highest-velocity signal. Color flow imaging is of limited value for locating the best continuous-wave signal because it provides only 2D information; jet direction in the elevational plane remains unknown. Temporal factors also affect data quality, and caution is needed in interpreting the shape of the velocity curve if jet direction (and thus Doppler-jet intercept angle) varies during the regurgitant flow period.

Again, the continuous-wave Doppler signal provides only a semiquantitative evaluation of stenosis severity. Signal intensity is judged subjectively and may underestimate regurgitant severity if ultrasound tissue penetration is suboptimal. Attempts to quantitate regurgitant severity based on the diastolic slope of the velocity curve have been frustrated by the numerous other physiologic abnormalities that affect this measurement (see below).

Calculation of regurgitant volume and regurgitant fraction from volume flow at two intracardiac sites has been shown to be accurate in animal models and in selected patient series. However, wide clinical application of this technique has been limited by the difficulty of measuring 2D diameters accurately, particularly from acoustic windows where the structure of interest is not perpendicular to the ultrasound beam. Small errors in diameter measurement lead to large errors in cross-sectional area calculations due to the quadratic relationship between the two ($CSA = \pi r^2$). Other potential pitfalls in volume flow measurement are discussed in detail in Chapter 4. This method clearly can provide accurate quantitation of regurgitant severity when image quality is excellent; in other cases, it is helpful to evaluate the ratio of velocity-time integrals (or peak velocities) across the regurgitant valve to that across a competent valve as an indicator of their relative stroke volumes.

Perhaps the most important problem with quantitation of regurgitant severity is the failure of *any* measure (Doppler or angiographic) to provide specific prognostic data or data that affect clinical decision making. Once a diagnosis of "hemodynamically significant" regurgitation is confirmed, it is the patient's symptoms and the left ventricular response to chronic volume overload that dictate medical therapy and the timing of surgical intervention rather than regurgitant severity per se. Given this situation, current Doppler methods remain valuable diagnostic tools mainly because they allow differentiation of mild, moderate, and severe aortic regurgitation. The diagnostic value of the echocardiographic study is increased when the interpretation integrates data from several potential measures of regurgitant severity into a summary statement. Rather than being redundant, the different approaches to regurgitant severity serve as cross-checks on each other. Errors or limitations of one approach will be recognized when other approaches, with better data quality, show discrepant results (Table 10–4). When echocardiographic data are suboptimal, other approaches, such as contrast angiography, should be considered (see Fig. 10–17).

AORTIC REGURGITATION

Diagnostic Imaging of the Valve Apparatus

Aortic regurgitation may be due either to abnormalities of the aortic root or to abnormalities of the leaflets themselves (Table 10–5). The disease processes that cause valvular aortic stenosis (*congenital bicuspid valve, calcific valve disease,* and *rheumatic disease*) also can result in aortic regurgitation due to alterations in leaflet flexibility or shape leading to inadequate diastolic coaptation of the leaflets. The 2D echocardiographic findings for these diagnoses are discussed in Chapter 9.

Other diseases that cause aortic regurgitation include *myxomatous valve disease,* which can affect the aortic valve as well as the mitral valve. The leaflets are thickened and redundant on 2D echocardiography with slight sagging of the leaflets into the left ventricular outflow tract in diastole (Fig. 10–15). The normal hemicylindrical configuration of each leaflet in diastole is distorted so that the short-axis view intersects the center of the leaflet *en face,* resulting in the false appearance of an ill-defined echogenic "mass."

Endocarditis results in aortic regurgitation either by leaflet perforation by the infectious process or by deformity of diastolic leaflet closure due to the presence of a valvular vegetation. Less common abnormalities of the aortic valve leaflets leading to aortic regurgitation include congenital leaflet fenestrations, involvement by nonbacterial thrombotic endocarditis (Libman-Sachs vegetations in systemic lupus erythematosus), infiltrative diseases (e.g., amyloid), and collagen-vascular disorders, mucopolysaccharidosis, or glycogen storage diseases.

Abnormalities of the aortic root can result in aortic regurgitation, even when the leaflets them-

TABLE 10–4. COMPARISON OF INFORMATION DERIVED AT CATHETERIZATION VERSUS ECHOCARDIOGRAPHY IN VALVULAR REGURGITATION

	CATHETERIZATION	ECHOCARDIOGRAPHY
Semiquantitative severity index	Angiographic (0–4+)	Flow mapping (0–4+)
Quantitative regurgitant stroke volume	Forward versus total stroke volume	Volume flow at two sites
Hemodynamics	Direct pressure measurement	Shape of continuous-wave Doppler curve
Left ventricular size and systolic function	Left ventricular angiography	2D echo

TABLE 10-5. ETIOLOGY OF AORTIC REGURGITATION (EXAMPLES)

Leaflet Abnormalities

Congenital bicuspid valve

Calcific valve disease

Rheumatic valve disease

Myxomatous valve disease

Endocarditis

Nonbacterial thrombotic endocarditis

Aortic Root Abnormalities

Hypertensive aortic root dilation

Cystic medial necrosis

Marfan's syndrome

Aortic dissection

selves are normal, by alterations in the geometry of the structures supporting the leaflets. The aortic annulus is not a discrete planar ring of fibrous tissue but rather a complex crown-shaped structure where the leaflets attach to the aortic valve with the three "points" of the crown at the commissures and the three lowest points at the midsection of each leaflet. Dilation of this area at the base of the aortic root—often termed *annular dilation*—results in aortic regurgitation due to inadequate coaptation of the stretched leaf-

lets. Note that adjacent leaflets normally overlap (apposition zone) so that mild degrees of annular dilation may not result in valvular incompetence. Annular dilation may be due to a variety of causes, including chronic *hypertension, cystic medial necrosis,* or *Marfan's syndrome.* Marfan's syndrome is characterized by effacement of the normal sinotubular junction with dilation of the annulus and sinuses of Valsalva (see Chap. 14). In cystic medial necrosis, the sinotubular junction usually is identifiable, although dilation may involve the base of the root as well as the ascending aorta. Many other diseases cause aortic root dilation, with consequent aortic regurgitation, including rheumatoid arthritis, Reiter's syndrome, syphilitic aortitis, and mycotic aneurysm.

Aortic dissection can result in aortic regurgitation either by annular dilation resulting in inadequate coaptation or by the false channel of the dissection undermining the aortic annulus and resulting in a flail leaflet (see Chap. 14). Aortic regurgitation due to syphilitic aortitis is rare in the United States. When present, it typically is characterized by extensive calcification of the dilated aortic root.

The *differential diagnosis* for the echocardiographer in evaluation of a patient referred for suspected aortic regurgitation depends on the specific indications for the examination. If a diastolic murmur has been noted on auscultation, different diagnoses include pulmonic regurgitation, mitral or tricuspid stenosis, and (rarely) a coronary arteriovenous fistula. In some cases, only the diastolic portion of a continuous murmur (e.g., a patent ductus arteriosus) may have been appreciated. If aortic regurgitation is suspected because of a concern for aortic dissection, the differential diagnosis should focus on examination of the ascending aorta.

The echocardiographic approach to the patient with aortic regurgitation focuses not only on the presence of regurgitation but also on the etiology, severity, functional consequences, and associated abnormalities (Table 10–6).

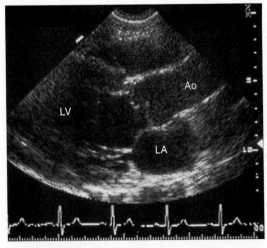

Figure 10–15. Parasternal long-axis view in a patient with aortic regurgitation due to a bicuspid aortic valve disease with prolapse of the right coronary cusp in diastole resulting in inadequate leaflet coaptation.

2D/M-Mode Findings in Aortic Regurgitation (Table 10–7)

In addition to anatomic abnormalities of the aortic valve and the secondary left ventricular dilation that occurs in response to volume overload, several 2D and M-mode echocardiographic findings are seen in patients with aortic regurgitation. If the regurgitant jet impinges on the

TABLE 10–6. ECHOCARDIOGRAPHIC APPROACH TO AORTIC REGURGITATION

1. Valve anatomy/etiology of regurgitation

2. Severity of aortic regurgitation
   a. Flow mapping (color or pulsed)
   b. Continuous-wave Doppler
   c. Descending aortic diastolic flow reversal
   d. Volume flow at 2 sites

3. Left ventricular response
   a. Left ventricular dilation (*end-systolic* dimension)
   b. Left ventricular systolic function

4. Associated abnormalities

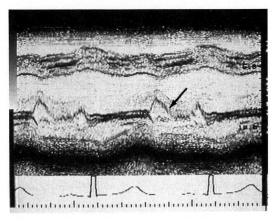

Figure 10–16. M-mode tracing showing increased *E* point–septal separation, and high-frequency fluttering of the anterior mitral leaflet (*arrow*) due to impingement by an aortic regurgitant jet.

anterior mitral valve leaflet, it causes impaired leaflet opening, resulting in an increased distance between the maximal anterior motion of the mitral valve in early diastole (the *E* point) and the most posterior motion of the interventricular septum (increased EPSS, or *E* point septal separation). High-frequency fluttering of the anterior mitral valve leaflet resulting from impingement of the regurgitant jet also may be appreciated on M-mode (with its high sampling rate), although it is rarely appreciated on 2D imaging (due to the relatively low frame rate) (Fig. 10–16).

On 2D long- and short-axis imaging, the anterior mitral leaflet may appear curved in diastole with the concavity toward the ventricular septum (Fig. 10–17). This contrasts with the normal linear appearance of the anterior leaflet in diastole in the long- and short-axis views with a curved appearance of the anterior leaflet with the convexity toward the ventricular septum when the valve is open. This observation has been termed *reverse doming*, since the curvature of the anterior leaflet is opposite to that seen in rheumatic mitral stenosis. In short-axis views, a discrete area of reversed curvature corresponding to the spatial location of the regurgitant jet may be seen.

With chronic regurgitation, the focal blood flow disturbance impinging on the septum or anterior mitral leaflet may result in a raised fibrotic lesion—identifiable by the pathologist postmortem as a jet lesion—which appears as an area of increased echogenicity on 2D imaging.

While none of these indirect signs of aortic regurgitation provides quantitative data, their presence may suggest a previously unsuspected diagnosis and prompt a directed Doppler examination. Recognition of the impact of aortic regurgitation on mitral leaflet motion and the appearance of jet lesions avoids misinterpretation of these findings.

TABLE 10–7. 2D AND M-MODE FINDINGS IN AORTIC REGURGITATION

Aortic valve and root anatomic abnormalities

Left ventricular dilation and sphericity

Indirect signs of aortic regurgitation
   Increased *E*-point septal separation
   High-frequency fluttering of the AMVL
   "Reverse doming" of the AMVL
   Jet lesion on septum or AMVL

AMVL = anterior mitral valve leaflet.

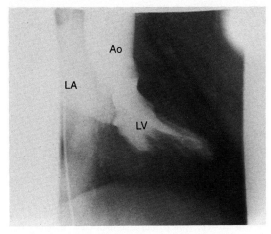

Figure 10–17. Left ventricular angiogram at end-systole showing severe mitral regurgitation with complete, dense opacification of the left atrium on the first beat.

Left Ventricular Response to Aortic Regurgitation

When exposed to chronic volume overload from aortic regurgitation, progressive dilation and increased sphericity of the left ventricle occur (Fig. 10–18). Initially, left ventricular systolic function remains normal. Note that ejection fraction remains normal (not hypernormal), since the total left ventricular stroke volume is ejected across the aortic valve into the high-impedance systemic vasculature (unlike the situation with chronic mitral regurgitation). With chronic, gradually increasing aortic regurgitation, the left ventricle remains compliant in diastole so that end-diastolic pressure remains normal. Typically, left ventricular size slowly increases over a period of years without impairment of systolic function. However, left ventricular systolic dysfunction eventually occurs in the presence of hemodynamically significant chronic volume overload, and in some individuals, irreversible left ventricular systolic dysfunction supervenes even in the absence of clinical symptoms.

In contrast to chronic regurgitation, in acute aortic regurgitation the short interval from onset of volume overload to clinical presentation means that significant left ventricular dilation has not yet occurred. The physiologic differences between acute and chronic aortic regurgitation are reflected both in the 2D echocardiographic findings and in the Doppler examination (Table 10–8).

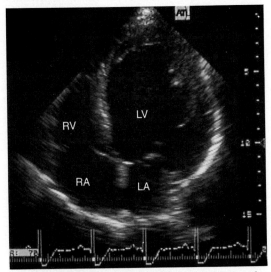

Figure 10–18. Apical four-chamber view showing that geometric changes, specifically increased sphericity, accompany the left ventricular dilation seen with chronic aortic regurgitation.

TABLE 10–8. CHRONIC VERSUS ACUTE AORTIC REGURGITATION

	CHRONIC	ACUTE
Etiology (examples)	Bicuspid valve Hypertension	Endocarditis Aortic dissection
Left ventricular size	Dilated	Normal
Left ventricular end-diastolic pressure	Normal	Elevated
Pulse pressure	Wide	Narrow
Continuous-wave Doppler slope	Flat	Steep

Evaluation of Aortic Regurgitant Severity (Table 10–9)

Doppler Flow Mapping

Flow mapping with conventional pulsed Doppler or with color flow imaging allows differentiation of mild, moderate, and severe aortic regurgitation. The 3D extent of the regurgitant jet is examined in multiple image planes to assess its length, width, and height. The aortic jet can be imaged in the apical long-axis view and in a four-chamber view angulated anteriorly, providing two nearly orthogonal views. This window is particularly helpful in assessing jet length.

Parasternal views in both long and short axis also are helpful and may allow identification of the exact origin of the regurgitant jet as well as assessment of its width, height, and direction. In fact, a short-axis view of the regurgitant jet immediately adjacent to the aortic valve may be the single most useful image plane. In this view, mild aortic regurgitation fills only a small area of the left ventricular outflow tract, moderate regurgitation fills one-third to two-thirds of the outflow tract area, and severe regurgitation nearly completely fills the cross-sectional area (Figs. 10–19 and 10–20).

Continuous-Wave Doppler

The continuous-wave Doppler spectral recording of aortic regurgitation has its onset at aortic valve closure (during isovolumic relaxation) with a rapid increase in velocity to a maximum of 3 to 5 m/s, followed by a gradual decline in velocity during diastole. The velocity abruptly decelerates during isovolumic contraction, reaching baseline at aortic valve opening. The intensity of the signal, relative to antegrade velocity, is an indicator of regurgitant severity. In moderate or severe regurgitation, the signal can easily be recorded throughout diastole, whereas mild regurgitation may not appear holodiastolic, with a recordable signal only at the beginning or end of diastole. This observation may be due to low signal strength or variation in jet direction during diastole resulting in significant intercept angle changes.

The shape of the continuous-wave Doppler time-velocity curve depends on the time-varying instantaneous pressure gradient across the valve in diastole, thus reflecting both severity and chronicity of regurgitation. Chronic severe aortic regurgitation results in an increased aortic pulse pressure with a low end-diastolic aortic pressure. The rapid rate of decline in aortic pressure is reflected in a more rapid decline in the Doppler velocity—i.e., a steeper diastolic deceleration slope even if end-diastolic left ventricular pressure remains low (Fig. 10–21). This observation led to the suggestion that the diastolic deceleration slope may provide a quantitative measure of aortic regurgitant severity. While this hypothesis is valid to some extent, other factors that affect either left ventricular or aortic diastolic pressure also affect the course of the pressure difference (and velocity) across the regurgitant valve. With *acute* regurgitation, even if only moderate in severity, the compliance of the left ventricle has not adapted to chronic volume overload, so a significant increase in end-diastolic pressure is seen. In extreme cases, aortic and left ventricular end-diastolic pressure may equalize at end-diastole, resulting in a triangular-shaped continuous-wave spectral output with a linear deceleration slope from maximum velocity to the baseline. Other factors that affect left ventricular diastolic pressure (e.g., systolic dysfunction, ischemia) or aortic diastolic pressure (e.g., sepsis, patent ductus arteriosus) also will affect the shape of the aortic regurgitant velocity curve.

The continuous-wave signal for aortic regurgitation most often is best recorded from an apical window in order to obtain a parallel intercept angle between the jet and the blood flow direction. Occasionally, an eccentric jet, directed either anteriorly or posteriorly, will be recorded best from a parasternal approach. If signal strength from the suprasternal notch is ade-quate, a signal similar to that recorded from the apex (but, of course, inverted) is seen.

Holodiastolic Flow Reversal in the Descending Aorta

With severe aortic regurgitation, holodiastolic flow reversal is seen in the proximal abdominal aorta, recorded from the subcostal window (Fig. 10–22). This observation is analogous to the physical examination finding of diastolic reversal in the femoral arteries (DeRosier's sign). Holodiastolic flow reversal in the abdominal aorta is sensitive (100 percent) and specific (97 percent) for diagnosing severe aortic regurgitation. False-positive results may be due to the presence of a patent ductus arteriosus, where the diastolic flow is from aorta to pulmonary artery rather than to the left ventricle. More proximal holodiastolic flow reversal, in the descending thoracic aorta, also is sensitive for detection of severe aortic regurgitation but is less specific, also being seen in some subjects with only moderate regurgitation (Fig. 10–23).

Volume Flow at Two Intracardiac Sites

As described above, aortic regurgitant volume and fraction can be calculated as the difference between transaortic and transmitral volume flow (Fig. 10–24). In addition, in the specific case of aortic regurgitation, both forward and total stroke volume can be calculated at a single anatomic site: the proximal descending thoracic aorta. When aortic regurgitation is present, significant systolic expansion of the aorta occurs, so the antegrade flow velocity integral must be multiplied by the systolic cross-sectional area. The flow velocity integral of the reversed flow in diastole is multiplied by diastolic cross-sectional area. Either 2D short-axis imaging or an M-mode through the aortic arch can be used for measurement of systolic and diastolic cross-sectional areas. Note that this quantitative approach is the logical extension of the semiquantitative approach which relies on the *presence* and spatial extent of holodiastolic flow reversal in the aorta in patients with aortic regurgitation.

Clinical Utility

Diagnostic Utility for Aortic Regurgitation

An echocardiogram may be requested either to confirm or exclude a clinical diagnosis of aor-

TABLE 10–9. SELECTED STUDIES VALIDATING QUANTITATIVE EVALUATION OF REGURGITANT SEVERITY USING DOPPLER ECHOCARDIOGRAPHY

FIRST AUTHOR, YEAR	METHOD	STANDARD OF REFERENCE	N	R VALUE	SEE
Downstream Flow Reversal					
Boughner, 1975	Diastolic flow reversal in descending Ao	Angio LV, Fick CO	15 AR pts	0.91 (RF)	—
Touche, 1985	Diastolic flow reversal in descending Ao	Angio LV, TD-CO	30 AR pts	0.92 (RF)	8.8%
Volume Flow at Two Sites					
Ascah, 1985	Transmitral vs transaortic SV	EM-flow	30 flow rates in canine model	0.83 (RF)	—
Kitabatake, 1985	Transaortic vs transpulmonic SV	Angio LV, TD-CO	20 AR pts	0.94 (RF)	—
Rokey, 1986	Transmitral vs transaortic SV	Angio LV, TD-CO	19 MR and 6 AR pts	0.91 (RF)	7%
Continuous-Wave Doppler					
Teague, 1986	AR half-time	Angio LV, Fick CO	32 AR pts	−0.88 (RF)	11%
Masuyama, 1986	AR half-time	Angio LV, ID-CO	20 AR pts	−0.89 (RF)	—
Jenni, 1989	CW Doppler Amplitude-weighted velocity	Angio LV, Fick CO	25 MR pts	0.96 (RF)	6.1%
Color Flow Imaging (Regurgitant Jet)					
Spain, 1989	Color jet area	Angio LV, TD-CO	15 MR pts	0.62 (RF)	—
Tribouilloy, 1992	Regurgitant jet width at origin	Angio LV, TD-CO	31 MR pts	0.85 (RSV)	—
Enriquez-Sarano, 1993	Color jet area	Doppler SV at two sites	80 MR pts	0.69 (RF)	4.4 cm²
Proximal Acceleration (Color Flow)					
Recusani, 1991	PISA (hemispherical)	Rotometer	In vitro, constant flow	0.94–0.99 (flow rate)	1–1.6 liters/min
Utsunomiya, 1991	PISA (hemispherical)	Actual flow rate stopwatch and cylinder	In vitro, pulsatile flow	0.99 (flow rate)	0.53 liters/min
Vandervoort, 1993	PISA	Actual flow rate	In vitro, steady flow	0.98–0.99 (flow rate)	—
Giesler, 1993	PISA	LV angio, Fick CO	16 MR pts	0.88 (RSV)	17 ml
Chen, 1993	PISA	Doppler SV at two sites	46 MR pts	0.94 (RSV)	18 ml

TABLE 10-9. SELECTED STUDIES VALIDATING QUANTITATIVE EVALUATION OF REGURGITANT SEVERITY USING DOPPLER ECHOCARDIOGRAPHY
Continued

FIRST AUTHOR, YEAR	METHOD	STANDARD OF REFERENCE	N	R VALUE	SEE
Jet Momentum					
Cape, 1989	Conservation of momentum	EM-flow	In vitro, constant flow	0.98	0.18 liters/min

Abbreviations: Ao = aortic; AR = aortic regurgitation; CO = cardiac output; EM-flow = volume flow rate measured by electromagnetic flowmeter; ID = indicator dilation; LV = left ventricle; MR = mitral regurgitation; PISA = proximal isovelocity surface area method; RF = regurgitant fraction; RSV = regurgitant stroke volume; SV = stroke volume; TD = thermodilution.

Data from Boughner et al: Circ 52:874–79, 1975; Touche et al: Circ 72:819–24, 1985; Ascah et al: Circ 72:377–83, 1985; Kitabatake et al: Circ 72:523–29, 1985; Rokey et al: JACC 7:1273–78, 1986; Teague et al: JACC 8:592–99, 1986; Masuyama et al: Circ 73:460–66, 1986; Jenni et al: Circ 79:1294–99, 1989; Spain et al: JACC 13:585–90, 1989; Tribouilloy et al: Circ 85:1248–53, 1992; Enriquez-Sarano et al: JACC 21:1211–19, 1993; Rescusani et al: Circ 83:594–604, 1991; Utsunomiya et al: J Am Soc Echo 4:338–48, 1991; Vandervoort et al: JACC 22:535–41, 1993; Giesler et al: AJC 71:217–24, 1993; Chen et al: JACC 21:374–83, 1993; Cape et al: Circ 79:1343–53, 1989.

tic regurgitation. Given the high sensitivity and specificity of this approach, the resulting diagnostic data are highly reliable. In addition, information on the etiology of valve disease, associated conditions, and the degree of left ventricular dilation is obtained.

If aortic regurgitation is detected in the course of an echocardiogram ordered for some other indication, it is incumbent upon the echocardiographer to search carefully for the etiology of regurgitation. The finding of regurgitation may be the first clue that aortic root disease or a disease process affecting the aortic leaflets is present.

Sequential Evaluation of Chronic Asymptomatic Aortic Regurgitation

Several studies examining outcome after valve replacement for aortic regurgitation have shown that a left ventricular end-systolic dimension of less than 55 mm is predictive of preserved (or improved) left ventricular systolic function and an excellent prognosis after valve replacement. While a prospective, randomized trial of surgical intervention in the asymptomatic patient has not been performed, a carefully performed decision-analysis model (Suggested Reading 22) based on

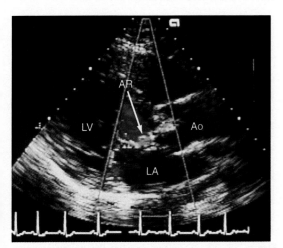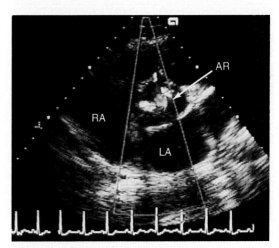

Figure 10-19. Color Doppler images in parasternal long- (*left*) and short-axis (*right*) views in a patient with mild aortic regurgitation. In long axis, an eccentric jet is seen, which in short axis has a small cross-sectional area at the regurgitant orifice relative to the area of the outflow tract.

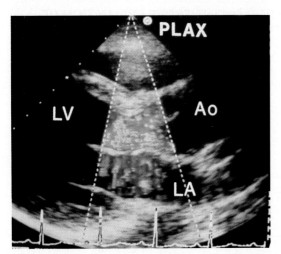

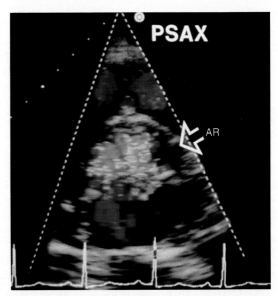

Figure 10–20. Color Doppler images in parasternal long- and short-axis views in a patient with severe aortic regurgitation. The flow disturbance fills the outflow tract in both views.

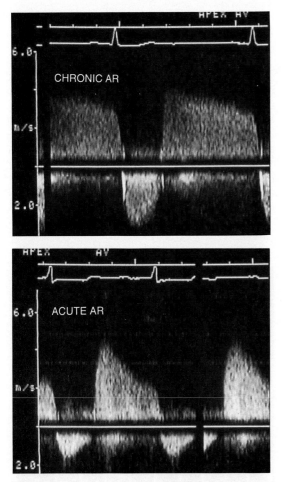

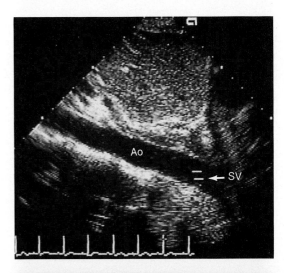

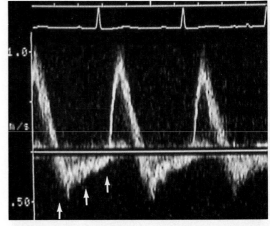

Figure 10–21. Continuous-wave Doppler recording in two patients, one with chronic aortic regurgitation (AR) due to calcific aortic valve disease (*above*) and one with acute regurgitation due to aortic dissection (*below*) showing the differences in the deceleration slope in these clinical situations.

Figure 10–22. 2D image showing the pulsed Doppler sample volume (SV) position in the descending aorta from a subcostal approach (*above*). The Doppler velocity curve (*below*) shows holodiastolic flow reversal (*arrows*) consistent with severe aortic regurgitation.

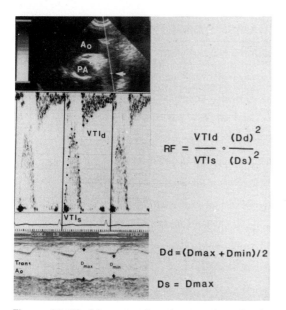

$$RF = \frac{VTI_d}{VTI_s} \cdot \frac{(Dd)^2}{(Ds)^2}$$

$$Dd = (Dmax + Dmin)/2$$

$$Ds = Dmax$$

Figure 10–23. Measures of aortic regurgitant fraction from diastolic and systolic flow in the descending thoracic aorta. (*Above*) Suprasternal 2D echo image showing the aortic arch (Ao) passing over the pulmonary artery (PA). The pulsed-Doppler sample volume (*white arrow*) is positioned in the descending thoracic aorta. (*Center*) Inverted flow velocity tracing showing systolic anterograde flow as an upward deflection from the baseline, while diastolic retrograde flow appears as an aliased downward deflection from the baseline. The diastolic velocity-time integral (VTI_d) is proportional to regurgitant stroke volume, while the systolic velocity-time integral (VTI_s) is proportional to total (i.e., forward plus reverse) stroke volume. (*Below*) M-mode recording of transverse aortic (Trans Ao) diameter during the cardiac cycle. Mean diastolic diameter is taken as the average of maximum (D_{max}) and minimum (D_{min}) diameters; mean systolic diameter is taken as D_{max}. Aortic regurgitant fraction (RF) then can be calculated as the product of the ratios (VTI_d/VTI_s) and (D_d^2/D_s^2). (*Reprinted with permission from Pearlman AS, Otto CM: Echocardiography 4:271, 1987.*)

the expected probabilities of each event (e.g., symptom development, operative mortality, heart failure), the utility of different outcomes (stroke, life on anticoagulation), and expected quality-adjusted life years over a 10-year time frame convincingly supports these data. Many clinicians use echocardiography sequentially (usually annually) to evaluate changes in left ventricle size and systolic function and optimize the timing of valve replacement in the asymptomatic patient. Clearly, end-systolic dimension is not an ideal measure of the left ventricular response to chronic volume overload (since it is afterload-dependent), and continued evaluation of better measures of ventricular contractility is needed. Of note, the relationship between quantitative measures of regurgitant severity (by any diagnostic modality) and clinical outcome has rarely been addressed.

MECHANISMS OF MITRAL REGURGITATION

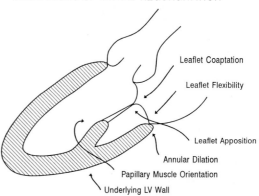

Figure 10–24. Schematic diagram illustrating how abnormalities of any part of the complex mitral valve apparatus can result in mitral regurgitation.

In sequential studies, the accuracy of detecting a change in left ventricular dimension is greatest when similar examination techniques are used and when the studies are compared "side by side." With slow disease progression, similar directional changes on serial studies at several time points are more reliable than a single-interval change.

Alternate approaches to follow-up in patients with chronic aortic regurgitation include resting and exercise radionuclide ventriculography, magnetic resonance imaging, and cardiac catheterization.

MITRAL REGURGITATION

Diagnostic Imaging of the Mitral Valve Apparatus (Table 10–10)

Functionally, the mitral valve apparatus has several components: the left atrial wall, the mitral annulus, the anterior and posterior leaflets, the chordae, the papillary muscles, and the left ventricular myocardium underlying the papillary muscles. Dysfunction or altered anatomy of any one of these components can result in mitral regurgitation (see Fig. 10–24).

Mitral annular dilation may be due to either left atrial or left ventricular dilation and results in mitral regurgitation because of incomplete leaflet coaptation. The normal mitral apparatus is a saddle-shaped ellipse with its most apical points seen in the apical four-chamber view and its most basal points seen in the long-axis view. As noted for the aortic valve, the mitral leaflets have a normal area of overlap (or apposition) so

TABLE 10–10. ETIOLOGY AND PRESUMED MECHANISMS OF MITRAL REGURGITATION

ETIOLOGY	PRESUMED MECHANISM
Annular dilation	Inadequate leaflet coaptation
Mitral annular calcification	Increased rigidity of annulus impairing systolic contraction
Myxomatous mitral valve disease	Inadequate coaptation and apposition, flail segments
Rheumatic mitral valve disease	Increased rigidity of leaflets
Endocarditis	Leaflet perforation or deformity
Marfan's syndrome	Anterior leaflet redundancy
Age-related degenerative leaflet changes	Abnormal coaptation
Hypertrophic cardiomyopathy	Abnormal leaflet motion and anatomy
Chordae disruption or elongation	Inadequate systolic support of leaflet
Regional left ventricle dysfunction	Inadequate systolic support of leaflets
Left ventricular dilation	Abnormal papillary muscle orientation
Papillary muscle rupture	Inadequate systolic support of leaflets

that some degree of mitral annular dilation may be tolerated without significant regurgitation.

The mitral annulus area normally is smaller in systole than in diastole. Increased rigidity of the annulus, as seen with *mitral annular calcification*, impairs systolic contraction of the annulus leading to mitral regurgitation. Mitral annular calcification has a typical appearance on 2D imaging as areas of increased echogenicity on the left ventricular side of the annulus immediately adjacent to the attachment point of the posterior leaflet (Fig. 10–25). Acoustic shadowing, due to the presence of calcium, is seen. In short-axis views, the annular calcium may be focal or extensive, involving the entire U-shaped posterior annulus. The region of anterior mitral leaflet–aortic root continuity is involved only rarely. Mitral annular calcification is commonly seen as an incidental finding in elderly subjects. "Premature" annular calcification is seen in patients with renal failure or hypertension.

Diseases of the mitral valve leaflets include myxomatous disease, rheumatic disease, endocarditis, Marfan's syndrome, and rare disorders such as infiltrative diseases (amyloid, sarcoid, mucopolysaccharidosis) and collagen-vascular disorders (systemic lupus erythematosus, rheumatoid arthritis). *Myxomatous* mitral valve disease is characterized by thickened, redundant leaflets and chordae with sagging of portions of the leaflets into the left atrium in systole (Figs. 10–26 and 10–27). The severity of disease is variable, ranging from mitral valve prolapse, in

which there is only minimal displacement of the leaflets into the left atrium in systole, to severe involvement of both leaflets by myxomatous disease with frankly prolapsed or flail leaflet segments.

Rheumatic mitral regurgitation, like rheumatic mitral stenosis, is characterized by some degree of commissural fusion and thickening of the leaflet tips. *Endocarditis* results in mitral regurgitation by leaflet destruction, perforation, or deformity. *Marfan's syndrome* is associated with a long redundant anterior leaflet that sags into the left atrium in systole. Infiltrative diseases result in irregular leaflet thickening and inadequate coaptation. Of note, *age-related degenerative changes* in the mitral leaflets often are seen (with or without associated mitral annular calcification) and appear as irregular areas of thickening and increased echogenicity of the mitral leaflets. Obviously, while some conditions with unique anatomic features can be reliably diagnosed by 2D imaging (rheumatic or myxomatous disease), there is considerable overlap in the anatomic features of other conditions (degenerative versus infiltrative leaflet abnormalities). In these cases, the echocardiographer can describe the valve anatomy and indicate the possible etiologies of the findings even though the specific tissue diagnosis remains unknown.

Abnormalities of leaflet motion also can result in mitral regurgitation. The best known example of this phenomenon is *hypertrophic cardiomyopathy*. As the anterior leaflet obstructs the left

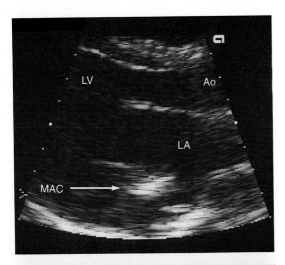

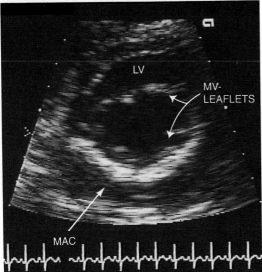

Figure 10–25. 2D parasternal long- (*top*) and short-axis (*bottom*) views of mitral annular calcification (MAC).

Regional left ventricular dysfunction with abnormal contraction of either papillary muscle or the underlying ventricular wall results in mitral regurgitation, presumably due to inadequate support of the closed leaflets in systole. *Abnormal orientation of the papillary muscles,* as seen with dilated cardiomyopathy, also results in mitral regurgitation. Other etiologies of abnormal papillary muscle function or orientation include coronary artery disease, chronic volume overload leading to left ventricular dilation, and systolic dysfunction secondary to other conditions.

Papillary muscle rupture can occur as a complication of acute myocardial infarction. If the entire papillary muscle is disconnected from the underlying left ventricular wall, few patients survive due to acute severe mitral regurgitation. Echocardiographic evaluation in those who do survive shows a mass (the ruptured papillary muscle) attached to flail segments of anterior and posterior leaflets (since each papillary muscle attaches to both leaflets). The ruptured papillary muscle head is seen in the left atrium in systole and in the left ventricle in diastole. Severe mitral regurgitation is present on Doppler examination. Partial rupture of a papillary muscle, defined as rupture of one of several "heads" or as partial disconnection of the base of the papillary muscle, is seen more often. In this situation, the echocardiogram shows a thin, attenuated, excessively mobile papillary muscle and, if one head has ruptured, a mass attached to the leaflet with prolapse into the left atrium in systole (see Fig. 6–25).

Response of the Left Ventricle, Left Atrium, and Pulmonary Vasculature to Mitral Regurgitation (Table 10–11)

When mitral regurgitation is present, the left ventricle ejects blood both forward into the aorta against systemic vascular resistance and backward into the low-resistance left atrium. Since the left ventricle effectively pumps against a low afterload early in the disease course, the increase in left ventricular stroke volume is achieved mainly by more complete left ventricular emptying (an increased ejection fraction) rather than by left ventricular dilation. Thus the left ventricle is expected to appear hyperdynamic on 2D imaging when mitral regurgitation is present.

With chronic regurgitation, progressive left ventricular dilation eventually occurs as the regurgitant volume (and thus total left ventricular stroke volume) increases. As with aortic regurgitation, an irreversible decline in left ventricu-

ventricular outflow tract in systole, coaptation of the anterior and posterior leaflets is disrupted, resulting in a posteriorly directed mitral regurgitant jet. In addition, mitral valve anatomy is abnormal in patients with hypertrophic cardiomyopathy (see Chap. 7).

Chordal disruption or elongation leads to mitral regurgitation because of inadequate tensile support of the closed leaflets in systole. Chordal elongation results in severe bowing of the leaflet, or leaflet segment, into the left atrium, with the tip of the leaflet still directed toward the ventricular apex. With chordal rupture, there is a flail segment of the leaflet such that the leaflet is displaced into the left atrium in systole, with the tip of the leaflet pointing away from the ventricular apex.

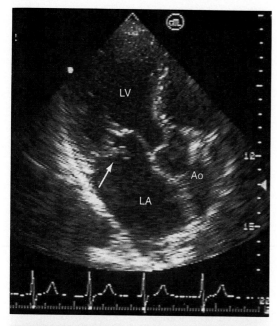

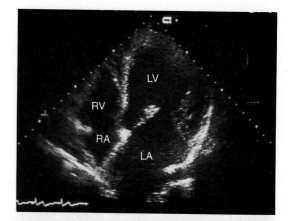

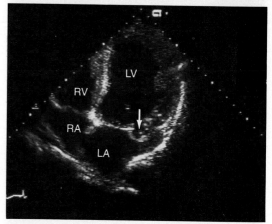

Figure 10–27. Diastolic and systolic apical four-chamber views in a patient with myxomatous mitral valve disease and severe prolapse of the posterior leaflet (*arrow*).

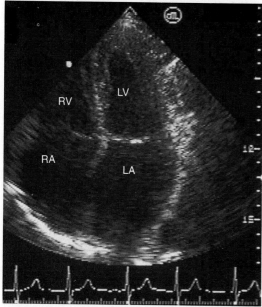

Figure 10–26. 2D apical long-axis and apical four-chamber views of myxomatous mitral valve disease. Posterior leaflet prolapse and partial flail (*arrow*) are appreciated best in the long-axis view. Left atrial dilation due to chronic mitral regurgitation is evident.

lar contractility can occur in the absence of symptoms. Given the low left ventricular afterload, apparent "normal" left ventricular systolic function, as assessed qualitatively by 2D imaging or by quantitation ejection fraction measurement, raises the possibility of impaired contractility.

With chronic mitral regurgitation, the left atrium gradually dilates to accommodate the regurgitant volume while maintaining a normal left atrial pressure. Left atrial compliance increases; that is, the left atrial pressure-volume relationship is shifted downward and to the right. With acute mitral regurgitation, the regurgitant volume is delivered into a small, noncompliant left atrium, resulting in a significant increase in left atrial pressure and a *v* wave in the left atrial pressure curve.

Pulmonary artery pressure rises passively in response to both the chronic mildly elevated left atrial pressure seen with chronic mitral regurgitation and the acute severe elevation seen with acute regurgitation. When left atrial pressure is chronically elevated, pulmonary vascular resistance may increase. Echocardiographic evaluation of the patient with mitral regurgitation includes noninvasive measurement of pulmonary artery pressure from the tricuspid regurgitant jet velocity and an estimate of right atrial pressure.

TABLE 10–11. ECHOCARDIOGRAPHIC APPROACH TO MITRAL REGURGITATION

1. Mitral valve apparatus anatomy, etiology of regurgitation

2. Severity of mitral regurgitation
   a. Flow mapping
   b. Continuous-wave Doppler
   c. Pulmonary vein systolic flow reversal
   d. Volume flow at two sites

3. Left atrial dilation

4. Left ventricle
   a. Dilation (*end-systolic* dimension)
   b. Systolic function

5. Pulmonary artery pressures

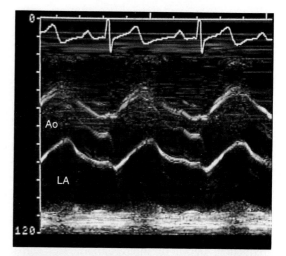

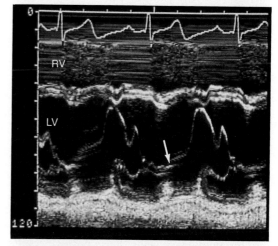

Other 2D/M-Mode Findings in Mitral Regurgitation

The anteroposterior motion of the aortic root, as seen on M-mode recordings, reflects left atrial emptying and filling. The left atrium lies between the rigid spinal column posteriorly and the aortic root anteriorly so that an increase in left atrial volume displaces the aortic root anteriorly, while a decrease in left atrial volume allows the aortic root to move posteriorly. Since mitral regurgitation results in increased left atrial volume in systole (due to the regurgitant volume) followed by an abrupt decrease in left atrial volume in diastole (due to the elevated transmitral stroke volume), an increase in aortic root motion is seen on the M-mode recording (Fig. 10–28).

Evaluation of Mitral Regurgitant Severity

Doppler Flow Mapping

Flow mapping of the mitral regurgitant jet is performed with either conventional pulsed or color flow Doppler in several tomographic planes in order to build a mental 3D reconstruction of the extent of the flow disturbance. Based on this evaluation, regurgitation is graded on an 0 to 4+ scale, where 1+ is mild, 2 to 3+ is moderate, and 4+ is severe regurgitation. Apical four-chamber and long-axis views are useful because they are nearly orthogonal to each other, but signal attenuation at the depth of the left atrium may limit their utility if ultrasound penetration is suboptimal. Parasternal long- and short-axis views can be used for flow mapping

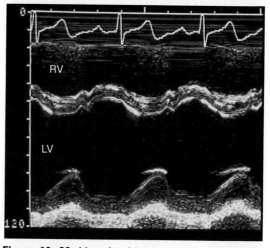

Figure 10–28. M-mode of increased aortic root motion (*above*), the mitral valve (*center*) with late-systolic prolapse (*arrow*), and the hyperdynamic left ventricle (*below*) in a patient with severe mitral regurgitation due to myxomatous mitral valve disease.

and may allow identification of the anatomic origin of the regurgitant jet.

The shape and direction of the mitral regurgitant jet depend on the regurgitant orifice geometry and thus the etiology of mitral regurgitation. Abnormalities of the posterior leaflet tend to result in an anteriorly directed jet (Fig. 10–29), while papillary muscle dysfunction tends to result in a posteriorly directed jet (Fig. 10–30). Dilation of the left ventricle or mitral annulus results in a central, symmetrical regurgitant jet (Fig. 10–31).

When evaluation of mitral valve anatomy or the severity of regurgitation is suboptimal from a transthoracic approach, transesophageal imaging may be helpful. Since the transducer frequency, depth of interrogation, and signal strength are quite different for these two approaches, the influence of these factors on the appearance of the regurgitant jet must be considered in the overall evaluation of regurgitation severity (see Chap. 1).

Pulmonary Vein Flow Reversal

As the mitral regurgitant jet enters the left atrium, it necessarily displaces blood that was already in the chamber. When severe regurgitation is present, systolic flow reversal in the pulmonary veins is seen. False-negative results occur when the left atrium is severely enlarged and compliant so that all the excess volume is contained in the left atrium without displacement into the pulmonary veins. False-positive results occur when an eccentric jet is directed into a pulmonary vein, causing flow reversal even when regurgitation is not severe.

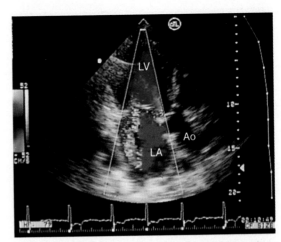

Figure 10–30. A posteriorly directed mitral regurgitant jet due to papillary muscle dysfunction seen in an apical long-axis view.

Continuous-Wave Doppler Evaluation

The continuous-wave Doppler spectral recording of mitral regurgitation shows a rapid rise in velocity (at a rate proportional to the rise in left ventricular dP/dt) from baseline during isovolumic contraction to a maximum velocity of 5 to 6 m/s. The velocity stays high throughout systole with a curve paralleling the rise and fall of left ventricular pressure given a normal left atrial pressure. During isovolumic relaxation, the velocity rapidly returns to baseline.

With acute mitral regurgitation (Table 10–12), a rise in left atrial pressure during late systole—a v wave—may be present due to a steep pressure-volume relationship of the nondilated left atrium. In this situation, the pressure gradient between the left ventricle and the left atrium is

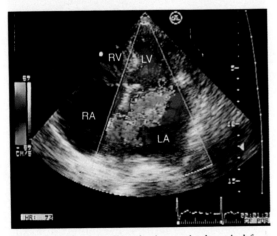

Figure 10–29. Color Doppler images in the apical four-chamber view in moderate mitral regurgitation due to myxomatous disease with an anteriorly directed jet.

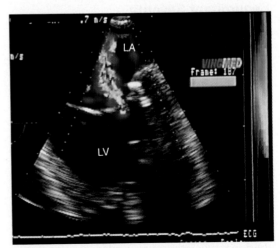

Figure 10–31. On transesophageal images, a central mitral regurgitant jet due to dilated cardiomyopathy is seen.

TABLE 10–12. CHRONIC VERSUS ACUTE MITRAL REGURGITATION

	CHRONIC	ACUTE
Etiology (examples)	Myxomatous valve disease Annular dilation	Endocarditis Papillary muscle rupture Chordal rupture
Left ventricular size	Dilated	Normal
Left ventricular systolic function	Hyperdynamic early, may be normal or depressed with long-standing disease	Hyperdynamic
Left atrial size	Enlarged	Normal
Continuous-wave Doppler curve	High velocity throughout systole	Late systolic velocity decline (*v* wave)

high initially but then begins to equalize in late systole as left atrial pressure rises. The corresponding Doppler velocity curve shows a high initial velocity with a more rapid fall in velocity in middle to late systole. This pattern of Doppler velocities also is termed a *v* wave (Figs. 10–8 and 10–32).

Signal intensity of the mitral regurgitant signal, in comparison with antegrade flow, is related to mitral regurgitation severity. In addition, significant regurgitation is associated with an increase in the antegrade velocity due to increased transmitral volume flow.

Volume Flow at Two Intracardiac Sites

Mitral regurgitant stroke volume can be calculated from transmitral stroke volume (total left ventricular stroke volume) and transaortic stroke volume (forward stroke volume) as (Fig. 10–33):

$$\text{Mitral regurgitant volume} = \text{Transmitral stroke volume} - \text{Transaortic stroke volume}$$

Alternate sites for measurement of forward stroke volume are the tricuspid valve and the pulmonary artery.

Clinical Utility

Diagnosis and Severity of Mitral Regurgitation

Determination of the etiology of mitral regurgitation using 2D imaging often has important clinical implications. Evaluation of regurgitant severity also is of clinical importance, although a high degree of sophistication in echocardiographic interpretation is needed for this application. In assessing the severity of regurgitation,

the echocardiographer should first describe the individual findings and then integrate these findings into a consistent overall interpretation. In addition, the degree of pulmonary hypertension, left atrial size, left ventricular size and systolic function, and any associated abnormalities are added to the Doppler findings before arriving at a final interpretation.

Examples of clinical situations in which decisions can be based on echocardiographic and Doppler data include acute mitral regurgitation after myocardial infarction, mitral valve endocarditis, and chronic mitral regurgitation due to myxomatous mitral valve disease. The decision whether or not to perform valve surgery (repair or replacement) usually can be made based on clinical and echocardiographic data without invasive studies in these patient groups. Only in cases where there is a discrepancy between the clinical impression and the echocardiographic findings (or when coronary angiography is indicated) are further diagnostic tests warranted.

Mitral Valve "Prolapse" Versus Myxomatous Mitral Valve Disease

Myxomatous mitral valve disease is a pathologic condition characterized histologically by increased mucopolysaccharides, thickening, and disarray of the mitral valve leaflet. Grossly, the leaflets and chordae are thick and redundant but with reduced tensile strength so that they are prone to progressive elongation or rupture. 2D imaging demonstrates thick, redundant leaflets and chordae with systolic displacement of the leaflets into the left atrium in systole. Patients with this disease have a high incidence of significant mitral regurgitation and often go on to require mitral valve surgery. Patients with myxomatous mitral valve disease also may have aortic or tricuspid valve involvement.

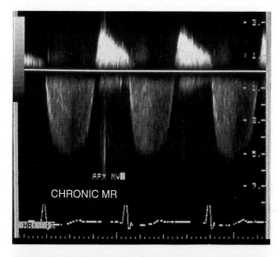

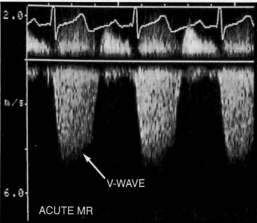

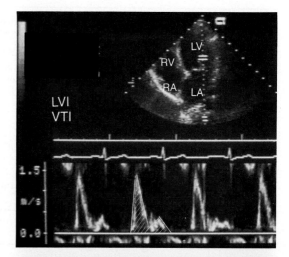

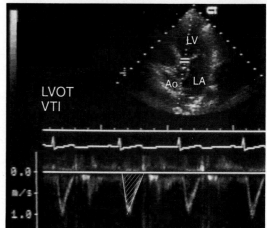

Figure 10–32. Continuous-wave Doppler recordings in a patient with chronic mitral regurgitation (*above*) and a patient with more acute regurgitation (*below*) showing a *v* wave (*arrows*).

Figure 10–33. Quantitative evaluation of mitral regurgitant severity by calculation of transmitral and transaortic volume flow rates. Mitral annulus diameter and the velocity-time integral (VTI) of flow across the mitral annulus are used to calculate total stroke volume. Forward stroke volume is determined from the cross-sectional area and velocity-time integral of left ventricular outflow tract flow.

In contrast, mitral valve prolapse is a less clearly defined condition. The current diagnostic criteria are in flux but will be refined as more data on the pathology and genetics of this condition become available. Possibly, this condition simply represents one end of a spectrum that includes myxomatous mitral valve disease. On 2D imaging, the closure plane of the mitral leaflets may appear "flat" relative to the mitral annulus, especially in the apical four-chamber view where the most apical points of the annulus are seen. Obviously, even a normal leaflet closure plane may appear displaced in oblique image planes. Instead of arbitrarily defining *prolapse* as movement of the leaflets beyond the annulus, it is more helpful to describe the valve anatomy (leaflet size, thickness, redundancy, chordal involvement) and pattern of valve motion qualitatively.

The clinician then can interpret these findings in conjunction with the patient's symptoms and physical findings. While a few echocardiographic findings are independently diagnostic of mitral valve prolapse, others only support the diagnosis in the appropriate clinical setting. Yet other findings simply represent the range of normal variation in mitral valve anatomy and dynamics (Table 10–13).

Follow-Up of Chronic Asymptomatic Mitral Regurgitation

Sequential echocardiographic studies can be used to follow asymptomatic patients with mi-

TABLE 10–13. GUIDELINES FOR THE CLINICAL DIAGNOSIS OF MITRAL VALVE PROLAPSE

Major Criteria*

Auscultation
  Mid- to late systolic clicks and late systolic murmur or whoop alone or in combination at the cardiac apex

Two-dimensional echocardiogram
  Marked superior systolic displacement of mitral leaflets with coaptation point at or superior to annular plane
  Mild to moderate superior systolic displacement of mitral leaflets with
    Chordal rupture
    Doppler mitral regurgitation
    Annular dilatation

Echocardiogram plus auscultation
  Mild to moderate superior systolic displacement of mitral leaflets with
    Prominent mid- to late systolic clicks at the cardiac apex
    Apical late systolic or holosystolic murmur in the young
    Late systolic "whoop"

Minor Criteria

Auscultation
  Loud first heart sound with an apical holosystolic murmur

Two-dimensional echocardiogram
  Isolated mild to moderate superior systolic displacement of the posterior mitral leaflet
  Moderate superior systolic displacement of both mitral leaflets

Echocardiogram plus history
  Mild to moderate superior systolic displacement of mitral leaflets with
    Focal neurologic attacks or amaurosis fugax in the young
    First-degree relatives with major criteria

Reprinted with permission from Perloff JK et al: New guidelines for the clinical diagnosis of mitral valve prolapse. Am J Cardiol 57:1124–1129, 1986.
*Major criteria establish the diagnosis. Minor criteria are supportive but not diagnostic.

tral regurgitation. While mitral regurgitation severity and mitral valve anatomy are important data, the most important factor in patient evaluation is left ventricular size and systolic function. Current data suggest that evidence of progressive ventricular dilation, an end-systolic dimension ≥45 mm, or any reduction in left ventricular systolic function should prompt consideration of surgical intervention regardless of the symptomatic status of the patient to prevent irreversible ventricular dysfunction postoperatively.

Decision Making Concerning Mitral Valve Repair or Replacement

Once the decision has been made that surgical intervention is needed, the echocardiographic images are invaluable in considering whether mitral valve repair or reconstruction is possible. The study should be reviewed with the surgeon, focusing on the exact etiology of mitral regurgitation, the degree of annular dilation, the rela-

tive involvement of anterior and posterior leaflets, the chordal and papillary muscle structural integrity, and overall ventricular size and systolic function. Typically, posterior leaflet prolapse and annular dilation are most amenable to repair, while more complex or extensive disease requires more complex procedures with a lower likelihood of successful repair.

Intraoperative Evaluation of Mitral Valve Repair

In the patient undergoing surgical mitral valve repair, transesophageal echocardiography is used to assess results after the procedure. Baseline transesophageal images are obtained in the operating room to reconfirm regurgitant severity under the loading conditions of general anesthesia and to serve as a baseline for comparison to the postrepair echocardiogram. After valve repair, the patient is weaned from cardiopulmonary bypass, and valve anatomy and mitral regurgitant severity are reassessed. Preferably, regurgitant severity is evaluated under physiologic loading conditions with similar hemodynamics to those recorded during the baseline study (Fig. 10–34). If significant residual mitral regurgitation is present, a second bypass pump run may be done as part of the same procedure to allow a second attempt at repair or mitral valve replacement. Other complications of the valve repair also may be identified, including dynamic left ventricular outflow tract obstruction (Figs. 10–35 and 10–36), functional mitral stenosis, and worsening of left ventricular systolic dysfunction.

TRICUSPID REGURGITATION

Diagnostic Imaging of the Tricuspid Valve Apparatus

Tricuspid regurgitation occurs with abnormalities of the supporting structures (annulus, right ventricle) or the leaflets themselves. Tricuspid regurgitation secondary to *annular dilation* often is due either to primary right ventricular dilation and systolic dysfunction or to *pulmonary hypertension*. Left-sided heart disease leading to pulmonary hypertension—especially

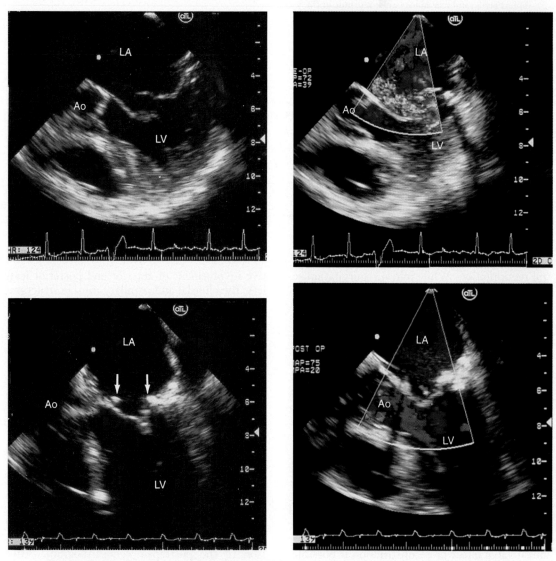

Figure 10–34. 2D (*left*) and color Doppler (*right*) intraoperative transesophageal images in a patient with myxomatous mitral valve disease before (*above*) and after (*below*) mitral valve repair. Before repair, severe mitral prolapse with a partial flail leaflet segment and moderate to severe mitral regurgitation are present. After repair, only minimal regurgitation is detected at similar loading conditions. A mitral annuloplasty ring (*arrows*) is seen.

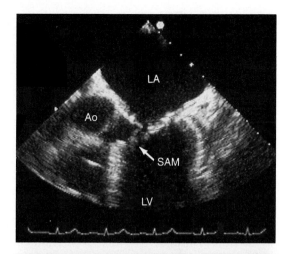

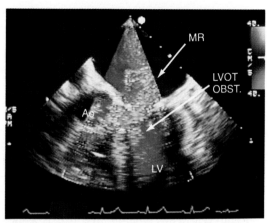

Figure 10–36. Color flow imaging in the same patient as in Figure 10–35 shows systolic turbulence in the left ventricular outflow tract distal to the obstruction and persistent severe mitral regurgitation due to the systolic anterior motion of the mitral leaflet.

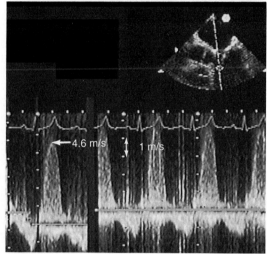

Figure 10–35. Dynamic left ventricular outflow tract obstruction seen on intraoperative transesophageal imaging immediately after mitral valve repair. The anterior leaflet demonstrates systolic anterior motion (SAM, *arrow*), while a guided continuous-wave Doppler recording (despite a possibly nonparallel intercept angle) shows high-velocity flow across this region which was confirmed by direct manometric measurement of left ventricular and aortic pressures.

mitral stenosis or regurgitation—often results in significant tricuspid regurgitation, presumably on the basis of right ventricular dilation and systolic dysfunction.

Abnormalities of the tricuspid valve leaflets also are a cause of tricuspid regurgitation. *Rheumatic disease* involves the tricuspid valve in about 20 to 30 percent of cases, nearly always occurring in conjunction with mitral valve involvement and usually with aortic valve involvement as well. Rheumatic tricuspid disease typically is mild and may be difficult to appreciate on 2D echocardiography unless careful attention is directed toward imaging the valve leaflets and searching for evidence of commissural fusion. Rheumatic tricuspid regurgitation is more common than rheumatic tricuspid stenosis.

Carcinoid heart disease is a rare condition, but the echocardiographic findings are pathognomonic. Carcinoid heart disease (seen with metastatic carcinoid tumor to the liver) is characterized by thickened, shortened, and immobile tricuspid valve leaflets with resultant tricuspid regurgitation or, less often, tricuspid valve stenosis. The pulmonic valve also may be involved. *Endocarditis* may involve the tricuspid valve, resulting in tricuspid regurgitation, and is most common in patients with a history of intravenous drug abuse.

Ebstein's anomaly of the tricuspid valve is a congenital abnormality in which one or more leaflets of the tricuspid valve are displaced from the tricuspid annulus toward the ventricular apex (see Figs. 15–8 and 15–9). Most often, the septal leaflet is involved, either in isolation or in association with apical displacement of posterior and anterior leaflets. The degree of apical displacement is extremely variable. The normal tricuspid valve insertion plane is slightly more apical than the mitral valve attachment plane, but Ebstein's anomaly should be considered when the separation between mitral and tricuspid valve planes is greater than 10 mm. The portion of the right ventricle excluded from the pumping chamber is said to be *atrialized*, since it effectively functions as part of the right atrium. The right atrium may appear severely enlarged due to "atrialization" of the base of the ventricle *plus* dilatation of the atrium due to tricuspid regurgitation. Right ventricular enlargement is seen as well if significant tricuspid regurgitation is present.

Right Ventricular and Right Atrial Dilation

Hemodynamically significant tricuspid regurgitation results in progressive right ventricular and right atrial enlargement due to volume overload. This dilation may complicate assessment of the etiology of regurgitation because the dilation itself may further increase regurgitant severity.

Right ventricular volume overload is associated with a pattern of abnormal septal motion characterized on M-mode recording by posterior motion of the septum in diastole (since right ventricular filling exceeds left ventricular filling) and anterior motion of the septum in systole, often referred to as *paradoxical septal motion*. On 2D short-axis imaging, the ventricular septum appears "flattened" in diastole as the increased transtricuspid stroke volume fills the right ventricle. In systole, the ventricular septum moves toward the center of gravity of the heart (normally toward the middle of the left ventricle), which is the midline of the right ventricle if severe right ventricular dilation is present.

The differential diagnosis of 2D findings of right ventricular dilation and paradoxical septal motion includes other causes of right ventricular volume overload such as an atrial septal defect, partial anomalous pulmonary venous return, pressure overload due to pulmonic valve disease, or pulmonary hypertension either due to left-sided heart disease or intrinsic lung disease.

Evaluation of Tricuspid Regurgitation Severity

Tricuspid regurgitation can be evaluated with Doppler flow mapping in a manner similar to that described for mitral regurgitation. Mild regurgitation is characterized by a flow disturbance in systole localized to the area adjacent to the valve closure plane (less than a third of the atrial area). Moderate regurgitation fills between one-third and two-thirds of the right atrium, while severe regurgitation fills more than two-thirds of an enlarged right atrium (Figs. 10–37 and 10–38). Multiple views are needed to fully "map" the flow disturbance because 3D anatomy of the jet may be asymmetrical. Useful views include the right ventricular inflow view, the apical four-chamber view, and the subcostal four-chamber view. Mild to moderate tricuspid re-

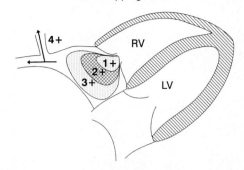

Flow Mapping for TR

subcostal approach

Figure 10–37. Schematic diagram of flow mapping for semiquantitative evaluation of tricuspid regurgitant severity. Severe (4+) tricuspid regurgitation is associated with systolic reversal in the hepatic veins.

gurgitation often is directed along the interatrial septum and must be distinguished from normal caval inflow or from atrial septal defect flow.

Severe tricuspid regurgitation results in systolic flow reversal in the inferior and superior vena cava, analogous to the physical finding of a systolic pulsation in the neck veins. Inferior vena caval flow is best recorded in the central hepatic vein, which provides a flow channel parallel to the ultrasound beam from a subcostal approach and has no venous valves between the recording site and the right atrium.

The absolute value of the maximum velocity in the tricuspid regurgitant continuous-wave Doppler spectral recording reflects the maximum pressure difference across the tricuspid valve and *not* the severity of regurgitation. Severe regurgitation with a normal right ventricular systolic pressure (as seen with tricuspid valve endocarditis) has a low maximum velocity. Mild tricuspid regurgitation in the presence of pulmonary hypertension (as seen with primary pulmonary hypertension) has a high maximum velocity. However, the intensity of the continuous-wave signals relative to the antegrade flow signal intensity does relate to regurgitant severity. In addition, the shape of the velocity-time curve indicates the time course of the instantaneous pressure differences across the valve (Fig. 10–39). A right atrial v wave seen in acute regurgitation results in a more rapid decline in velocity in late systole similar to that seen in acute mitral regurgitation.

Clinical Utility

Evaluation of tricuspid regurgitation by Doppler echocardiography is the standard clinical

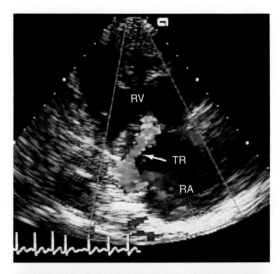

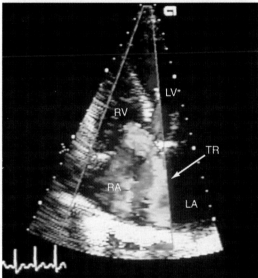

Figure 10–38. Color flow imaging in parasternal right ventricular inflow (*top*) and apical four-chamber (*bottom*) views in a patient with moderate tricuspid regurgitation (TR).

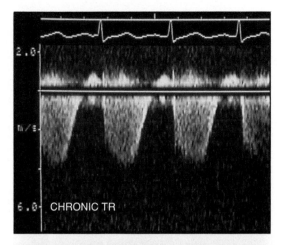

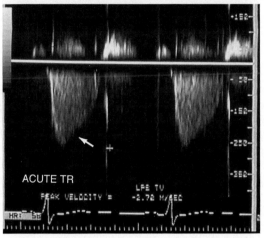

Figure 10–39. Continuous-wave Doppler recording of tricuspid regurgitation in a patient with chronic (*above*) and acute (*below*) tricuspid regurgitation. Note the late systolic velocity decline (*v* wave) in the acute case (*arrow*).

esophageal echocardiography can be used to optimize the surgical approach and assess the functional consequences of the repair procedure.

PULMONIC REGURGITATION

Pulmonic regurgitation most often is a normal finding, with a small amount of diastolic backflow across the pulmonic valve seen in most normal individuals (Fig. 10–40). Pathologic pulmonic regurgitation usually is a result of congenital pulmonic valve disease, either untreated mild disease or residual regurgitation after pulmonic valve surgery. Acquired pulmonic regurgitation is rare, being due to endocarditis, carcinoid syndrome, or myxomatous valve disease.

Evaluation of pulmonic valve anatomy may be limited in adult patients by poor acoustic access.

approach to this problem. Even cardiac catheterization is of limited value, since the catheter placed across the tricuspid valve to perform the right ventricular angiogram may itself induce regurgitation.

Evaluation of tricuspid regurgitant severity is particularly important in the patient undergoing mitral valve surgery. Many of these patients have significant coexisting tricuspid regurgitation, and many of the clinical symptoms will persist postoperatively if this condition is not recognized and treated (with tricuspid annuloplasty) at the time of surgery.

In patients undergoing tricuspid valve repair or surgery for endocarditis, intraoperative trans-

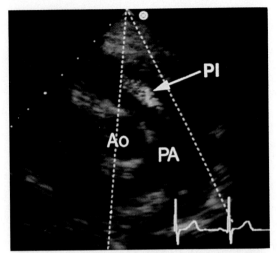

Figure 10–40. Color flow imaging in a right ventricular outflow view showing the degree of pulmonic insufficiency (PI) seen in normal individuals.

With congenital disease, thickened, deformed leaflets are seen. In endocarditis, a valvular vegetation may be identified, although the pulmonic valve is involved least often. Carcinoid syndrome results in shortening and thickening of the pulmonic valve leaflet, similar to the involvement of the tricuspid valve, and may lead to stenosis and/or regurgitation. Myxomatous valve disease is rare, resulting in thickening, redundancy, and systemic sagging of the pulmonic valve leaflets.

Pulmonic regurgitation is diagnosed by documenting a diastolic flow disturbance in the right ventricular outflow tract with conventional pulsed or color Doppler flow imaging. The extent of the flow disturbance provides a semiquantitative index of pulmonic regurgitant severity. The intensity and shape of the continuous-wave Doppler velocity-time spectral output also provide an indication of regurgitant severity, analogous to the findings in aortic regurgitation. Holodiastolic flow reversal may be noted in the main pulmonary artery when significant regurgitation is present and must be distinguished from diastolic flow reversal due to a patent ductus arteriosus.

In adults, evaluation of pulmonic regurgitation is of most importance in patients with uncorrected or residual congenital heart disease. In these patients, the severity of pulmonic regurgitation may be a factor in deciding whether to perform further surgical procedures and in the specific design of the surgical procedure.

When pulmonic regurgitation is present, even if only mild in degree, the velocity in the pulmonic regurgitant curve reflects the pulmonary artery to right ventricular diastolic pressure difference. The instantaneous end-diastolic pulmonary artery to right ventricular gradient (calculated as $4v^2$) can be added to an estimate of right ventricular diastolic pressure (from inferior vena cava size and respiratory variation) to provide an estimate of diastolic pulmonary artery pressure. This approach to estimation of pulmonary artery pressure complements systolic pressure estimation from the tricuspid regurgitant jet and serves as an internal validity check when both can be recorded accurately.

SUGGESTED READING

BASIC PRINCIPLES AND QUANTITATIVE APPROACHES

1. Perloff JK, Roberts WC: The mitral apparatus: Functional anatomy of mitral regurgitation. Circulation 46:227–239, 1972.
   Classic detailed description of the anatomy of the mitral valve apparatus with correlations between the valve anatomy and the mechanism of mitral regurgitation for differing etiologies of mitral valve disease.

2. Bolger AF, Eigler NL, Maurer G: Quantifying valvular regurgitation. Limitations and inherent assumptions of Doppler techniques. Circulation 78:1316–1318, 1988.
   Editorial reviewing limitations of Doppler evaluation of regurgitant severity.

3. Rokey R, Sterling LL, Zoghbi WA, et al: Determination of regurgitant fraction in isolated mitral or aortic regurgitation by pulsed Doppler two-dimensional echocardiography. J Am Coll Cardiol 7:1273–1278, 1986.
   Calculation of regurgitant volume and regurgitant fraction by Doppler at two intracardiac sites (mitral and aortic) was compared with invasive determinations in 25 patients (r = 0.91, SEE = 7 percent).

4. Recusani F, Bargiggia GS, Yoganathan AP, et al: A new method for quantification of regurgitant flow rate using color Doppler flow imaging of the flow convergence region proximal to a discrete orifice: An in vitro study. Circulation 83:594–604, 1991.
   The proximal isovelocity surface area method was used to calculate volume flow rate and then combined with continuous-wave Doppler data to calculate orifice areas in an in vitro study (r = 0.75–0.96).

5. Utsunomiya T, Ogawa T, Doshi R, et al: Doppler color flow "proximal isovelocity surface area" method for estimating volume flow rate: Effects of orifice shape and machine factors. J Am Coll Cardiol 17:1103–1111, 1991.
   The proximal isovelocity surface area method is applicable to noncircular orifices and is insensitive to changes in ultrasound system color flow settings, including gain, wall filters, frame rate, transmit power, packet size, and aliasing velocity.

6. Reimold SC, Ganz P, Bittl JA, et al: Effective aortic regurgitant orifice area: Description of a method based on the conservation of mass. J Am Coll Cardiol 18:761–768, 1991.
   Description of a method for calculating regurgitant orifice area based on the continuity equation using a Doppler cath-

eter system (for regurgitant volume flow measurement) and continuous-wave Doppler recordings of the regurgitant jet (for transvalvular mean velocity measurement) in an in vitro model and in 23 patients.

7. Takenaka K, Dabestani A, Gardin JM, et al: A simple Doppler echocardiographic method for estimating severity of aortic regurgitation. Am J Cardiol 57:1340–1343, 1986.
   Holodiastolic flow reversal in the proximal abdominal aorta is a sensitive (100 percent) and specific (97 percent) method for separating subjects with 3–4+ from those with 0–2+ aortic regurgitation. The single false-positive result was a patient with a patent ductus arteriosus.

8. Touche T, Prasquier R, Nitenberg A, et al: Assessment and follow-up of patients with aortic regurgitation by an updated Doppler echocardiographic measurement of the regurgitant fraction in the aortic arch. Circulation 72:819–824, 1985.
   Quantitative method for calculating aortic regurgitant fraction based on diastolic flow reversal (and aortic diameters) in the descending thoracic aorta.

9. Grayburn PA, Handshoe R, Smith MD, et al: Quantitative assessment of the hemodynamic consequences of aortic regurgitation by means of continuous wave Doppler recordings. J Am Coll Cardiol 10:135–141, 1987.
   Relationship between the shape of the aortic regurgitant jet on continuous-wave Doppler recordings and intracardiac dynamics is explored. All 10 patients with a diastolic decay slope >3.0 m/s² had 3+ to 4+ aortic regurgitation, although 9 of 21 (43 percent) of those with a slope <3.0 m/s² also had severe aortic regurgitation.

10. Labovitz AJ, Ferrara RP, Kern MJ, et al: Quantitative evaluation of aortic insufficiency by continuous wave Doppler echocardiography. J Am Coll Cardiol 8:1341–1347, 1986.
    An aortic regurgitant diastolic slope on the continuous-wave Doppler recording >2 m/s² indicated moderate or severe aortic regurgitation.

COLOR FLOW MAPPING OF VALVULAR REGURGITATION

11. Reimold SC, Maier SE, Fleischmann KE, et al: Dynamic nature of the aortic regurgitant orifice area during diastole in patients with chronic aortic regurgitation. Circulation 89:2085–2092, 1994.
    Using 2D/Doppler echocardiography (continuity equation) and cine phase contrast magnetic resonance imaging, regurgitant orifice area was found to vary directly with regurgitant fraction (r = 0.86) in 17 patients with chronic aortic regurgitation. However, the regurgitant orifice area decreased during diastole in 88 percent of patients. This dynamic component decreased with increasing regurgitant fraction (r = −0.90).

12. Krabill KA, Sung H-W, Tamura T, et al: Factors influencing the structure and shape of stenotic and regurgitant jets: An in vitro investigation using Doppler color flow mapping and optical flow visualization. J Am Coll Cardiol 13:1672–1681, 1989.
    Jet shape depends on orifice size, driving pressure, viscosity, and interfering flowstreams.

13. Simpson IA, Valdes-Cruz LM, Sahn DJ, et al: Doppler color flow mapping of simulated in vitro regurgitant jets: Evaluation of the effects of orifice size and hemodynamic variables. J Am Coll Cardiol 13:1195–1207, 1989.
    In vitro simulation of color flow regurgitant jet areas showed a strong relation to flow rates for any given orifice size and shape but a less strong relation to the absolute volume of regurgitant flow. The power mode depiction of jet areas with color flow Doppler may have potential advantages.

14. Spain MG, Smith MD, Grayburn PA, et al: Quantitative assessment of mitral regurgitation by Doppler color flow imaging: Angiographic and hemodynamic correlations. J Am Coll Cardiol 13:585–590, 1989.
    In 47 patients with mitral regurgitation, maximal color Doppler jet area showed only modest correlation (r = 0.62) with regurgitant fraction at catheterization, but a jet area >8 cm² predicted severe regurgitation (sensitivity 82 percent, specificity 94 percent), while a maximal jet area <4 cm² predicted mild regurgitation (sensitivity 85 percent, specificity 75 percent).

15. Stevenson JG: Two-dimensional color Doppler estimation of the severity of atrioventricular valve regurgitation: Important effects of instrument gain setting, pulse repetition frequency, and carrier frequency. J Am Soc Echocardiogr 2:1–10, 1989.
    Low color Doppler gain settings can reduce apparent jet areas by 29 percent, higher transducer frequencies result in a smaller apparent jet area, and higher pulse-repetition frequencies also reduce apparent jet area. In addition, the area of a given jet will appear different on different ultrasound systems. Careful adjustment and annotation of instrument settings are needed.

16. Taylor AL, Eichhorn EJ, Brickner ME, et al: Aortic valve morphology: An important in vitro determinant of proximal regurgitant jet width by Doppler color flow mapping. J Am Coll Cardiol 16:405–412, 1990.
    In an in vitro model using simulated degenerative, rheumatic, and bicuspid aortic valves, although jet width was related to valve area (p = 0.0001), bicuspid shapes had a smaller proximal jet width than circular, rheumatic, or degenerative orifices.

17. Chen C, Thomas JD, Anconina J, et al: Impact of impinging wall jet on color Doppler quantification of mitral regurgitation. Circulation 84:712–720, 1991.
    For the same regurgitant fraction, mitral regurgitant jets that impinge on a left atrial wall have smaller color Doppler jet areas (by 40 percent) than jets that are "free" within the chamber.

18. Thomas JD, O'Shea JP, Rodriguez L, et al: Impact of orifice geometry on the shape of jets: An in vitro Doppler color flow study. J Am Coll Cardiol 17:901–908, 1991.
    Jet momentum, defined as the product of the volume flow rate across the orifice, and velocity predict the appearance of jets in vitro. However, this approach assumes axial symmetry of the jet. In this paper, the authors use an in vitro model to show that jets from irregular orifices became nearly axisymmetrical within a few orifice diameters of jet origin.

19. Cape EG, Yoganathan AP, Weyman AE, Levine RA: Adjacent solid boundaries alter the size of regurgitant jets on Doppler color flow maps. J Am Coll Cardiol 17:1094–1102, 1991.
    Influence of impinging walls on jet geometry and area is described. Jets deflected toward adjacent walls have smaller jet areas than jets that are centrally located in the receiving chamber.

20. Smith MD, Harrison MR, Pinton R, et al: Regurgitant jet size by transesophageal compared with transthoracic Doppler color flow imaging. Circulation 83:79–86, 1991.
    Color Doppler regurgitant jet areas appear larger from a transesophageal than from a transthoracic approach.

CLINICAL APPLICATIONS OF ECHO DOPPLER IN PATIENTS WITH VALVULAR REGURGITATION

21. Szlachcic J, Massie BM, Greenberg B, et al: Intertest variability of echocardiographic and chest x-ray measurements: Implications for decision making in patients with aortic regurgitation. J Am Coll Cardiol 7:1310–1317, 1986.

Excellent discussion of the factors affecting intertest variability in sequential examinations of cardiac size. The 95 percent level prediction limits were ± 8 mm for left ventricular dimensions and 12 percent for fractional shortening, so a difference greater than these limits indicates an interval change between studies.

22. Bonow RO, Lakatos E, Maron BJ, Epstein SE: Serial long-term assessment of the natural history of asymptomatic patients with chronic aortic regurgitation and normal left ventricular systolic function. Circulation 84:1625–1635, 1991.

Clinical study in 104 asymptomatic patients with aortic regurgitation demonstrating that the initial end-systolic dimensions, rate of change in end-systolic dimension, and resting ejection fraction are predictive of long-term outcome.

23. Biem HJ, Detsky AS, Armstrong PW: Management of asymptomatic chronic aortic regurgitation with left ventricular dysfunction: A decision analysis. J Gen Intern Med 5:394–401, 1990.

Review of the literature on timing of aortic valve replacement in chronic asymptomatic aortic regurgitation emphasizing echo parameters. Convincing decision analysis suggests that an "early surgical approach" (when end-systolic dimension exceeds 55 mm or onset of left ventricular systolic dysfunction) is preferable to "late surgery" (onset of symptoms) based on quality-adjusted life years.

24. Reed D, Abbott RD, Smucker ML, Kaul S: Prediction of outcome after mitral valve replacement in patients with symptomatic chronic mitral regurgitation: The importance of left atrial size. Circulation 84:23–24, 1991.

Clinical study in 176 patients who underwent mitral valve replacement shows that preoperative pulmonary rales, left atrial size, and the ratio of end-systolic left ventricular wall thickness to chamber dimension are predictive of mortality postoperatively (follow-up 3.8 ± 0.5 years).

25. Sheikh KH, Bengtson JR, Rankin JS, et al: Intraoperative transesophageal Doppler color flow imaging used to guide patient selection and operative treatment of ischemic mitral regurgitation. Circulation 84:594–604, 1991.

Use of intraoperative transesophageal echo in 246 patients undergoing surgery for coronary artery disease resulted in a change in operative management in 27 patients (11 percent) due to finding less mitral regurgitation by echo versus cath-eterization (n = 22) so that valve replacement was not needed or to finding more severe mitral regurgitation (n = 5) necessitating valve replacement.

26. Stewart WJ, Currie PJ, Salcedo EE, et al: Intraoperative Doppler color flow mapping for decision-making in valve repair for mitral regurgitation: Technique and results in 100 patients. Circulation 81:556–566, 1990.

Intraoperative echo in 100 patients undergoing mitral valve repair showed a satisfactory repair in 92, persistent significant mitral regurgitation in 4, dynamic outflow obstruction in 3, and a persistent flail leaflet in 1 patient. Further mitral valve surgery was performed at the same operation in 6 of the 8 patients with unsatisfactory results; the other 2 required reoperation for persistent regurgitation.

27. Weisenbaugh T, Skudicky D, Sareli P: Prediction of outcome after valve replacement for rheumatic mitral regurgitation in the era of chordal preservation. Circulation 89:191–197, 1994.

In 61 patients with rheumatic mitral regurgitation, preoperative end-systolic diameter was the only independent predictor of postoperative death. There was an increased probability of death or severe heart failure with a preoperative end-systolic diameter greater than 50 mm, with a 98 percent accuracy of this breakpoint for predicting outcome.

28. Tischler MD, Cooper KA, Rowen R, LeWinter MM: Mitral valve replacement versus mitral valve repair: A Doppler and quantitative stress echocardiographic study. Circulation 89:132–137, 1994.

Exercise Doppler and quantitative 2D echocardiographic studies were performed in 10 patients pre- and postmitral valve repair and in 10 matched subjects undergoing mitral valve replacement. In patients with mitral valve repair, end-systolic circumferential wall stress was lower at rest and with exercise, ejection fraction was higher, and the left ventricle was less spherical than in patients with mitral valve replacement.

ALTERNATE APPROACHES TO EVALUATION OF VALVULAR REGURGITATION

29. Kandath D, Nanda NC, Miller DD, et al: Aortic regurgitation: The role of echocardiography, radionuclide imaging, and nuclear magnetic resonance imaging in its assessment (Parts I–III). Curr Prob Cardiol 15:39–114, 1990.

Review of assessment of aortic regurgitation by radionuclide and MRI, as well as echo Doppler techniques.

30. Grossman W, Baim DS: Cardiac Catheterization, Angiography and Interventions, 4th ed. Lea & Febiger, Philadelphia, 1991.

Textbook of cardiac catheterization techniques emphasizing clinical applications. Chapters on hemodynamic principles and profiles in valvular heart disease are especially helpful.

CHAPTER 11

ECHOCARDIOGRAPHIC EVALUATION OF PROSTHETIC VALVE DYSFUNCTION

INTRODUCTION

Echocardiographic evaluation of prosthetic valves is similar, in many respects, to evaluation of native valvular disease. However, there are some important dissimilarities. First, there are several different types of prosthetic valves with differing fluid dynamics for each basic design and differing flow velocities for each valve size. Second, the mechanisms of valve dysfunction are somewhat different from those for native

valve disease. Third, the technical aspects of imaging artificial devices—specifically the problem of acoustic shadowing—significantly affect the diagnostic approach when prosthetic valve dysfunction is suspected (Table 11–1).

Echocardiographers increasingly are asked to evaluate prosthetic valve function, given the increasing number of prosthetic valves implanted annually and the increasing longevity of patients with prosthetic valves. Both an understanding of the basic approach to echocardiographic evalua-

279

TABLE 11–1. COMPARISON OF DIFFERENT VALVE TYPES

	NORMAL NATIVE VALVE	BIOPROSTHESIS	MECHANICAL VALVE
Fluid dynamics	Central orifice, laminar flow, blunt flow profile	Central orifice, laminar flow, blunt flow profile	Complex fluid dynamics depending on valve type
Antegrade velocity	Normal	Increased	Increased
Normal regurgitation	Mild, central	Mild, central	Mild, oblique jets
Mechanisms of dysfunction	Multiple	Tissue degeneration, endocarditis, pannus ingrowth, sewing ring dehiscence	Mechanical failure, endocarditis, pannus ingrowth, thrombus, sewing ring dehiscence
Technical aspects of imaging	Calcification may cause acoustic shadows in some cases	Acoustic shadow from sewing ring	Extensive reverberations and acoustic shadowing

tion (as outlined in this chapter) and detailed knowledge of the specific flow dynamic for the size and type of prosthesis in an individual patient (which may require additional reference sources) are needed for appropriate patient management.

BASIC PRINCIPLES

Types of Prosthetic Valves and Fluid Dynamics (Fig. 11–1)

The three basic types of prosthetic valves are (1) tissue valves, or bioprostheses, (2) homograft valves, and (3) mechanical valves (Table 11–2).

Bioprosthetic Valves

Tissue valves are composed of three biologic leaflets with an anatomic structure similar to the native aortic valve. Valve leaflets (heterografts, typically porcine), or pericardium (usually bovine) shaped to mimic normal leaflets are mounted on a cloth-covered metal support that functions as the crown-shaped aortic annulus with a raised "stent" at each of the three commissures. Variations in the support structure and leaflet types abound in commercially available valves. Examples include Carpentier-Edwards porcine valves, Hancock porcine valves, Ionescu-Shiley bovine pericardial valves, and Carpentier-Edwards pericardial valves. However, all these tissue valves are similar in that the trileaflet valve opens to a circular orifice (in systole in the aortic position or in diastole in the

mitral position). The normal flow pattern is similar to that of a native valve, specifically laminar flow with a relatively blunt flow profile. Regardless of valve type, the orientation of a mitral prosthesis valve results in the inflow stream being directed anteriorly and medially toward the ventricular septum in most patients instead of toward the ventricular apex, as is seen for normal native valves (Fig. 11–2). This results in a reversed vortex of blood flow in middiastole, as seen in an apical four-chamber view (Fig. 11–3).

Tissue valves also differ from native valves in the presence of the support structure, which both (1) limits acoustic access and (2) results in a "normal" valve area that is smaller than the native valve (with corresponding higher "normal" antegrade flow velocities) due to limitation of the flow area by the supporting structure. As is seen with native valves, a small degree of valve regurgitation is found in a high percentage of normally functioning bioprosthetic valves.

Homograft Valves

Homograft valves are cryopreserved human aortic valves harvested at autopsy. Typically, the valve, ascending aorta, and anterior mitral leaflet are preserved as a block, to be trimmed appropriately at the time of implantation. Aortic homografts are used in the aortic or pulmonic position and in valved conduits but are rarely utilized for an atrioventricular valve replacement (since a supporting prosthetic structure would be needed). While the fluid dynamics of a homograft are similar to those of a native valve, flow velocities are slightly higher and valve areas slightly smaller than for a normal native valve

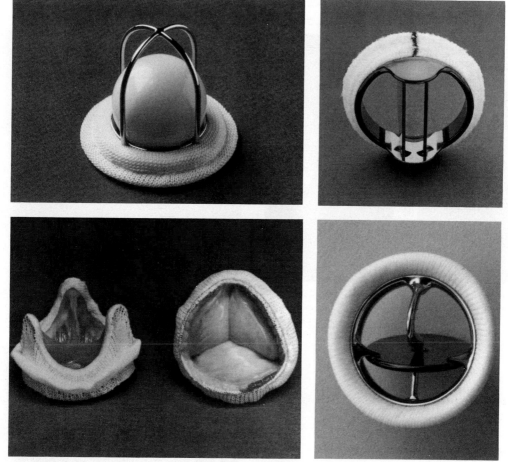

Figure 11–1. Photographs of four different prosthetic valves: a ball-cage type valve (Starr-Edward mitral, *above, left*), a tissue valve (Carpentier-Edward™ aortic, *below, left*), a bileaflet mechanical valve (St. Jude Medical™ heart valve, *above, right*), and a tilting-disk valve (Medtronic Hall™ valve, *below, right*). (*Photographs supplied courtesy of Baxter Healthcare Corporation, Santa Ana, CA; St. Jude Medical, St. Paul, MN; and Medtronic, Inc. Minneapolis, MN.*)

TABLE 11–2. EXAMPLES OF VALVE TYPES AND NAMES

I.	Homografts	Cryopreserved by tissue bank
II.	Heterografts	
	A. Porcine	Carpentier-Edwards Hancock
	B. Bovine pericardium	Ionescu-Shiley
	C. Pericardial	Carpentier-Edwards
III.	Mechanical	
	A. Ball-cage	Starr-Edwards
	B. Floating-disk	Beall (no longer used)
	C. Tilting-disk	Omniscience Bjork-Shiley
	D. Bileaflet	St. Jude

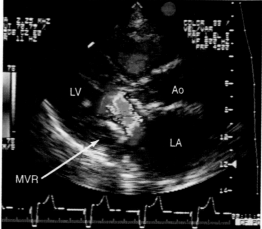

Figure 11–2. Normal left ventricular inflow pattern across a porcine mitral valve replacement (MVR) in the parasternal long-axis view. The flowstream is directed toward the ventricular septum. The flow velocity is greater than the Nyquist limit, so flow toward the transducer is displayed in blue.

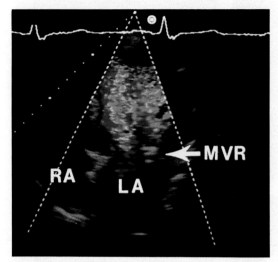

Figure 11–3. Apical four-chamber view in a patient with a porcine mitral valve replacement (MVR) showing color flow toward the apex along the ventricular septum with flow toward the base along the lateral wall—the opposite of the normal pattern shown in Figure 2–41.

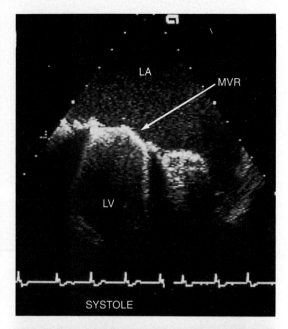

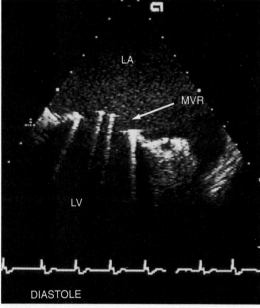

Figure 11–4. Bileaflet mitral valve prosthesis seen in systole (*above*) and diastole (*below*) from a transesophageal approach. In systole, the two leaflets close with a slightly obtuse closure angle. In diastole, the sewing ring and two parallel open leaflets are seen. Reverberations from the leaflets and shadowing from the sewing ring are prominent in both systole and diastole.

due to the space occupied by the homograft annulus in the patient's outflow tract.

Mechanical Valves

A wide variety of mechanical valves currently are available. In addition, several other types of valves, which were implanted in the past, are still in site in some patients. The basic types of mechanical valves are (1) a ball-cage valve in which a spherical occluder is contained by a metal "cage" when the valve is open and fills the orifice in the closed position (like on a snorkle), (2) a tilting-disk valve where a single circular disk opens at an angle to the annulus plane, being constrained in its motion by a smaller "cage," a central strut, or a slanted slot in the valve ring, and (3) a bileaflet valve where two hemicircular disks hinge open to form two large lateral orifices and a smaller central orifice (Fig. 11–4).

Antegrade Flow Profiles. As might be expected, the spatial flow profiles across each of these valve types vary substantially, and none is analogous to flow across the normal native valve. With a ball-cage valve in the open position, blood flows across the sewing ring and around the ball occluder on all sides. When the valve closes, a small amount of regurgitation is seen circumferentially around the ball as it seats in the sewing ring.

The fluid dynamics of a tilting-disk valve are characterized by two orifices in the open position, one larger than the other (major versus minor), with an asymmetrical flow profile as blood accelerates along the tilted surface of the open disk. Subtle variations in this flow pattern depend on the shape of the disk (convex versus concave surface) as well as the sewing ring design.

Bileaflet mechanical valves have complex fluid dynamics which affect the Doppler echocardiographic evaluation of these valves. With the leaflets open, there are two large lateral valve orifices with a small narrow central "slitlike" orifice. The flow velocity profile shows three peaks corresponding to these three orifices, with higher velocities in the center of each orifice. Of note, the local acceleration forces within the narrow central orifice result in localized high-pressure gradients in this region of the valve. These local gradients often are substantially higher than the overall pressure gradient across the valve.

Normal Mechanical Valve Regurgitation. With a tilting-disk valve, when the disk closes to occlude the valve annulus, regurgitation occurs at the closure line with the major regurgitant jet directed away from the sewing ring at the edge of the major orifice (Fig. 11–5). Note that the orientation of the prosthetic valve in the annulus can be variable, depending on surgical preference, so that the open disk position and the orientation of the regurgitant jet may be variable. Additional smaller regurgitant jets circumferentially around the annulus also may be present normally. With a single-disk valve and a central strut (e.g., Medtronic-Hall), a small central jet of regurgitation also occurs around the central hole of the disk, as might be expected. When a bileaflet valve closes, two crisscross jets of regurgitation are seen in the plane parallel to the leaflet opening plane. In the perpendicular plane, two smaller diverging regurgitant jets are seen. The total volume of regurgitation is small with normal prosthetic valve function.

Valved Conduits

Valved conduits are used in congenital heart surgery and in ascending aortic repairs when both a new passageway for blood flow and a valve are needed. The conduit may be biologic (i.e., a homograft) or artificial (i.e., Gore-Tex or Dacron) material. A conduit may incorporate either a tissue or a mechanical valve with fluid dynamics similar to those for a valve implanted in the native annulus.

Mechanisms of Prosthetic Valve Dysfunction

The types of disease processes that affect prosthetic valves are distinctly different from native valvular heart disease.

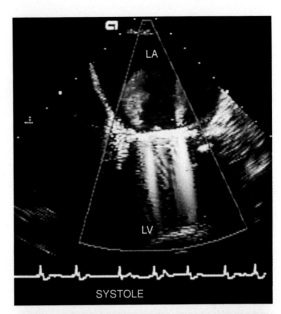

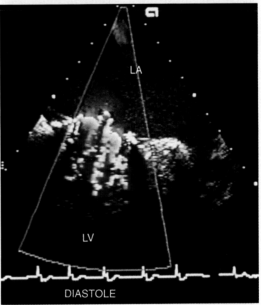

Figure 11–5. Color flow image in systole (*above*) of a bileaflet mitral valve prosthesis showing two normal jets of regurgitation. In diastole (*below*), acceleration of flow across the valve is seen with two large lateral orifices and a small central orifice.

Tissue Degeneration

Failure of a bioprosthetic valve to open or close properly (mechanical failure) usually is the result of slowly progressive tissue degeneration with fibrocalcific changes of the leaflets resulting in increased resistance to opening (stenosis) or failure to coapt during valve closure (regurgitation). Acute bioprosthetic valve stenosis is rare. Acute bioprosthetic regurgitation can occur with a leaflet tear, usually adjacent to a region of calcification. Occasionally, these patients present with the sudden onset of a "honking noise in my chest" and no other symptoms.

Mechanical Failure

Failure of a mechanical valve can occur due to faulty design or wear and tear of the prosthetic material resulting in disk escape or incomplete valve closure. More often, mechanical valve stenosis or regurgitation is due to thrombus formation or pannus ingrowth around the valve, impairing disk excursion or closure.

Paraprosthetic Regurgitation

With both bioprosthetic and mechanical valves, paravalvular regurgitation can occur around the sewing ring due to loss of suture material postoperatively, most often related to fibrocalcific disease in the valve annulus. The new onset of paravalvular regurgitation late after surgery raises the possibility of an infectious process (endocarditis) resulting in valve dehiscence.

Prosthetic Valve Endocarditis

Infection of a valve prosthesis is a serious clinical problem, so suspected endocarditis is a frequent indication for echocardiography in patients with prosthetic valves. Endocarditis on a bioprosthesis may result in vegetations similar to those seen on a native valve. However, with a mechanical valve, the infection often is paravalvular, and no vegetation may be present.

Technical Aspects of Echo Evaluation

The most technically limiting aspect of echocardiographic evaluation of prosthetic valves is the problem of acoustic shadowing. The sewing rings of both bioprosthetic and mechanical valves and the occluders of mechanical valves are strong echo reflectors, resulting in acoustic shadows and reverberations (Fig. 11–6). These reverberations and shadows obscure the motion of the valve structures themselves and block visualization of two-dimensional (2D) or Doppler abnormalities in the acoustic shadow region. During the examination, considerable effort is directed toward utilizing windows and views that avoid these imaging artifacts. Transesophageal echocardiography is particularly useful in evaluation of prosthetic mitral valves because it provides

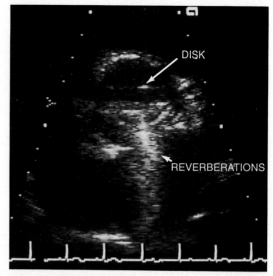

Figure 11–6. Parasternal short-axis view of a bileaflet mechanical aortic valve in systole. The anterior disk is seen as a clear line. The posterior disk and posterior sewing ring are obscured by reverberations from the valve.

acoustic access from the left atrial side of the valve.

ECHOCARDIOGRAPHIC APPROACH

2D/M-Mode Imaging

Bioprosthetic Valves

Normal. An aortic homograft appears similar to a native aortic valve except for some increased thickness in the left ventricular outflow tract and the ascending aorta at the proximal and distal suture sites (Fig. 11–7). Typically, the homograft is positioned inside the patient's native aorta with appropriate trimming to maintain patency of the coronary ostia. Less often a segment of aortic root is resected and replaced by the homograft with reimplantation of the coronary arteries. In patients with endocarditis, the attached anterior mitral leaflet of the homograft may be used to patch a ventricular septal defect or abscess cavity. The echocardiographic appearance of a homograft on 2D and M-mode evaluations is very similar to that of a native aortic valve, except for the associated surgical changes. Standard parasternal long- and short-axis image planes provide optimal visualization of valve leaflet anatomy and motion.

Heterograft leaflet or pericardial tissue prosthetic valves have a trileaflet structure similar to a native aortic valve. However, the echogenic

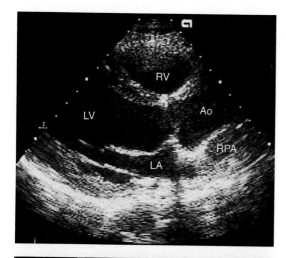

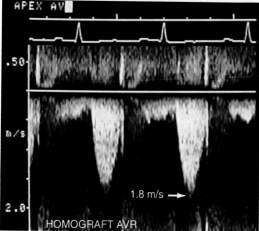

Figure 11–7. Aortic valve homograft in a parasternal long-axis view showing an appearance similar to a native valve other than thickening and increased echogenicity of the aortic root. Continuous-wave Doppler shows a mildly increased antegrade velocity across the homograft compared with a native valve. RPA = right pulmonary artery.

sewing ring and struts may limit visualization of the leaflets on 2D imaging. An M-mode through the leaflets shows the typical "boxlike" opening in systole (for the aortic position) or diastole (for the mitral position) as is seen with a normal native aortic valve. Particularly in the mitral position, improved images of the valve leaflets can be obtained from a transesophageal approach, since the ultrasound beam has a perpendicular orientation to the leaflets with no intervening structures from this approach. Transesophageal imaging of aortic prostheses is less rewarding because the posterior part of the sewing ring shadows the valve leaflets. Conversely, the anterior part of the sewing ring shadows the leaflets from a transthoracic approach. When images of the leaflets themselves are suboptimal, Doppler data

can provide valuable information. The specific 2D echo appearance of the supporting structures of bioprosthetic valves varies with the specific model. Since there is marked variability in surgeons' valve preferences, it is helpful to obtain photographs of the valves most commonly encountered at your institution. For example, a Carpentier-Edwards porcine valve has three prominent struts on 2D short-axis imaging (Fig. 11–8).

Leaflet Degeneration. Bioprosthetic valves have an average longevity of 10 years, with slowly progressive tissue failure being the primary reason for reoperation. Typically, the leaflet develops fibrocalcific changes which result in leaflet deformity (resulting in regurgitation) and/or increased stiffness (resulting in stenosis). Echocardiographically, increased echogenicity and irregularity of the leaflets may be noted, although images of the leaflets often are suboptimal due to shadowing and reverberation.

Mechanical Valves

2D and M-mode imaging of mechanical valves from a transthoracic approach is frustrating because of severe reverberations and acoustic shadowing. While the 2D images may provide clues as to the type of valve prostheses (e.g., "low-profile" bileaflet or tilting-disk valve versus "high-profile" ball-cage valve), obviously it is simpler to ascertain the exact valve type and size from the patient's medical record or valve ID card. Assessing motion of the valve occluder often is

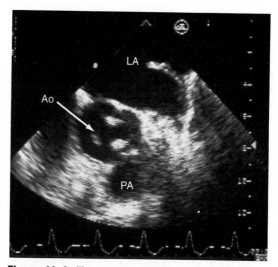

Figure 11–8. Transesophageal view of a porcine aortic valve replacement in a short-axis view showing the three normal stents that support the valve leaflets.

difficult. For example, the leading edge of a tilting-disk valve results in a strong reverberation across the 2D image obscuring motion of the disk itself. In addition, an oblique image plane often is obtained relative to the prosthetic valve, since orientation of the prosthesis within the annulus is not standard. With a tomographic plane perpendicular to the open bileaflet valve, the two leaflets can be identified clearly, but this image plane may be difficult to achieve.

Technical limitations make identification of prosthetic valve endocarditis or thrombosis problematic because the abnormalities may be obscured by reverberations or hidden by acoustic shadowing. Transesophageal imaging can be helpful in identifying thrombus or infected vegetations on the atrial side of a mitral prosthesis, since the left atrium is "masked" by the prosthetic valve from both parasternal and apical windows. In a patient with a mechanical aortic valve, the subaortic region can be evaluated well from a transthoracic approach from parasternal and apical windows. In this situation, transesophageal images are less helpful due to shadowing of the outflow tract by the posterior aspect of the prosthesis.

While M-mode patterns of occluder motion have been described for both normally and abnormally functioning mechanical valves, the use of M-mode largely has been supplanted by evaluation of prosthetic valve hemodynamics with Doppler echocardiography. M-mode tracings remain helpful in verifying rapid independent motion of structures attached to the prosthetic valve seen on 2D imaging that may represent vegetations or thrombus formation.

Valved Conduits

The 2D and M-mode evaluation of a bioprosthetic or mechanical valve in a conduit (e.g., right ventricular to pulmonary artery) may be difficult due to ultrasound attenuation by the conduit prosthetic material. Of note, stenosis in a valved conduit can occur as a result of stenosis of the valve prosthesis or fibrotic ingrowth along the length of the conduit. In addition, residual or progressive stenosis at the proximal or distal anastomosis site can occur. Evaluation of narrowing in the conduit is difficult with 2D imaging, but a careful Doppler examination may allow detection of this diagnosis. Continuous-wave Doppler is used to assess the maximum flow velocity, while pulsed Doppler or high-pulse-repetition-frequency (HPRF) Doppler is used to localize the level of obstruction along the length of the conduit.

Doppler Evaluations

Normal Doppler Findings

Prosthetic Valve "Clicks." The motion of the occluder of a mechanical valve (or the tissue leaflets of a biologic valve) creates a brief intense Doppler signal that appears as a dark narrow band of short duration on the spectral display (Fig. 11–9). Audibly, this signal is similar to the valve "click" appreciated on auscultation. However, unlike on auscultation, usually both opening and closing valve clicks are seen on spectral Doppler analysis. The Doppler signals associated with valve opening and closing are similar to those seen with native valves but are of greater intensity. The motion of the occluder also may result in color flow artifacts, with color signals covering large areas of the 2D sector that are inconsistent from beat to beat.

Antegrade Velocities/Pressure Gradients. Compared with a normal native valve, all prosthetic valves are inherently stenotic to some extent. Specifically, the expected antegrade velocities and pressure gradients across a normally functioning prosthetic valve are higher than the corresponding values for a native valve. Similarly, the effective orifice area of a prosthetic valve is smaller than the orifice area of a normal native valve.

The expected velocities, pressure gradients, and valve areas depend on the specific type, size, and position of the prosthetic valve. While manufacturers have data on in vitro flow characteristics for each valve, in vivo echocardiographic

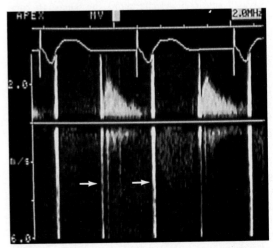

Figure 11–9. Left ventricular inflow across a mechanical mitral valve replacement showing an increased antegrade velocity (compared with a native valve) and prominent valve clicks (*arrows*).

TABLE 11–3. NORMAL DOPPLER DATA FOR PROSTHETIC AORTIC VALVES

VALVE TYPE	SIZE (mm)	V_{max} (m/s)	MEAN GRADIENT (mmHg)	VELOCITY RATIO	AVA (cm²)
Bileaflet (St. Jude)	19	3.0 (2.0–4.5)	20 (10–30)	0.37	1.0
	21	2.7 (2.5–3.5)	14 (10–30)	0.40	1.3
	23	2.5 (2.0–3.5)	12 (10–30)	0.37	1.3
	25	2.4 (2.0–3.5)	12 (5–30)	0.42	1.8
	27	2.2 (2.0–3.1)	11 (5–20)	0.46	2.4
	29	2.0 (2.0–2.5)	10 (5–15)	0.49	2.7
	31	2.1 (1.5–2.5)	10 (5–15)	0.49	3.1
Tilting-disk (Bjork-Shiley, Medtronic Hall)	19		21 ± 7		
	21	2.8 ± 0.9	16		
	23	2.6 ± 0.4	14 ± 5		
	25	2.1 ± 0.3	13 ± 3		
	27	1.9 ± 0.2	10 ± 3		
	29	1.9 ± 0.2	7 ± 6		
Ball-cage (Starr-Edwards)		3.1 ± 0.5	24 ± 4		
Porcine tissue (Hancock or Carpentier-Edwards)	19	2.8 ± 0.7	16 ± 2		1.5 ± 0.1
	21	2.6 ± 0.4	15 ± 6		1.8 ± 0.2
	23	2.6 ± 0.4	13 ± 6		2.1 ± 0.2
	25	2.5 ± 0.4	11 ± 2		
	27	2.4 ± 0.4	10 ± 1		
	29	2.4 ± 0.4	12		
Homograft		1.8 ± 0.4	7 ± 3		2.2 ± 0.8

Note: Values shown are mean ± 1 SD or mean (range). Velocity ratio = LV outflow velocity/aortic jet velocity.
References: Reisner et al: JASE 1:201, 1988; Zabalgoitia et al: Curr Prob Cardiol 5:271, 1992; Sagar et al: JACC 7:68, 1986; Baumgartner et al: Circ 82:1467, 1990; Chafizadeh et al: Circ 83:213, 1991; Jaffe et al: AJC 63:1466, 1989.

data are sparse owing to the large number of valve types and sizes. Even in a large study, only a few patients have the same valve type, position, and size. In the available Doppler studies of normal prosthetic valves, data often are presented in various ways. Some studies report the mean ± 1 SD for each variable; others include the range as well. While compilation of the normal values from all these studies is not possible from the published data, estimates of the expected normal velocities, pressure gradients, and valve areas for several commonly seen prosthetic valves are shown in Tables 11–3 and 11–4.

TABLE 11–4. NORMAL DOPPLER DATA FOR PROSTHETIC MITRAL VALVES

VALVE TYPE	V_{max} (m/s)	MEAN GRADIENT (mmHg)	$T_{1/2}$ (m/s)	MVA (cm²)
Bileaflet (St. Jude)	1.6 ± 0.3	4 ± 1	77 ± 17	2.9 ± 0.6
Tilting-disk (Bjork-Shiley)	1.6 ± 0.3	3 ± 2	90 ± 22	2.4 ± 0.6
Ball-cage (Starr-Edwards)	1.9 ± 0.5	5 ± 2	110 ± 27	2.0 ± 0.5
Porcine Tissue				
Ionescu-Shiley	1.5 ± 0.3	3 ± 1	93 ± 25	2.4 ± 0.8
Carpentier-Edwards	1.8 ± 0.2	6 ± 2	90 ± 25	2.5 ± 0.7
Hancock	1.5 ± 0.3	4 ± 2	129 ± 31	1.7 ± 0.4

Note: Values shown are mean ± 1 SD.
References: Reisner & Meltzer: JASE 1:201, 1988; Zabalgoitia: Curr Prob Cardiol 5:271, 1992.

Note that, in general, the larger the valve size, the lower are the velocities and gradients and the larger is the effective orifice area. In fact, many of the smaller prosthetic valves have hemodynamics that are consistent with clinical stenosis even with normal valve function. Also note the different expected velocities with different valve types. Typically, mechanical valves have better hemodynamics at small valve sizes (the apparent discrepancies in the data for bileaflet valves are discussed below) than do bioprosthetic valves. The significant exception is the aortic homograft valve, which has excellent hemodynamics over the entire size range. Finally, note that mitral valve prostheses have lower velocities and pressure gradients than aortic valve prostheses due, in part, to larger valve sizes but also to passive flow at a lower pressure gradient from the atrium and ventricle in diastole compared with active ejection and a higher left ventricular to aortic pressure gradient in systole.

As indicated by the ranges and standard deviations in the tables, there is a wide range of reported "normal" values for a given prosthetic valve type and size. Anatomic features and the details of implantation in each patient may account for some of this variability. However, the impact of transvalvular volume flow rate on transvalvular velocities and pressure gradients should not be underestimated. Even with a normally functioning prosthesis, a high cardiac output (e.g., postoperative, pregnancy, or sepsis) results in a high velocity and pressure gradient. This variability in "normal" velocities can be compensated for by calculating effective orifice area to "correct" for volume flow rate. Alternatively, a pragmatic approach is to obtain a baseline Doppler echo study in each patient after valve replacement (but not in the immediate postoperative period). The values obtained then serve as the "normal" reference for that patient. This facilitates detection of changes in prosthetic valve function over time, with each patient serving as his or her own control.

Normal Regurgitation. Normal prosthetic valve function implies a small degree of valvular regurgitation in virtually all mechanical valves and in a high percentage (30 to 50 percent) of bioprosthetic valves. The patterns of regurgitation detected correspond to the fluid dynamics of each valve type (see above). Color flow imaging shows the spatial distribution of normal prosthetic regurgitation with patterns specific to each valve type. On a transthoracic study, it may be difficult to separate normal from pathologic prosthetic regurgitation, especially for the mitral position. Transesophageal imaging may

be needed if pathologic regurgitation is suspected. On color flow imaging, normal prosthetic regurgitation tends to be a uniform color with little variance, whereas pathologic regurgitation shows aliasing and variance with a "confetti-like" appearance to the flow pattern. On pulsed and continuous-wave Doppler examination, normal prosthetic regurgitation has a low signal strength, may persist through only part of the cardiac cycle, and is spatially localized (see Fig. 11–12).

Prosthetic Valve Stenosis

Pressure Gradients. The principles applied to evaluation of native valve stenosis also have been utilized for suspected stenosis of prosthetic valves. From a continuous-wave Doppler recording of the antegrade velocity across the valve, obtained at a parallel intercept angle, maximum instantaneous and mean pressure gradients can be calculated using the Bernoulli equation ($4v^2$). Although the maximum velocity across a prosthetic valve is higher than that for a native valve, the shape of the velocity curve is triangular (in contrast to the rounded contour seen in aortic stenosis). Thus the calculated mean gradient typically is less for a prosthetic valve than for a native valve with the same maximum antegrade velocity (Fig. 11–10).

Maximum and mean pressure gradients across bioprosthetic valves calculated by Doppler echo compare well with directly measured pressure gradients (Table 11–5). The situation is more complex for mechanical valves because of the

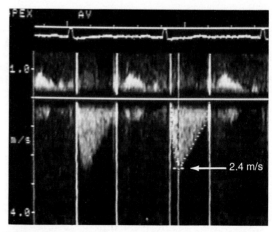

Figure 11–10. Antegrade velocity across a normal aortic valve replacement. The antegrade velocity is increased compared with a native valve, the shape of the flow curve is triangular, and prominent prosthetic valve clicks are present.

TABLE 11–5. VALIDATION OF DOPPLER ECHO PROSTHETIC MEAN VALVE GRADIENTS COMPARED WITH INVASIVE DATA (SELECTED SERIES)

FIRST AUTHOR, YEAR	VALVE TYPE/ POSITION	*n*	*r*	SEE (mmHg)	MEAN DIFFERENCE
Sagar, 1986	Hancock & B.S./ mitral	19	0.93	2.5	
Sagar, 1986	Hancock & B.S./ aortic	11	0.94	7.4	
Wilkins, 1986	Starr-Edwards, B.S./porcine/ mitral	11	0.96	—	
Burstow, 1989	Mixed/aortic	20	0.94	3	
	Mixed/mitral	20	0.97	1.2	
Baumgartner, 1990	St. Jude	In vitro	0.98	1.9	10 ± 3 mmHg
	Hancock	In vitro	0.98	1.4	2 ± 1 mmHg
Stewart, 1991	Bioprosthetic/aortic	In vitro	0.78–0.98		Overestimation by Doppler
Baumgartner, 1992	St. Jude	In vitro	0.98	2.0	13 ± 8 mmHg
	Medtronic-Hull	In vitro	0.99	0.5	0.8 ± 0.6
	Starr-Edwards	In vitro	0.97	2.0	8 ± 4 mmHg
	Hancock	In vitro	0.99	1.5	1.9 ± 1.6

B.S. = Bjork-Shiley tilting-disk mechanical valve.
References as in Suggested Reading.

differing fluid dynamics of each type of prosthesis. In theory, the pressure gradient across a given degree of stenosis will be identical whether the stenosis consists of a single orifice or multiple orifices, with the Bernoulli relationship being valid for each orifice. Thus a maximum pressure gradient of 36 mmHg will correspond to a single or multiple 3 m/s jets across the valve. However, while this theory holds true when local acceleration and viscous forces can be ignored, local higher-pressure gradients do occur with some valve types. This phenomenon has been studied most thoroughly for the bileaflet valve.

With the valve leaflets open, the bileaflet valve has a narrow, slitlike central orifice flanked by two larger semicircular orifices (Fig. 11–11). The walls of this narrow central orifice are formed by the parallel valve disks, which are nearly perpendicular to the sewing ring of the valve. Within this narrow central flowstream, acceleration forces result in a localized high-pressure gradient (and corresponding high velocity) with rapid pressure recovery distal to the valve. Thus, the pressure difference measured between the upstream side of the valve and this central orifice is greater than the pressure difference between the upstream and downstream sides of the valve. Since continuous-wave Doppler ultrasound records the highest velocity along the length of the ultrasound beam, it is this higher localized velocity that is recorded. While this high localized gradient is measured correctly, the gradient of interest is the upstream-to-downstream valve gradient. Thus, even though the correlation between Doppler and invasive pressure gradient measurements is

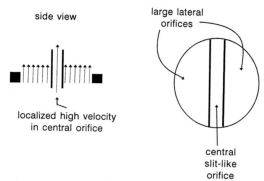

Bi-leaflet Mechanical Valve

Figure 11–11. Schematic drawing of a bileaflet mechanical valve in the open position in side (*left*) and frontal (*right*) views. Two large lateral orifices flank a central slit-like orifice which is associated with localized high-velocity flow (and a localized pressure gradient).

high, the slope of the regression line indicates that the Doppler approach consistently "overestimates" the overall transvalvular gradient. This overestimation is large enough that an erroneous diagnosis of severe stenosis might be made if this phenomenon is not recognized.

Interestingly, the overestimation of pressure gradients across bileaflet valves becomes less significant in the presence of prosthetic valve stenosis. The proposed mechanism for this observation is a gradual reduction in the size of the central orifice as leaflet opening is reduced. Clinically, this poses a dilemma in that a high velocity across a bileaflet valve might represent overestimation of the pressure gradient with normal valve function or a correct estimate of a high gradient with a stenotic valve. Again, a baseline study in the postoperative period provides a standard of comparison when subsequent valve dysfunction is suspected.

Valve Areas. Even when accurately measured, the physiologic limitation of transvalvular velocities across prosthetic valves is that velocities vary with volume flow rate for a given orifice area. A normally functioning valve prosthesis in an individual patient may have a high transvalvular velocity if cardiac output is elevated (e.g., with exercise, anemia, fever) or a low transvalvular velocity if cardiac output is depressed (e.g., left ventricular dysfunction). For these reasons, a flow-independent measure of prosthetic valve function is more useful clinically.

AORTIC. Bioprosthetic aortic valves have fluid dynamics similar to those of a native aortic valve, and it is logical to assume that continuity equation valve area calculations are valid in this situation (Fig. 11–12). In fact, direct comparisons of Doppler echo (AVA_{prost}) and invasive valve areas in patients with suspected stenosis of bioprosthetic aortic valves have shown a reasonable correlation. As for a native aortic valve, the components of the continuity equation are the left ventricular outflow tract velocity-time integral (VTI_{LVOT}), the left ventricular outflow tract cross-sectional area (CSA_{LVOT}), and the aortic jet velocity-time integral (VTI_{Ao}). The continuity equation, then, is

$$AVA_{prost} = \frac{CSA_{LVOT} \times VTI_{LVOT}}{VTI_{Ao}}$$

Left ventricular outflow tract velocity is recorded from an apical approach using pulsed Doppler echo with the sample volume positioned proximal to the prosthetic valve, avoiding the small region of flow acceleration immediately adjacent to the valve. Aortic jet velocity is

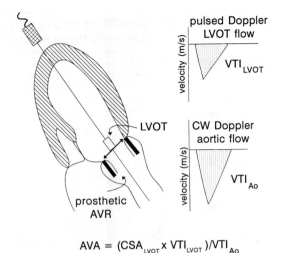

$$AVA = (CSA_{LVOT} \times VTI_{LVOT})/VTI_{Ao}$$

Figure 11–12. The continuity equation can be used for calculation of aortic valve area (AVA) for an aortic valve replacement (AVR). Left ventricular outflow tract (LVOT) flow is recorded from an apical approach using pulsed Doppler with the sample volume positioned just proximal to the prosthetic valve. LVOT diameter is measured from a parasternal long-axis view for calculation of a circular cross-sectional area (CSA) of flow. Continuous-wave (CW) Doppler is used to record the flow signal across the prosthetic valve from whichever window yields the highest-velocity jet.

recorded with continuous-wave Doppler from whichever window gives the highest-velocity signal, as for native valve stenosis. Left ventricular outflow tract diameter is measured in a parasternal long-axis view in midsystole from the septal endocardium to the anterior mitral leaflet parallel to and immediately adjacent to the aortic valve (Fig. 11–13). Direct measurement of outflow tract diameter is preferable to use of the implanted prosthetic valve size, since valve size relates to the external diameter of the sewing ring, not the effective diameter of the subvalvular flow region. As usual, a circular cross-sectional left ventricular outflow tract area is calculated as $\pi(D/2)^2$ from this diameter measurement.

The use of the continuity equation for mechanical aortic valves is more problematic. Presumably, if the transvalvular velocity-time integral is an accurate reflection of transvalvular volume flow rate, then calculated valve areas should be accurate. Remember that the continuity equation assumes a flat flow velocity profile *in* the stenotic orifice (or vena contracta) as well as proximal to the valve. Clearly, this assumption is not true for bileaflet valves. The local high velocities in the central orifice will result in a significant error in measurement of volume

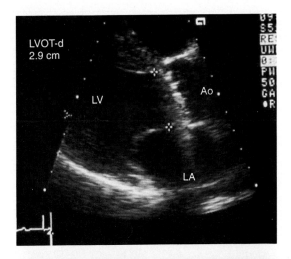

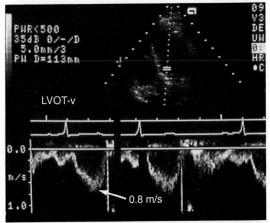

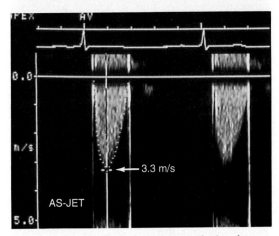

Figure 11–13. Continuity equation prosthetic valve area is calculated from a parasternal long-axis midsystolic diameter (2.9 cm) measurement (*above*), the pulsed Doppler left ventricular outflow tract velocity (0.8 m/s) recorded from an apical approach (*center*), and the continuous-wave Doppler signal of flow across the valve (3.3 m/s) recorded from whichever window gives the highest velocity (*below*). Even though the antegrade velocity is increased compared with a native valve, the calculated valve area is 1.6 cm².

flow rate across the valve orifice, with a consequent underestimation of valve area. However, for tilting-disk and ball-cage valves, limited data suggest that the continuity equation may be reasonably accurate, despite complex fluid dynamics, because the continuous-wave velocity signal provides an approximation of the spatial mean flow velocity across the valve (Table 11–6).

Another approach to evaluation of suspected prosthetic aortic valve stenosis is to measure the "step-up" in velocity across the valve. The ratio of the outflow tract velocity to aortic jet velocity reflects the degree of stenosis—if no obstruction is present, these velocities will be nearly equal with a ratio close to 1; as the degree of narrowing increases, the aortic jet velocity will increase with no change in outflow tract velocity resulting progressively in a ratio <1. Since all prosthetic valves are inherently stenotic to some degree, the "normal" velocity ratio across an aortic prosthesis ranges from 0.35 to 0.50, compared with 0.75 to 0.90 for a normal native aortic valve.

The advantages of the use of the velocity ratio are (1) it takes volume flow rate into account, (2) it does not require an outflow tract diameter measurement, (3) a baseline "normal" value can be established for comparison on follow-up studies, and (4) it is easily measured and reproducible. Some investigators advocate measuring the velocity ratio with increases in flow rate (e.g., with exercise) to increase its specificity in excluding prosthetic valve stenosis.

Pragmatically, even if Doppler velocities and continuity equation valve areas overestimate the degree of prosthetic valve stenosis, in an individual patient a *change* in velocity or valve area is valuable in patient management decisions. Again, a baseline study at a time when valve function is normal provides a reference point for subsequent studies.

MITRAL. Prosthetic mitral valve areas can be estimated using the pressure half-time approach as for native mitral valve stenosis (Fig. 11–14). The expected normal half-time for a prosthetic valve is longer than for a native valve, with the specific value depending on valve type and size. For bioprosthetic mitral valves, valve area can be estimated from the same formula as for native valves:

$$\text{MVA} = \frac{220}{T_{1/2}}$$

where the pressure half-time ($T_{1/2}$) is measured in milliseconds, as described in Chapter 9.

Somewhat surprisingly, the empirical con-

TABLE 11–6. VALIDATION OF DOPPLER ECHO PROSTHETIC VALVE AREAS (SELECTED SERIES)

FIRST AUTHOR, YEAR	VALVE TYPE/ POSITION	n	COMPARISON	r	SEE	MEAN DIFFERENCE
Sagar, 1986	Hancock & B.S./ mitral	12	$T_{1/2}$ vs. Gorlin	0.98	0.1 cm^2	
Wilkins, 1986	Porcine/mitral	8	$T_{1/2}$ vs. Gorlin	0.65	—	
Rothbart, 1990	Bioprosthetic/aortic	22	Cont eq vs. Gorlin at cath	0.93	—	—
Chafizadeh, 1991	St. Jude/aortic	67	Cont eq vs. actual orifice area	0.83	Doppler effective orifice area less than actual orifice area	
Baumgartner, 1992	St. Jude	In vitro	Cont eq vs.	0.99	0.08	0.4–0.6 cm^2
	Medtronic-Hall	In vitro	Gorlin	0.97	0.10	0–0.25 cm^2
	Hancock aortic	In vitro		0.93	0.10	0–0.25 cm^2

Note: B.S. = Bjork-Shiley tilting-disk mechanical valve; Cont eq = continuity equation valve area with Doppler and 2D echo data; Gorlin = Gorlin formula valve area using invasive data; $T_{1/2}$ = Doppler pressure half-time method.
References as in Suggested Reading.

stant 220 also appears to provide a reasonable approximation of mitral valve area for mechanical prostheses. With a bileaflet valve, the higher localized velocities in the central slitlike orifice affect the accuracy of pressure gradient calculations. However, the pressure half-time measurement is less affected because it depends on the *time course* of the velocity decline relative to the maximum velocity rather than on the velocities themselves.

Continuity equation valve area also can be calculated for a mitral prosthesis (in the absence of

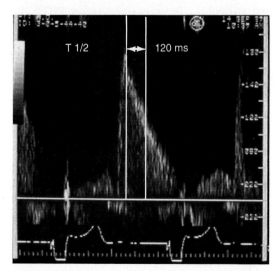

Figure 11–14. Pressure half-time for a mitral prosthetic valve is calculated as for a native valve. In this case, the $T_{1/2}$ is 120 ms.

mitral regurgitation) using the antegrade stroke volume across the aortic or pulmonic valve in the equation.

The antegrade velocity curve across a mitral bioprosthesis may be recorded from an apical approach using pulsed, high pulse-repetition frequency, or continuous-wave Doppler ultrasound. Care in positioning the transducer is needed because inflow may be directed obliquely into the ventricular chamber. Some echocardiographers find it helpful to use the color flow image to aid in alignment of the Doppler beam parallel to the inflow stream. In many patients after mitral valve replacement, the inflow stream is directed anteriorly and medially toward the ventricular septum. In these patients, a low parasternal window may provide an optimal intercept angle for recording antegrade velocity. As for native mitral valve stenosis, Doppler acquisition parameters are adjusted to show a smooth velocity deceleration slope and a band of velocity signals along the edge of the curve.

Prosthetic Valve Regurgitation

Detection of Regurgitation. The echocardiographic approaches described for evaluation of native valve regurgitation in Chapter 10 also apply to evaluation of prosthetic valve regurgitation. The major differences between evaluation of native or prosthetic valves are (1) the prosthetic valve has a higher antegrade velocity,

(2) the degree of normal prosthetic regurgitation is greater than the trivial amounts of native valve regurgitation seen in normal individuals, and (3) acoustic shadowing, reverberations, and beam width artifact make evaluation of a prosthetic valve more difficult and decrease the sensitivity of transthoracic echocardiography for detection of prosthetic regurgitation

Conventional pulsed Doppler can be used to detect prosthetic regurgitation, but a meticulous examination is needed with persistent repositioning of the sample volume in multiple views to detect the regurgitant signal. For the aortic valve, both parasternal and apical views are helpful because the sample volume is proximal to the valve prosthesis, avoiding the problem of acoustic shadowing. For the mitral valve, the parasternal approach is most helpful if a view can be obtained with the sample volume on the left atrial side of the valve but without the ultrasound beam transversing the prosthetic valve itself. Apical views may be limited due to acoustic shadowing, but occasionally, a paraprosthetic jet can be identified from this approach. If a suspicious signal is obtained, its timing should be assessed carefully (Fig. 11–15). Mitral regurgitation starts immediately after mitral valve closure, whereas aortic outflow starts slightly later (after isovolumic contraction). With loud prosthetic valve clicks and a low signal-to-noise ratio, it is easy to mistake normal left ventricular outflow for mitral regurgitation if signal timing is not examined.

Continuous-wave Doppler has the advantage of a wide beam size at the depth of a prosthetic valve and a high signal-to-noise ratio, enhancing the likelihood that a weaker signal or eccentric jet (i.e., paraprosthetic regurgitation) will be identified. Again, the timing of the presumed regurgitant signal is extremely important for correct identification of the origin of the Doppler signal. Many laboratories find it helpful to examine the prosthetic valve with continuous-wave Doppler starting with the ultrasound beam aligned in the flow direction of the valve and then slowly scanning in progressively larger circles to identify any potential paraprosthetic jets (Fig. 11–16).

Color Doppler flow imaging for prosthetic valve regurgitation can be helpful, particularly if a view can be obtained where the ultrasound beam has access to the chamber receiving the regurgitant flow without first transversing the valve prosthetic. Evaluation of an aortic valve prosthesis from a transthoracic approach often is diagnostic. The left ventricular outflow tract can be interrogated from both parasternal and apical approaches without shadowing by the valve prosthesis. However, color artifacts are prominent in patients with prosthetic valves, and transesophageal echocardiography may provide more accurate evaluation of prosthetic valve regurgitation (Fig. 11–17).

Especially for the mitral position, the transesophageal approach provides not only improved image quality but the opportunity to in-

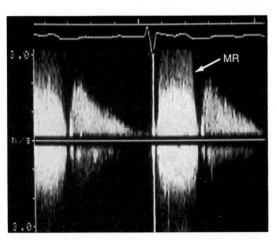

Figure 11–15. Continuous-wave Doppler recording of prosthetic mitral regurgitation obtained from an apical window. The regurgitant signal starts immediately following the mitral closure clock and continues up to the onset of antegrade flow across the prosthesis in diastole. The jet is eccentric and not parallel with the ultrasound beam, so flow signals appear as both sides of the baseline.

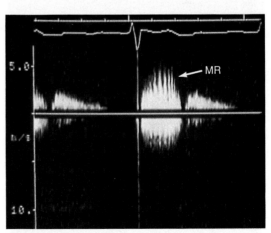

Figure 11–16. Continuous-wave Doppler signal from the same patient as in Figure 11–15 from a parasternal window. Again, a high-velocity signal is seen on both sides of the baseline due to an eccentric jet orientation. The patient's presenting complaint was a "honking noise in my chest." The prominent systolic striations in the Doppler signal were due to fluttering of a ruptured porcine valve cusp adjacent to a calcific nodule.

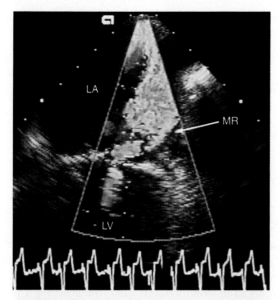

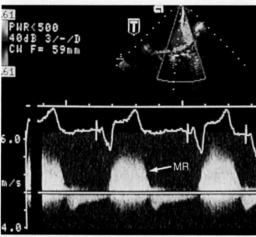

Figure 11–17. Transesophageal view of prosthetic mitral regurgitation with an eccentric jet seen on color flow imaging. Continuous-wave Doppler shows an intense, high-velocity regurgitant jet.

terrogate the valve from the left atrial side—i.e., the acoustic shadow now will obscure the left ventricle rather than the left atrium. Thus, when prosthetic mitral valve regurgitation is suspected, a transesophageal study should be considered. A transthoracic study showing prosthetic regurgitation can be clinically useful (high positive predictive value) but rarely allows for accurate quantitation of mitral regurgitant severity. A transthoracic study that does not show prosthetic regurgitation does not exclude this possibility (low negative predictive value).

Severity and Etiology of Prosthetic Regurgitation. When prosthetic regurgitation is detected, the first step in evaluation and inter-

pretation is whether "normal" or pathologic prosthetic regurgitation is present. While the normal backflow across the valve represents a small volume of blood, the color jets on transesophageal imaging can be fairly large in area. Distinguishing features are the characteristic pattern for each valve type, a uniform color pattern rather than the mosaic flow disturbance seen with pathologic regurgitation, and the absence of other features (increased antegrade velocity, chamber sizes and function, pulmonary hypertension) to suggest significant regurgitation (Figs. 11–18, 11–19, and 11–20).

Regurgitation of bioprosthetic valves most often is due to degenerative changes of the leaflets. This can be slowly progressive, with gradually increasing severity of a central regurgitant stream, or can occur abruptly, with cusp rupture adjacent to a fibrocalcific nodule. Regurgitant severity is graded as for a native valve by (1) the extent of the flow disturbance in the receiving chamber with color flow imaging, (2) evidence for distal flow reversal (e.g., descending aorta diastolic flow in aortic regurgitation), (3) the intensity and shape of the continuous-wave Doppler signal, and (4) associated Doppler and 2D findings (see below).

Mechanical valves can have prosthetic regurgitation due to incomplete closure resulting from pannus ingrowth around the sewing ring or from thrombus formation. Again, the flow disturbance will be larger than that seen with "normal" regurgitation, and severity can be quantitated by the usual approaches. Transesophageal imaging is helpful in identifying the etiology as well as the severity of regurgitation for prosthetic valves in the mitral position.

Paraprosthetic regurgitation is most common with mechanical valves but also can occur with bioprosthetic valves. Distinguishing prosthetic from paraprosthetic regurgitation is difficult on transthoracic imaging; in most cases, transesophageal echocardiography is needed. The etiology of paraprosthetic regurgitation may be a scarred and/or calcified annulus resulting in disruption of the sutures securing the valve or a paravalvular abscess with tissue destruction. The regurgitant jet originates external to the sewing ring, with an eccentric jet extending into the receiving chamber (see Figs. 11–18 to 11–20). A single or multiple paraprosthetic jets may be present. Color flow imaging may show proximal flow acceleration (on the left ventricular side of the mitral valve) into the regurgitant orifice, facilitating identification of the paraprosthetic origin of the signal. Immediately after implantation, a small degree of paraprosthetic

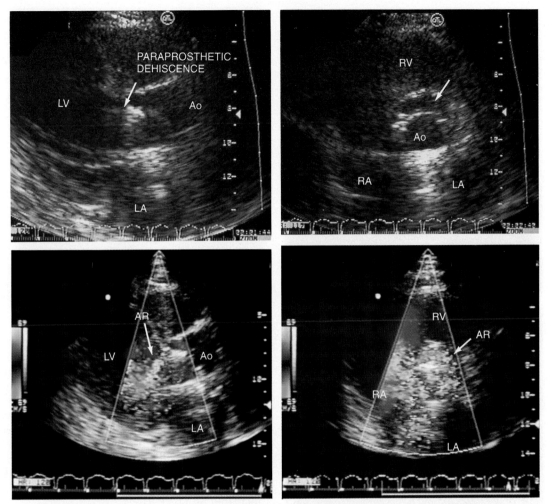

Figure 11–18. 2D (*above*) and color flow (*below*) images in parasternal long-axis (*left*) and short-axis (*right*) views in a patient with aortic valve dehiscence due to endocarditis and paraprosthetic aortic regurgitation. 2D imaging shows an echo-lucent space anterior to the sewing ring. Color flow imaging shows flow anterior to the prosthesis in a long-axis view with a circumferential pattern of regurgitation seen in the short-axis view.

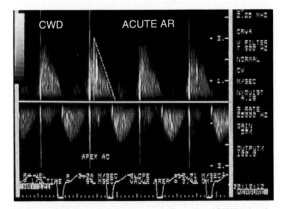

Figure 11–19. Continuous-wave Doppler (CWD) in the same patient as in Figure 11–18 shows an aortic regurgitant signal of equal intensity to antegrade flow with a steep deceleration slope consistent with acute, severe aortic regurgitation (AR).

regurgitation may be normal on intraoperative transesophageal echocardiography.

Other Echocardiographic Findings in Prosthetic Valve Dysfunction
(Table 11–7)

In addition to direct imaging or Doppler interrogation of the prosthetic valve itself, several other findings on the echocardiographic examination are integrated in the overall interpretation of prosthetic valve function.

1. The response of the cardiac chambers in terms of size, hypertrophy, and systolic function should be considered. For example, persistent

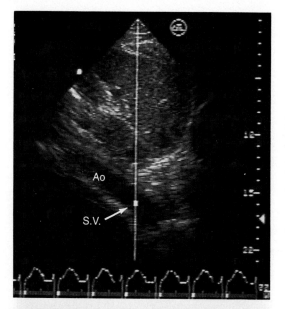

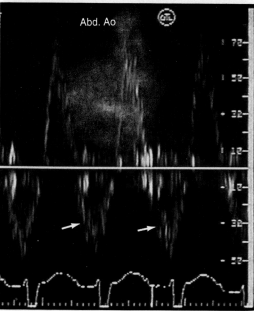

Figure 11–20. With a pulsed Doppler sample volume (SV) in the proximal abdominal aorta (*above*) in the same patient as in Figure 11–18, prominent holodiastolic (*arrow*) flow reversal (*below*) is seen, again consistent with severe aortic regurgitation.

TABLE 11–7. ECHOCARDIOGRAPHIC SIGNS OF PROSTHETIC VALVE DYSFUNCTION

Increased antegrade velocity across the valve

Decreased valve area (continuity equation or $T_{1/2}$)

Increased regurgitation on color flow

Increased intensity of continuous-wave Doppler regurgitant signal

Progressive chamber dilation

Persistent left ventricular hypertrophy

Recurrent pulmonary hypertension

---

ficult in some patients to separate persistent postoperative abnormalities from new pathologic findings, a change between examinations is of concern.

2. The antegrade velocity across the prosthetic valve is evaluated. An increase in antegrade velocity may be due to increased volume flow as a result of prosthetic regurgitation rather than prosthetic stenosis. In this case, while the calculated gradient will be higher, the valve area will be unchanged. Alternatively, an increased flow velocity across the prosthetic valve may be due to a high cardiac output state (such as fever, anemia, or anxiety). In this situation, antegrade velocities across the other cardiac valves will be increased proportionately.

3. Pulmonary artery pressures are estimated and compared with previous studies in that patient. While pulmonary hypertension can persist after successful mitral valve surgery, *recurrent* pulmonary hypertension (after an initial postoperative decline) may relate to prosthetic valve dysfunction.

An incidental finding in some patients with a prosthetic valve is the phenomenon of *spontaneous contrast*. This phenomenon is similar to the spontaneous left atrial contrast seen in patients with an enlarged left atrium and low-velocity flow, which has been reported to be associated with a high propensity for thrombus formation. With a prosthetic valve, the appearance of echogenic particles downstream from the valve can occur even in the absence of a low flow state. The presumed mechanism of spontaneous contrast with a prosthetic valve is microcavitation due to impact of the occluder against the sewing ring and this phenomenon is more common with mechanical valves.

left ventricular hypertrophy after aortic valve replacement for aortic stenosis raises the possibility of prosthetic valve stenosis. In other cases, left ventricular dilation may suggest aortic or mitral prosthetic regurgitation with resultant volume overload. A hyperdynamic (but previously normal) left ventricle may indicate prosthetic mitral regurgitation. While it may be dif-

TECHNICAL ASPECTS/LIMITATIONS/ALTERNATE APPROACHES

Transthoracic Echocardiographic Approach to the Patient with a Prosthetic Valve

During the transthoracic echocardiographic examination of the patient with a prosthetic valve, attention is focused on

1. The antegrade velocity across the valve in relation to the size, type, and position of the implanted prosthesis.
2. Calculation of mean gradient and valve area when stenosis is suspected.
3. A careful search for prosthetic valve regurgitation using both color flow imaging and continuous-wave Doppler.
4. Evaluation of chamber sizes, wall thickness, and systolic function.
5. Estimation of pulmonary artery pressure.

These data then are evaluated in conjunction with clinical data and in comparison with previous examinations.

The echocardiographic windows and technical details of data recording are the same for prosthetic valves as for native valve disease. Thus the antegrade velocity curve across a prosthetic mitral valve typically is recorded from an apical approach with either pulsed or continuous-wave Doppler (although sometimes a parasternal approach provides a more parallel intercept angle), while an aortic prosthesis requires a meticulous examination with continuous-wave Doppler from multiple windows (apical, suprasternal, right parasternal) with careful transducer angulation to obtain the highest-velocity signal.

The approaches utilized for native valve regurgitation also apply to prosthetic valves. The major technical difference between examination of a native and a prosthetic valve is the problem of acoustic shadowing. This problem may be circumvented by careful image acquisition or the use of unusual image planes (e.g., mitral regurgitation from a suprasternal notch approach), but transesophageal echocardiography clearly is a more sensitive technique in this situation.

Limitations

As repeatedly emphasized in this chapter, the major limitation of transthoracic echocardiography for evaluation of prosthetic valves is technical, specifically reverberations, artifacts, and acoustic shadowing. The last of these problems can be circumvented to some extent with the transesophageal approach by casting the shadow in the opposite direction. Reverberations and other ultrasound artifacts remain a problem with both approaches.

Other limitations are overestimation of transvalvular pressure gradients with bileaflet mechanical valves, limited validation of valve area calculations for mechanical valves, and the problem of differentiating "normal" from pathologic prosthetic valve regurgitation.

Importantly, the same factors that can lead to errors in evaluation of native valves also are significant limitations in evaluation of prosthetic valves. Most notably, these factors include ultrasound tissue penetration, Doppler intercept-angle assumptions, accurate measurement of 2D images, correct image orientation, and correct identification of the origin of Doppler signals.

Alternate Approaches

When the echocardiographic examination is negative or yields results discordant with other clinical findings, other diagnostic procedures may be indicated. Cardiac catheterization can be performed with direct measurement of intracardiac pressures to confirm the pressure gradient across the valve and measure pulmonary artery pressures. In combination with cardiac output measurement, Gorlin formula valve area and pulmonary vascular resistance can be calculated. For some mechanical valves, catheterization may be complicated by a risk of inducing valve dysfunction if a catheter is passed retrograde across the valve. In these cases, evaluation of a mechanical aortic valve requires transseptal catheterization with measurement of left ventricular pressures by advancing the catheter across the mitral valve into the left ventricle. With a mitral valve prosthesis, transseptal catheterization is more reliable than the pulmonary wedge pressure in evaluating the left atrial to left ventricular pressure gradient. In a patient with both a mechanical aortic and mitral valve, measurement of left ventricular pressure may require direct left ventricular puncture.

Angiographic evaluation (left ventricle for mitral regurgitation, aortic root for aortic regurgitation) is helpful in evaluating prosthetic regurgitation on a semiquantitative (0 to 4+) scale or for calculating regurgitant volumes and fractions in conjunction with other quantitative cardiac output data.

Fluoroscopy of the valve is important for some valve types. For bileaflet and single-disk mechanical valves, the angle of opening can be measured from a view oriented perpendicular to the plane of the open leaflet(s). In a small number of valve models, the occluder undergoes degeneration, resulting in a smaller size that can be detected by fluoroscopic measurements. None of the valves prone to this type of wear (and subsequent leaflet escape) are currently implanted, and there are few patients with these prostheses still in place.

Neither MRI nor CT imaging has proven particularly helpful in evaluation of prosthetic valves. Newer approaches to imaging regurgitant jets with these techniques may yield useful data in the future.

CLINICAL UTILITY

Prosthetic Valve Stenosis

Echocardiography is the initial diagnostic approach to evaluation of suspected prosthetic valve stenosis. The antegrade velocity and mean gradient across the prosthetic valve, particularly in comparison with previous data in that patient, may be diagnostic. Valve area can be calculated by the continuity equation for valves in the aortic (Fig. 11–21) or pulmonic position and by the pressure half-time method for valves in the mitral or tricuspid (Fig. 11–22) position. Despite the overestimation of the average transvalvular gradient that occurs with Doppler evaluation of bileaflet mechanical valves, this approach still is helpful in assessing changes over time in an individual patient.

The differential diagnosis of an increased antegrade velocity across the valve includes a high cardiac output state or coexisting valvular regurgitation, as well as prosthetic valve stenosis. A significant prosthetic or paraprosthetic regurgitant jet can increase the antegrade volume flow rate across the valve substantially, resulting in a high velocity and a high transvalvular gradient. Valve area, however, remains relatively normal.

With careful examination techniques, the antegrade velocity across the prosthetic valve can be recorded in nearly all patients. When signal strength is suboptimal, invasive evaluation may be required. This is most likely for evaluation of a prosthetic valve in a conduit (typically right ventricle or right atrium to pulmonary artery). In this situation, the valve is difficult to image due to shadowing by the vascular graft, and it is

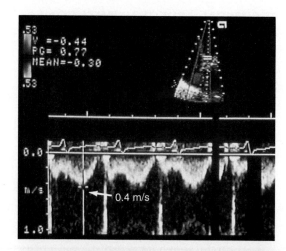

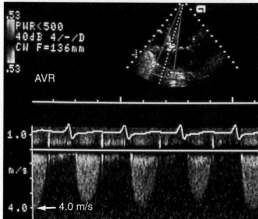

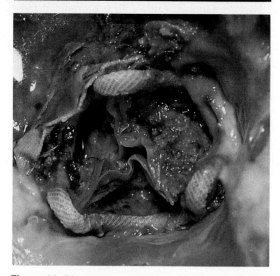

Figure 11–21. A 46-year-old man with chronic renal failure and a porcine valve replacement 8 years ago presented with presyncope. Echocardiography showed severely reduced left ventricular systolic function, a left ventricular outflow tract velocity of only 0.4 m/s, and an aortic jet of 4.0 m/s. Continuity equation valve area was 0.5 cm². At autopsy, the porcine valve leaflets were severely calcified and stiff.

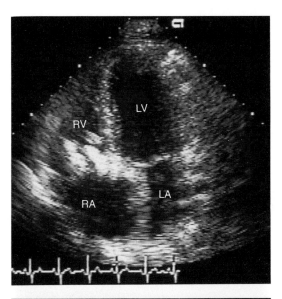

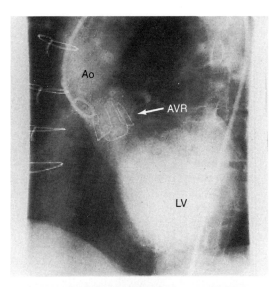

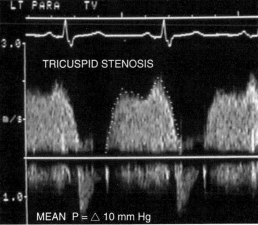

Figure 11–22. A 36-year-old man with a prior tricuspid valve replacement for endocarditis presented with right-sided failure. The apical four-chamber view showed a severely calcified porcine tricuspid valve replacement (*above*) with an increased antegrade velocity and prolonged pressure half-time (*below*).

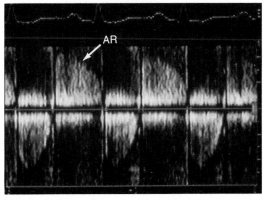

Figure 11–23. A 60-year-old man with a previous porcine aortic valve replacement presented with congestive heart failure. Angiography (*above*) showed severe prosthetic aortic regurgitation (the left ventricle is densely opacified with an aortic root contrast injection). Echocardiography was technically limited due to poor ultrasound tissue penetration, but the continuous-wave Doppler signal (*below*) is diagnostic for significant aortic regurgitation.

difficult to obtain a window where the Doppler beam is parallel to flow across the prosthetic valve.

Prosthetic Valve Regurgitation

Transthoracic echocardiography is accurate for the diagnosis of prosthetic aortic valve regurgitation and for the differentiation of normal from pathologic regurgitation (Fig. 11–23). Standard methods for evaluating regurgitant severity can be employed for aortic valve prostheses. Because of acoustic shadowing, the sensitivity for detection of mitral prosthetic re-

gurgitation is lower, and it is more difficult to distinguish normal from pathologic regurgitation. Transesophageal echocardiography imaging is needed when this diagnosis is suspected on clinical grounds. Transesophageal echocardiography has a high accuracy for detection of prosthetic regurgitation and reliably distinguishes transprosthetic from paraprosthetic regurgitation.

Prosthetic Valve Endocarditis

Detection of valvular vegetations on prosthetic valves is difficult with transthoracic echocardiography due to reverberations and acoustic shadowing. Features that might increase the suspicion of prosthetic valve endocarditis on a transthoracic echocardiographic examination include Doppler evidence of valve dysfunction (either regurgitation due to incomplete closure or stenosis due to an infected pannus on the inflow surface of the valve), evidence of valve instability (i.e., "rocking" on 2D images), an unexplained increase in pulmonary artery pressures, or an interval change in chamber dimensions. Prosthetic valve endocarditis often involves the sewing ring and annulus, resulting in formation of a paravalvular abscess ("ring" abscess) rather than the typical vegetation seen with native valve infection. Identification of an abscess may be limited on transthoracic echocardiography (Fig. 11–24).

Thus, given the technical and pathologic peculiarities of evaluation of suspected prosthetic valve endocarditis, transesophageal imaging is needed in the majority of these patients. Transesophageal echocardiography has a high sensitivity for detection of prosthetic valve endocarditis and/or abscess formation. As for native valve endocarditis (see Chap. 12), cardiac abscesses may be echo-dense or relatively echofree (Fig. 11–25).

Prosthetic Valve Thrombosis

In patients with embolic events presumed secondary to prosthetic valve thrombosis, even transesophageal echocardiography may be negative if the thrombi are small or if new thrombus has not formed since the embolic event. When thrombi are documented on transesophageal echocardiography, this may be important in patient management in some cases. However, an embolic event in a patient with a prosthetic valve (especially mechanical) presumably is related to the presence of a prosthetic valve even if transesophageal echocardiography is negative. Thus the potential clinical implications of the study results should be considered *before* the examination. If the treatment and subsequent management would be the same whether or not a thrombus is documented, then transesophageal echocardiography may be unnecessary. If documentation of thrombus or exclusion of other possible abnormalities would affect patient management, then transesophageal echocardiography examination is appropriate. Of course, infected pannus due to prosthetic valve endocarditis cannot be differentiated from thrombus on 2D imaging. Careful clinical and bacteriologic

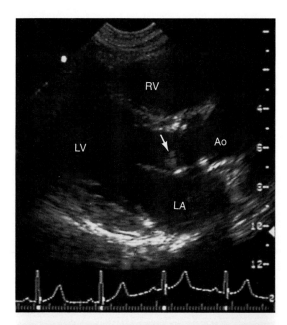

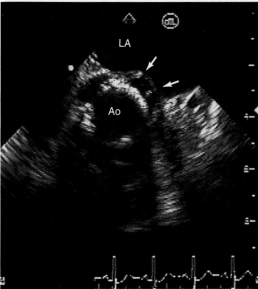

Figure 11–24. Prosthetic valve endocarditis of a porcine valve in the aortic position. The vegetation (*arrow*) is seen on the transthoracic parasternal long-axis view (*above*), but the paravalvular abscess (*arrows*) was diagnosed on transesophageal imaging (*below*).

correlation is needed whenever an abnormal valve-associated mass is observed (Fig. 11–26).

"Routine" Follow-Up of Prosthetic Valve Function

While it is difficult to justify routine periodic echocardiographic examinations of prosthetic

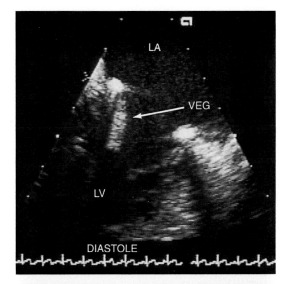

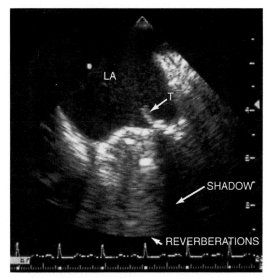

Figure 11–26. Transesophageal view of thrombus (T) on the left atrial side of a bileaflet mechanical valve in a 56-year-old woman who was noncompliant with Coumadin therapy.

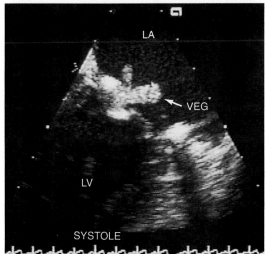

Figure 11–25. Prosthetic valve endocarditis of a mitral porcine valve seen on transesophageal imaging with a large vegetation prolapsing into the left ventricle in diastole (*above*) and into the left atrium in systole (*below*).

valve function in clinically stable patients, the importance of a baseline examination in each patient with a prosthetic valve should not be overlooked. There is wide variability in normal antegrade velocities and in the degree of "normal" regurgitation across prosthetic valves even for a given size, type, and position. Establishing baseline Doppler findings in each patient soon after implantation serves as a reference point should prosthetic valve dysfunction be suspected in the future. Approximately 6 to 8 weeks postoperatively is a reasonable time to obtain this baseline study because the patient has recovered from surgery, is returning to cardiology follow-up,

and has stable hemodynamics with a normal cardiac output. This timing of the examination also allows evaluation of regression of left ventricular hypertrophy or dilation, recovery of left ventricular systolic function, changes in pulmonary artery pressures, and other long-term effects of the valve surgery.

SUGGESTED READING

NORMAL DOPPLER FLOW PATTERNS

1. Reisner SA, Meltzer RS: Normal values of prosthetic valve Doppler echocardiographic parameters: A review. J Am Soc Echocardiogr 1:201–210, 1988.
   Summary of normal Doppler velocities across prosthetic valves, including data from 18 studies with a total of 1105 patients. Thirty-two references.

2. Zabalgoitia M: Echocardiographic assessment of prosthetic heart valves. Curr Prob Cardiol 17:269–325, 1992.
   Review of echocardiographic evaluation of prosthetic valve function. Two-hundred and three references.

3. Jones M, McMillan ST, Eidbo EE, et al: Evaluation of prosthetic heart valves by Doppler flow imaging. Echocardiography 3:513–525, 1986.
   Description of laser Doppler anemometry flow characteristics of prosthetic valves in comparison with color Doppler flow patterns. Flow velocity profiles and turbulence patterns are shown for several valve types.

4. Jaffe WM, Coverdale HA, Roche AHG, et al: Doppler echocardiography in the assessment of the homograft aortic valve. Am J Cardiol 63:1466–1470, 1989.
   Doppler echocardiographic findings in 27 patients with normal functioning aortic homograft valves and 30 patients

with suspected valve dysfunction. Significant regurgitation of the aortic homograft was unlikely with an antegrade velocity <2.0 m/s.

5. Sagar KB, Wann LS, Paulsen WHJ, Romhilt DW: Doppler echocardiographic evaluation of Hancock and Bjork-Shiley prosthetic valves. J Am Coll Cardiol 7:681–687, 1986.
   Doppler echocardiographic findings in 50 patients with clinically normal valve function and 46 patients with suspected prosthetic valve dysfunction.

6. Connolly HM, Miller FA Jr, Taylor CL, et al: Doppler hemodynamic profiles of 82 clinically and echocardiographically normal tricuspid valve prostheses. Circulation 88:2722–2727, 1993.
   In 41 patients with clinically normal heterograft tricuspid valves, Doppler-echo studies showed a mean early filling velocity of 1.3 ± 0.2 m/s, a mean gradient of 3.2 ± 1.1 mmHg, and a pressure half-time of 146 ± 39 ms. In 22 percent, mild prosthetic regurgitation was detected. Values were similar for ball-cage, bileaflet and tilting disk valve prostheses.

VALIDATION OF DOPPLER ECHO PRESSURE GRADIENTS

7. Baumgartner H, Khan S, DeRobertis M, et al: Discrepancies between Doppler and catheter gradients in aortic prosthetic valves in vitro. A manifestation of localized gradients and pressure recovery. Circulation 82:1467–1475, 1990.
   In vitro study emphasizing the importance of pressure recovery downstream from the valve as a cause of discrepancies between Doppler and invasive pressure gradient measurements, with an overestimation of 13 ± 11 percent for mean gradients across the Hancock bioprosthetic valve. High localized gradients in the narrow central orifice at the valve plane of the St. Jude (bileaflet) valve were measured accurately by Doppler echo. However, this localized gradient was greater than the gradient measured 30 mm downstream from the valve.

8. Wilkins GT, Gillam LD, Kritzer GL, et al: Validation of continuous-wave Doppler echocardiographic measurements of mitral and tricuspid prosthetic valve gradients: A simultaneous Doppler-catheter study. Circulation 74:786–795, 1986.
   Simultaneous Doppler and catheter pressure gradients were measured across prosthetic mitral valves in 12 patients, showing an excellent correlation for both porcine and mechanical valves.

9. Burstow DJ, Nishimura RA, Bailey KR, et al: Continuous wave Doppler echocardiographic measurement of prosthetic valve gradients. A simultaneous Doppler-catheter correlative study. Circulation 80: 504–514, 1989.
   Simultaneous Doppler and catheter pressure gradients were measured in 36 patients. Correlations for maximum and mean pressure gradients were excellent for both aortic and mitral prostheses and for bioprosthetic and mechanical valves.

10. Stewart SFC, Nast EP, Arabia FA, et al: Errors in pressure gradient measurement by continuous-wave Doppler ultrasound: Type, size and age effects in bioprosthetic aortic valves. J Am Coll Cardiol 18:769–779, 1991.
    Consistent overestimation of pressure gradients across prosthetic valves as measured by Doppler echocardiography was observed in detailed in vitro studies of 4 types of bioprosthetic

valves. *Pressure recovery downstream did not account for this overestimation. Instead, this error may be related to neglect of proximal velocities in the Bernoulli equation. For example, a mean proximal velocity of 0.66 ± 0.02 m/s at a mean flow rate of 5.6 liters/min would result in an error of 1.74 ± 0.10 mmHg for mean gradient and 3.48 ± 0.21 mmHg for maximum gradient. These differences are even larger at higher flow rates.*

11. Baumgartner H, Khan S, DeRobertis M, et al: Effect of prosthetic aortic valve design on the Doppler-catheter gradient correlation: An in vitro study of normal St. Jude, Medtronic-Hall, Starr-Edwards and Hancock valves. J Am Coll Cardiol 19:324–332, 1992.
    This in vitro study shows that smaller valve sizes have higher antegrade velocities and pressure gradients than larger valve sizes. The 19-mm-size St. Jude and Hancock valves can have velocities as high as 4.7 m/s with a gradient of 89 mmHg even with normal prosthetic valve function. Doppler gradients consistently overestimated catheter gradients for St. Jude and Starr-Edwards valves (differences as great as 44 mmHg were seen). Agreement was closer for Hancock and Medtronic-Hall valves.

PROSTHETIC VALVE AREA

12. Chafizadeh ER, Zoghbi WA: Doppler echocardiographic assessment of the St. Jude medical prosthetic valve in the aortic position using the continuity equation. Circulation 83:213–223, 1991.
    In 67 patients with recent implantation (and clinically normal valve function) of St. Jude aortic valve prostheses, continuity equation valve areas (0.73 to 4.23 cm²) correlated well with the reported actual orifice area (r = 0.83). The Doppler velocity index—the ratio of left ventricular outflow tract to aortic jet velocity—provides a useful simple index of valve function and is less dependent on valve size.

13. Baumgartner H, Khan SS, DeRobertis M, et al: Doppler assessment of prosthetic valve orifice area: An in vitro study. Circulation 85:2275–2283, 1992.
    Continuity equation valve areas correlated well with invasively derived Gorlin formula valve areas for St. Jude, Medtronic-Hall, and Hancock aortic valves in a pulsatile flow model. However, valve area of St. Jude valves was significantly underestimated due to the localized high velocities in the narrow central orifice. Valve areas decrease with low flow in Hancock valves consistent with incomplete opening of the leaflets at low flow rates.

14. Rothbart RM, Castriz JL, Harding LV, et al: Determination of aortic valve area by two-dimensional and Doppler echocardiography in patients with normal and stenotic bioprosthetic valves. J Am Coll Cardiol 15:817–824, 1990.
    In 22 patients undergoing catheterization for suspected dysfunction of bioprosthetic aortic valves, Doppler continuity equation valve areas agreed well with invasively determined Gorlin valve areas.

15. Dumesnil JG, Honos GN, Lemieux M, Beauchemin J: Validation and applications of indexed aortic prosthetic valve areas calculated by Doppler echocardiography. J Am Coll Cardiol 16:637–643, 1990.
    In 31 patients with a Medtronics Intact Bioprosthesis in the aortic position, both standard and simplified continuity equation valve areas correlated well with in vivo and known in vitro prosthetic valve areas (r = 0.86, SEE = 0.16 cm²).

16. Baumgartner H, Schima H, Kuhn P: Effect of prosthetic valve malfunction on the Doppler-catheter gra-

dient relation for bileaflet aortic valve prostheses. Circulation 87:1320–1327, 1993.

Malfunction of bileaflet mechanical valves was simulated in a pulsatile flow model by restricting opening of one leaflet. While Doppler and catheter gradients correlated well for each degree of prosthetic valve stenosis, the slope of the regression line progressively approached 1 with increasing stenosis. Thus, while Doppler overestimates bileaflet prosthetic valve gradients with normal valve function, the Doppler gradients are accurate when stenosis is present. The mechanism of this observation most likely is a reduction in the central orifice size. Clinically, these findings suggest that the development of stenosis of a bileaflet mechanical valve may not be reflected in increases in velocity across the prosthesis.

17. Chambers JB, Cochrane T, Black MM, Jackson G: The Gorlin formula validated against directly observed orifice area in porcine mitral bioprostheses. J Am Coll Cardiol 13:348–353, 1989.

In an in vitro pulsatile flow system, measured orifice area and the modified Gorlin relation (Q/V_{max}) correlated well (r = 0.88). Maximum valve orifice area, measured by a high-speed video camera, decreased at low flow rates for all four Carpentier-Edwards prostheses.

NATURAL HISTORY OF DOPPLER ECHO FINDINGS

18. Reimold SC, Yoganathan AP, Sung H-W, et al: Doppler echocardiographic study of porcine bioprosthetic heart valves in the aortic valve position in patients without evidence of cardiac dysfunction. Am J Cardiol 67:611–615, 1991.

Several studies over 5 years showed a decrease in Doppler-derived effective orifice area >0.20 cm² in 10 of 16 patients. The mean decrease in effective orifice area was 0.25 ± 0.29 cm² (at 34 ± 1 month follow-up) with an increase in mean gradient from 12 ± 4 to 15 ± 7 mmHg.

EXERCISE STUDIES WITH PROSTHETIC VALVES

19. Leavitt JI, Coats MH, Falk RH: Effects of exercise on transmitral gradient and pulmonary artery pressure in patients with mitral stenosis or a prosthetic mitral valve: A Doppler echocardiographic study. J Am Coll Cardiol 17:1520–1526, 1991.

The feasibility of measurements of transmitral mean gradient and pulmonary artery pressure immediately after exercise was demonstrated in 12 patients with mitral stenosis and 11 patients with a normally functioning prosthetic valve (10 of 11 mechanical). Mean gradient increased from 5 ± 2 to 8 ± 3 mmHg and pulmonary artery systolic pressure from 28 ± 8 to 39 ± 16 mmHg with an increase in heart rate from 79 ± 9 to 104 ± 21 beats per minute with exercise in the prosthetic valve patients.

20. van den Brink RB, Verhuel HA, Visser CA, et al: Value of exercise Doppler echocardiography in patients with prosthetic or bioprosthetic cardiac valves. Am J Cardiol 69:367–372, 1992.

In 61 asymptomatic patients with an aortic (n = 24) or mitral (n = 39) prosthetic valve, postexercise Doppler data could be obtained within 60 s in 92 percent. In the mitral group, heart rate increased from 80 ± 12 to 116 ± 14 beats per minute, mean gradient from 6 to 14 mmHg, and pulmonary artery systolic pressure from 34 to 57 mmHg. In the aortic group, heart rate increased from 74 ± 10 to 105 ± 18 beats per minute and mean gradient from 24 (range 12 to 50) to 39 (range 18 to 100) mmHg.

PROSTHETIC VALVE REGURGITATION

21. Baumgartner H, Khan S, DeRobertis M, et al: Color Doppler regurgitant characteristics of normal mechanical mitral valve prostheses in vitro. Circulation 85:323–332, 1992.

Patterns of normal regurgitation for bileaflet and tilting-disk mechanical mitral valves in a pulsatile flow model are described. Bileaflet valves showed two converging jets from the pivot points, a small central jet, and a variable number of peripheral jets. Normal bileaflet regurgitant jets showed little signal aliasing. Tilting-disk (with a central strut and hole) valves showed a large central jet and one or two small peripheral jets. The large central jet showed aliasing extending distally into the atrium.

22. Flachskampf FA, O'Shea JP, Griffin BP, et al: Patterns of normal transvalvular regurgitation in mechanical valve prostheses. J Am Coll Cardiol 18:1493–1498, 1991.

In an in vitro system, bileaflet valves showed peripheral convergent jets in a plane parallel to the two disk axes and several diverging jets in the orthogonal place. Tilting-disk (with central strut and hole) valves showed a prominent central jet with minor jets along the periphery of the disk.

23. Bargiggia GS, Tronconi L, Raisaro A, et al: Color Doppler diagnosis of mechanical prosthetic mitral regurgitation: Usefulness of the flow convergence region proximal to the regurgitant orifice. Am Heart J 120:1137–1142, 1990.

On transthoracic imaging, identification of flow acceleration on the left ventricular side of the prosthesis aids in identifying the presence and location of prosthetic regurgitation. Proximal acceleration was detected in 19 of 20 (95 percent) of the subgroup with mechanical prosthetic mitral regurgitation, whereas a jet in the left atrium was detected in only 12 of 20 (60 percent) due to acoustic shadowing of the left atrium.

TRANSESOPHAGEAL ECHOCARDIOGRAPHY

24. Khandheria BK, Seward JB, Oh JK, et al: Value and limitations of transesophageal echocardiography in assessment of mitral valve prostheses. Circulation 83:1956–1968, 1991.

In reviewing the clinical experience at the Mayo Clinic, 50 patients with a prosthetic mitral valve had a transesophageal study followed by confirmatory cardiac catheterization, surgery, or both. For mechanical valves, 10 of 25 (40 percent) were considered abnormal on transthoracic echocardiography, while 16 of 25 (64 percent) had abnormalities detected on transesophageal echocardiography. Findings were concordant at surgery in 20 of 23 (87 percent). For bioprosthetic valves, 9 of 25 (36 percent) had an abnormal prosthesis on transthoracic echocardiography, while 20 of 25 (80 percent) had an abnormal transesophageal echocardiography examination. Transesophageal echocardiographic findings were confirmed at surgery in all cases.

25. Alton ME, Pasierski TJ, Orsinelli DA, et al: Comparison of transthoracic and transesophageal echocardiography in evaluation of 47 Starr-Edwards prosthetic valves. J Am Coll Cardiol 20:1503–1511, 1992.

The high sensitivity of transesophageal echocardiography for detection of prosthetic valve vegetations, abscess formation, and thrombus is emphasized in this study of 37 patients with 47 Starr-Edwards valves. All the normal mitral valves (13) had a small degree of early systolic mitral regurgitation with a central jet directed posteriorly.

26. Karalis DG, Chandrasekaran K, Ross JJ Jr, et al: Single-plane transesophageal echocardiography for assessing function of mechanical or bioprosthetic valves in the aortic valve position. Am J Cardiol 69:1310–1315, 1992.
In 89 patients, with 69 mechanical and 20 bioprosthetic aortic valves, transesophageal echocardiography was superior to transthoracic echocardiography for evaluation of prosthetic aortic regurgitation only when transthoracic echocardiographic image quality was poor. Transesophageal echocardiography was superior for detection of perivalvular abscess, subaortic perforation, valve dehiscence, and abnormal bioprosthetic valve cusps, as well as in differentiating valvular from paravalvular regurgitation.

27. Daniel WG, Mugge A, Grote J, et al: Comparison of transthoracic and transesophageal echocardiography for detection of abnormalities of prosthetic and bioprosthetic valves in the mitral and aortic positions. Am J Cardiol 71:210–215, 1993.
In 126 patients with 148 prosthetic valves (35 mechanical, 113 bioprosthetic), transesophageal echocardiography had a higher sensitivity (35 of 41, 85 percent) than transthoracic echocardiography (13 of 41, 32 percent) for detection of prosthetic valve endocarditis and thrombi. Transesophageal echocardiography also had a higher sensitivity for anatomic bioprosthetic valve abnormalities (87 versus 65 percent).

28. Barbetseas J, Crawford ES, Safi HJ, et al: Doppler echocardiographic evaluation of pseudoaneurysms complicating composite grafts of the ascending aorta. Circulation 85:212–222, 1992.
Description of the echo Doppler findings in 8 patients with pseudoaneurysms of ascending aortic grafts. An echo-free space adjacent (often posterior) to the aortic graft with flow from the graft lumen into the pseudoaneurysm is seen. Identification is facilitated by transesophageal echocardiography imaging when image quality is suboptimal on a transthoracic echocardiographic approach.

CHAPTER 12

THE ROLE OF ECHOCARDIOGRAPHY IN SUSPECTED OR DEFINITE ENDOCARDITIS

INTRODUCTION

While echocardiographic evaluation has become an essential tool in management of patients with endocarditis, the diagnosis of endocarditis rests on clinical and microbiologic findings. Any imaging technique, including echocardiography, cannot provide a definite diagnosis of active infection nor can it exclude the diagnosis with certainty when it is clinically suspected. It is only by integrating the echocardiographic findings with clinical and microbiologic data that the echocardiogram is a useful diagnostic test.

BASIC PRINCIPLES

Numerous definitions of endocarditis have been proposed. All include evidence of systemic infection, manifested as fevers and positive blood cultures, and localized cardiac involvement, demonstrated by a new murmur, and/or embolic events. Minor criteria may be included as well, such as peripheral manifestations of endocarditis (splinter hemorrhages, Janeway lesions, Osler's nodes) and renal involvement (hematuria), both of which are thought to be due to immune-complex deposition. The clinical diagnosis of infectious endocarditis in the absence of positive blood cultures is problematic. In some cases, blood cultures are negative due to prior antibiotic treatment or inadequate culture techniques. Other cases may be noninfectious in etiology.

The pathologic criterion for endocarditis is the finding at autopsy or surgery of valvular vegetations with active infection, local tissue destruction, and/or paravalvular abscess formation. Echocardiography can identify an abnormal mass associated with a cardiac valves and may show certain features that increase the likelihood that this mass represents a valvular vegetation rather than a tumor, thrombus, or excess valve tissue (as in myxomatous disease); however, an old, "healed" vegetation or a noninfectious vegetation appears similar to a new actively infected lesion.

The goals of echocardiography in a patient with a clinical diagnosis of endocarditis are:

1. To identify the presence, location, size, and number of valvular vegetations.
2. To assess functional abnormalities of the affected valve(s), especially valvular regurgitation.
3. To identify the underlying anatomy of the affected valve(s) and any coincident valvular disease.
4. To assess the impact of valvular disease on chamber dimensions and function, most importantly left ventricular size and systolic function.
5. To identify other complications of endocarditis (e.g., paravalvular abscess, pericardial effusion).
6. To provide prognostic data on the anticipated clinical course, risk of systemic embolization, and potential need for surgical intervention.

In a patient with a lower likelihood of endocarditis on clinical grounds, an echocardiogram often is requested to "rule out" endocarditis. In this setting, the goals of the echocardiographic examination are:

1. Identification of any valvular vegetations.
2. Assessment of valve anatomy and function with respect to anatomic or physiologic factors that increase the likelihood of endocarditis (e.g., bicuspid aortic valve, myxomatous mitral valve, etc.).

If an abnormality is identified, complete evaluation is directed toward the goals listed above for clinical endocarditis.

ECHOCARDIOGRAPHIC APPROACH

Valvular Vegetations

Transthoracic Echocardiography

On two-dimensional (2D) echocardiography, a valvular vegetation typically appears as an abnormal echogenic, irregular mass attached to the upstream side of the valve leaflet with a pattern of motion that is dependent on, but more chaotic than, normal valve motion. For example, an aortic valve vegetation prolapses into the left ventricular outflow tract in diastole and extends into the aortic root in systole (Fig. 12–1). The mass is attached to the left ventricular side of the valve leaflet but shows motion in excess of normal valve excursion with rapid oscillations in diastole (best appreciated on M-mode recordings). A mitral valve vegetation is attached on the atrial side of the valve, prolapses into the left atrium in systole, and moves into the left ventricle, beyond the normal range of mitral valve opening, in diastole (Fig. 12–2).

Valvular vegetations vary in size from so small as to be undetectable with current imaging techniques to greater than 3 cm in length. Vegetations may be attached at any area of the leaflet, although lesions at the coaptation line are most common. More than one valve can be involved, either by direct extension of infection or

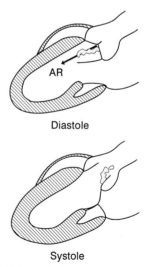

Aortic Valve Vegetation

Diastole

Systole

Figure 12–1. Schematic diagram of an aortic valve vegetation attached to the ventricular side of the leaflet with prolapse into the left ventricular outflow tract in diastole. AR = aortic regurgitation.

Mitral Valve Vegetation

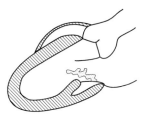

Diastole

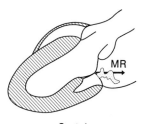

Systole

Figure 12–2. Schematic diagram of a mitral valve vegetation attached to the atrial side of the leaflet with prolapse into the left atrium in systole. MR = mitral regurgitation.

as a separate process, emphasizing the caveat that each valve requires careful examination even if a vegetation has been identified on another valve. In most cases, endocarditis occurs on a previously abnormal valve.

Multiple acoustic windows and 2D views are needed for detection of a valvular vegetation. First, since the vegetation is a discrete structure, it may be seen only in certain tomographic planes. Slow scanning between the standard image planes—for example, between the parasternal long-axis view and the right ventricular inflow view—increases the likelihood of identifying a valvular vegetation. Orthogonal views further ensure that all segments of the valve leaflets are examined. In a patient with suspected endocarditis, a complete examination is needed with scanning from parasternal, apical, subcostal, and suprasternal notch views for careful evaluation of each valve. The reported sensitivity of transthoracic echocardiography for detection of valvular vegetations ranges from less than 50 percent to as high as 90 percent (Table 12–1). To some extent, the reported sensitivity

TABLE 12–1. ACCURACY OF ECHOCARDIOGRAPHIC DIAGNOSIS OF VALVULAR VEGETATIONS (SELECTED STUDIES)

FIRST AUTHOR, YEAR	STUDY ENTRY CRITERIA/ STANDARD OF REFERENCE	NO. OF VALVES	PERCENT PROSTHETIC	TRANSTHORACIC ECHO		TRANSESOPHAGEAL ECHO	
				Sensitivity	Specificity	Sensitivity	Specificity
1. Mügge, 1989	Definite endocarditis *plus* surgery/autopsy	91	24%	53/91 (58%)	—	82/91 (90%)	—
2. Jaffe, 1990	Definite endocarditis *plus* surgery/autopsy	38	16%	38/44 (86%)	—	Not done	
3. Burger, 1991	Suspected endocarditis and clinical outcome	101	—	35/39 (90%)	61/62 (98%)	Not done	
4. Shively, 1991	Suspected endocarditis and clinical outcome	66	18%	7/16 (44%)	49/50 (98%)	15/16 (94%)	50/50 (100%)
5. Pedersen, 1991	Suspected endocarditis and clinical outcome	24	42%	5/10 (50%)	13/14 (93%)	10/10 (100%)	14/14 (100%)
6. Daniel, 1993	Prosthetic valve with surgically confirmed endocarditis	33	100%	12/33 (36%)	—	27/33 (82%)	—
7. Sochowski, 1993	Suspected endocarditis with initially negative TTE study	65	32%	—	—	Negative predictive value = 56/65 (86%)	
8. Shapiro, 1994	Suspected endocarditis	68	—	23/34 (68%)	31/34 (91%)	33/34 (97%)	31/34 (91%)

Data from Mügge et al: JACC 14:631–638, 1989; Jaffe et al: JACC 15:1227–1233, 1990; Burger et al: Angiology 42:552–560, 1991; Shiveley et al: JACC 18:391–397, 1991; Pedersen et al: Chest 100:351–356, 1991; Daniel et al: AJC 71:210–215, 1993; Sochowski and Chan: JACC 21:216–221, 1993; Shapiro et al: Chest 105:377, 1994.

of transthoracic echocardiography increased between the advent of 2D instruments in the late 1970s and the improved image quality with advances in instrumentation in the 1980s.

Aortic Valve. Aortic valve vegetations most often are detected in parasternal long- and short-axis views. Careful angulation from medial to lateral in the long-axis plane and from inferior to superior in the short-axis plane is needed because vegetations often are eccentrically located. Image quality is optimized by use of a minimum depth setting and adjustment of gain and processing parameters. An echogenic mass attached to the ventricular side of the leaflet with independent motion and prolapse into the outflow tract in diastole is diagnostic for a valvular vegetation (Fig. 12–3). Rapid oscillating motion may be best appreciated on an M-mode recording.

Less typically, a vegetation may be attached to the aortic side of the leaflet or may show little independent motion. A definitive diagnosis may be difficult if the underlying valve anatomy is abnormal. For example, a vegetation on a calcified aortic valve may be difficult to visualize. In these cases, the findings of independent motion and prolapse into the left ventricle in diastole are particularly helpful signs. Comparison with previous echocardiograms may allow recognition of recent changes, increasing the likelihood of valve infection, or may show no significant difference, decreasing the likelihood of an acute process.

Findings that may be mistaken for an aortic valve vegetation include beam-width artifact related to either a calcified nodule, a prosthetic valve, the normal leaflet opposition zone, or the normal leaflet thickening at the central coaptation region (the nodule of Arantius). Occasionally, a linear echo representing a normal variant called a *Lambl's excrescence* is seen. These small fibroelastic protrusions from the ventricular side of the leaflet closure zone occur with increasing frequency with age and are present in a high percentage of patients. As image quality improves, these normal structures are seen more frequently (Fig. 12–4).

Apical views of the aortic valve, both from an anteriorly angulated four-chamber view and from an apical long-axis view, may show an aortic valve vegetation. The finding of an abnormality in both parasternal and apical views decreases the likelihood of an ultrasound artifact, since the relationship of the ultrasound beam and aortic valve are entirely different from these two windows.

2D imaging of a definite or suspected aortic valve vegetation is accompanied by evaluation of

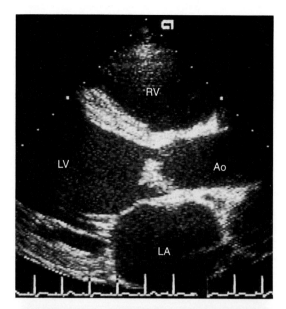

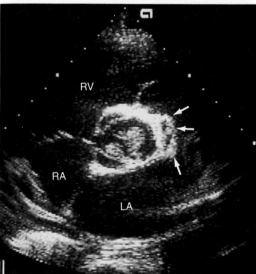

Figure 12–3. In a 29-year-old IV drug abuser with *S. aureus* endocarditis, aortic valve vegetations are seen in a transthoracic parasternal long-axis (*above*) and short-axis (*below*) views. Irregularly shaped echogenic masses are attached to the ventricular side of the aortic valve leaflets with prolapse into the outflow tract in diastole (seen in the long-axis view) and extension into the aortic root in systole (seen in the short-axis view). Severe aortic regurgitation was present. The short-axis view also shows a paravalvular abscess (*three arrows*).

the functional abnormalities due to valve destruction, as discussed below.

Mitral Valve. Mitral valve vegetations typically are located on the atrial side of the leaflets. Diagnostic features include rapid independent motion, prolapse into the left atrium in systole,

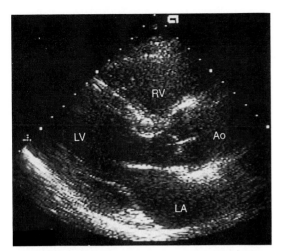

Figure 12–4. Lambl's excrescence or beam-width artifact at the aortic closure line that might be mistaken for a valvular vegetation.

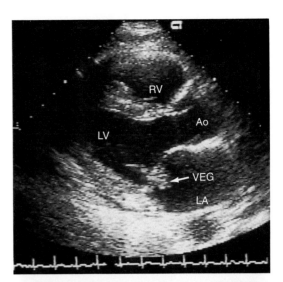

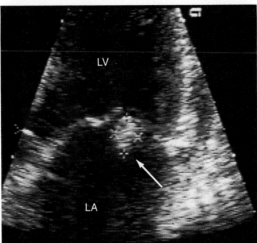

Figure 12–5. A 31-year-old woman with a history of intravenous drug abuse and *S. aureus* endocarditis has a typical appearing mitral valve vegetation (VEG) seen in a parasternal long-axis view (*above*) and in a focused apical four-chamber view (*below*). The mass is attached to the atrial side of the leaflets near the coaptation line with prolapse into the left atrium in systole and extension into the left ventricle in diastole.

and functional evidence of valve dysfunction. Parasternal long- and short-axis views with careful scanning across the valve apparatus in both image planes allows assessment of the presence, size, and location of any vegetation (Fig. 12–5). Apical four-chamber, two-chamber, and long-axis views again are helpful both in visualizing valve and vegetation anatomy and in distinguishing a true valve mass from an ultrasound artifact.

As for the aortic valve, beam-width artifacts can be mistaken for a vegetation. A particular artifact to be aware of is the appearance of a "mass" on the atrial side of the anterior mitral leaflet in the apical four-chamber view due to beam-width artifact from a calcified or prosthetic aortic valve. Other types of mitral valve pathology may be difficult to distinguish from a valvular vegetation, including a severely myxomatous leaflet, a partial flail leaflet, or a ruptured papillary muscle (Fig. 12–6).

Again, comparison with previous studies may help differentiate an acute process from chronic underlying valve disease. With mitral valve endocarditis, mitral regurgitation typically, but not invariably, is present.

Tricuspid Valve. Tricuspid valve endocarditis occurs most often in intravenous drug abusers, is associated with large vegetations due to *Staphylococcus aureus* infection, and tends to have a better prognosis than left-sided valvular involvement.

The right ventricular inflow view often is diagnostic, showing a large, mobile mass of echos attached to the atrial side of the leaflet with prolapse into the right atrium in systole (Fig. 12–7). Given the range of excursion and mobility of these vegetations, it is not surprising that septic pulmonary emboli are a frequent complication of tricuspid valve endocarditis.

The apical and subcostal four-chamber views allow further evaluation of the presence and extent of tricuspid valve infection. Assessment of tricuspid regurgitant severity and consequent right atrial and right ventricular dilation also can be performed from these windows.

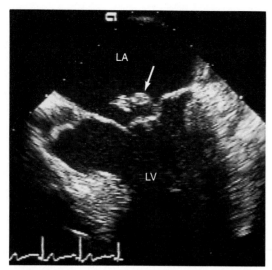

Figure 12–6. Abnormal valve (myxomatous) with flail leaflet (*arrow*) but no vegetation on transesophageal imaging. Angulation showed this "mass" to be a flail leaflet. The patient had no clinical evidence of endocarditis.

Transesophageal Imaging

Transesophageal imaging clearly has a greater sensitivity for detection of vegetations. Some echocardiographers propose that transesophageal echocardiography should be performed whenever endocarditis is suspected. It is generally agreed that transesophageal echocardiography should be considered when transthoracic imaging is suboptimal or when the level of clinical suspicion is high and the presence of a valvular vegetation would affect therapy. It is noteworthy that the reported sensitivity of transthoracic echocardiography is highest from laboratories that did not have transesophageal echocardiography at the time of the study (2 and 3 in Table 12–1). This supports the view that the sensitivity of the echocardiographic examination is directly related to the completeness and care with which the examination is performed. However, transesophageal echocardiography clearly has a higher diagnostic accuracy and should be used in appropriate clinical settings.

From the transesophageal approach, the aortic valve is examined in both long- and short-axis planes. As for transthoracic imaging, careful scanning from medial to lateral in the longitudinal plane and from superior to inferior in the short-axis plane is needed to fully evaluate valve anatomy and to achieve a high sensitivity for detection of valvular vegetations (Figs. 12–8 and 12–9). When the image plane is oblique, an aortic leaflet may be seen *en face*, mimicking an aortic valve mass. Evaluation in more than one im-

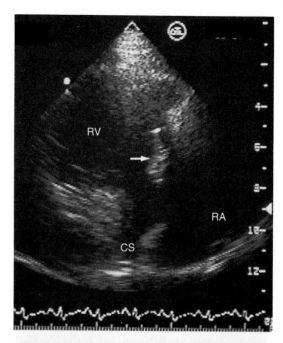

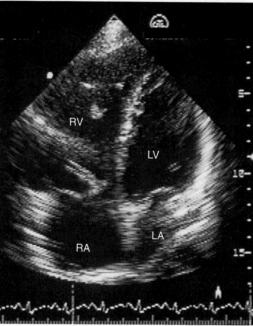

Figure 12–7. Transthoracic imaging in a 27-year-old woman with a history of intravenous drug use and *S. aureus* tricuspid valve endocarditis. In the right ventricular inflow view (*above*), a mobile mass attached to the atrial side of the anterior leaflet is seen (*arrow*). In the apical four-chamber view (*below*), right ventricular and right atrial enlargement secondary to volume overload from tricuspid regurgitation can be appreciated. The patient underwent tricuspid annuloplasty for severe, symptomatic tricuspid regurgitation. CS = coronary sinus.

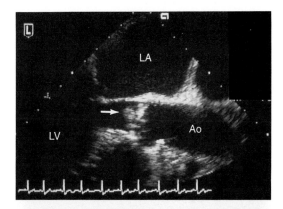

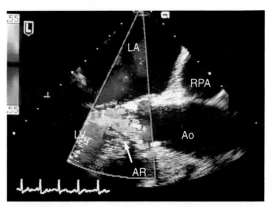

Figure 12–9. Color flow imaging in the same view as 12–8 (*bottom panel*) shows acute severe aortic regurgitation (AR) due to the flail leaflet in this patient. RPA = right pulmonary artery.

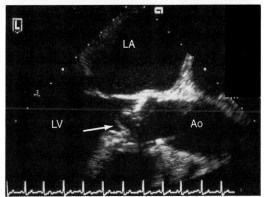

Figure 12–8. Transesophageal long-axis view of the aortic valve showing valvular vegetations (*above*) and a flail aortic leaflet (*below*) with slight angulation of the image plane in a 75-year-old woman with endocarditis who died after emergency aortic valve replacement for severe acute aortic regurgitation.

age plane and assessment of the pattern of motion (rapid oscillating independent motion versus motion *with* the valve) avoid this potential error. Since image quality tends to be superior from the transesophageal approach, small normal variants of valve anatomy may be appreciated and should not be overinterpreted as abnormalities. When a transgastric apical view can be obtained, the aortic valve may be evaluated from this view as well. However, images from this view may be no better than from a transthoracic approach due to the distance from the transducer to the aortic valve.

The mitral valve is well seen from a high esophageal position. The mitral valve is imaged in transverse and longitudinal planes with careful angulation from superior to inferior in the transverse plane and rotation from lateral to medial in the longitudinal plane. The degree of mitral regurgitation can be assessed with color flow imaging in these same views. Given the distance of the normal valve from the chest wall in

both parasternal and apical transthoracic views, transesophageal imaging often provides dramatically better images and important clinical data (Fig. 12–10).

The tricuspid valve is seen in the transesophageal four-chamber view and from a transgastric approach. Since the tricuspid valve lies closer to the chest wall than the mitral valve, transthoracic imaging often is diagnostic, and information that would change patient therapy or management may not be obtained on transesophageal imaging (Fig. 12–11).

Diagnostic Accuracy of Echocardiography for Detection of Vegetations

While numerous studies have evaluated the sensitivity of echocardiography for diagnosis of valvular vegetation by comparing the echo findings with subsequent surgical or autopsy findings, there are fewer data on the specificity of echocardiography for valvular vegetations. This stems from two study design problems: (1) Most studies only include subjects with a definite diagnosis of endocarditis. Thus there are no subjects without the disease in the study group. (2) When surgical or autopsy inspection of the valve is the standard of reference, only patients who are sick enough to need surgery or who have died are included in the study group. Direct inspection of valves that appeared normal on echocardiography rarely is available.

A few studies (for example, 3 through 5 in Table 12–1) have circumvented these study design problems by including all patients with *suspected* endocarditis (some have the disease and some do not) and using clinical outcome rather than di-

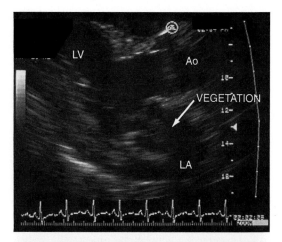

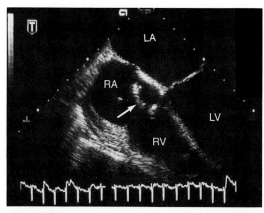

Figure 12–11. Transesophageal view of a tricuspid valve vegetation (*arrow*) attached to the atrial side of the septal leaflet of the tricuspid valve in a 38-year-old woman undergoing tricuspid valve repair for *S. aureus* endocarditis.

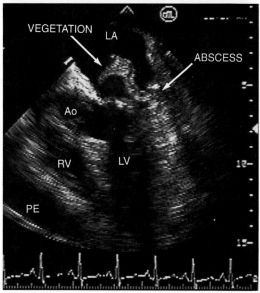

Figure 12–10. Transthoracic (*above*) and transesophageal (*below*) imaging in a 61-year-old man with group B streptococcal endocarditis. The valvular vegetation (*arrow*) is seen on transthoracic imaging but is better defined on transesophageal imaging. In addition, there was evidence for a mitral annular abscess. There was no detectable mitral regurgitation. At surgery, the patient had an extensive mitral annular abscess and purulent pericarditis. PE = pericardial effusion.

artifacts (Table 12–2). In a patient with abnormal valve leaflets (e.g., myxomatous, calcified), it may be difficult to distinguish the abnormal tissue from a valvular vegetation unless a study performed before onset of the illness is available for comparison. Mistaking ultrasound artifacts for a vegetation can be avoided by identification of the characteristic findings in more than one view. Note that not all valvular vegetations are "typical." Some may be on the downstream side of the valve or may show little independent motion. These atypical findings further decrease the sensitivity and specificity of echocardiography for valvular vegetations.

Endocarditis most often occurs on a previously abnormal valve or a prosthetic valve. Eval-

rect valve inspection as the standard of reference. All these studies demonstrate a high specificity of transthoracic (93 to 98 percent) and transesophageal (100 percent) echocardiography in excluding the diagnosis of endocarditis. Another study (7 in Table 12–1) found that the negative predictive value of a negative transesophageal study also is high (86 percent).

The specificity of echocardiography depends on distinguishing a valvular vegetation from other intracardiac masses and from ultrasound

TABLE 12–2. ANATOMIC ABNORMALITIES THAT MAY MIMIC INFECTIOUS ENDOCARDITIS ON ECHOCARDIOGRAPHY

Papillary fibroma

Myxomatous mitral valve disease (especially with partial flail leaflet or ruptured chordae)

Old, "healed" vegetation

Nonbacterial thrombotic endocarditis

Systemic lupus cardiac involvement

Thrombus (especially with prosthetic valve)

Beam-width artifact from calcific valve disease or prosthesis

Aortic valve Lambl's excrescence or nodule of Arantius

uation of the underlying valve disease is an important aspect of the ultrasound examination.

Functional Valvular Abnormalities Due to Endocarditis

Valve leaflet destruction by the infectious process plus the distortion of leaflet closure by the vegetation mass result in valvular regurgitation. Regurgitation can occur at the closure line or through a perforation in the leaflet itself. The degree of regurgitation varies from none through mild-moderate to severe.

Assessment of valvular regurgitation in endocarditis is performed using the pulsed, color flow, and continuous-wave Doppler approaches described in Chapter 10 with careful attention to the features that distinguish acute from chronic regurgitation. Since endocarditis often affects a previously abnormal valve, acute regurgitation may be superimposed on chronic regurgitation, resulting in mixed findings on echocardiography.

Valvular stenosis due to endocarditis is rare. Occasionally, a large vegetation will partially obstruct the orifice of the open valve, resulting in some degree of functional stenosis.

Note that not *all* patients with endocarditis have a new murmur (about 10 percent do not) and a few have *no* regurgitation detectable on Doppler examination. This is most likely to occur if the vegetation is located at the base of the leaflet, resulting in little distortion of leaflet closure. Echocardiographic recognition of the diagnosis in this subgroup is all the more important in that endocarditis often is not suspected clinically. In these cases, the echocardiogram may have been ordered for other reasons.

Other Echocardiographic Findings

In addition to direct assessment of valvular disease, the examination includes evaluation of cardiac chamber size and function. Acute aortic regurgitation results in only mild left ventricular dilation, but a subacute or acute course superimposed on mild to moderate chronic disease may result in significant ventricular dilation. Severe valve destruction may result in a flail aortic leaflet (see Figs. 12–8 and 12–9). Mitral regurgitation results in left atrial and left ventricular enlargement. Left ventricular systolic dysfunction may be seen either due to long-standing valvular disease or due to the acute infectious process.

Pulmonary pressures may be elevated due to mitral regurgitation directly resulting in an elevated left atrial pressure or to aortic regurgitation with a high end-diastolic left ventricular pressure.

A small pericardial effusion often is seen with endocarditis. A larger effusion raises the concern of purulent pericarditis due to direct extension from a paravalvular abscess.

Diagnosis of Paravalvular Abscess and Intracardiac Fistula

Unlike abscesses elsewhere in the body, a cardiac abscess may be either echolucent or echodense on ultrasound examination. Typically, abscesses occur in the valve annulus adjacent to the infected leaflet tissue. For diagnosis of aortic annular abscess, findings include increased echogenicity or an echolucent area in the base of septum or increased thickness of the posterior aortic root (Figs. 12–12 to 12–14). Involvement of the aortic annulus may extend into the contiguous anterior mitral valve leaflet with evidence of increased thickness of the leaflet tissue, a valvular vegetation, and/or leaflet perforation (Figs. 12–15 and 12–16). A sinus of Valsalva aneurysm can occur due to infection of the sinus wall and may be detected by echocardiography, before rupture occurs, as a dilated and distorted sinus. In effect, this represents an abscess that is in direct communication with the bloodstream.

Rupture of an aortic annular abscess can occur in several fashions. The region of the noncoronary cusp can rupture into the right ventricular outflow tract either in the sinus of Valsalva (an aortic to right ventricular connection) or from the left ventricular outflow tract through the septum into the right ventricle (a ventricular septal defect). An aortic to right ventricular fistula shows both systolic and diastolic left to right flow on Doppler interrogation, while a ventricular septal defect shows predominantly systolic flow (see Fig. 14–3).

The right coronary sinus region can rupture into the right ventricle or right atrium and can lead to involvement of the adjacent septal leaflet of the tricuspid valve. Again, rupture can occur either from the aorta or from the left ventricular outflow tract into the right side of the heart. Note that a small segment of ventricular septum (the atrioventricular septum) actually separates the left ventricle from the right *atrium* so that a ventriculoatrial communication can occur. The left coronary sinus can rupture into the left or right atrium, or infection may extend directly into the interatrial septum.

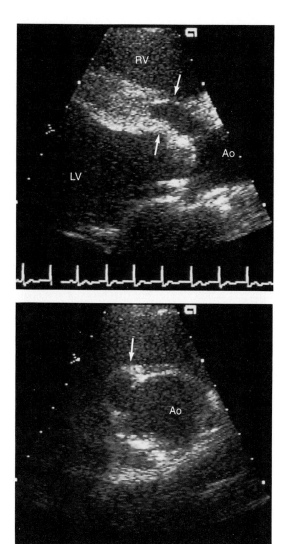

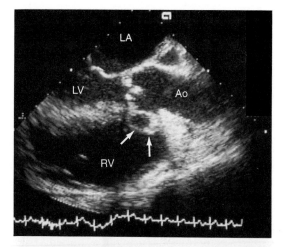

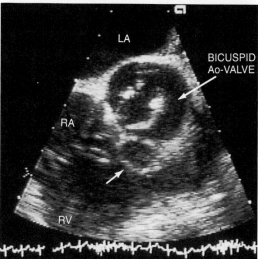

Figure 12–12. Transthoracic parasternal long-axis (*above*) and short-axis (*below*) views in a 34-year-old man with a bicuspid aortic valve and suspected endocarditis. Definite evidence for valvular vegetations and a paravalvular abscess (*arrows*) is seen. Doppler allowed assessment of the severity of aortic regurgitation.

Figure 12–13. Transesophageal long- (*top*) and short-axis (*bottom*) views of the aortic valve in the same patient as in Figure 12–3. While the bicuspid valve, valvular vegetations, and paravalvular abscess (*arrows*) are more clearly seen, no additional diagnostic information was obtained compared with the transthoracic study. At surgery, a paravalvular abscess due to α-hemolytic *Streptococcus* was found.

A mitral annular abscess occurs less often than an aortic ring abscess. It appears as increased thickening and echogenicity in the posterior aspect of the mitral annulus. Infection may extend into the basal segments of the ventricular myocardium or into the pericardial space. Again, identification may be difficult on echocardiographic imaging, and the diagnosis should be pursued with transesophageal echocardiography when suspected on clinical grounds. An unusual complication of mitral valve endocarditis is a persistent contour abnormality, in effect a pseudoaneurysm of the valve leaflet, which persists even after the infection is treated (Figs. 12–17 and 12–18).

Tricuspid valve endocarditis may be associated with a ring abscess, again manifested as increased thickening and echogenicity in the annulus region.

Diagnosis of paravalvular abscess by transthoracic echocardiography has a markedly lower sensitivity and specificity (Table 12–3), compared with transesophageal imaging, due to poor ultrasound tissue penetration resulting in suboptimal image quality. A high index of suspicion is needed by the echocardiographer, and subtle

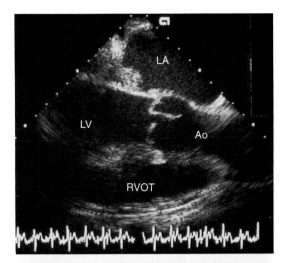

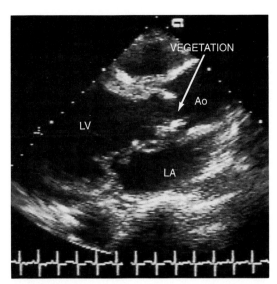

Figure 12–15. Aortic valve endocarditis with vegetations and with extension into the base of the anterior mitral valve leaflet resulting in mitral leaflet perforation.

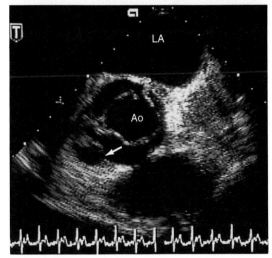

Figure 12–14. TEE long- (*top*) and short-axis (*bottom*) views showing a contour abnormality of the right coronary sinus of Valsalva (*arrows*) suggestive of a paravalvular abscess in a 43-year-old man with *S. aureus* endocarditis on a congenital bicuspid valve. This patient suffered an embolic cerebrovascular event and died of acute congestive heart failure.

abnormalities that may suggest a valve abscess should not be ignored. However, even with careful imaging from several acoustic windows in multiple tomographic planes, a definite diagnosis may not be possible. Paravalvular abscess is more likely to complicate prosthetic valve endocarditis. Shadowing and reverberations from the valve prosthesis further compromise the examination (see Chap. 11).

The superior image quality of transesophageal echocardiography is associated with a higher sensitivity (87 percent) and specificity (96 percent) for diagnosis of paravalvular abscess. In addition to 2D findings of abnormal areas of in-

creased echogenicity or abnormal echolucent areas adjacent to the valve, color flow imaging and conventional pulsed Doppler may allow demonstration of flow into and out of these abnormal areas consistent with an abscess that partially communicates with the bloodstream.

Usually, both transthoracic and transesophageal approaches are needed for patient evaluation in

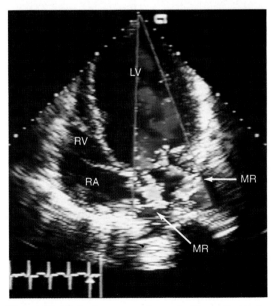

Figure 12–16. In the same patient as in Figure 12–13, the apical four-chamber color flow image showed two jets of mitral regurgitation—one through the leaflet perforation and one through the valve coaptation zone.

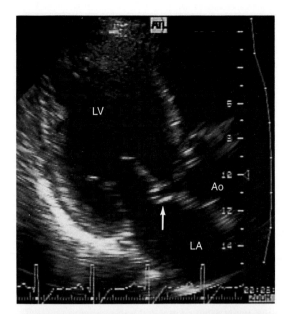

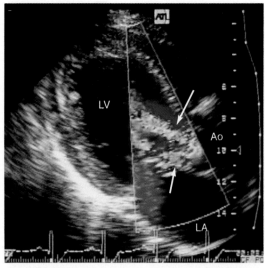

Figure 12–18. In the same patient as Figure 12–17, color flow imaging shows two aortic regurgitant jets (*arrow*) with one jet directed at the pseudoaneurysm of the anterior mitral valve leaflet.

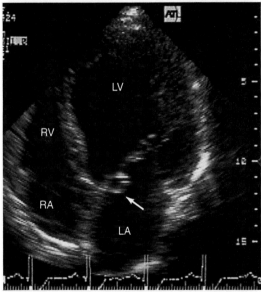

Figure 12–17. Chronic mitral valve pseudoaneurysm in a 69-year-old man with a remote history of bacterial endocarditis. In the apical long-axis (*above*) and four-chamber (*below*) views, a circular echolucent structure is seen at the base of the anterior mitral leaflet (*arrow*).

endocarditis. One advantage of transthoracic imaging is the ability to align a continuous-wave Doppler beam parallel to high-velocity flows of interest. When abnormal intracardiac communications complicate endocarditis due to abscess rupture, identification of an abnormal high-velocity jet may be the first clue to the diagnosis. The transthoracic approach also allows measurement of chamber dimensions in standard views, quantitation of left ventricular sys-

tolic function, and measurement of pulmonary artery pressures.

LIMITATIONS/TECHNICAL CONSIDERATIONS (Table 12–4)

Active Versus Healed Vegetations

Sequential echocardiographic studies in a patient undergoing treatment for endocarditis may show a gradual reduction in size, decreased mobility, and increased echogenicity of the valvular vegetation. However, vegetations may either abruptly "disappear" from the heart due to embolization or may remain unchanged in size or appearance long after the acute episode. Thus a patient with active endocarditis may have no visible vegetation if recent embolization has occurred. Conversely, a patient with prior endocarditis may have a persistent vegetation without active infection. Echocardiography, by itself, can neither exclude nor establish a diagnosis of endocarditis. Correlation of the echocardiographic findings with the patient's clinical presentation (fevers, systemic emboli, new murmur, peripheral manifestation of endocarditis) plus the results of microbiologic cultures is needed for diagnosis. Obviously, echocardiography provides no information regarding the causative organism. While certain etiologic agents (fungal endocarditis, *Hemophilus influenzae*) are associated with larger vegetations, this

TABLE 12–3. ACCURACY OF ECHOCARDIOGRAPHIC DIAGNOSIS OF PARAVALVULAR ABSCESS (SELECTED SERIES)

FIRST AUTHOR, YEAR	STUDY ENTRY CRITERIA	NO. OF VALVES	PERCENT PROSTHETIC	TRANSTHORACIC ECHO		TRANSESOPHAGEAL ECHO	
				Sensitivity	Specificity	Sensitivity	Specificity
1. Daniel, 1991	Endocarditis with surgery or autopsy	137	25%	13/46 (28%)	90/91 (99%)	40/46 (87%)	87/91 (96%)
2. Jaffe, 1990	Endocarditis with surgery or autopsy	7		5/7 (71%)			
3. Karalis, 1992	Endocarditis with surgery or autopsy	55	46%	13/24 (54%)		24/24 (100%)	

Data from Daniel et al: NEJM 324:795–800, 1991; Jaffe et al: JACC 15:1227–1233, 1990; Karalis et al: Circ 86:353–362, 1992.

observation is not diagnostically useful in an individual patient.

Nonbacterial Thrombotic Endocarditis

The echocardiographic appearance of nonbacterial thrombotic endocarditis, as has been described in patients with malignancy and in patients with systemic lupus erythematosus, is similar to that of infectious endocarditis. Although the vegetations of nonbacterial thrombotic endocarditis tend to be smaller, to be located near the leaflet base, and to show variable echo density and less independent motion, again, clinical and bacteriologic correlation is needed for a correct diagnosis.

Diagnosis of Vegetations with Underlying Valve Disease

Endocarditis most often occurs on a previously abnormal valve, since the local flow disturbance increases the likelihood of bacterial deposition. When the underlying disease is anatomically straightforward, such as a bicuspid aortic valve, this poses little problem in diagnosing superimposed valvular vegetations. Often, however, the presence of an abnormal valve makes exclusion or confirmation of a valvular vegetation more difficult. For example, with calcific aortic stenosis, the irregular areas of increased echogenicity on the valve leaflets could represent a vegetation or chronic fibrocalcific changes. Findings of independent rapid motion and prolapse into the outflow tract on diastole increase the likelihood of a vegetation, but the

absence of these findings does not allow a definite conclusion as to the absence of a vegetation.

Again, in the example of myxomatous mitral valve disease, an independently mobile mass of echos attached to the leaflet and prolapsing into the left atrium in systole could represent either a valvular vegetation or a flail leaflet segment and attached chordae. When underlying valve disease is present, the improved images obtained by the transesophageal approach may increase the certainty of diagnosis. In any case, careful integration with other clinical findings usually leads to a correct diagnosis.

Endocarditis of Prosthetic Valves

Evaluation of prosthetic valves for suspected endocarditis is problematic for two reasons. First, infection often involves the area around the sewing ring of the prosthetic valve rather than resulting in a discrete valvular vegetation. Second, reverberations and shadowing by the prosthesis limit the ability of echocardiography

TABLE 12–4. LIMITATIONS OF ECHOCARDIOGRAPHY IN EVALUATION OF PATIENTS WITH ENDOCARDITIS

1. Active versus healed vegetation

2. Noninfectious endocarditis

3. Abnormal underlying valve anatomy

4. Prosthetic valve

5. Detection of abscess

6. Need for clinical and microbiologic correlation

to detect abnormalities. This is a particular problem with transthoracic imaging of mitral prostheses, where the left atrial side of the valve is "masked" by the prosthesis so that neither the paravalvular infection in the mitral annulus nor the resulting valvular incompetence can be detected (see Chap. 11). Acoustic shadowing is less of a problem with aortic valve prostheses because aortic regurgitation can be evaluated from both apical and parasternal windows without "masking" by the valve prosthesis. However, since the anterior part of the valve prosthesis shadows the more posterior portions, images of the valve leaflets may be suboptimal.

With suspected prosthetic valve endocarditis, the transthoracic examination may provide clues that suggest the diagnosis even when definitive findings are not present. For example, if color flow imaging is nondiagnostic due to shadowing and color flow artifacts, a careful continuous-wave Doppler examination may show a regurgitant signal. Care is needed in assessment of the *severity* of regurgitation in this situation, and it may be prudent to state only that regurgitation is present but cannot be quantitated. Other clues to prosthetic valve dysfunction include an increased antegrade flow velocity across the prosthesis (reflecting increased antegrade volume flow due to prosthetic regurgitation) and an elevated tricuspid regurgitant jet velocity due to pulmonary hypertension.

Whenever prosthetic valve endocarditis is suspected, transesophageal imaging should be strongly considered. If the transthoracic images are diagnostic, or if the results of transesophageal imaging will not change patient management, it may not be needed. Otherwise, this technique is warranted given its higher sensitivity and specificity for detection of prosthetic valve endocarditis, paravalvular abscess, and prosthetic mitral regurgitation.

Endocarditis rarely can result in prosthetic valve stenosis due to impingement of the infected mass on leaflet opening or to an infected pannus on the upstream side of the valve. Again, visualization of the infected mass may not be possible on transthoracic imaging. Prosthetic valve stenosis is recognized by findings of an increased transvalvular pressure gradient and a decreased valve area (by pressure half-time or by continuity equation).

In an individual patient, a *change* in the appearance or flow characteristics of a prosthetic valve is more diagnostic than an observation at one point in time. Review of previous studies (if available) performed when the patient clinically was well can improve the diagnostic yield of echocardiography.

Clinical and Microbiologic Correlation

Despite the potential limitations of echocardiography for diagnosis of endocarditis, the only other useful diagnostic tests are clinical presentation, physical examination, and microbiologic studies. No other imaging techniques have been shown to have clinical utility in evaluation of endocarditis.

CLINICAL UTILITY

"Rule Out" Endocarditis

In Figure 12–19, the posttest likelihood of endocarditis has been calculated using Bayesian analysis based on the reported sensitivities and specificities of transthoracic and transesophageal echocardiography. In the setting of a low pretest likelihood of disease—the echocardiogram ordered to "rule out" endocarditis—although the posttest likelihood of disease appears to be high, the studies these data are based on may not have included the findings of old, healed vegetations, artifacts, or abnormal (but not infected) valve tissue being mistaken for active endocarditis.

When the pretest likelihood of disease is high (>80 percent), even a "negative" transthoracic echocardiogram decreases the posttest likelihood of disease only modestly (still >50 percent). In some patients, when endocarditis is present, a repeat echocardiogram after several days may show vegetations when the initial study was negative. A negative transesophageal echocardiogram results in a much lower posttest likelihood of disease even when the pretest likelihood is high. Thus transesophageal echo is most useful when the clinical findings support a diagnosis of endocarditis, especially if the transthoracic study is "negative".

Cardiac Evaluation of the Patient with Endocarditis

In a patient with endocarditis, an echocardiogram is an invaluable adjunct to clinical decision making concerning potential surgical intervention and prediction of short- and long-term prognosis. Echocardiography often allows clear definition of which (and how many) valves are affected.

Diagnosis of acute severe valvular regurgitation or a paravalvular abscess is a clear indication for surgical treatment. Associated left ventricu-

Diagnostic Utility of Echo for Endocarditis

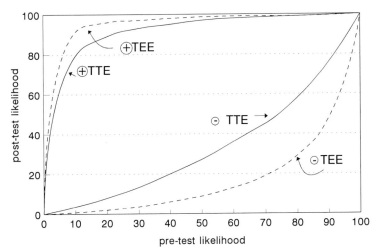

Figure 12–19. Bayesian analysis of the posttest likelihood of endocarditis for transthoracic (TTE) and transesophageal (TEE) echocardiography, using the overall sensitivity and specificity determined from the data in Table 12–1 (TTE sens = 64 percent, spec = 98 percent; TEE sens = 90 percent, spec = 99 percent).

lar dysfunction, involvement of more than one valve, and secondary pulmonary hypertension as evaluated by echocardiography are important determinants of the surgical approach and timing of intervention.

The occurrence of a systemic embolic event generally is accepted as an indication for valve replacement; however, the importance of vegetation size and appearance by echocardiography remains controversial. If patients with emboli-

zation prior to echocardiography are excluded, several studies have shown a trend toward a higher incidence of systemic embolization with a vegetation diameter greater than 1 cm (Table 12–5). However, other studies (see Suggested Reading 11) contest this conclusion. Infection with *H. influenzae* and mitral valve involvement also have been shown to predict a higher rate of systemic emboli. Recent studies have suggested that sequential transesophageal echocar-

TABLE 12–5. SIZE OF VEGETATION BY TWO-DIMENSIONAL ECHOCARDIOGRAPHY VERSUS RISK OF EMBOLISM

| STUDY | n | TOTAL NO. OF EMBOLI | EMBOLISM | | p VALUE |
			No Veg or <10 mm	Veg >10 mm	
Lutas et al.	76	17	16% (8/50)	45% (9/26)	0.06‡
Buda et al.*	42	14	26% (8/31)	55% (6/11)	0.08‡
Wann et al.†	21	7	21% (3/14)	57% (4/7)	0.16§
Wong et al.	31	6	20% (3/15)	19% (3/16)	0.64§
Jaffe et al.	50	10	11% (2/18)	26% (8/32)	0.19§
TOTAL	251	56	19% (24/128)	33% (30/92)	0.018‡

*Excludes patients with right-sided endocarditis.
†Vegetation size graded qualitatively on 1+ to 3+ scale; 3+ was considered >10 mm.
‡Chi-square analysis.
§Fisher's exact test.
Reproduced with permission from Jaffe WM, Morgan DE, Pearlman AS, Otto CM: Infective endocarditis, 1983–1988: Echocardiographic findings and factors influencing morbidity and mortality. J Am Coll Cardiol 15:1227–1233, 1990.
Data from Lutas et al: Am Heart J 112:107, 1986; Buda et al: Am Heart J 112:1291, 1986; Wann et al: Circulation 60:728, 1979; Wong et al: Arch Intern Med 143:1874, 1983.

diographic evaluation of patients with endocarditis can predict whether antimicrobial therapy is effective by demonstrating progressive decreases in vegetation size. However, the cost-effectiveness (and patient acceptance) of this approach remains unclear.

In the current era, with aggressive and prompt surgical intervention, severe regurgitation and heart failure do *not* predict mortality, since these patients undergo early valve replacement. With antibiotic therapy and appropriate surgical intervention, risk factors for in-hospital death are prosthetic valve infection, systemic embolism, and infection with *S. aureus*. Long-term outcome in survivors is related to the residual degree of valve damage, the effects of chronic valvular regurgitation on ventricular function and pulmonary artery pressures, and the risk of recurrent episodes of endocarditis.

SUGGESTED READING

1. Mügge A, Daniel WG, Frank G, Lichtlen PR: Echocardiography in infective endocarditis: Reassessment of prognostic implications of vegetation size determined by the transthoracic and the transesophageal approach. J Am Coll Cardiol 14:631–638, 1989.
   In 105 patients with endocarditis, a vegetation size >10 mm on TTE or TEE was predictive of embolic events (22 of 47 with vegetation ≤10 mm, p < 0.01). Mitral valve endocarditis also was associated with a higher likelihood of embolism. Heart failure and survival were not related to vegetation size.

2. Jaffe WM, Morgan DE, Pearlman AS, Otto CM: Infective endocarditis, 1983–1988: Echocardiographic findings and factors influencing morbidity and mortality. J Am Coll Cardiol 15:1227–1233, 1990.
   In 70 patients with endocarditis, predictors of in-hospital mortality were prosthetic valve endocarditis, occurrence of a systemic embolic event, and infection with S. aureus. Abnormal (≥2+) valvular regurgitation was noted on transthoracic Doppler examination in 88 percent of patients.

3. Burger AJ, Peart B, Jabi H, Touchon RC: The role of two-dimensional echocardiography in the diagnosis of infective endocarditis. Angiology 42:552–560, 1991.
   In 106 patients with suspected endocarditis, vegetations were present on echocardiography in 36 patients, 35 of whom had active infective endocarditis. Of the 65 patients with no vegetation on the initial echo, only 4 patients had clinical endocarditis.

4. Shiveley BK, Gurule FT, Roldan CA, et al: Diagnostic value of transesophageal compared with transthoracic echocardiography in infective endocarditis. J Am Coll Cardiol 18:391–397, 1991.
   Transesophageal echocardiography was more sensitive and specific than transthoracic echocardiography for diagnosis of endocarditis. A negative TEE study resulted in a low probability of disease in patients with an intermediate pretest likelihood of disease.

5. Pedersen WR, Walker M, Olson JD, et al: Value of transesophageal echocardiography as an adjunct to transthoracic echocardiography in evaluation of native and prosthetic valve endocarditis. Chest 100:351–356, 1991.
   In 24 consecutive patients with possible endocarditis (10 with prosthetic valves), transesophageal echocardiography was more sensitive than transthoracic echocardiography for diagnosing vegetations or abscesses.

6. Daniel WG, Mügge A, Grote J, et al: Comparison of transthoracic and transesophageal echocardiography for detection of abnormalities of prosthetic and bioprosthetic valves in the mitral and aortic positions. Am J Cardiol 71:210–215, 1993.
   Detection of prosthetic valve endocarditis was enhanced by TEE. Of 148 prosthetic valves, 124 were abnormal at surgery or autopsy (33 endocarditis, 8 thrombi, and 83 degeneration). Endocarditis was correctly identified in 12 of 36 (36 percent) by TTE and 27 of 33 (82 percent) by TEE.

7. Sochowski RA, Chan K-L: Implication of negative results on a monoplane transesophageal echocardiographic study in patients with suspected infective endocarditis. J Am Coll Cardiol 21:216–221, 1993.
   In 65 patients with a negative TEE study for suspected endocarditis, 56 remained free of clinical evidence of endocarditis, 4 were treated empirically, and 5 had infective endocarditis either on repeat TEE study (3), at autopsy (1), or based on the subsequent clinical course (1). Factors associated with endocarditis and a negative initial TEE study were gram-positive bacteremia and an aortic valve prosthesis.

8. Shapiro SM, Young E, DeGuzman, et al: Transesophageal echocardiography in diagnosis of infective endocarditis. Chest 105:377–382, 1994.
   In 64 patients with suspected endocarditis, transesophageal echocardiography (TEE) was more sensitive (97 percent) than transthoracic echocardiography (TTE 68 percent) for detection of valvular vegetations. Based on strict clinical criteria, 30/64 (47 percent) had acute infective endocarditis. Both TTE and TEE were highly specific (91 percent) for this diagnosis with false-positive echocardiographic findings in 3 patients, 2 of whom had a prior history of endocarditis. All 9 perivalvular abscesses were diagnosed by TEE versus 2/9 on TTE.

9. Daniel WG, Mügge A, Martin RP, et al: Improvement in the diagnosis of abscesses associated with endocarditis by transesophageal echocardiography. N Engl J Med 324:795–800, 1991.
   In 118 consecutive patients with endocarditis, 44 (37 percent) had surgical or autopsy evidence of abscess formation. Abscesses were more common with infection with Staphylococcus (52 percent of cases) and with aortic valve involvement. Hospital mortality in patients with an abscess was 23 versus 14 percent in the remainder of the study group. TEE was much more sensitive than TTE for diagnosis of paravalvular abscess.

10. Karalis DG, Bansal RC, Huack AJ, et al: Transesophageal echocardiographic recognition of subaortic complications in aortic valve endocarditis: Clinical and surgical implications. Circulation 86:353–362, 1992.
    Detailed description (with illustrations) of the patterns of paravalvular and subaortic abscess formation in patients with aortic valve endocarditis. The authors note that eccentric jets of mitral regurgitation in patients with aortic valve endocarditis raise the possibility of involvement (perforation) of the anterior mitral leaflet by the infectious process.

11. Steckelberg JM, Murphy JG, Ballard D, et al: Emboli in infective endocarditis: The prognostic value of echocardiography. Ann Intern Med 114:635–640, 1991.
    In 207 patients with endocarditis, the likelihood of first embolic events was 6.2 per 1000 patient days (95 percent con-

fidence interval, 4.2 to 9.2). The risk of embolic events was related to infection with viridens streptococcal infections but not to vegetation size. The likelihood of embolization decreased over time, falling to 1.2 per 1000 patient days after 2 weeks of therapy.

12. Sanfilippo AJ, Picard MH, Newell JB, et al: Echocardiographic assessment of patients with infectious endocarditis: Prediction of risk for complications. J Am Coll Cardiol 18:1191–1199, 1991.
In 204 patients with endocarditis, multivariate predictors of complications (persistent fever, congestive heart failure, systemic emboli, surgery, and mortality) were vegetation size, extent, and mobility. The authors propose an echo score for vegetation appearance to predict the likelihood of complications.

13. Rohmann S, Erbel R, Darius H, et al: Prediction of rapid versus prolonged healing of infective endocarditis by monitoring vegetation size. J Am Soc Echocardiogr 4:465–474, 1991.
Increasing vegetation size during antibiotic therapy was associated with a higher rate of valve replacement, embolic events, paravalvular abscess formation, and mortality in 83 patients with echocardiographic evidence of endocarditis.

14. Hecht SR, Berger M: Right-sided endocarditis in intravenous drug users: Prognostic features in 102 episodes. Ann Intern Med 117:560–566, 1992.
Clinical study of 132 patients with right-sided endocarditis emphasizes the high prevalence of S. aureus infection (82 percent), tricuspid valve involvement (96 percent), large vegetation size (>10 mm in 80 percent), and low mortality (7 percent) in right-sided (versus left-sided) endocarditis.

15. Lopez JA, Ross RS, Fishbein MC, Siegel RJ: Nonbacterial thrombotic endocarditis: A review. Am Heart J 113:773–784, 1987.
Review of nonbacterial thrombotic endocarditis. Diagnosis often is missed antemortem but, if suspected, may be seen on echocardiography. Advocates use of heparin to prevent embolization.

16. Roldan CA, Shively BK, Lau CC, et al: Systemic lupus erythematosus valve disease by transesophageal echocardiography and the role of antiphospholipid antibodies. J Am Coll Cardiol 20:1127–1134, 1992.
In 54 patients with lupus erythematosus, diffuse leaflet thickening was common (50 percent) in those with antiphospholipid antibody and was associated with valve regurgitation in 64 percent and/or a valve mass in 41 percent. Even in lupus erythematosus patients without antiphospholipid antibody, 47 percent had leaflet thickening, 25 percent had valve masses, and 59 percent had valve regurgitation. In contrast to infective endocarditis, lupus-associated valve lesions tended to occur near the leaflet bases, were heterogeneous in echo density, and showed little independent motion.

17. Yvorchuk KJ, Chan KL: Application of transthoracic and transesophageal echocardiography in the diagnosis and management of infective endocarditis. J Am Soc Echocardiogr 14:294–308, 1994.
Review article on the utility of echocardiography in patients with known or suspected endocarditis. An excellent synthesis of the literature with tables summarizing data, clear examples, and a proposed diagnostic approach. 61 references.

18. Lowry RW, Zoghbi WA, Baker WB, et al: Clinical impact of transesophageal echocardiography in the diagnosis and management of infective endocarditis. Am J Cardio 73:1089–1091, 1994.
In 93 consecutive patients undergoing transesophageal echocardiography (TEE) for suspected endocarditis, the negative predictive value of TEE was 100 percent for native valves and 90 percent for prosthetic valves. TEE resulted in a change in the subsequent diagnostic or therapeutic plan in >90 percent of patients.

CHAPTER 13

ECHOCARDIOGRAPHIC EVALUATION OF CARDIAC MASSES AND POTENTIAL CARDIAC "SOURCE OF EMBOLUS"

INTRODUCTION

A cardiac mass is defined as an abnormal structure within a cardiac chamber, attached to a cardiac structure, or immediately adjacent to the heart. There are three basic types of cardiac masses: tumor, thrombus, and vegetation. Abnormal mass lesions must be distinguished from the occasional unusual appearance of a normal cardiac structure, which may be mistakenly considered as an apparent "mass." Echocardiography allows dynamic evaluation of intracardiac masses with the advantage, compared with other tomographic techniques, that both the anatomic extent and the physiologic consequences of the mass can be evaluated. In addition, associated abnormalities (e.g., valvular regurgitation associated with a vegetation) and conditions that predispose to development of a mass (e.g., apical aneurysm leading to left ventricular thrombus or rheumatic mitral stenosis resulting in left atrial thrombus) can be evaluated. Disadvantages of echocardiography include suboptimal image quality in some patients, a relatively narrow field of view compared with computed tomography or magnetic resonance imaging, and the possibility of mistaking an ultrasound artifact for an anatomic mass.

323

BASIC PRINCIPLES

The first step in assessing a possible cardiac mass is to ensure that the echocardiographic findings represent an actual mass rather than an ultrasound artifact. As discussed in detail in Chapter 1, artifacts can be caused by electrical interference, characteristics of the ultrasound transducer/system, or various physical factors influencing image formation from the reflected ultrasound signals. These include beam-width artifact, near-field "ring-down," and multipath artifact. Appropriate transducer selection, scanning technique, and evaluation from multiple examining windows will help to distinguish artifacts from actual anatomic structures.

Besides ultrasound artifacts, several normal structures and normal variants may be mistaken for a cardiac mass (Table 13–1). In the ventricles, normal trabeculae, aberrant trabeculae or chordae (ventricular "webs" or false tendons) (Fig. 13–1), muscle bundles (such as the moderator band), or the papillary muscles may be mistaken for abnormal structures.

Valvular anatomy includes a wide range of normal variation, and the appearance of a normal (but often unrecognized) structure such as a nodule of Arantius on the aortic valve may be considered incorrectly to represent a cardiac mass. The belly of a valve leaflet, if cut tangentially, may appear as a "mass" when it actually is a portion of the leaflet itself seen *en face*. In the atrium, normal ridges adjacent to the venous entry sites (Figs. 13–2 and 13–3), normal trabeculations (Fig. 13–4), postoperative changes (Fig.13–5), and distortion of the free wall contour by structures adjacent to the atrium (Fig. 13–6) all may be diagnosed erroneously as a cardiac mass.

Definitive diagnosis of an intracardiac mass by echocardiography is based on:

1. Excellent image quality, which may require use of a high frequency (5- or 7.5-MHz) short-focus transducer to evaluate the left ventricular apex from the transthoracic approach and the use of transesophageal imaging to evaluate posterior cardiac structures (e.g., left atrium, mitral valve).

TABLE 13–1. STRUCTURES THAT MAY BE MISTAKEN FOR AN ABNORMAL CARDIAC MASS

Left atrum	Dilated coronary sinus (persistent left superior vena cava)
	Raphe between left superior pulmonary vein and left atrial appendage
	Atrial suture line after cardiac transplant
	Beam-width artifact from calcified aortic valve, aortic valve prosthesis, or other echogenic target adjacent to the atrium
	Interatrial septal aneurysm
Right atrium	Crista terminalis
	Chiari network (Eustachian valve remnants)
	Lipomatous hypertrophy of the interatrial septum
	Trabeculation of right atrial appendage
	Atrial suture line after cardiac transplant
	Pacer wire, Swan-Ganz catheter, or central venous line
Left ventricle	Papillary muscles
	Left ventricular web (aberrant chordae)
	Prominent apical trabeculations
	Prominent mitral annular calcification
Right ventricle	Moderator band
	Papillary muscles
	Swan-Ganz catheter or pacer wire
Aortic valve	Nodules of Arantius
	Lambl's excrescences
	Base of valve leaflet seen *en face* in diastole
Mitral valve	Redundant chordae
	Myxomatous mitral valve tissue
Pulmonary artery	Left atrial appendage (just caudal to pulmonary artery)
Pericardium	Epicardial adipose tissue
	Fibrinous debris in a chronic organized pericardial effusion

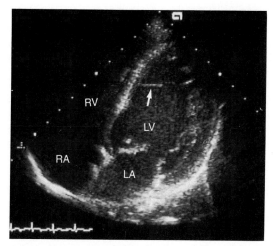

Figure 13–1. Left ventricular aberrant trabeculation or "web" seen in an apical four-chamber view in a 35-year-old woman with a normal echo.

2. Identification of the mass throughout the cardiac cycle, in the same anatomic region of the heart, from more than one acoustic window. This decreases the likelihood of an ultrasound artifact.

3. Knowledge of the normal structures, normal variants, and postoperative changes that may simulate a cardiac mass.

4. Integration of other echocardiographic findings (e.g., rheumatic mitral stenosis and left atrial enlargement in a patient with suspected left atrial thrombus) and clinical data in the final echocardiographic interpretation.

ECHOCARDIOGRAPHIC APPROACH
(Table 13–2)

Once it is clear that a cardiac mass is present, the next step is to determine whether that mass most likely is a tumor, a vegetation, or a thrombus. A definitive diagnosis generally cannot be made from the echocardiographic images alone, since the microscopic and bacteriologic characteristics of the structure cannot be determined. However, a reasonably secure diagnosis often can be made by integrating the clinical data, echocardiographic appearance, and associated echo Doppler findings.

Infectious Cardiac Masses

Infectious cardiac masses include valvular vegetations, which are seen in patients with endocarditis (bacterial or fungal). Noninfectious vegetations also occur in patients with nonbacterial thrombotic endocarditis (NBTE, or *marantic* endocarditis). Vegetations typically are irregularly shaped, attached to the upstream side

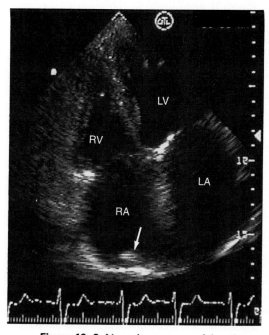
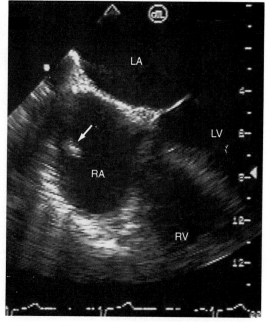

Figure 13–2. Normal appearance of the crista terminalis (*arrow*) in the right atrium in a transthoracic apical four-chamber view (*left*) and in a transesophageal view (*right*) in two different patients.

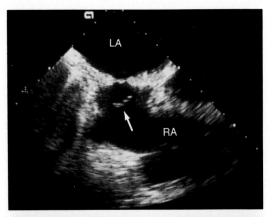

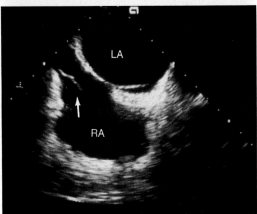

Figure 13–3. Prominent valve at the entrance of the inferior vena cava into the right atrium seen obliquely on transesophageal imaging (*above*) might be mistaken for a cardiac mass. A more longitudinal view (*below*) shows the inferior vena cava and valve more clearly.

of the valve leaflet (e.g., left atrial side of the mitral valve, left ventricular side of the aortic valve), and exhibit chaotic motion that differs from that of the leaflets themselves (see Figs. 12–1 and 12–2). Valvular regurgitation is a frequent but not invariable accompaniment of endocarditis. Valvular stenosis *due* to the vegetation is rare. Paravalvular abscess, which also presents as a cardiac mass, may be difficult to recognize on transthoracic imaging but can be diagnosed with a high sensitivity and specificity on transesophageal echocardiography. Infectious cardiac masses are discussed in detail in Chapter 12.

Cardiac Tumors (Table 13–3)

Nonprimary

Nonprimary cardiac tumors are about 20 times more common than primary cardiac tumors. Tumors can involve the heart by direct invasion from adjacent malignancies (lung, breast), by lymphatic spread, or by metastatic spread of distant disease (lymphoma, melanoma). In autopsy series of patients with a malignancy, cardiac involvement is present in approximately 10 percent of cases, although clinical recognition of cardiac involvement occurs less frequently. Melanoma has the highest rate of pericardial metastases, but since there are relatively few patients with melanoma, a cardiac tumor is more likely to represent a more preva-

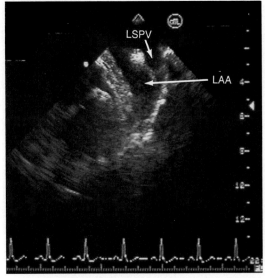

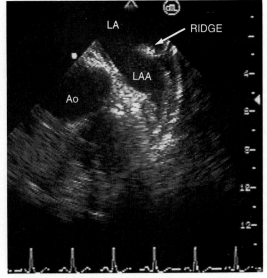

Figure 13–4. The normal ridge between the left atrial appendage (LAA) and left superior pulmonary vein (LSPV) may be mistaken for an abnormal mass (*left*). Slight angulation of the image plane shows a more typical appearance (*right*).

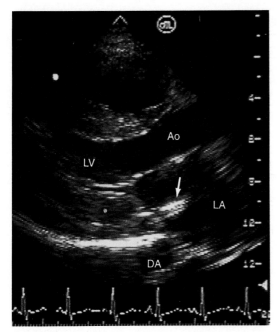

Figure 13–5. Postcardiac transplant patient with a prominent suture line (*arrow*) in the left atrium in a parasternal long-axis view.

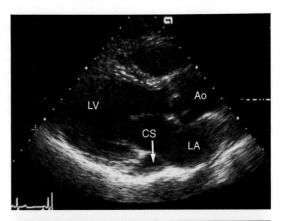

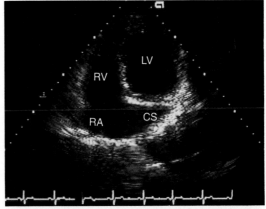

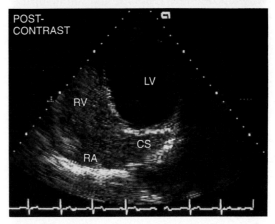

Figure 13–6. Persistent left superior vena cava resulting in a dilated coronary sinus (CS) posterior to the left atrium seen in a parasternal long-axis view (*top*). If there is ultrasound "drop-out" from the wall of the coronary sinus, the abnormal contour of the left atrium may be mistaken for a mass. In the posteriorly angulated apical four-chamber view, the dilated coronary sinus connects to the right atrium (*center*). Contrast injection in a left arm vein results in opacification of the coronary sinus, confirming the diagnosis (*below*).

lent malignancy, as shown in Table 13–4. Almost three-quarters of cardiac metastases are due to lung, breast, or hematologic malignancies. It is noteworthy that lymphomas associated with acquired immunodeficiency syndrome (AIDS) have frequent and extensive cardiac involvement.

Tumors can affect the heart by (1) invasion of the pericardium, epicardium, myocardium, or endocardium, (2) production of biologically active substances, or (3) toxic effects of treatment on the heart (e.g., radiation or chemotherapy).

Cardiac malignancies most often involve the pericardium and epicardium (about 75 percent of metastatic cardiac disease), presenting as a pericardial effusion, with or without tamponade physiology (Fig. 13–7). Since echocardiographic diagnosis of the *cause* of a pericardial effusion rarely is possible, the diagnosis of a pericardial effusion (and particularly tamponade) in a patient with a known malignancy should alert the clinician to the possibility of cardiac involvement. Confirmation of the diagnosis requires examination of pericardial fluid and, if necessary, pericardial biopsy. The differential diagnosis of a pericardial effusion in a patient with a known malignancy includes radiation pericarditis and idiopathic pericarditis (which is common in cancer patients), as well as metastatic disease. The prognosis of a patient with a malignant pericar-

TABLE 13–2. DISTINGUISHING CHARACTERISTICS OF INTRACARDIAC MASSES

CHARACTERISTIC	THROMBUS	TUMOR	VEGETATION
Location	LA (especially when enlarged or associated with MV disease) LV (in setting of reduced systolic function or segmental wall abnormalities)	LA (myxoma) Myocardium Pericardium Valves	Usually valvular Occasionally on ventricular wall or Chiari network
Appearance	Usually discrete and somewhat spherical in shape *or* laminated against LV apex or LA wall	Various: may be circumscribed or may be irregular	Irregular shape, attached to the proximal (upstream) side of the valve with motion independent from the valve
Associated findings	Underlying etiology usually evident LV systolic dysfunction or segmental wall motion abnormalities (exception: eosinophilic heart disease) MV disease with LA enlargement	Intracardiac obstruction depending on site of tumor	Valvular regurgitation usually present Clinically: fevers, systemic signs of endocarditis, positive blood cultures

MV = mitral valve, LV = left ventricle, LA = left atrium.

dial effusion is extremely poor, with a predicted 1-year survival less than 50 percent. Repeat echocardiographic evaluation of these patients often is needed for initial diagnosis, assessment of therapeutic interventions, and follow-up for recurrent effusion.

Myocardial involvement by metastatic disease is less common than pericardial involvement, but does occur, particularly with lymphoma or melanoma. Intramyocardial masses can project into or compress cardiac chambers, resulting in hemodynamic compromise. Endocardial involvement is rarely seen.

A specific type of cardiac involvement by tumor that should be recognized by the echocardiographer is extension of *renal cell carcinoma* up the inferior vena cava (Fig. 13–8). A "finger-like" projection of tumor may protrude into the right atrium from the inferior vena cava, and the tumor can be followed retrograde (from a subcostal approach) back to the kidney. Collaboration with the abdominal ultrasound laboratory may be needed for full delineation of the tumor extent. Identification is important, since curative en bloc resection may be possible. *Uterine tumors* occasionally present in this fashion as well.

TABLE 13–3. PRIMARY CARDIAC TUMORS IN ADULTS

Benign	Myxoma	27%
	Lipoma	10%
	Papillary fibroelastoma	10%
	Hemangioma	3%
	Mesothelioma of the AV node	1%
Malignant	Angiosarcoma	9%
	Rhabdomyosarcoma	5%
	Mesothelioma	4%
	Fibrosarcoma	3%
	Malignant lymphoma	2%
	Extraskeletal osteosarcoma	1%
Cysts	Pericardial	18%
	Bronchogenic	2%

Data from McAllister HA, Fenoglio JJ: Tumors of the cardiovascular system. *In:* Fasicle 15, Second Series, Atlas of Tumor Pathology, Armed Forces Institute of Pathology, 1978.

TABLE 13–4. ORIGIN OF METASTATIC CARDIAC TUMORS IN ADULTS (in order of frequency)

Lung
Lymphoma
Breast
Leukemia
Stomach
Melanoma
Liver
Colon

Data from Abraham KP, Reddy V, Gattuso P: Neoplasms metastatic to the heart: Review of 3314 consecutive autopsies. Am J Cardiovas Pathol 3:195–198, 1990.

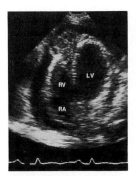
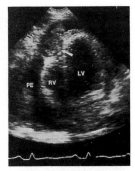

Figure 13-7. Metastatic tumor to the heart with an irregular epicardial mass invading the myocardium at the right ventricular apex and an associated pericardial effusion.

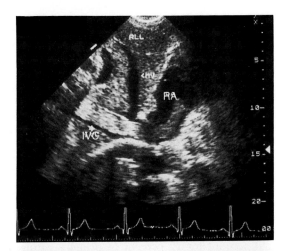

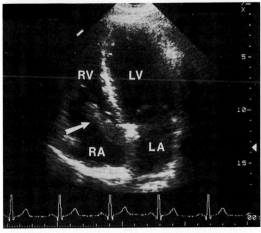

Tumors also can affect the cardiac structures indirectly, as is seen in *carcinoid heart disease* (Fig. 13-9). Metastatic carcinoid tissue in the liver produces biologically active substances, including serotonin, which cause abnormalities of the right-sided cardiac valves and endocardium. Typical changes include thickening, retraction, and increased rigidity of the tricuspid and pulmonic valve leaflets, resulting in valvular regurgitation or, less often, valvular stenosis. Left-sided valvular involvement is rarely seen, possibly due to a lower concentration of the active molecules after passage through the lungs. While metastatic carcinoid disease is rare, the echocardiographic findings are pathognomonic and may lead to the diagnosis in a patient in whom it was not considered previously. Although only a third of patients with carcinoid tumors have cardiac involvement, half the deaths in carcinoid patients are due to heart failure secondary to severe tricuspid regurgitation.

Figure 13-8. Renal cell carcinoma extending up the inferior vena cava (IVC) is seen on a subcostal view (*above*) and in an apical four-chamber view (*below*) protruding into the right atrium and across the tricuspid valve into the right ventricle. This tumor was resected *en bloc* at the time of surgery.

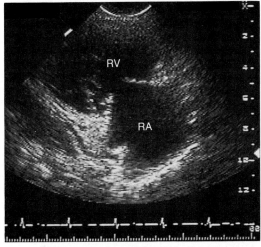
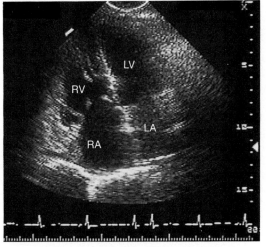

Figure 13-9. Carcinoid heart disease with thickening and shortening of the tricuspid leaflets seen in a right ventricular inflow view (*left*) and an apical four-chamber view (*right*). Mild stenosis and severe regurgitation of the tricuspid valve were present.

Primary

As for tumors elsewhere in the body, the distinction between benign and malignant primary cardiac tumors is based on pathologic examination of tissue and its tendency to invade adjacent tissue or metastasize to distant sites. Although 75 percent of primary cardiac tumors are benign, a pathologically benign cardiac tumor can have "malignant" hemodynamic consequences if it obstructs the normal pattern of blood flow. Thus the echocardiographic examination includes definition of both the anatomic extent of a cardiac tumor and its physiologic consequences.

Benign Primary Cardiac Tumors. Myxomas account for 27 percent of primary cardiac tumors. Cardiac myxomas most often are single, arising from the fossa ovalis of the interatrial septum and protruding into the left atrium (in about 75 percent of cases) (Fig. 13–10). Other sites of origin include the right atrium (18 percent), the left ventricle (4 percent), and the right ventricle (4 percent). More than one site can occur in an individual patient (5 percent of cases).

The clinical presentation of a cardiac myxoma can include constitutional symptoms (fever, malaise), clinically evident embolic events, and symptoms of mitral valve obstruction. A myxoma also may be an unexpected finding on a study requested for other clinical indications.

A left atrial myxoma may nearly fill the left atrial chamber (Fig. 13–11), with prolapse of the

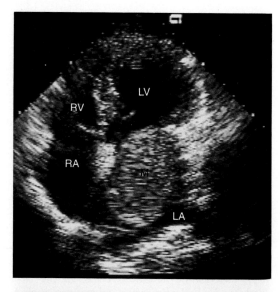

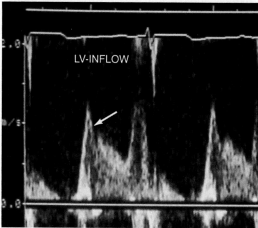

Figure 13–11. Large left atrial myxoma (M) in an 84-year-old woman with prolapse across the mitral annulus in diastole (*above*) in an apical four-chamber view. Doppler left ventricular filling (*below*) shows normal filling at valve opening (*arrow*) followed by obstruction as the myxoma obstructs the mitral orifice.

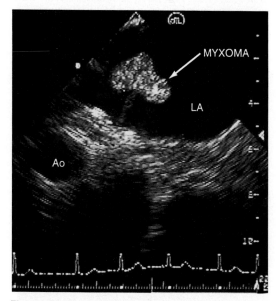

Figure 13–10. Left atrial myxoma arising from a thin stalk attached to the fossa ovalis of the interatrial septum seen in a transesophageal view.

tumor mass across the mitral annulus into the left ventricle in diastole (accounting for the tumor "plop" on auscultation). The mass often has an irregular shape characterized by protruding "fronds" of tissue or a "grape cluster" appearance. The echogenicity of the mass may be nonhomogeneous, and sometimes areas of calcification are noted.

The degree to which the tumor causes functional obstruction to left ventricular diastolic filling can be evaluated qualitatively by color flow imaging and quantitatively by the pressure half-time method (Fig. 13–12). Careful echocardiographic evaluation from multiple views,

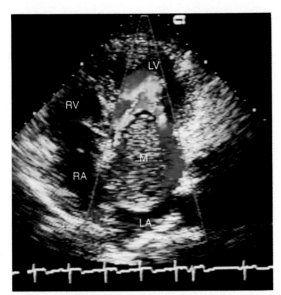

Figure 13–12. Color flow imaging also shows the partial obstruction to left ventricular diastolic filling due to the atrial myxoma (M) in the same patient as Figure 13–11.

often including transesophageal, is needed in planning the surgical approach. Important goals of the echo examination are to identify the site of tumor attachment, to ensure that the tumor does not involve the valve leaflets themselves, and to exclude the possibility of multiple masses. Postoperatively, complete excision should be documented by echocardiography. Sequential long-term follow-up may be indicated, since recurrent myxomas have been reported, particularly with a familial form of this disease, with multiple myxomas, or with a less than full-thickness excision.

The echocardiographic approach to myxomas arising in other locations is similar to that described for left atrial myxomas, except that the two-dimensional (2D) views and Doppler examination should be tailored toward evaluating the specific region of tumor involvement in that patient. Again, it should be emphasized that the diagnosis of a myxoma, based on the clinical features, anatomic location, and echocardiographic appearance of the tumor, is only presumptive until confirmed histologically. A "typical" myxoma may turn out to be a metastatic malignancy or a primary cardiac malignancy on pathologic examination. Hence the echocardiographic examination should be as complete as possible to exclude tissue invasion by the tumor, multiple sites of involvement, or atypical features.

A *papillary fibroelastoma* is a benign cardiac tumor that arises on valvular tissue, thus mimicking the appearance of a valvular vegetation. These small masses are attached to the mitral or (less often) aortic valve, and they show independent motion (Fig. 13–13). Unlike a vegetation, they are more often found on the downstream side of the valve (left ventricular side of mitral valve, aortic side of aortic valve). On histologic examination, papillary fibroelastomas are very similar to the smaller Lambl's excrescences, which can be seen on normal valves in the elderly. Usually papillary fibroelastomas are of no clinical significance, but they may cause consternation on the part of the physicians caring for the patient and lead to further diagnostic tests with their associated costs and complications. Occasional cases of superimposed thrombus formation resulting in systemic embolic events have been described.

Other benign cardiac tumors seen in adults include hemangiomas, and mesotheliomas of the atrioventricular node.

Lipomatous hypertrophy of the interatrial septum presents as a cardiac mass that may be mistaken

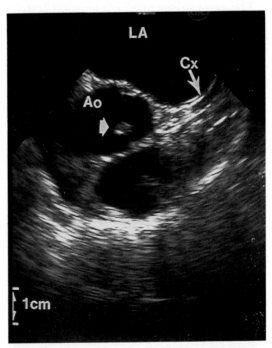

Figure 13–13. Small papillary fibroelastoma attached to the left coronary cusp of the aortic valve (with independent motion) as seen on transesophageal imaging (*arrow*). This mass was not seen on transthoracic imaging. In this patient with increased thrombogenicity, this benign valve tumor had associated thrombus which resulted in embolic events (Cx = circumflex coronary artery). (*From Huth M, Gordon D, Verner ED, Otto CM. Aortic valvular fibroma as a source of systemic emboli in POEMS syndrome. J Am Soc Echocardiogr 4:401, 1991.*)

for a tumor. Lipomatous hypertrophy typically involves the superior and inferior fatty portions of the atrial septum, sparing the fossa ovalis region (Fig. 13–14). However, symmetrical ellipsoid-shaped enlargements of the interatrial septum also have been described. If the etiology of atrial septal hypertrophy is unclear on echocardiography, CT scanning may establish the diagnosis of lipomatous hypertrophy by showing the characteristic radiographic density of adipose tissue.

Malignant Primary Cardiac Tumors. Malignant primary cardiac tumors are rare. In adults, angiosarcomas, rhabdomyosarcomas (Fig. 13–15), mesotheliomas, and fibrosarcomas are seen (see Table 13–3). The clinical presentation is variable, ranging from an "incidental" finding on echocardiography or nonspecific systemic symptoms (fever, malaise, fatigue) to signs and symptoms of cardiac tamponade. Since metastatic disease is far more likely than a primary cardiac origin, thorough evaluation must include a search for potential primary sites. Ultimately, the diagnosis depends on examination of tissue from the cardiac mass.

The echocardiographic examination focuses on the anatomic location and extent of the tumor involvement, the physiologic consequences of the tumor (e.g., valve regurgitation, chamber obliteration, obstruction), and associated findings (pericardial effusion, evidence of tamponade physiology). Along with other imaging techniques, the echocardiographic examination may help guide therapy by determining whether the tumor is resectable or whether palliative cardiac procedures are likely to be beneficial. Specific attention also is directed toward possible involvement of the valves, coronary arteries, or conducting system.

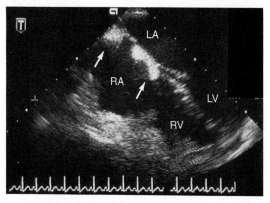

Figure 13–14. Lipomatous hypertrophy (*arrows*) of the interatrial septum seen on transesophageal imaging with typical sparing of the thin fossa ovalis.

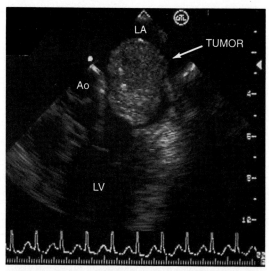

Figure 13–15. Large, recurrent left atrial rhabdomyosarcoma attached to the ridge between the left atrial appendage and left superior pulmonary vein. Note that this malignant tumor appears similar on echocardiography to a benign myxoma.

Technical Considerations/Alternate Imaging Techniques

While echocardiography has definite advantages for evaluating cardiac tumors, it has significant disadvantages as well. These include (1) poor acoustic access, resulting in suboptimal image quality, which limits the confidence with which tumor location and extent can be defined or results in a missed diagnosis (transesophageal imaging may obviate this limitation in some patients), (2) the need for a careful and meticulous examination to detect and fully evaluate the cardiac tumor (as for other applications, echocardiography is operator-dependent, and a significant learning curve for obtaining optimal data can be observed), and (3) the limited "field of view" inherent in echocardiography (i.e., structures adjacent to the heart in the mediastinum and lung are difficult to evaluate). Other tomographic imaging techniques, specifically computed tomography and magnetic resonance imaging, have the advantage of a wide field of view so that the relationship between cardiac and extracardiac tumor involvement can be evaluated. Often judicious use of both echocardiographic techniques (to assess cardiac involvement in detail and to evaluate the physiologic consequences of the tumor mass) and computed tomography or magnetic resonance imaging (to assess potential extracardiac involvement) may be needed in an individual patient for optimal clinical decision making. Both computed tomography and magnetic resonance imaging may provide data on the tissue characteristics of the abnormal mass, which currently cannot be obtained with echocardiography (Fig. 13–16).

Left Ventricular Thrombus

Predisposing Conditions

Thrombus formation in the left ventricle tends to occur in regions of blood stasis or low velocity blood flow. The most familiar example of blood flow stasis in the left ventricle is a ventricular aneurysm, in which low-velocity swirling blood flow patterns are seen. Stasis also may occur with less severe segmental wall motion abnormalities (e.g., apical akinesis) and with diffuse left ventricular dysfunction (e.g., dilated cardiomyopathy). Left ventricular thrombus formation is extremely rare in the absence of an akinetic or dyskinetic apex or diffuse left ventricular dysfunction. Thrombus formation also often accompanies a left ventricular pseudoaneurysm. In this case, the thrombus lines an area of left ventricular rupture that has been contained by the pericardium.

Even when a definite left ventricular thrombus is not seen on an echocardiographic examination, the likelihood of thrombus formation remains high in patients with left ventricular aneurysm, apical akinesis, or diffuse left ventricular systolic dysfunction with an ejection fraction of less than 20 percent. Doppler analysis of apical flow patterns has been suggested to help identify which of these patients are at highest risk of thrombus formation. Evidence of apical flow stasis, or of continuous swirling of flow around the apex is thought to identify patients at particular risk for apical thrombus.

Identification of Left Ventricular Thrombi

The sensitivity of echocardiography for detecting left ventricular thrombi is extremely operator-dependent (Table 13–5). A careful and thorough examination requires not only standard views but also angulated apical views and the use of higher-frequency short-focus transducers to improve near-field resolution. It is advantageous to use a 5.0- or 7.5-MHz transducer from the standard apical four-chamber window and also to move the transducer slightly laterally while angulating it medially to obtain an apical short-axis view. Scanning across the apex in several views usually allows distinction of prominent apical trabeculations or false tendons—which are bright linear structures that attach to mural trabeculae—from apical thrombi. Thrombus is often (though not always) somewhat more echogenic than the underlying myocardium, and it has a contour distinct from the endocardial border.

The diagnosis of left ventricular thrombus is most secure when an echogenic mass is seen with a convex surface (e.g., spherical) that is not a ring-down artifact, is clearly distinct from the endocardium, and is located in a region of abnormal wall motion (Fig. 13–17). The diagnosis of laminated thrombus is more problematic unless a clear demarcation between the thrombus and the underlying myocardium is seen, but it can be suspected when the apex appears "rounded" and akinetic with apparent excessively thick apical myocardium (Fig. 13–18).

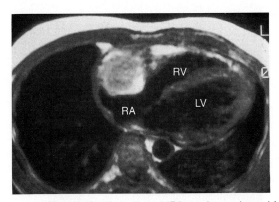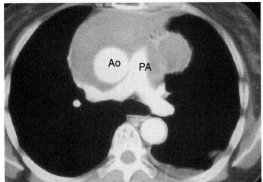

Figure 13–16. (*Left*) An MRI scan in a patient with angiosarcoma shows a large nonhomogeneous right atrial mass. (*Right*) A CT scan at the level of the pulmonary artery and ascending aorta in a different patient (who also had an angiosarcoma) shows extensive intrapericardial tumor involvement. These cases illustrate the advantage of the wide field of view of MRI and CT techniques compared with the narrow field of view of echocardiography.

TABLE 13–5. SENSITIVITY AND SPECIFICITY OF DIAGNOSTIC TESTS FOR INTRACARDIAC THROMBUS FORMATION

	SENSITIVITY	SPECIFICITY
LA thrombus		
Echo-TTE[a]	59–63%	95–99%
Echo-TEE[b]	100%	100%
Radionuclide angiography	67%	54%
CT[c]	100%	91%
Angiography[c]	70%	88%
LV thrombus		
Echo-TTE[d]	92–95%	86–88%
Radionuclide angiography[e]	77%	88%
MRI[f]	93%	85%
Indium-111 platelet scintigraphy[g]	71%	100%

[a]Shrestha et al: Am J Cardiol 48:954–960, 1981; Chiang et al: J Ultrasound Med 6:525–529, 1987; Bansal et al: Am J Cardiol 64:243–246, 1989.
[b]Aschenberg et al: JACC 7:163–166, 1986; Olson et al: JASE 5:52–56, 1992.
[c]Tomoda et al: Am Heart J 100:306, 1980.
[d]Visser et al: Chest 83:228–232, 1983; Stratton et al: Circulation 66:156–165, 1982.
[e]Stratton et al: Am J Cardiol 48:565–572, 1981.
[f]Sechtem et al: Am J Cardiol 64:1195–1199, 1989.
[g]Stratton et al: Am J Cardiol 47:874–881, 1981; Seabold et al: JACC 9:1057–1066, 1987.
LA = left atrium, LV = left ventricle, MRI = magnetic resonance imaging, TEE = transesophageal echocardiography, TTE = transthoracic echocardiography.

Clinical Implications

In some cases, apical images are suboptimal despite careful examination technique. In this situation, definite exclusion of apical thrombus may not be possible. Even so, clinical management (e.g., chronic anticoagulation) may depend more on assessment of overall left ventricular function or the presence of an apical aneurysm than on the presence or absence of an echocardiographically documented thrombus.

The presence of a left ventricular thrombus on echocardiographic examination is a strong predictor of subsequent embolic events, particularly when the thrombus protrudes into the ventricular cavity or shows independent mobility. Sessile, nonprotruding thrombi may have lower embolic potential.

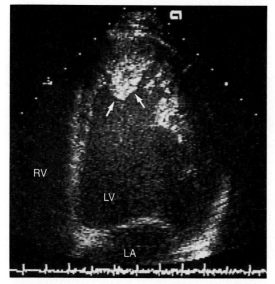

Figure 13–17. Protruding thrombus (*arrows*) in an akinetic apex in a 53-year-old man with a dilated cardiomyopathy seen in an apical four-chamber view.

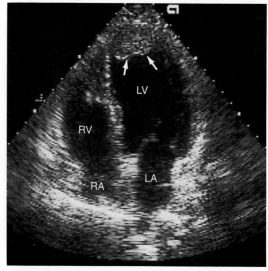

Figure 13–18. Apical thrombus "obliterating" the left ventricular apex in a 53-year-old woman with an old anterior myocardial infarction.

Alternate Approaches

Transthoracic echocardiography is the clinical procedure of choice for identification of left ventricular thrombi. Transesophageal imaging rarely is helpful and may be less sensitive, as the apex may not be visualized in standard image planes and since the left ventricular apex is at considerable distance from the transducer, thereby limiting resolution of structural detail. Left ventricular contrast angiography and radionuclide ventriculography both have a low sensitivity and specificity for diagnosing left ventricular thrombus. In the research setting, indium 113–labeled platelets with gamma-camera imaging have shown a high specificity, but this approach is not available for routine clinical use.

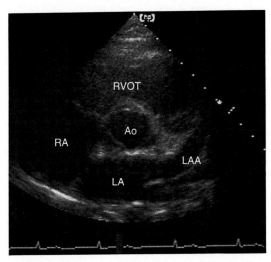

Figure 13–19. Transthoracic parasternal short-axis view of the left atrial appendage (LAA).

Left Atrial Thrombus

Predisposing Factors

Left atrial thrombi tend to form when there is stasis of blood flow in the left atrium. In general, low-velocity flow in the left atrium is associated with atrial enlargement, mitral valve disease, and atrial fibrillation. The highest incidence of left atrial thrombus is in patients with rheumatic mitral stenosis and atrial fibrillation. However, in the presence of mitral stenosis or poor left ventricular function, even patients in sinus rhythm and those with only modest left atrial enlargement can have left atrial thrombi.

Left atrial thrombi are less common in patients with mitral regurgitation, presumably because the high-velocity regurgitant jet mechanically disrupts the area of blood stasis within the left atrium.

Identification of Left Atrial Thrombi

Visualization of left atrial thrombi using transthoracic echocardiography is limited by two factors:

1. The left atrium is in the far field of the image from both parasternal and apical windows, thus limiting resolution of left atrial structures and possible thrombi.
2. A large percentage of left atrial thrombi are found in the left atrial appendage, which is difficult to image from the transthoracic approach.

In some patients, the left atrial appendage can be visualized from a parasternal approach (Fig. 13–19), starting in the short-axis view at the aor-

tic valve level and angulating the transducer inferiorly and laterally to demonstrate the triangular appendage just inferior to the pulmonary artery. From the apical two-chamber view, the left atrial appendage may be visualized by slight superior angulation of the transducer. If a discrete echogenic mass is seen in the left atrium of a patient with mitral stenosis and atrial fibrillation, the specificity of this finding for left atrial thrombi is very high (Fig. 13–20). Of course, the differential diagnosis includes tumor, but this possibility is much less likely in this setting. Nonetheless, the sensitivity of transthoracic

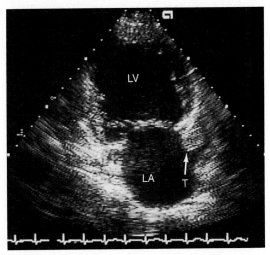

Figure 13–20. Transthoracic apical two-chamber view showing a definite thrombus (T) in the left atrial appendage in a 51-year-old man with dilated cardiomyopathy.

echocardiography for detection of left atrial thrombus remains modest at best. If *no* left atrial thrombus is seen in a patient in whom the diagnosis is suspected, a transthoracic echo study certainly does *not* exclude this possibility.

Transesophageal imaging has a much greater sensitivity and a high negative predictive value for the diagnosis of left atrial thrombi. Hence transesophageal evaluation should be considered when the presence or absence of left atrial thrombus is important for patient management. From the transesophageal approach, the left atrium lies close to the transducer, and usually it can be visualized clearly with a 5-MHz transducer. The left atrial appendage and the body of the left atrium can be evaluated most thoroughly by using both transverse and longitudinal imaging planes (Fig. 13–21).

Stasis of blood flow may be seen on transesophageal imaging as "spontaneous" echo contrast, that is, echogenic reflections from the low-velocity blood flow appearing as white swirls on the 2D echocardiographic image (Fig. 13–22). While the appearance of "spontaneous" contrast depends on technical factors such as transducer frequency and instrument gain as well as the pattern of blood flow, it clearly is associated with an increased risk of left atrial thrombus formation. An increased risk of embolic complications that appears to be independent of associated atrial thrombus also has been reported.

Prognosis/Clinical Implications

The importance of a left atrial thrombus depends on the clinical setting. In a patient with new atrial fibrillation and an embolic stroke, the most likely cause of the stroke is a left atrial thrombus whether or not one is actually imaged, and thus the demonstration of a left atrial thrombus would be unlikely to change clinical management. In contrast, in a patient with rheumatic mitral stenosis, the presence of a left atrial thrombus is a contraindication to mitral balloon commissurotomy.

Alternate Approaches

While few direct comparisons of echocardiography versus computed tomographic or magnetic resonance imaging have been performed, these imaging modalities have been reported to have a high sensitivity for detection of left atrial thrombus.

Right Heart Thrombi

Formation of thrombi in the right side of the heart is rare, although it has been reported in cases of severe right ventricular dilation and systolic dysfunction. A more likely source of thrombi seen within the right side of the heart is

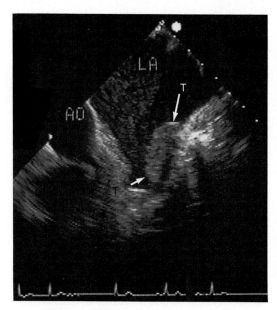 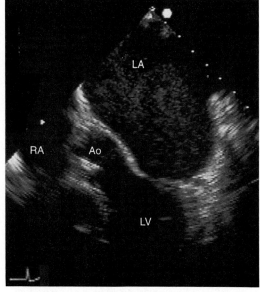

Figure 13–21. Thrombus (*left*) in the left atrial appendage seen on transesophageal imaging in a 42-year-old man with severe rheumatic mitral stenosis. "Spontaneous" contrast (*right*), with a swirling motion in real time, is seen in the body of the enlarged left atrium.

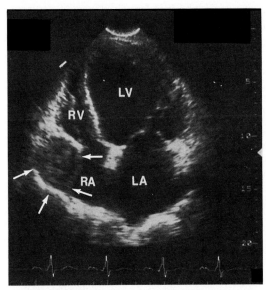

Figure 13–22. Extracardiac localized thrombus after coronary artery surgery is seen indenting the right atrium in a four-chamber view.

venous thrombi that have embolized and become entrapped in the tricuspid valve apparatus or right ventricular trabeculations during passage from the peripheral veins toward the pulmonary artery. Thrombi also can form on indwelling catheters or pacer wires. While thrombi in the right side of the heart can sometimes be demonstrated by meticulous transthoracic imaging (Figs. 13–22 and 13–23), trans-

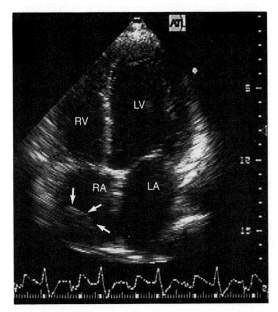

Figure 13–23. Right atrial thrombus (*arrows*) in a patient with a dilated cardiomyopathy.

esophageal echo is better able to resolve the presence, extent, and attachment of right-sided heart thrombi.

When mobile echogenic targets are seen within the right heart chambers, it is important to distinguish thrombi from Eustachian valve remnants, microbubbles, or reverberation artifacts. Eustachian valve remnants, which are unresorbed portions of the embryologic valves of the sinus venosus, are typically mobile, thin linear structures attached at the junction of the inferior or superior cavae and the right atrial cavity. They may be extensive and can cross the atrium, attaching to the fossa ovalis. They do not extend antegrade to cross the tricuspid valve in diastole, however. Microbubbles, which are encapsulated gas bubbles that can be seen in patients with indwelling venous access, appear as discrete echogenic targets that are usually located in different parts of the heart during successive cycles.

CARDIAC SOURCE OF EMBOLUS

Basic Principles

In a patient with a suspected cardiac origin of a systemic embolic event, echocardiographic evaluation is directed toward:

1. Identification of an abnormal intracardiac mass (e.g., left ventricular thrombus, left atrial tumor, valvular vegetation), and/or

2. Identification of an abnormality that may predispose the patient to development of intracardiac thrombi (e.g., left ventricular aneurysm, mitral stenosis, atrial flow stasis), and/or

3. Identification of a cardiac abnormality that may serve as a potential source for systemic embolism (patent foramen ovale, atrial septal aneurysm, atheromatous aortic debris).

Note that echocardiographic evaluation *after* an index embolic event may fail to demonstrate a cardiac thrombus even if it was the etiology of the clinical event, since now the thrombus has embolized and is no longer in the heart. Recurrent intracardiac thrombus formation may not yet have occurred.

Identifiable Cardiac Sources of Emboli

In patients with an echocardiographically demonstrated abnormal intracardiac mass in the aftermath of a recent systemic embolic event, the likelihood is very high that a portion of the mass embolized, thereby causing the clinical event. Cardiac masses known to be associated with clinical systemic embolic events include valvular vegetations, left ventricular and atrial thrombi, and cardiac tumors (especially left atrial myxomas). Other potential pathways for systemic embolization (patent foramen ovale) and possible cardiac sources (atrial septal aneurysm, aortic atherosclerosis) are discussed below. In patients with suspected systemic embolic events, a definite cardiac source is documented by transthoracic echocardiography in approximately 10 to 15 percent of sequential cases. To some extent, the low prevalence of a definite source may relate to imaging *after* the event (when the mass is no longer in the heart). On the other hand, in many patients the source of embolus may have been noncardiac (e.g., atheromas with or without superimposed thrombus in the carotids or ascending aorta), or the intracardiac thrombi may have embolized soon after formation. In this latter group, it is especially important to search for conditions that predispose to intracardiac thrombus formation, even though an intracardiac thrombus is not identified at the time of the examination.

Predisposing Conditions

Apical aneurysms have a high incidence of associated thrombus formation. Other segmental wall motion abnormalities and diffuse left ventricular systolic dysfunction also predispose to left ventricular thrombus formation. A left ventricular pseudoaneurysm is almost invariably accompanied by thrombus lining the pseudoaneurysm cavity.

Rheumatic mitral stenosis is associated with left atrial thrombus formation. Atrial fibrillation, even when it occurs without coexisting mitral valve disease, is strongly associated with systemic embolic events, presumably due to left atrial thrombi. In a patient with a systemic embolic event and either paroxysmal or sustained atrial fibrillation, left atrial thrombus formation is so likely that even if transesophageal echocardiography fails to demonstrate a left atrial clot, it still may be appropriate to treat the patient with systemic anticoagulants in order to prevent recurrent atrial thrombus formation.

Intracardiac thrombi may occur in congenital heart disease patients, particularly those with atrial dilation or ventricular dysfunction. Patients with a large atrial septal defect are at risk for "paradoxical" systemic embolization of peripheral venous thrombi. Thrombi can pass from the right to the left atrium even when the shunt is predominantly left to right, owing to flowstreaming or transient shifts in the right-to-left atrial pressure gradient. While patients with Eisenmenger's physiology and a large ventricular septal defect are at risk of systemic embolization from peripheral venous thrombus formation, such paradoxical embolization is unlikely when the ventricular septal defect is small and there is a large pressure difference between the left and right ventricles.

Prosthetic valves are another potential source of embolic events; the incidence of clinical events is higher with mechanical compared with tissue valves. Demonstration of small thrombi on prosthetic valves is difficult even with transesophageal imaging, owing to shadowing and reverberations from the prosthetic leaflets and sewing ring. Hence the diagnosis often is presumptive when there is evidence of suboptimal anticoagulation at the time of the event or when other causes for the clinical event have been excluded even if the level of anticoagulation appears to have been adequate. In these patients, the primary goals of the echocardiographic examination are to assess prosthetic valve function (since significant thrombus may result in stenosis and/or regurgitation) and to exclude other intracardiac sources of thrombus formation (e.g., associated left ventricular systolic dysfunction).

The advent of transesophageal echocardiography has made it possible to image atrial structures in more detail and has led to the recognition of other anatomic variants that may be associated with systemic embolic events: (1) patent foramen ovale, (2) interatrial septal aneurysm, (3) a swirling pattern of blood flow in the left atrium in the absence of an exogenous "contrast" agent (thought to represent flow stasis and often called *spontaneous contrast*), and (4) atherosclerotic debris in the aorta.

A patent foramen ovale is present in 25 to 35 percent of unselected patients at necropsy. During fetal development, incomplete closure of the interatrial septum shunts oxygenated placental blood from the right to left atrium and then to the brain. This potential interatrial communication fuses within the first few days after birth in most individuals. If the flap valve covering the fossa ovalis remains unfused, there usually is no passage of blood across the interatrial septum. The "flap" is functionally closed because left atrial pressure normally exceeds right atrial pressure. However, if right atrial pressure transiently exceeds left atrial pressure (as during a cough or the Valsalva maneuver), or if right atrial pressure chronically exceeds left atrial pressure (e.g., after pulmonary embolization or with chronic lung disease), there can be right-to-left passage of blood (or thrombi) across the interatrial septum.

Echocardiographic demonstration of a patent foramen ovale is possible with color flow Doppler imaging from a transesophageal approach in only about 5 to 10 percent of patients, with a lesser number detected by transthoracic color Doppler imaging. Detection of a patent foramen is enhanced by intravenous injection of echo contrast material (such as agitated saline) providing opacification of the right-sided heart structures. Passage of contrast across the interatrial septum is seen as bright echo contrast in the left atrium within 1 to 3 beats of its appearance in the right atrium (Fig. 13–24). Often the site of origin of the contrast in the left atrium can be identified on frame-by-frame analysis. Using echo contrast, a patent foramen is detectable at rest in about 5 percent of the general population. When maneuvers to transiently increase right atrial pressure are performed simultaneously with contrast injection, the prevalence of detectable patent foramen ovale by contrast transesophageal echocardiography increases to approximately 25 percent—similar to the incidence at autopsy.

Accurate detection of a patent foramen ovale is more likely on transesophageal imaging due to improved image quality. However, contrast injections still are needed to detect all cases. Passage of very small microbubbles through the pulmonary capillaries can occur; these typically appear in the left atrium via the pulmonary veins late after the appearance of contrast material in the right atrium. The examiner should evaluate whether contrast material in the left atrium detected on transesophageal imaging passed across the interatrial septum or reflects transpulmonary passage. Meticulous evaluation using biplane transesophageal echocardiography often is helpful.

In young patients (<45 years of age) with transient ischemic attacks or cerebrovascular events, a higher incidence of patent foramen ovale is found than in the general population, suggesting that passage of thrombi across the atrial septum may be a significant cause of systemic embolic events in these patients. This diagnosis is most secure in a patient with a patent foramen ovale when a peripheral venous source of thrombi is also identified.

An *interatrial septal aneurysm* is defined as a transient bulging of the fossa ovalis region of the

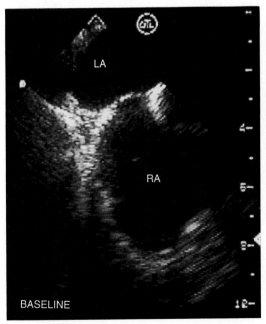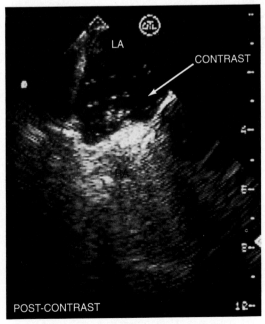

Figure 13–24. Patent foramen ovale demonstrated on transesophageal echocardiography by injection of echo contrast in a peripheral vein. Small microbubbles are seen traversing the defect from the opacified right into the unopacified left atrium.

interatrial septum (total excursion from the septal plane) greater than 15 mm in the absence of chronically elevated left or right atrial pressure (Fig. 13–25). Septal aneurysms are associated with a high likelihood (up to 90 percent) of associated fenestration. Until recently, the diagnosis rarely was made from transthoracic echo imaging due to suboptimal image quality, and this finding was thought to be of little clinical significance. The excellent views of the interatrial septum on transesophageal echocardiography have resulted in an increasing recognition of this anatomic variant. Several investigators have suggested a possible relationship between the presence of an atrial septal aneurysm and an increased risk of systemic embolic events.

"Spontaneous" contrast is seen in the left atrium when there is stasis of blood flow. It is seen more often on transesophageal than transthoracic imaging due to the higher transducer frequency and the closer proximity of the left atrium when interrogated from the esophagus but can be seen on transthoracic imaging in some patients. Spontaneous contrast is associated with left atrial enlargement and left atrial thrombus formation, and it may be a marker for a "prethrombotic" state when definite atrial thrombi are not seen. In extreme cases of spontaneous contrast in mitral stenosis patients, the jet of diastolic blood flow across the stenotic mitral orifice can be seen on 2D imaging due to the "contrast" effect.

Spontaneous contrast can be seen in the left ventricle when there is stasis of blood flow, such as in the region of an apical aneurysm. Spontaneous contrast also is observed frequently in patients with mechanical prosthetic valves. Here the mechanism of spontaneous contrast formation may be different, relating to the mechanical impact of the valve occluder during closure and resulting in microcavitation or liberation of gas from solution. Of course, patients with mitral prosthetic valves also may have stasis of blood flow in the left atrium if long-standing disease has resulted in left atrial enlargement and atrial fibrillation.

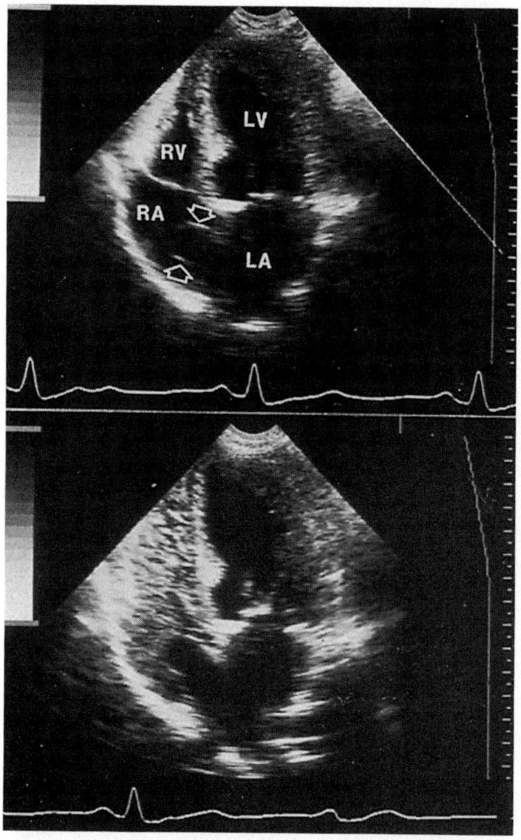

Indications for Echocardiography in Patients with Systemic Embolic Events

Our current understanding of potential cardiac etiologies for systemic embolism is incomplete, and there is considerable controversy as to the indications for transthoracic and transesophageal echocardiography in patients with suspected systemic embolic events. Transthoracic echocardiography rarely demonstrates abnormalities in patients without clinical evidence of heart disease, and most authorities do not recommend transthoracic echo evaluation unless there is clinically apparent heart disease. The proper role of transesophageal echo is more controversial. At one extreme, some clinicians advocate echocardiography in nearly all patients on the principle that even if a cardiac abnormality is unlikely, the risk of echocardiography is so low that evaluation still is warranted. At the other extreme, some clinicians argue that echocardiography is indicated only if there is definite evidence for cardiac disease by history or physical examination.

In young patients (<45 years of age) with a systemic embolic event, an intracardiac source of embolus should be strongly considered given the low prevalence of significant carotid atherosclerosis in this age group. If transthoracic studies are unrevealing, transesophageal imaging

Figure 13–25. Incidental finding of an atrial septal aneurysm (*arrows*) in an elderly patient with aortic stenosis seen in a transthoracic apical four-chamber view with contrast injection to opacify the right atrium and right ventricle (*below*).

should be performed, given its higher sensitivity for diagnosis of a patent foramen ovale, left atrial thrombus, interatrial septal aneurysm, valvular vegetation, and small intracardiac tumors.

In older patients, the yield of echocardiographic imaging is highest in those without evidence for an extracardiac source (e.g., those without carotid disease) and with evidence (or risk factors) for underlying cardiac disease. The possibility that atheromas of the ascending aorta may lead to embolic events also should be considered in this age group (see Chap. 14).

Currently accepted definite indications for echocardiography in patients with suspected cerebral embolism include clinical evidence of heart disease or age under 45 years. Opinion is divided on the appropriateness of echocardiography in patients over age 45 with suspected cerebral embolism but no clinical evidence of heart disease. Most cardiologists agree that echocardiography is not indicated in patients with known noncardiac causes of cerebral embolism.

SUGGESTED READING

1. Meltzer RS, Visser CA, Fuster V: Intracardiac thrombi and systemic embolization. Ann Intern Med 104:689–698, 1986.
   Review of the utility of transthoracic echocardiography in evaluation of intracardiac thrombi. Ninety-six references.

2. Shrestha NK, Moreno FL, Narciso FV, et al: Two-dimensional echocardiographic detection of intraatrial masses. Am J Cardiol 48:954–960, 1981.
   One of the few studies comparing detection of left atrial thrombi by transthoracic echo with surgical results. Of the 51 patients with left atrial thrombus at surgery, 30 were detected by 2D echo (sensitivity 59 percent). Of the 242 patients without thrombus at surgery, in 239 the 2D echo did not show a thrombus (3 false-positives, specificity 99 percent).

3. Herzog CA, Bass D, Kane M, Asinger R: Two-dimensional echocardiographic imaging of left atrial appendage thrombi. J Am Coll Cardiol 3:1340–1344, 1984.
   Description of visualization of the left atrial appendage on transthoracic imaging in the parasternal short-axis view by slight superomedial angulation of the transducer.

4. Manning WJ, Silberman DI, Gordon SPF, et al: Cardioversion from atrial fibrillation without prolonged anticoagulation with the use of transesophageal echocardiography to exclude the presence of atrial thrombi. N Engl J Med 328:750–755, 1993.
   Transesophageal echocardiography was performed in 119 patients with atrial fibrillation longer than 2 days in duration, who were not on long-term anticoagulants and had no contraindications to the transesophageal procedure. Left atrial thrombi were identified in 12 (13 percent) patients. In the 78 patients without detectable atrial thrombi and successful conversion to sinus rhythm, none had an embolic event. Most of these patients received short-term heparin before cardioversion and warfarin for 1 month after cardioversion.

5. Grimm RA, Stewart WJ, Black IW, et al: Should all patients undergo transesophageal echocardiography before electrical cardioversion of atrial flutter? J Am Coll Cardiol 23:533–541, 1994.
   Review article proposing that transesophageal echocardiography can be used to allow early cardioversion if atrial thrombus is absent (although anticoagulation at the time of cardioversion and for 4 weeks postcardioversion is recommended in all patients). In patents with thrombus identified on transesophageal echocardiography, cardioversion is delayed to avoid risk of embolization. Seventy-one references.

6. Stratton JR, Lighty GW Jr, Pearlman AS, Ritchie JL: Detection of left ventricular thrombus by two-dimensional echocardiography: Sensitivity, specificity, and causes of uncertainty. Circulation 66:156–165, 1982.
   In 78 patients with surgical, autopsy, or indium-111 platelet imaging evidence of left ventricular thrombus, the 2D transthoracic echo was positive or equivocal in 21 of the 22 patients with a thrombus (sensitivity 95 percent) and was negative in 48 of 56 without a thrombus (specificity 86 percent). A definitely positive echo had a positive predictive accuracy of 86 percent, while an equivocal study had a positive predictive value of only 29 percent.

7. Ezekowitz MD, Wilson DA, Smith EO, et al: Comparison of indium-111 platelet scintigraphy and two-dimensional echocardiography in the diagnosis of left ventricular thrombi. N Engl J Med 306:1509–1513, 1982.
   In 53 patients with autopsy or surgical proof of left ventricular thrombus, 2D echo had a sensitivity of 77 percent and specificity of 93 percent, while indium-111 platelet scintigraphy had a sensitivity of 71 percent and a specificity of 100 percent.

8. Stratton JR, Ritchie JL, Hammermeister KE, et al: Detection of left ventricular thrombi with radionuclide angiography. Am J Cardiol 48:565–572, 1981.
   Radionuclide angiography had a sensitivity of 77 percent (10 of 13) and a specificity of 88 percent (23 of 26) for detection of left ventricular thrombi. In a subset of these patients (n = 13), 2D echo had a sensitivity and specificity of 100 percent for detection of left ventricular thrombus.

9. Delemarre BJ, Visser CA, Bot H, Dunning AJ: Prediction of apical thrombus formation in acute myocardial infarction based on left ventricular spatial flow pattern. J Am Coll Cardiol 15:355–360, 1990.
   Data are presented supporting the hypothesis that abnormal left ventricular apical flow patterns can be used to predict the risk of thrombus formation. A normal apical flow pattern is characterized by simultaneous onset of flow at the mitral valve and apex with a discontinuous (diastolic toward and systolic away from the transducer) Doppler signal along the lateral wall and septum in the apical four-chamber view. Accompanying editorial.

10. Visser CA, Kan G, Meltzer RS, et al: Embolic potential of left ventricular thrombus after myocardial infarction: A two-dimensional echocardiographic study of 119 patients. J Am Coll Cardiol 5:1276–1280, 1985.
    In 119 acute myocardial infarction patients (98 anterior), systemic embolization occurred in 26 patients (22 percent). Embolization was more likely with protrusion or free mobility of the thrombus.

11. Reeder GS, Khandheria BK, Seward JB, Tajik AJ: Transesophageal echocardiography and cardiac masses. Mayo Clin Proc 66:1101–1109, 1991.
    Descriptive paper of the Mayo Clinic's experience with transesophageal echo for detection of cardiac masses over a 2-year period (83 masses were identified). Several illustrative 2D echocardiograms.

12. Salcedo EE, Cohen GI, White RD, Davison MB: Cardiac tumors: Diagnosis and management. Curr Prob Cardiol 17:75–137, 1992.
    Review of the clinical aspects of diagnosis and management of cardiac tumors. One hundred and seventy-four references.

13. Hancock EW: Neoplastic pericardial disease. Clin Cardiol 8:673–682, 1990.
    Review article focusing on the presentation and management of malignant pericardial disease. Forty-three references.

14. Abraham KP, Reddy V, Gattuso P: Neoplasms metastatic to the heart: Review of 3314 consecutive autopsies. Am J Cardiovasc Pathol 3:195–198, 1990.
    Autopsy study (n = 3314) with malignant disease in 24 percent (n = 806) and cardiac involvement in 12 percent of these cases (n = 95). Analysis of frequency of primary tumors. Used as the source of data for Table 13–4.

15. Klatt EC, Heitz DR: Cardiac metastases. Cancer 65:1456–1459, 1990.
    A large autopsy series of patients with a malignancy (n = 1029) with a rate of cardiac involvement of 11 percent. In this study, lung was the most common primary site (36 percent). Over 75 percent of metastatic cardiac disease involved the epicardium, and 34 percent of these had a pericardial effusion.

16. Waller BF (ed): Pathology of the Heart and Great Vessels. Churchill-Livingstone, New York, 1988.
    Multiauthor textbook of cardiac pathology in the current era emphasizing surgical findings. Chapters are included on prosthetic valve dysfunction, endomyocardial biopsy, and diseases of the great vessels, as well as valvular heart disease and cardiac tumors.

17. Becker AE, Anderson RH: Cardiac Pathology: An Integrated Text and Colour Atlas. Raven Press, New York, 1982.
    An atlas of cardiac pathology with excellent illustrations and concise descriptions.

18. Pearson AC, Labovitz AJ, Tatineni S, Gomez CR: Superiority of transesophageal echocardiography in detecting cardiac source of embolism in patients with cerebral ischemia of uncertain etiology. J Am Coll Cardiol 17:66–72, 1991.
    In 79 patients with unexplained cerebrovascular events, TTE detected a potential cardiac source of embolus in only 15 percent compared with 57 percent by TEE. Abnormalities detected included atrial septal aneurysms with a patent foramen ovale (9), left atrial thrombus or tumor (6), and left atrial "spontaneous" contrast (13).

19. DeRook FA, Comess KA, Albers GW, Popp RL: Transesophageal echocardiography in the evaluation of stroke. Ann Intern Med 117:922–931, 1992.
    Review of the utility of transesophageal echo in evaluation of patients with cerebrovascular events possibly due to cardiogenic emboli. Sixty-six references.

20. Black IW, Hopkins AP, Lee LCL, Walsh WF: Left atrial spontaneous echo contrast: A clinical and echocardiographic analysis. J Am Coll Cardiol 18:398–404, 1991.
    Spontaneous left atrial contrast was found in 75 of 400 patients (19 percent) undergoing TEE. Atrial fibrillation or mitral stenosis was present in 71 (95 percent) of the patients with "spontaneous" contrast. In the 60 patients with nonvalvular atrial fibrillation, the only independent predictors of left atrial thrombus or systemic embolism were spontaneous left atrial contrast and age.

21. Fatkin D, Kelly RP, Feneley MP: Relations between left atrial appendage blood flow velocity, spontaneous echocardiography contrast and thromboembolic risk in vivo. J Am Coll Cardiol 23:961–969, 1994.
    In 140 patients with atrial fibrillation, left atrial spontaneous contrast was present in 78 (56 percent) patients and left atrial thrombus was present in 15 (11 percent) patients. On multivariate analysis, spontaneous echo contrast was the only significant predictor for the presence of thrombus. Left atrial appendage velocity was negatively associated with the degree of spontaneous contrast and an appendage velocity < 35 cm/s was associated with a 30 times higher risk of spontaneous contrast.

22. Pearson AC, Nagelhout D, Castello R, et al: Atrial septal aneurysm and stroke: A transesophageal echocardiographic study. J Am Coll Cardiol 18:1223–1229, 1991.
    In 410 patients undergoing TEE, an atrial septal aneurysm (defined as a base width ≥1.5 cm with ≥1.1 cm total excursion) was found in 32 (8 percent) patients. Atrial septal aneurysm was diagnosed more frequently in patients with stroke (15 versus 4 percent; p < 0.05).

23. Karalis DG, Chandrasekaran K, Victor MF, et al: Recognition and embolic potential of intraaortic atherosclerotic debris. J Am Coll Cardiol 17:73–78, 1991.
    In 556 patients undergoing TEE, intraaortic atherosclerotic debris was identified in 7 percent. The incidence of embolism was higher with pedunculated and mobile versus layered and immobile debris (8 of 11 versus 3 of 25; p < 0.002).

24. Katz ES, Tunick PA, Rusinek H, et al: Protruding aortic atheromas predict stroke in elderly patients undergoing cardiopulmonary bypass: Experience with intraoperative transesophageal echocardiography. J Am Coll Cardiol 20:70–77, 1992.
    Protruding atheromas were identified in 23 of 130 (18 percent) of patients undergoing TEE. Strokes occurred in 3 of 12 patients with mobile atheroma versus 2 of 118 without a mobile atheroma (p = 0.001).

25. Fatkin D, Kelly RP, Feneley MP: Relations between left atrial appendage blood flow velocity, spontaneous echocardiographic contrast and thromboembolic risk in vivo. J Am Coll Cardiol 23:961–969, 1994.
    In 140 patients with atrial fibrillation, left atrial spontaneous contrast was seen in 56 percent on transesophageal echocardiography. Increasing grades of spontaneous contrast were associated with decreasing atrial appendage blood flow velocities. On multivariate analysis, spontaneous contrast was the cardiac factor most strongly associated with left atrial thrombus (identified in 11 percent of patients) and a history of embolic events (36 percent of patients)

26. Tunick PA, Rosenzweig BP, Katz ES, et al: High risk for vascular events in patients with protruding aortic atheromas: a prospective study. J Am Coll Cardiol 23:1085–1090, 1994.
    Of 521 consecutive patients undergoing transesophageal echocardiography, 42 had protruding atheromas and no other potential source of emboli. Compared with 42 age- and gender-matched control subjects, multivariate analysis identified protruding atheromas as the only independent predictor of subsequent vascular events (odds ratio 4.3, 95 percent, confidence intervals 1.2 to 15).

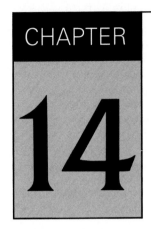

CHAPTER 14

CLINICAL ECHOCARDIOGRAPHY FOR DISEASES OF THE GREAT VESSELS

INTRODUCTION

Echocardiographic evaluation of the aortic root and main pulmonary artery is a routine part of the standard echocardiographic examination. In addition, further evaluation of the ascending aorta, arch, and descending aorta can be performed when disease is suspected clinically. Transthoracic images often are suboptimal due to overlying or adjacent air-filled structures, so transesophageal imaging has greatly enhanced the diagnostic utility of echocardiography for diseases of the aorta.

BASIC PRINCIPLES

The most common abnormality of the aorta is *dilation*, or an increase in diameter greater than expected for age and body size. Dilation of the ascending aorta occurs in a wide variety of diseases. Most cases of ascending aortic dilation are due to hypertension, atherosclerosis, cystic medical necrosis, or are poststenotic in etiology. In addition, aortic root dilation is seen in collagen-vascular and inflammatory disorders such as Marfan's syndrome, rheumatoid arthritis, systemic lupus erythematosus, and Reiter's syn-

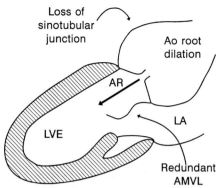

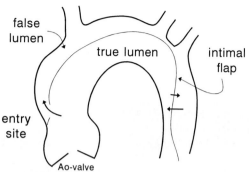

Figure 14–1. Schematic diagram of the typical 2D echo findings in Marfan's syndrome as seen in a long-axis view. The aortic root is markedly dilated with effacement of the sinotubular junction. Aortic annular dilation results in inadequate aortic leaflet apposition with a central jet of aortic regurgitation (AR) and consequent left ventricular enlargement (LVE). Often the anterior mitral leaflet (AMVL) is long and redundant.

Figure 14–2. Schematic diagram of an aortic dissection showing an entry site above the sinotubular junction into a false lumen. In real time, the intimal flap shows rapid undulating motion, independent of the cardiac cycle. As indicated by the arrows across the intimal flap in the descending aorta, multiple flow communications between the true and false lumens may be seen with color flow imaging.

drome. With poststenotic dilation or with dilation due to hypertension or atherosclerosis, the contours of the sinuses of Valsalva and the normal narrowing at the sinotubular junction typically are preserved. In contrast, Marfan's syndrome is characterized by effacement of the sinotubular junction and enlargement of the sinuses of Valsalva, as well as dilation of the ascending aorta, resulting in a "water balloon" appearance of the aortic root (Fig. 14–1).

When aortic dilation is severe, the term *aneurysm* is used. Aneurysms can involve one or more segments of the aorta (ascending, arch, descending) and may be tubular or saccular in configuration. Aortic aneurysms most often are due to cystal medial necrosis, Marfan's syndrome, hypertension, atherosclerosis, collagen-vascular, or inflammatory diseases. Aneurysms also may be seen in tertiary syphilis (with a characteristic pattern of calcification), aortic arteritis (such as Takayasu's arteritis), and as a result of blunt or penetrating chest trauma. Aortic aneurysms are prone to rupture, so prophylactic repair often is recommended.

An *aortic dissection* is a life-threatening situation in which an intimal tear in the aortic wall allows passage of blood into a "false" channel between the intima and the media (Fig. 14–2). This false channel may be localized or may propagate downstream, often in a spiral fashion, due to the pressure of blood flow in the channel. The false lumen may (1) expand, compressing the true aortic lumen (which supplies major branch vessels), (2) propagate down major branch vessels, (3) thrombose, or (4) rupture. An accurate, rapid diagnosis of the presence or ab-

sence of aortic dissection and the site of the entry tear is crucial in management of patients with suspected dissection. Aortic dissection is associated with aortic valve disease, with a risk of aortic dissection of approximately five times normal in individuals with congenital bicuspid or unicuspid aortic valve. Dissection also is more likely in patients with a preexisting aneurysm, although dissection can occur in the absence of dilation in patients with Marfan's syndrome.

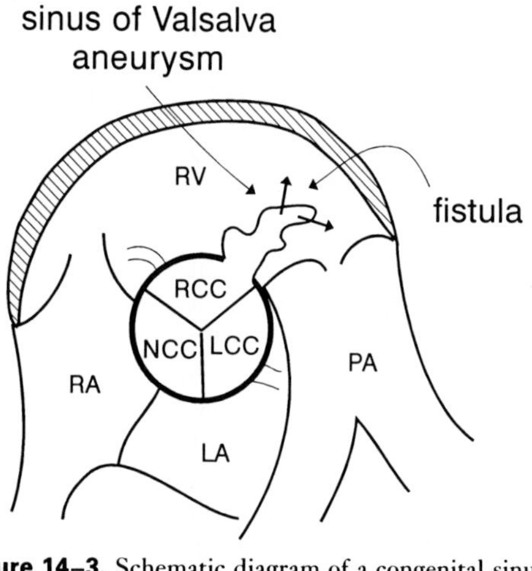

Figure 14–3. Schematic diagram of a congenital sinus of Valsalva aneurysm. A long "wind sock"–like membranous outpouching of the right coronary cusp (RCC) protrudes into the right ventricular (RV) outflow tract. If there are fenestrations in the aneurysm, an aortic to right ventricular fistula is seen. Note that an aneurysm of the left coronary cusp (LCC) would protrude into the left atrium (LA), while an aneurysm of the right coronary cusp (RCC) would protrude into the right atrium (RA).

The most prevalent risk factor for aortic dissection is chronic hypertension.

Sinus of Valsalva aneurysms (Fig. 14–3) may be congenital or may be due to infection, Marfan's syndrome, or previous surgical procedures. A sinus of Valsalva aneurysm protrudes into adjacent chambers and may be associated with a fistula. Specifically, an aneurysm of the right coronary sinus protrudes into the right ventricular outflow tract, the left coronary sinus into the left atrium, and the noncoronary sinus into the right atrium.

Atherosclerosis of the aorta may lead to dilation, aneurysm, or dissection. In addition, the presence of atheroma may be important as a marker for coexisting coronary artery disease and as a potential source of embolic cerebrovascular events.

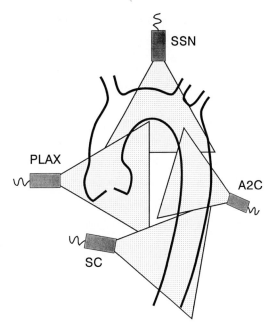

Figure 14–4. The use of several acoustic windows for complete evaluation of the aorta from a transcutaneous approach is shown. From a parasternal long-axis (PLAX) window, the root and a segment of the ascending aorta are seen. From the suprasternal notch (SSN) window, the arch and proximal descending thoracic aorta are seen; from a posteriorly angulated apical two-chamber (A2C) approach, the midsegment of the descending thoracic aorta is seen; and from a subcostal (SC) approach, the distal thoracic and proximal abdominal aortae are seen. In some individuals, the segment of ascending aorta between the standard PLAX and SSN views can be imaged from a high parasternal position. However, in other patients, this segment of the aorta is "missed" on transthoracic imaging.

ECHOCARDIOGRAPHIC APPROACH

Transthoracic Imaging of the Aorta
(Fig. 14–4)

2D and Doppler Echo

On transthoracic imaging, the *aortic root* is well seen in parasternal long- and short-axis views. Depending on ultrasound penetration, images of further cephalad segments of the ascending aorta may be obtained by moving the transducer cephalad one or more interspaces. Image quality is enhanced by positioning the patient in a steep left lateral decubitus position, bringing the aorta in contact with the anterior chest wall (Figs. 14–5 and 14–6). Doppler interrogation of the ascending aorta from the parasternal approach is limited to qualitative evaluation of the flow pattern in the proximal root and assessment of aortic regurgitation severity (if present) given the nonparallel intercept angle from this position. The aortic root also may be imaged from the apical approach in an anteriorly angulated four-chamber view and in an apical long-axis view. While two-dimensional (2D) image quality may be limited at the depth of the ascending aorta from the apical approach, this view does allow a parallel intercept angle between the Doppler beam and the direction of blood flow. In some individuals, images of the ascending aorta can be obtained from the subcostal approach.

The *aortic arch* is imaged from a suprasternal notch or supraclavicular approach with the patient in a supine position with the neck extended. Both longitudinal (Fig. 14–7) and transverse (Fig. 14–8) views of the arch are obtainable in nearly all individuals. Usually only a short segment of the ascending aorta is visible from the suprasternal notch window, but this is variable between patients. Also note that the descending aorta appears to taper due to an oblique image plane with respect to its curvature; i.e., the descending aorta is only partially in the image plane.

Pulsed or continuous-wave Doppler recordings of descending aortic flow from the suprasternal notch show systolic flow away from the transducer at a velocity of about 1 m/s. Normally, there is (1) brief, low-velocity, early diastolic flow reversal, (2) low-velocity antegrade flow in mid-diastole, and (3) low-velocity flow reversal at end-diastole. The use of low wall filter settings is needed to appreciate this normal flow pattern (Fig. 14–9).

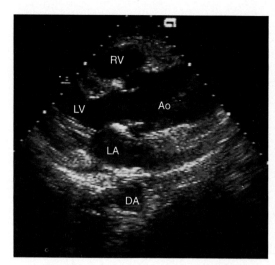 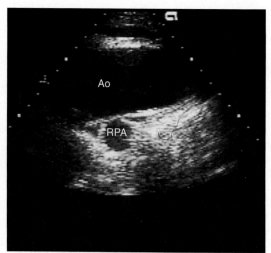

Figure 14–5. Example of a parasternal long-axis view of the ascending aorta (*left*) and the same image plane with the transducer moved cephalad 1 to 2 interspaces (*right*) in a 56-year-old man with hypertension and mild to moderate aortic dilation (DA = descending aorta; RPA = right pulmonary artery).

Even though 2D imaging of the ascending aorta is suboptimal from the suprasternal approach, high quality Doppler flow signals may be obtained because the Doppler beam is aligned parallel to flow. Antegrade flow toward the transducer in systole is seen, the reciprocal of the ascending aortic flow signal recorded from the apex.

The *descending thoracic aorta* is seen in cross section posterior to the left atrium in the parasternal long-axis view. A longitudinal section of this segment of the descending aorta may be obtained by clockwise rotation and lateral angulation of the transducer. From the suprasternal notch approach, a small portion of the descending thoracic aorta is seen. From the apical two-chamber view, a longitudinal section of a segment of the descending aorta is seen by lateral angulation and clockwise rotation of the transducer (Fig. 14–10). Doppler interrogation of de-

Figure 14–6. Parasternal long-axis view in a patient with Marfan's syndrome showing a dilated root with effacement of the sinotubular junction. A dissection flap is present (*arrow*) just cephalad to the noncoronary cusp of the aortic valve.

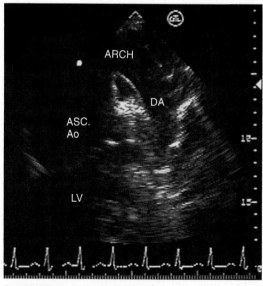

Figure 14–7. Long-axis suprasternal notch view of the aorta in the patient with Marfan's syndrome shown in Figure 14–6 (DA = descending aorta).

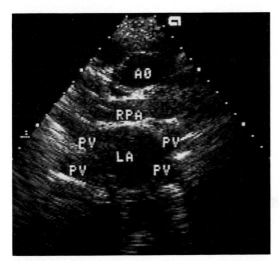

Figure 14–8. Short-axis suprasternal notch view in a normal individual showing the aortic arch (Ao), right pulmonary artery (RPA), left atrium (LA), and four pulmonary veins (PV).

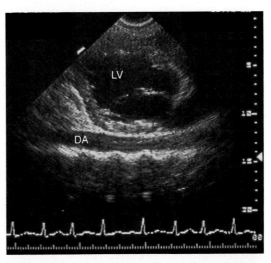

Figure 14–10. Posteriorly angulated apical two-chamber view showing the descending thoracic aorta (DA) along its long axis in the patient with Marfan's syndrome.

scending thoracic aortic flow is most easily performed from the suprasternal notch long-axis view. Flow abnormalities may be related to aortic disease (e.g., coarctation), shunts (e.g., patent ductus arteriosus), or aortic valve disease (e.g., regurgitation).

From the subcostal approach, the *distal thoracic* and *proximal abdominal aorta* is seen as it traverses the diaphragm. From this approach, the angle between the transducer and the aorta allows Doppler interrogation of antegrade flow (Fig. 14–11).

Thus, by combining images from multiple acoustic windows, visualization of much of the aortic root, ascending aorta, arch, and descending thoracic aorta is possible.

In patients with a left pleural effusion, images of the aorta can be obtained by imaging through

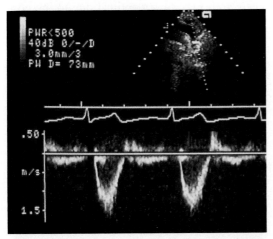

Figure 14–9. Normal pulsed Doppler recording of flow in the descending thoracic aorta from a suprasternal notch long-axis view. Antegrade flow in systole has a maximum velocity of 1.4 m/s with a normal systolic ejection curve. In diastole, there is brief early diastolic flow reversal, followed by low-velocity antegrade flow in mid-diastole and absence of flow (or low-velocity reversal) in end-diastole.

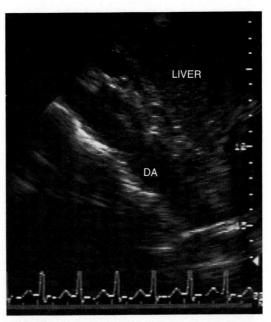

Figure 14–11. Subcostal view of the distal thoracic and proximal abdominal aorta. Although a nonparallel intercept angle from this window limits the quantitative velocity data, velocity recordings are helpful for evaluation of blood flow patterns.

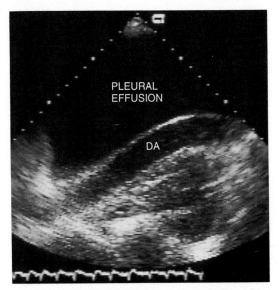

Figure 14–12. Descending thoracic aorta (DA) recorded through a large left pleural effusion with the patient lying on his left side and transducer positioned on the left posterior chest wall.

the fluid from the left posterior chest (paraspinal) with the patient in a right lateral decubitus position (Fig. 14–12).

Limitations of Transthoracic Imaging of the Aorta

The major limitations of the transthoracic approach to ultrasound evaluation of the aorta are acoustic access and image quality. In many individuals, acoustic access is suboptimal or minimal from one or more of the windows needed

for full evaluation of the aorta, leaving "gaps" in the echocardiographic examination. Even when acoustic access is adequate, image quality often is poor due to beam width at the depth of the aorta—particularly the descending thoracic aorta from apical and parasternal windows. Beam-width artifact, noise, and poor lateral resolution make differentiation of intraluminal defects from artifacts difficult. Because of these limitations, there has been increasing enthusiasm for transesophageal echocardiography in patients with suspected aortic disease.

Transesophageal Imaging

2D Echo

The aortic valve, *aortic root*, and proximal few centimeters of the ascending aorta are seen in the transverse plane at the aortic valve level from a high esophageal probe position. In the transverse plane, evaluation of more distal segments of the ascending aorta is obscured by the position of the air-filled trachea between the esophagus (and transducer) and the ascending aorta. However, in the longitudinal plane, a long-axis view of the aortic valve, sinus of Valsalva, and ascending aorta can be obtained in most patients (Fig. 14–13). Further cephalad segments of the ascending aorta may be seen by moving the transducer to a higher esophageal position.

The *aortic arch* is best seen in the transverse plane from a high esophageal position, angulated medially and inferiorly. However, images of the aortic arch may be suboptimal due to the positions of the trachea and bronchi. In many cases,

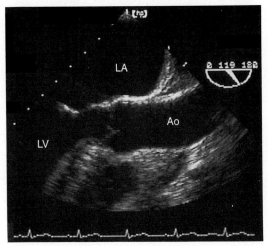
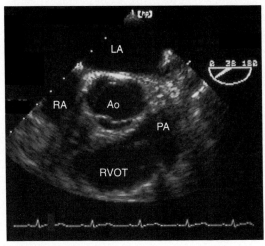

Figure 14–13. Normal ascending aorta seen on transesophageal imaging in long-axis (*left*) and short-axis (*right*) views using a multiplane probe to align the image plane appropriately relative to the aortic long axis.

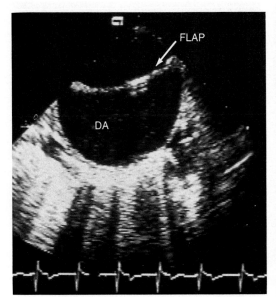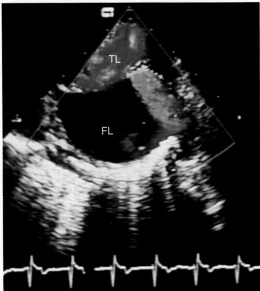

Figure 14–14. On transesophageal imaging, a 2D view (*left*) of the descending thoracic aorta shows a dissection flap (*arrow*), with flow between the true (TL) and false lumens (FL) seen on color flow imaging (*right*).

transthoracic suprasternal notch views of the arch provide superior image quality.

The *descending thoracic* and *proximal abdominal aorta* are well seen by the transesophageal approach. The descending thoracic aorta lies immediately lateral and slightly posterior to the esophagus so that posterior rotation of the probe provides excellent images in either a cross-sectional (transverse plane) or long-axis (longitudinal plane) view (Fig. 14–14). Slight rotational adjustments in transducer position are needed at different esophageal levels as the aorta curves relative to the esophagus. From a transgastric position, the proximal abdominal aorta is seen posterior to the stomach. Many examiners prefer to examine the length of the aorta in sequential cross-sectional views as the probe is slowly withdrawn from the stomach and esophagus, with imaging of the aortic arch just prior to probe removal. Any areas of abnormality are examined in both long- and short-axis views.

Doppler Flows

Color flow imaging of the aorta shows the normal antegrade flow pattern in the ascending aorta and arch. For the descending aorta, the ultrasound beam is nearly perpendicular to the direction of blood flow. In addition, normal flow shows a hemicylindrical swirling pattern so that normal flow appears red in one half and blue in

the other half of a cross-sectional view of descending aorta. Given the constraints of the probe position, alignment of the Doppler beam parallel to aortic flow is difficult from a transesophageal approach. It may be possible to obtain ascending aortic flow from a transgastric "apical" view, but underestimation of flow velocity due to a nonparallel intercept angle should be considered. Quantitative evaluation of aortic flow velocity from other transgastric or transesophageal views rarely is feasible. Aortic flow signals preferably are recorded from a transthoracic approach.

CLINICAL UTILITY

Chronic Aortic Dilation

Aortic dilation often is first recognized on the chest radiograph (Fig. 14–15) or on an echocardiographic examination requested for other reasons. In specific clinical settings, such as Marfan's syndrome, aortic dilation is an expected consequence of a systemic disease. In these cases, echocardiography is requested to assess the presence and degree of aortic abnormality.

Measurements of aortic diameter on echocardiography are accurate and reproducible when care is taken to obtain a true short-axis dimension (nonoblique), gain settings are appropriate,

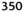

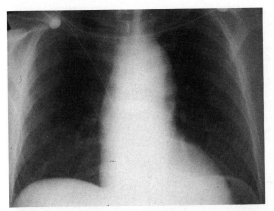

Figure 14–15. Chest radiography showing a dilated ascending aorta and wide mediastinum raising the diagnostic possibility of aortic dissection (same patient as in Figure 14–17).

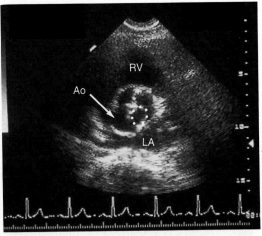

Figure 14–17. A 36-year-old man with known aortic valve disease presented with severe chest pain. Echocardiography showed a unicuspid stenotic aortic valve in the parasternal short-axis view in systole with the orifice indicated by the dots.

and standard measurement conventions (leading edge to leading edge) are used. In patients with aortic dilation, it is important to measure aortic diameter at several locations and to specify the measurement sites. Typical measurements include (1) the aortic annulus (the site used for left ventricular outflow tract diameter measurement), (2) the aortic leaflet tip level (the standard position of an M-mode of the aortic valve), (3) the sinotubular junction, (4) the ascending aorta, (5) the aortic arch, and (6) the descending thoracic aorta (Fig. 14–16). While all

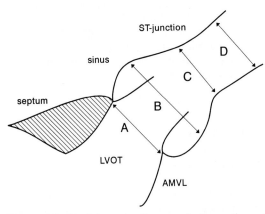

Figure 14–16. Schematic diagram of the aortic root and ascending aorta showing the possible measurement sites for "aortic" diameter. Left ventricular outflow tract (LVOT) diameter (*A*) is used for transaortic stroke volume calculations in the continuity equation. The aortic leaflet tips (*B*) in systole define the usual site for M-mode measurements and also usually indicate maximum diameter of the sinuses of Valsalva. The sinotubular (ST) junction typically is the narrowest segment of the ascending aorta (*C*), with variable degrees of dilation in the ascending aorta itself (*D*). The site of measurement should be specified in the echocardiographic report.

these measurements are not needed in every patient, quantitative evaluation of the extent and severity of aortic dilation is extremely useful in follow-up and management of patients with chronic, progressive aortic dilation. With discrete aneurysms, maximum diameter and length also are measured.

Sequential transthoracic studies of the degree of aortic dilation are used to follow patients with Marfan's syndrome. Prophylactic aortic root and valve replacement may be recommended when the degree of ascending aortic dilation reaches a critical range (some authorities suggest a value between 50 and 60 mm maximum diameter). For other etiologies of aortic dilation, sequential studies also may be utilized to assess whether the dilation is progressive or stable over time. Transesophageal evaluation of chronic aortic dilation is reserved for patients with inadequate transthoracic images.

Aortic Dissection

Transthoracic Imaging

Evaluation of the Aorta. A transthoracic echocardiographic examination for aortic dissection includes evaluation of the ascending aorta from the standard and high parasternal windows, the aortic arch from the suprasternal notch window, the descending aorta from parasternal and apical windows, and the proximal abdominal aorta from a subcostal approach. When a left pleural effusion is present, the de-

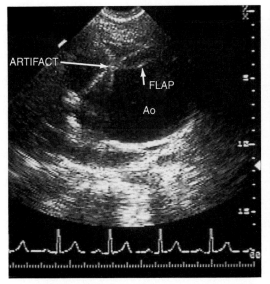 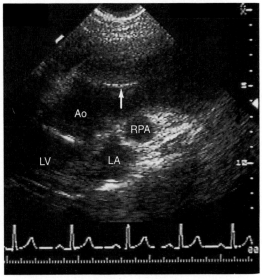

Figure 14–18. In a long-axis view, a dilated aorta with a dissection flap (*arrow*) was seen (*left*). Moving the transducer cephalad 2 interspaces provided better separation of the dissection flap (*arrow*) from a reverberation artifact (*right*) (RPA = right pulmonary artery).

scending thoracic aorta can be imaged through the effusion with the transducer positioned on the left posterior chest wall.

The echocardiographic diagnosis of aortic dissection is most secure when a linear, mobile echogenic structure is seen within a dilated aortic lumen (Figs. 14–17 and 14–18). When a definite, undulating intimal flap is seen, the specificity of transthoracic echocardiography for diagnosis of dissection is high (Table 14–1). However, beam-width artifact and reverberations can be mistaken for intraluminal structures by an inexperienced observer, resulting in a specificity of less than 100 percent, particularly when the images are not "classic" or image quality is suboptimal.

TABLE 14–1. DIAGNOSIS OF AORTIC DISSECTION

FIRST AUTHOR, YEAR	N	APPROACH*	SENSITIVITY	SPECIFICITY	STANDARD OF REFERENCE
Victor, 1981	42	TTE	80% (12/15)	96% (26/27)	Angiography
Erbel, 1987	21	TTE	29% (6/21)	(All had	Surgery or angiography
		TEE	100% (21/21)	dissection)	
Hashimoto, 1989	22	TTE	71% (15/21)	(All had	Angiography (17) and/or
		TEE	100% (22/22)	dissection)	surgery (12)
		CT	100% (8/8)		
Ballal, 1991	61	TEE	97% (33/34)	100% (27/27)	Angiography, surgery, or
		CT	67% (16/24)	100% (7/7)	autopsy
Nienaber, 1992	53	TTE	83% (26/31)	63% (14/22)	Surgery, autopsy, or
		TEE	100% (31/31)	66% (15/22)	angiography
		MRI	100% (31/31)	100% (22/22)	
Nienaber, 1993	110	TTE	59% (37/62)	83% (39/48)	Surgery (62), autopsy (7),
		TEE	98% (43/44)	98% (25/26)	and/or angiography
		MRI	98% (58/59)	87% (27/31)	(64)
		CT	94% (45/48)	83% (38/46)	

*TTE = transthoracic echocardiography; TEE = transesophageal echocardiography; CT = computed tomography; MRI = magnetic resonance imaging.

Data from Victor et al: Am J Cardiol 48:1155–1159, 1981; Erbel et al: Br Heart J 58:45–51, 1987; Hashimoto et al: JACC 14:1253–1262, 1989; Ballal et al: Circ 84:1903–1914, 1991; Neinaber et al: Circ 85:434–447, 1992; Neinaber et al: NEJM 328:1–9, 1993.

TABLE 14-2. COMPLICATIONS OF THORACIC AORTIC DISSECTION

I. Aortic valve regurgitation
   A. Due to aortic root dilation
   B. Due to leaflet flail

II. Coronary artery occlusion due to dissection at the orifice
   A. Ventricular fibrillation
   B. Acute myocardial infarction

III. Distal vessel obstruction or occlusion
   A. Carotid (stroke)
   B. Subclavian (upper limb ischemia)

IV. Aortic rupture
   A. Into the pericardium
     1. Pericardial effusion
     2. Pericardial tamponade
   B. Into the mediastinum
   C. Into the pleural space
     1. Pleural effusion
     2. Exsanguination

Conversely, the sensitivity of transthoracic echocardiography for aortic dissection is quite low; i.e., the inability to demonstrate an internal flap does not reliably exclude the diagnosis. This low sensitivity is due to poor image quality, particularly of the segment of ascending aorta between the sinotubular junction and the aortic arch, and the poor far-field resolution of the descending thoracic aorta from the transthoracic approach.

Complications of Aortic Dissection (Table 14–2). Indirect signs of aortic dissection on transthoracic imaging include aortic root dilation, the presence of aortic regurgitation, or evidence of complications of aortic dissection (Fig. 14–19). While the presence of these abnormalities does not confirm the diagnosis (since there

are many other etiologies for these findings), their presence or absence may weight the clinical evidence toward or away from a diagnosis of dissection. Complications of aortic dissection can be recognized on echocardiography and have important clinical implications both for diagnosis and therapy. Aortic regurgitation is nearly always present. Chronic regurgitation is due to aortic root dilation and/or associated anatomic valve abnormalities. Acute regurgitation (often superimposed on chronic) is due to further root dilation or to inadequate leaflet support due to retrograde extension of the dissection. In extreme cases, a flail aortic leaflet is seen.

Coronary artery ostial occlusion can occur as a result of the dissection flap separating the coronary artery from normal blood flow or by compression of the vessel. The resultant wall motion abnormalities—inferior for right coronary obstruction, anterolateral for left main obstruction—are easily recognized on echocardiography. The diagnostic difficulty in this situation is recognizing that the wall motion abnormalities are a secondary event due to aortic dissection rather than the primary event (e.g., acute myocardial infarction due to coronary thrombosis).

Distal vessel obstructions rarely will be recognized during the cardiac ultrasound examination. However, the possibility of aortic dissection should be considered in patients with distal vessel obstructions referred for echocardiography to "rule out" a cardiac source of embolus. The correct diagnosis of distal vessel obstruction due to a dissection flap (rather than an embolus) may be made by the astute echocardiographer.

Aortic dissections can rupture in one of several ways. *External* rupture into the mediastinum or pleural space often results in exsangui-

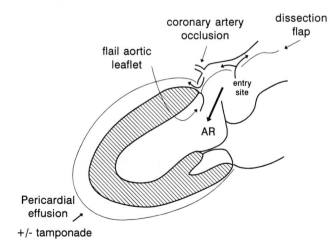

Figure 14-19. Potential complications of dissection of the ascending aorta are shown schematically. If the dissection proceeds retrograde (as well as antegrade) from the entry site, the false lumen can cause (1) occlusion in the coronary artery ostium with resultant myocardial infarction, (2) loss of support of an aortic leaflet with consequent severe aortic regurgitation (AR), or (3) rupture into the pericardium, which may result in tamponade physiology.

nation with acute hemodynamic collapse. If the rupture *thromboses*, the patient may exhibit a mediastinal hematoma and/or pleural effusion (more often left than right). Alternatively, the dissection can rupture at the aortic annulus into the pericardial space. Again, uncontrolled rupture leads to an acute pericardial effusion with tamponade and rapid hemodynamic collapse. However, a partial rupture or a leak may result in a smaller pericardial effusion. Obviously, the presence of any amount of pericardial fluid in a patient with an aortic dissection is an alarming sign and should prompt rapid intervention.

Echocardiographic Differential Diagnosis. In most cases where transthoracic echocardiography is requested to "rule out" aortic dissection, the differential diagnosis is broad, with aortic dissection being one of many (and often the least likely) possible diagnoses. Thus, if the echocardiographic appearance of the aorta is normal, echocardiographic examination for other possible etiologies of chest pain is needed, including coronary artery disease (e.g., wall motion abnormalities), valvular disease (e.g., aortic stenosis), pulmonary embolus, and pericarditis.

When the clinical suspicion of aortic dissection is low to intermediate, a normal aorta on echocardiography further decreases the posttest likelihood of disease, so other diagnoses might be pursued. However, when the clinical suspicion is moderate to high, a "negative" transthoracic echocardiogram does *not* substantially decrease the posttest likelihood of disease, so prompt further evaluation is needed. In fact, when the clinical suspicion is high, many clinicians would argue that transthoracic echocardiography is inappropriate; either transesophageal echocardiography, magnetic resonance imaging, computed tomography, or angiographic evaluation should be performed promptly.

Transesophageal Imaging

Transesophageal images of the aorta are far superior to transthoracic images in most patients due to (1) the shorter distance between the transducer and aorta, (2) the use of a higher-frequency transducer, and (3) better ultrasound tissue penetration (higher signal-to-noise ratio). The descending thoracic aorta can be examined in its entirety from the diaphragm to the arch in both long- and short-axis planes. A dissection flap appears as a linear, bright echogenic structure in the aortic lumen with erratic motion compared with normal systolic pulsations (Fig. 14–20). Color flow imaging may show blood flow in both true (bounded by endothelium) and

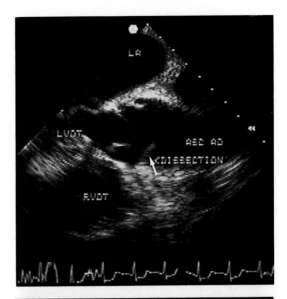
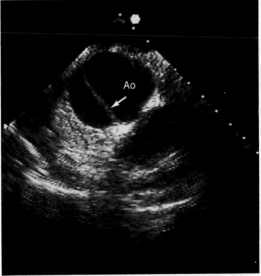

Figure 14–20. Transesophageal long-axis (*above*) and short-axis (*below*) views of an aortic dissection localized to the sinus of Valsalva in a 37-year-old woman with renal failure, hypertension, and acute chest pain. The flap is indicated by the arrow.

false (bounded by media) lumens. Both the entry site into the false lumen and other communications between the two channels are seen as high-velocity turbulent flow jets on color flow imaging. The false lumen may be thrombosed, which is more difficult to appreciate than a false lumen with blood flow. In some cases, hematoma in the wall of the aorta is seen rather than an initial flap, reflecting an impending dissection or rupture of a thrombosed false lumen. This area of hematoma appears as an echogenic mass adjacent to the aortic lumen and bounded by the bright adventitial echo signal (Fig. 14–21).

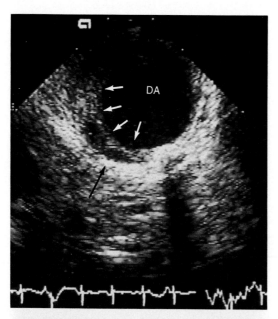

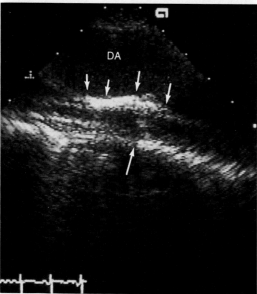

Figure 14–21. In a transesophageal short-axis view of the descending thoracic aorta (DA), a "thick" or double-walled appearance is seen (*above*) suggestive of an intramural hematoma. In a long-axis view, the atherosclerotic plaque (*small arrows*) is "lifted" off the posterior aortic wall (*large arrow*). This patient was treated medically and has done well.

The aortic root is seen on transesophageal imaging in the transverse plane at the aortic valve level. Evaluation of the ascending aorta depends on use of a longitudinal plane—this aortic segment cannot be adequately assessed with a single-plane transesophageal probe. Evaluation of the ascending aorta is particularly important be-

cause the decision between emergent surgical intervention and medical therapy hinges on whether the dissection originates in (or involves) the ascending aorta. Note that even a localized dissection flap in the ascending aorta carries a grim prognosis and warrants surgical treatment. Again, color flow imaging may further define the entry site and demonstrate flow in true and false lumens.

The sensitivity of transesophageal echocardiography for the diagnosis of aortic dissection is high (>97 percent; see Table 14–1) with a similarly high specificity in most studies. Specificity is less than 100 percent due to misinterpretation of ultrasound artifacts, such as reverberations, beam-width artifacts, and oblique imaging planes. Careful evaluation from multiple views with adjustment of instrument settings helps avoid these false-positive diagnoses.

Alternate Approaches (Table 14–3)

Several centers have suggested that transesophageal echocardiography is the procedure of choice for evaluation of acute aortic dissections given its high sensitivity/specificity plus the ability to perform the study quickly at the patient's bedside. Alternate techniques for evaluation of possible acute aortic dissection include contrast aortic root angiography (Fig. 14–22), chest computed tomography (Fig. 14–23), and magnetic resonance imaging (Fig. 14–24).

The choice of a particular procedure in an individual patient depends not only on availability of these tests but also on the differential diagnosis in the individual patient. Contrast angiography may be most appropriate when acute myocardial infarction is a likely diagnosis, since evaluation (and treatment) of coronary artery obstruction can be performed quickly if dissection is not present. Wide-angle tomographic imaging procedures (computed tomography, magnetic resonance imaging) may be most helpful in cases where the differential diagnosis includes mediastinal tumor. Echocardiography has the advantage of allowing evaluation of aortic valve anatomy and function, overall and regional left ventricular systolic function, and the presence and significance of a pericardial effusion.

Alternatively, the choice of imaging procedures may be driven by the specific additional information needed in an individual patient. Examples include distal vessel anatomy (angiography), adjacent mediastinal disease (computed tomography or magnetic resonance imaging), or valvular function (echocardiography).

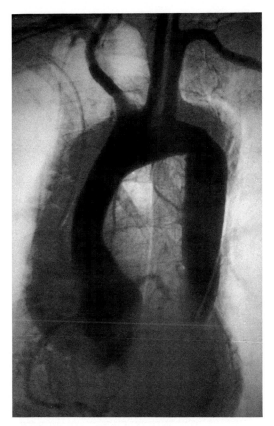

Figure 14–22. Subtracted contrast angiogram shows an aortic dissection extending from the aortic valve level to the proximal descending thoracic aorta. The true lumen is more densely opacified than the false lumen.

Sinus of Valsalva Aneurysm

A sinus of Valsalva aneurysm can be congenital or due to an acute infectious or inflammatory process. Echocardiographically, a dilated and distorted sinus of Valsalva is seen both in long- and short-axis views at the aortic valve level either from a transesophageal or transthoracic approach. A congenital aneurysm often is complex in shape with a "wind sock" appearance of a mass of irregular, mobile echos protruding from the aortic sinus into adjacent cardiac structures (Fig. 14–25). If the aneurysm is not fenestrated, Doppler flow examination is unremarkable. More commonly, multiple fenestrations are present, with high-velocity turbulent flow from the high-pressure aorta to the low-pressure adjacent chambers detectable by continuous-wave, pulsed-wave, and color flow Doppler techniques. Note that infection of a previously competent congenital sinus of Valsalva aneurysm may result in flow across a necrotic area of infection.

Acquired sinus of Valsalva aneurysms tend to be less irregular in shape. The dilation of the sinuses that occurs in Marfan's syndrome symmetrically involves all three sinuses with a rounded smooth pattern of root dilation. Because of persistent sinus of Valsalva dilation in Marfan's patients, ascending aorta root replacements are performed with a composite valve and graft (with reimplantation of the coronaries) to avoid sinus dilation and rupture with separate root and valve replacements. A sinus of Valsalva aneurysm due to endocarditis tends to result in a more spherical, but still irregular-appearing dilation of the sinus (Fig. 14–26). Again, the aneurysm protrudes and may rupture into adjacent cardiac structures depending on which sinus is involved.

Pre- and Postoperative Evaluation of Aortic Disease

Preoperative Evaluation

In some cases, the suspicion of aortic dissection is so high that transesophageal echocardiographic examination may be performed initially in the operating room with the patient anesthetized and undergoing preparation for surgery. In these cases, the echocardiographer aims to rapidly confirm or exclude the suspected diagnosis. If a dissection is present, evaluation of the entry site and extent of dissection is helpful in planning the surgical approach. Recognition of complications such as aortic regurgitation, coronary ostial occlusion, or pericardial effusion also may affect acute patient management.

Residual Dissection Flaps

Transesophageal echocardiography may be utilized intraoperatively to assess for residual dissection following surgical repair. A residual dissection flap, with flow in both true and false lumens, may persist in many patients (possibly as high as 70 to 80 percent) following emergent surgery for acute dissection. The usual operative procedure is to close the entry site by replacing a segment of the involved aorta with a prosthetic graft. At the distal graft anastomosis, the flap may persist. Often this persistence is intentional since some branch vessels may be supplied by the false lumen and other vessels by the true lumen. Thus the finding of a dissection flap in the aortic arch or descending aorta of a patient with a prior ascending aortic dissection and graft repair may represent stable residual disease or a

TABLE 14–3. DIAGNOSTIC IMAGING PROCEDURES IN AORTIC DISEASE

PROCEDURE	ADVANTAGES	DISADVANTAGES
Transthoracic echocardiography	Portable, rapid Inexpensive Evaluation of LV function Evaluation of aortic valve function Evaluation of pericardial effusion	Moderate sensitivity/specificity due to poor acoustic access and suboptimal image resolution
Transesophageal echocardiography	High sensitivity/specificity Portable, rapid Evaluation of LV fx, valve fx, PE Can assess proximal coronary arteries	Some risks (esp. if esophageal disease is present) Cannot evaluate distal coronary arteries
Chest computed tomography	High sensitivity/specificity Wide field of view	Site of intimal tear not well defined Not portable Ionizing radiation Little data on LV, aortic valve Cannot evaluate coronary involvement
Magnetic resonance imaging	High sensitivity/specificity Wide field of view Evaluation of pericardial effusion	High cost, not portable, limited availability Limited evaluation of valvular and ventricular function Cannot evaluate coronary involvement
Contrast aortography	High sensitivity/specificity Branch vessel anatomy Evaluation of AR Can assess and intervene for coronary artery disease	Expensive, invasive Ionizing radiation Limited availability Not portable No evaluation for pericardial effusion

LV = left ventricle; fx = function; PE = pericardial effusion; AR = aortic regurgitation.

second acute process. These conditions are differentiated by comparison with previous imaging studies (when available) and careful clinical evaluation. Some investigators have suggested that persistence of an intimal flap and flow in the false lumen are poor prognostic signs.

In patients with ascending aortic grafts, echocardiographic follow-up is warranted to assess for late complications. In patients with a valved conduit, a baseline study is indicated postoperatively to allow comparison with future studies in terms of prosthetic valve function (see Chap. 11). The prosthetic aortic graft itself appears as an echo-dense, cylindrical structure with a uniform diameter (Fig. 14–27). Irregular areas of thickening anterior and posterior to the graft may represent the native aorta "wrapped around" the prosthetic graft, as well as postop-

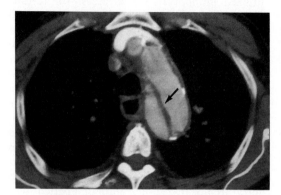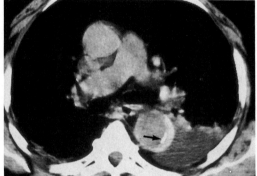

Figure 14–23. On chest CT, a clear dissection flap (*arrow*) is seen in the aortic arch (*left*). In a second patient, an atypical dissection is seen with displacement of intimal calcification (*arrow*) by an intramural thrombus in the descending thoracic aorta (*right*).

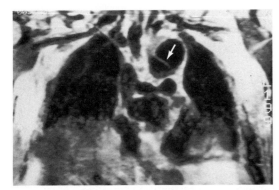

Figure 14–24. In a 61-year-old man with cystic medial necrosis and prior ascending aortic dissection and graft placement, an MRI scan in the coronal plane shows persistent dilation and a chronic dissection flap (*arrow*) in the aortic arch.

erative scar tissue. The coronary arteries retain their normal insertions if a segment of the native aorta has been preserved. In these cases, careful examination for dilation of the remaining aortic tissue and the sinuses of Valsalva is needed. When the graft extends to the aortic valve level, the right and left coronary ostia are reimplanted into the graft along with a small "button" of native aortic tissue. Dilation or loss of structural integrity of this aortic tissue or dehiscence of the coronary reimplantation suture line results in myocardial infarction due to disruption of coronary blood flow. In addition, this complication can lead to aortic rupture or pseudoaneurysm formation.

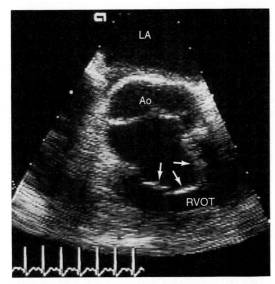

Figure 14–25. Congenital sinus of Valsalva aneurysm of the right coronary cusp (*arrows*) protruding into the right ventricular outflow tract on a transesophageal short-axis view.

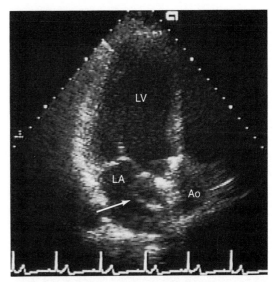

Figure 14–26. Acquired sinus of Valsalva aneurysm (*arrow*) after aortic valve replacement in an apical long-axis view protruding into the left atrium.

Aortic Graft Pseudoaneurysms

A pseudoaneurysm, escape of blood from the graft lumen into an area contained by surrounding scar tissue or the native aorta, can occur at the proximal or the distal graft anastomoses to the aorta or at the coronary reimplantation sites. Rarer instances of rupture of the graft material itself have been reported. A pseudoaneurysm appears as an echolucent area adjacent to the aortic graft (Fig. 14–28). Flow into this region can be demonstrated with color flow imaging, although a transesophageal study often is nec-

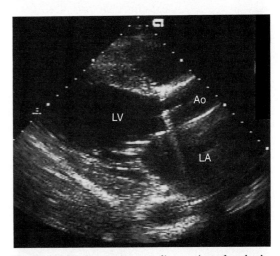

Figure 14–27. Composite ascending aortic graft and valve replacement postoperatively in the patient with Marfan's syndrome shown in Figure 14–6.

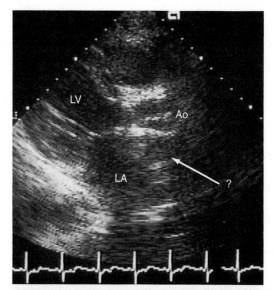

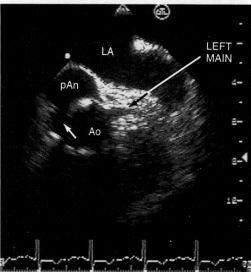

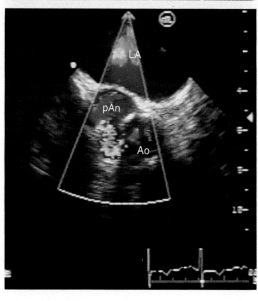

essary for adequate image quality. The pseudo-aneurysm may rupture into the mediastinum or pleural spaces (both of which are likely to be fatal) or back across the aortic annulus into the left ventricle. This pseudo-aortic regurgitation consists of flow from the pseudoaneurysm into the left ventricle in diastole, with flow from the left ventricle into the pseudoaneurysm in systole. The characteristics of this flow signal on pulsed and continuous-wave Doppler are similar to those of transvalvular aortic regurgitation. Color flow imaging shows the flow around, rather than through, the prosthetic aortic valve.

Atherosclerotic Aortic Disease

Aortic Atherosclerosis as a Potential Source of Embolus

The excellent-quality images of the aorta obtained by transesophageal echocardiography have led to the observation of extensive atherosclerotic plaque in many individuals, with mobile thrombus attached to the atheroma in some cases. These observations have generated the hypothesis that atherosclerosis of the ascending aorta and arch may serve as a nidus for embolic material, resulting in cerebrovascular events. These areas of atherosclerosis rarely are seen on transthoracic imaging due to poor image quality related to acoustic access, the depth of the aorta from the transthoracic approach, and the use of a lower-frequency transducer.

Aortic Atherosclerosis as a Marker for Coronary Artery Disease

Recently, it has been suggested that the presence of detectable atherosclerotic plaques in the descending aorta on transesophageal echocardiography (Fig. 14–29) is a marker of coronary artery disease with a sensitivity of 90 percent. Conversely, the absence of detectable atherosclerosis in the descending thoracic aorta suggests that significant coronary artery disease is not present with a specificity of 90 percent.

◄Figure 14–28. In a patient with aortic graft placement 5 years previously for aortic dissection, the ascending aortic graft seen on transthoracic imaging shows an apparent echolucent space posterior to the graft. It was unclear if this was a reverberation artifact or anatomic abnormality (*above*). Transesophageal imaging showed a definite pseudoaneurysm (pAn) posterior to the graft (*center*) with a communication with the aortic graft (*arrow*). Color flow imaging showed flow from the aorta into the pseudoaneurysm (*below*). A paravalvular regurgitant jet from the pseudoaneurysm into the left ventricle also was present.

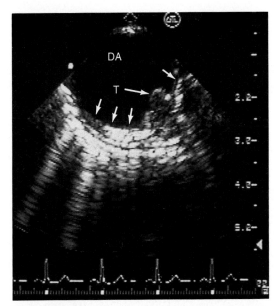

Figure 14–29. Transesophageal short-axis view of the descending thoracic aorta (DA) showing a large atherosclerotic plaque (*small arrows*) with attached thrombus (T), which showed independent motion in real time.

Pulmonary Artery Abnormalities

Most abnormalities of the pulmonary artery are congenital, including poststenotic dilation, branch pulmonary artery stenosis, and an abnormal position of the pulmonary artery, as in transposition of the great vessels. However, the pulmonary artery may be involved by systemic diseases that affect the aorta, such as Takayasu's arteritis. Pulmonary artery dissection is rare but has been reported in patients with chronic pulmonary hypertension.

The finding of a dilated pulmonary artery raises the possibility of right-sided volume overload (e.g., atrial septal defect) or pressure overload (e.g., pulmonary hypertension). Occasionally, a patient is seen with a dilated main pulmonary artery and no other cardiac abnormalities (*idiopathic* dilation of the pulmonary artery).

The pulmonary artery can be visualized on transthoracic echocardiography in a parasternal short-axis view at the aortic valve level or in a right ventricular outflow view. In adults, it may be difficult to visualize the anterior pulmonary artery wall due to overlying lung tissue. In younger patients, the pulmonary artery can be visualized from the anteriorly angulated apical four-chamber view by further anterior angulation. The subcostal short-axis view allows an alternate approach to visualize the pulmonary artery in most patients. From the suprasternal notch window, the right pulmonary artery is seen in cross section in the long-axis view of the aortic arch (see Fig. 14–7) and in its long axis in the orthogonal view (see Fig. 14–8). The left pulmonary artery can be imaged by slight lateral angulation and posterior rotation from the standard long-axis suprasternal notch view.

Alternate approaches to evaluation of the pulmonary artery include computed tomographic or magnetic resonance image scanning and contrast angiography.

LIMITATIONS/ TECHNICAL CONSIDERATIONS/ALTERNATE APPROACHES

The major limitations of echocardiographic evaluation of diseases of the great vessels are acoustic access and image quality. From the transthoracic approach, images of each segment of the aorta can be obtained, but image quality depends on the body habitus of the patient, the skill of the sonographer, and careful attention to the technical details of image acquisition. Interpretation of the images obtained must consider the likelihood of false-positive findings from beam-width artifacts, reverberations, and oblique image planes, as well as false-negative findings due to limited acoustic access and poor resolution.

Transesophageal imaging obviates many of these limitations by providing optimal acoustic access and excellent resolution. However, reverberations, beam-width artifacts, and oblique image planes still can result in apparent intraluminal "abnormalities," particularly in the ascending aorta, that in fact represent ultrasound artifacts. Use of a biplane or multiplane probe is essential, since the ascending aorta is visualized only at its base using the transverse image plane (single-plane probe). Even with a multiplane probe, a few centimeters of the ascending aorta at its junction with the arch may not be adequately visualized due to the interposed air-filled bronchial tree. Images of the ascending aorta are of particular importance in suspected aortic dissection because the entry site (ascending or descending aorta), rather than the simple presence or absence of disease, determines therapy.

Alternate approaches provide excellent-quality images of the aorta with sensitivities and specificities for diagnosis of aortic dissection at least comparable with those of transesophageal echocardiography. Chest computed tomography (CT) can be used to evaluate aortic disease with the advantages of a wide field of view, high accuracy, and wide availability. Disadvantages include the use of ionizing radiation and the non-portable nature of the study. Chest CT may identify associated pericardial effusion but is of limited value in evaluation of left ventricular or aortic valve function.

Magnetic resonance imaging (MRI) of the aorta has the advantages of high resolution, high diagnostic accuracy, wide field of view, and the ability to orient the images along the long axis of the aorta. Like chest CT, MRI is not portable. In addition, it is not as widely available, is expensive, and provides limited data on ventricular and valvular function in routine clinical use. However, both chest CT and MRI can provide data on branch vessel involvement, information that rarely is obtainable by echocardiography.

Contrast aortography allows accurate diagnosis of aortic disease, including aortic dissection, and may be the initial diagnostic procedure if the possibility of coronary artery disease is high on the differential diagnosis. Aortography allows evaluation of the degree of aortic regurgitation, involvement of branch vessels, and (by separate contrast injection) left ventricular systolic function. Cardiac catheterization, with contrast aortography, is the only diagnostic procedure that provides detailed coronary anatomy and allows rapid intervention should coronary artery obstruction be present. Disadvantages of contrast aortography are that it is not portable, uses ionizing radiation, is invasive, and is expensive.

Again, the choice of imaging procedures in a patient with suspected aortic disease depends largely in the differential diagnosis, the specific data needed in that patient, and procedure availability.

SUGGESTED READING

1. Roberts WC: Aortic dissection: Anatomy, consequences, and causes. Am Heart J 101:195–214, 1981.
   Excellent review of the pathology and anatomy of aortic dissection with clear diagrams and photographs. Emphasizes complications and etiology.

2. DeSanctis RW, Doroghazi RM, Austen WG, Buckley MJ: Aortic dissection. N Engl J Med 317:1060–1067, 1987.
   Review of pathogenesis, predisposing factors, clinical findings, diagnosis, and treatment of aortic dissection.

3. Roberts CS, Roberts WC: Dissection of the aorta associated with congenital malformation of the aortic valve. J Am Coll Cardiol 17:712–716, 1991.
   Of 186 patients with aortic dissection, 7.5 percent had a bicuspid aortic valve and 1.1 percent had a unicuspid aortic valve. The dissection entry site was in the ascending aorta in 100 percent of (16 of 16) patients with an abnormal aor-

tic valve but only 68 percent of those with a trileaflet aortic valve. A congenitally abnormal aortic valve is approximately five times more common in patients with (compared with patients without) aortic dissection.

4. Hahn RT, Roman MJ, Mogtader AH, Devereux RB: Association of aortic dilation with regurgitant, stenotic and functionally normal bicuspid aortic valves. J Am Coll Cardiol 19:283–288, 1992.
   In 83 adults with a bicuspid aortic valve, ascending aortic dilation was present in 50 percent of those with a functionally normal valve (n = 19), and 63 percent of those with aortic regurgitation or aortic stenosis, with mean aortic diameters of 3.6 ± 0.7 and 3.8 ± 0.7 cm, respectively, compared with 2.9 ± 0.7 cm in control subjects.

5. Goldstein SA, Mintz GS, Lindsay J Jr: Aorta: comprehensive evaluation by echocardiography and transesophageal echocardiography. J Am Soc Echocardiogr 6:634–659, 1993.
   Review of the use of transthoracic and transesophageal echocardiography for evaluation of diseases of the aorta. One hundred four references.

6. Kotler MN: Is transesophageal echocardiography the new standard for diagnosing dissecting aortic aneurysms? J Am Coll Cardiol 14:1263–1265, 1989.
   Editorial on transesophageal echocardiography for diagnosis of aortic dissection reviews previous studies of transthoracic echocardiography in which sensitivity ranged from 79 to 100 percent with a specificity of 90 percent. Emphasizes that transesophageal echocardiography allows evaluation of entrance sites, differentiation of true from false lumen, evaluation of aortic regurgitation, and detection of pericardial effusion in addition to identification of the intimal flap.

7. Cigarroa JE, Isselbacher EM, DeSanctis RW, Eagle KA: Diagnostic imaging in the evaluation of suspected aortic dissection. Old standards and new directions. N Engl J Med 328:35–43, 1993.
   Excellent review, with examples, of diagnostic imaging procedures for aortic dissection, including aortography, CT scanning, MRI, and echocardiography. Discusses the choice of imaging procedure in patients with suspected aortic dissection.

8. Victor MF, Mintz GS, Kotler MN, et al: Two-dimensional echocardiographic diagnosis of aortic dissection. Am J Cardiol 48:1155–1159, 1981.
   Transthoracic echocardiographic study of patients with suspected aortic dissection.

9. Erbel R, Borner N, Steller D, et al: Detection of aortic dissection by transesophageal echocardiography. Br Heart J 58:45–51, 1987.
   Evaluation of transthoracic and transesophageal echocardiography in 21 patients, all of whom had aortic dissection.

10. Hashimoto S, Kumada T, Osakada G, et al: Assessment of transesophageal Doppler echography in dissecting aortic aneurysm. J Am Coll Cardiol 14:1253–1262, 1989.
    Use of transesophageal echocardiography in aortic dissection emphasizing identification of sites of entry and detection of thrombus in the false channel.

11. Ballal RS, Nanda NC, Gatewood R, et al: Usefulness of transesophageal echocardiography in assessment of aortic dissection. Circulation 84:1903–1914, 1991.
    Besides diagnosis of dissection, TEE correctly identified the type of dissection in all 29 patients. Complications detected by TEE included involvement of the coronary arteries, communications between the true and false lumens, presence of thrombus in the false lumen, and localized rupture with pseudoaneurysm formation.

12. Nienaber CA, Spielmann RP, von Kodolitsch Y, et al: Diagnosis of thoracic aortic dissection. Magnetic resonance imaging versus transesophageal echocardiography. Circulation 85:434–447, 1992.
Comparison of MRI and TEE in suspected aortic dissection. False-positive results on TEE were related to reverberations, extensive plaque formation, and previous periaortic trauma. MRI was helpful in resolving these false-positive echocardiographic findings.

13. Nienaber CA, von Kodolitsch Y, Nicolas V, et al: The diagnosis of thoracic aortic dissection by noninvasive imaging procedures. N Engl J Med 328:1–9, 1993.
Further extension of the authors' study (12 above), including CT, MRI, TTE, and TEE diagnosis of aortic dissection. Again, the specificity of TEE was lowest (86 percent) for the ascending aorta due to echo reverberation and atherosclerotic plaque. MRI and TEE had the highest overall predictive value, and neither CT nor aortography provided further significant information in the patients in this series. The authors advocate that TTE should be followed by either MRI or TEE to provide a definitive diagnosis before surgical intervention.

14. Chan K-L: Usefulness of transesophageal echocardiography in the diagnosis of conditions mimicking aortic dissection. Am Heart J 122:495–504, 1991.
In 22 patients with suspected (but absent) aortic dissection, ischemic disease was present in 5. Of the remaining 17, transesophageal echocardiography demonstrated aortic disease in 16 patients with dilation in 10 (63 percent), atheromas in 7 (41 percent) (5 also had dilation), an extrinsic aortic mass in 2, a posttraumatic clot in the descending aorta in 1, and an anastomotic leak at a coronary reimplantation site in 1 patient. Thus transesophageal echocardiography provided valuable clinical data, even when aortic dissection was excluded.

15. Mohr-Kahaly S, Erbel R, Rennollet H, et al: Ambulatory follow-up of aortic dissection by transesophageal two-dimensional and color-coded Doppler echocardiography. Circulation 80:24–33, 1989.
Persistent dissection flaps were observed in 5 of 7 (71 percent) patients with aortic dissection treated surgically and 9 of 11 (82 percent) treated medically. Flow in the false lumen was present in 14 patients, and multiple persistent communications between the true and false lumens were detected frequently.

16. Erbel R, Oelert H, Meyer J, et al for the European Cooperative Study Group on Echocardiography: Effect of medical and surgical therapy on aortic dissection evaluated by transesophageal echocardiography: Implications for prognosis and therapy. Circulation 87:1604–1615, 1993.
Of 168 patients treated for acute aortic dissection, a persistent patent false lumen was seen at follow-up in 93 percent (28 of 30) after surgery for ascending aortic dissection that extended into the descending aorta but in only 11 percent (2 of 18) with dissection confined to the ascending aorta. The authors propose that thrombus formation in the false lumen is a good prognostic sign which is associated with a lower rate of complications and reoperation.

17. Barbetseas J, Crawford ES, Safi HJ, et al: Doppler echocardiographic evaluation of pseudoaneurysms complicating composite grafts of the ascending aorta. Circulation 85:212–222, 1992.
Description of the echocardiographic appearance of pseudoaneurysm formation after ascending aortic graft surgery in 8 cases. Periannular and coronary artery dehiscences were detected by echocardiography utilizing both 2D imaging (transthoracic and/or transesophageal) and Doppler flow studies.

18. Pyeritz RE, McKusick VA: The Marfan syndrome: Diagnosis and management. N Engl J Med 300:772–777, 1979.
Concise review article on the clinical manifestations of Marfan's syndrome. Nearly all patients with Marfan's syndrome have (or develop) aortic root dilation as seen on echocardiography. Annual echocardiographic examination is advocated.

19. Roman MJ, Devereux RB, Kramer-Fox R, Spitzer MC: Comparison of cardiovascular and skeletal features of primary mitral valve prolapse and Marfan syndrome. Am J Cardiol 63:317–321, 1989.
Of the 59 subjects with Marfan's syndrome, 39 (66 percent) had mitral valve prolapse on echocardiography. The average aortic root dimension in Marfan's patients was 4.1 ± 0.9 cm (at the sinuses of Valsalva) compared with 3.1 ± 0.5 cm in 59 age- and gender-matched mitral valve prolapse subjects ($p < 0.001$).

20. Simpson IA, de Belder MA, Treasure T, et al: Cardiovascular manifestations of Marfan's syndrome: Improved evaluation by transesophageal echocardiography. Br Heart J 69:104–108, 1993.
TEE studies in 11 patients with Marfan's syndrome, suspected aortic dissection, and inadequate TTE images revealed evidence for dissection in 6 subjects with surgical confirmation in all 6 cases.

21. Fazio GP, Redberg RF, Winslow T, Schiller NB: Transesophageal echocardiographically detected atherosclerotic aortic plaque is a marker for coronary artery disease. J Am Coll Cardiol 21:144–150, 1993.
In 61 patients (31 females) with previous coronary angiography, TEE showed atherosclerotic plaque in the descending thoracic aorta in 37 of 41 (sensitivity 90 percent) with documented coronary artery disease (>50 percent left main or >70 percent LAD, RCA, or circumflex). Of the 20 patients without significant coronary disease, 18 (specificity 90 percent) had no evidence for atherosclerosis in the descending aorta on TEE.

22. Mohr-Kahaly S, Erbel R, Kearney P, et al: Aortic intramural hemorrhage visualized by transesophageal echocardiography: findings and prognostic implications. J Am Coll Cardiol 23:658–664, 1994.
Localized intramural hemorrhage results in a layered appearance of the aorta on transesophageal imaging. This variant of aortic dissection was seen in 15/114 patients. The length of the intramural hematoma ranged from 3 to 20 cm with a thickness of 0.7 to 3 cm. At 11-month follow-up, mortality rate was 8/15 (53 percent)—5 (33 percent) patients developed classic aortic dissection, 4 (27 percent) had aortic rupture, and 5 (33 percent) became asymptomatic on medical therapy.

23. Shores J, Berger KR, Murphy EA, Pyeritz RE: Progression of aortic dilatation and the benefit of long-term beta-adrenergic blockade in Marfan's syndrome. N Engl J Med 330:1335–13341, 1994.
Echocardiography was used to follow the rate of aortic root dilation in 70 Marfan's patients in a randomized trial of beta-blockade therapy. Maximal measured aortic root diameter was divided by the predicted diameter for the patient's age, height, and weight. This "aortic ratio" was comparable both between patients and in the same patient during growth of the body. The rate of progression, measured as the slope of the aortic ratio regression line, was significantly lower in the treatment group compared with controls ($p <0.001$).

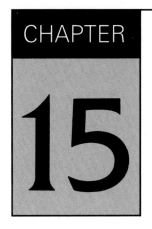

CHAPTER 15

INTRODUCTION TO ECHOCARDIOGRAPHIC EVALUATION OF THE ADULT WITH CONGENITAL HEART DISEASE

INTRODUCTION

There are two basic categories of congenital heart disease in adults:

1. The initial clinical presentation of previously undiagnosed and untreated congenital defects.

2. Survival into adulthood of patients with known congenital heart disease and previous surgical procedures.

In adult patients with no prior diagnosis of heart disease, a congenital defect often is not considered as a potential cause of symptoms, and thus the initial diagnosis may be made at the echocardiographic examination. In these patients, the diagnostic challenge is to recognize and correctly evaluate the congenital abnormality. In patients with known congenital disease and prior surgical procedures, the diagnostic challenge for the echocardiographer is to identify the postoperative anatomy and assess the physiologic consequences of residual defects in each patient. With "corrective" surgery, as well as with "palliative" procedures, many patients have significant residual or progressive abnormalities.

Both these challenges can be met by a logical and methodical approach to the echocardiographic examination with application of the basic principles of two-dimensional (2D) imaging and Doppler ultrasound described throughout this text. Unusual imaging planes and careful integration of imaging and Doppler data may be needed for complete assessment of congenital heart disease. In addition, the physician must have a thorough understanding of the three-dimensional (3D) anatomic relationships for each type of congenital defect.

Obviously, a comprehensive discussion of the echocardiographic findings in adult congenital heart disease is beyond the scope of this text. Instead, an overview of the echocardiographic approach to these patients and examples of the more common abnormalities will be presented. The reader is referred to the specialized references listed at the end of the chapter for more detailed information.

ECHOCARDIOGRAPHIC APPROACH

(Table 15–1)

Congenital Stenotic Lesions

Congenital stenotic lesions are common, including obstruction to right or left ventricular outflow (either subvalvular, valvular, or supravalvular), obstruction to left ventricular inflow (congenital mitral stenosis, cor triatiatum), and narrowings in the great vessels (aortic coarctation, branch pulmonary artery stenosis).

The anatomy of a congenital stenotic lesion is specific for each condition (as discussed below), although, in adult patients, 2D images of the stenotic region may be suboptimal. The physiology and fluid dynamics of congenital stenosis are identical to those seen in acquired disease. There is laminar, normal-velocity flow upstream and a flow disturbance downstream from the narrowing. In the narrowed region itself, a high-

---

TABLE 15–1. CATEGORIES OF CONGENITAL HEART DISEASE

Congenital stenotic lesions
  Subvalvular
  Valvular
  Supravalvular
  Peripheral great vessels

Congenital regurgitant lesions

Abnormal intracardiac communications
  Atrial septal defect
  Ventricular septal defect
  Patent ductus arteriosus

Abnormal chamber and great vessel connections

---

velocity laminar jet of flow is present, with velocity (V, in m/s) related to the pressure difference (ΔP, in mmHg) across the narrowing as stated in the simplified Bernoulli equation:

$$\Delta P = 4V^2$$

When a parallel intercept angle can be obtained between the jet and the ultrasound beam, quantitative data on stenosis severity and intracardiac hemodynamics can be derived. For example, if the maximum velocity across a subpulmonic stenosis is 4.5 m/s, then the maximum right ventricular to pulmonary artery systolic pressure difference is approximately 80 mmHg. Quantitative evaluation of stenosis severity for a congenitally stenotic lesion includes calculation of maximum and mean pressure gradients as for acquired valve stenosis. Similarly, when possible, valve area calculations are performed using either the continuity equation (aortic valve) or the pressure half-time method (mitral valve).

Several significant differences between congenital and acquired stenosis should be noted. First, congenital stenosis of ventricular outflow, for both right and left ventricles, may involve the subvalvular or supravalvular region rather than (or in addition to) stenosis of the valve itself. Careful evaluation with conventional pulsed Doppler or color flow imaging to identify the poststenotic flow disturbance is helpful in determining the exact site of obstruction. Second, when serial stenoses are present, quantitation of the contribution of each level of obstruction to the overall degree of stenosis can be difficult using Doppler echo methods. Third, the proximal flow pattern in congenital stenosis often is characterized by a greater increase in velocity due to anatomic tapering of the proximal flow region (e.g., in aortic coarctation or in the congenitally stenotic pulmonic valve). In these situations, accurate pressure gradient calculations should include the proximal velocity (V_{prox}) as well as the jet velocity (V_{jet}) in the Bernoulli equation:

$$\Delta P = 4(V^2_{jet} - V^2_{prox})$$

Otherwise, evaluation of congenital stenosis is similar to evaluation of acquired stenosis in adults, and the methods described in detail in Chapter 9 can be applied in this patient group.

Congenital Regurgitant Lesions

Careful 2D imaging of a congenitally regurgitant valve may reveal the specific mechanism of regurgitation in that patient. For the atrioventricular valves, particular attention is focused on the number and position of papillary muscles; the chordal attachments (especially aberrant ones); leaflet size, shape, thickness, redundancy, and motion; and annulus size and shape. Malformations can include myxomatous changes of the leaflets, abnormal leaflet position (Ebstein's anomaly), and abnormal chordal attachments (atrioventricular canal defect). The semilunar valves may be regurgitant due to great vessel dilation or a leaflet fenestration.

The physiology of regurgitation is no different from that of acquired regurgitation. There is a flow disturbance in the chamber receiving the regurgitant flow with progressive dilation (and eventual dysfunction) of the volume-overloaded cardiac chambers. Evaluation of congenital regurgitation is similar to evaluation of acquired regurgitation, as detailed in Chapter 10.

Abnormal Intracardiac Communications (Shunts)

An abnormal intracardiac communication is characterized by blood flow across the defect, with the direction, timing, and volume of flow determined by the size of the orifice, the pressure gradient across the defect, and the relative resistance to flow of the vascular beds on each side of the defect. If left-sided heart pressures exceed right-sided pressures—pulmonary vascular resistance is low—left-to-right flow across the defect predominates. Small degrees of right-to-left shunting may be present briefly during the cardiac cycle, since right-sided pressures may transiently exceed left-sided pressures.

With conventional pulsed Doppler ultrasound or with color flow imaging, a flow disturbance is found downstream from the defect: on the right side of the interventricular septum for a ventricular septal defect, in the right atrium for an atrial septal defect, and in the pulmonary artery for a patent ductus arteriosus.

Analogous to a stenotic or regurgitant orifice, the velocity of blood flow through the shunt orifice is related to the pressure gradient across the defect, as stated in the Bernoulli equation. Thus a small ventricular septal defect results in a high-velocity systolic flow signal (about 5 m/s), since left ventricular systolic pressure greatly exceeds right ventricular systolic pressure (by about 100 mmHg). Conversely, flow across an atrial septal defect typically is low in velocity because only a modest left atrial to right atrial pressure difference is present.

A left-to-right intracardiac shunt imposes a chronic volume overload on the receiving chamber(s) with consequent dilation of the affected chamber(s). With an atrial septal defect, both right atrial and right ventricular dilation, along with paradoxical septal motion, are seen. With a patent ductus arteriosus, the volume overload is imposed on the left atrium and left ventricle. Although it might seem that a ventricular septal defect would cause right ventricular volume overload, in fact, right ventricular size usually is normal since the left ventricle effectively ejects the shunt flow across the defect directly into the pulmonary artery in systole. Instead, left atrial and left ventricular dilation are seen, since these chambers receive the increased pulmonary blood flow as it returns to the left side of the heart via the pulmonary veins.

The volume of blood flow (Q) across an intracardiac shunt—the ratio of pulmonary to systemic blood flow (Q_p:Q_s)—can be quantitated by Doppler echo measurements of stroke volume at two intracardiac sites (Fig. 15–1). In the case of an atrial septal defect, transpulmonic volume flow (Q_p) is calculated from pulmonary artery (PA) cross-sectional area (CSA) and velocity-time integral (VTI), while systemic volume flow (Q_s) is calculated from measurements of left ventricular outflow tract (LVOT) cross-sectional area and velocity-time integral:

Shunt ratio

$$Q_p = CSA_{PA} \times VTI_{PA}$$
and $$Q_s = CSA_{LVOT} \times VTI_{LVOT}$$
so that $$Q_p{:}Q_s = (CSA_{PA} \times VTI_{PA}){:}$$
$$(CSA_{LVOT} \times VTI_{LVOT})$$

This approach is accurate when 2D images are of adequate quality for precise diameter measurements (for calculation of a circular cross-sectional area) and when Doppler velocity data are recorded at a parallel intercept angle to flow. Po-

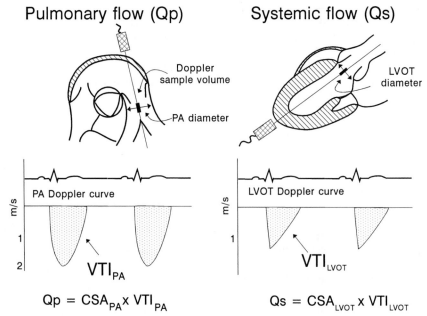

Figure 15–1. Schematic diagram of Doppler echo shunt ratio calculation. Primary flow (Q_p) is calculated from transpulmonic stroke volume calculation using pulmonary artery (PA) diameter measured at the site of the Doppler sample position and the velocity-time integral (VTI) of pulmonary artery flow. A circular cross-sectional area (CSA) is assumed. Similarly, systemic flow (Q_s) is calculated from left ventricular outflow tract (LVOT) diameter and the velocity-time integral of left ventricular outflow tract.

tential errors in estimation of the $Q_p{:}Q_s$ ratios may arise as for any Doppler echo stroke volume measurement (see Chap. 4).

With significant left-to-right shunting, pulmonary pressures become elevated, and irreversible pulmonary hypertension may develop over time. When pulmonary vascular resistance equals or exceeds systemic vascular resistance, the direction of shunt flow reverses, resulting in decreased systemic oxygen saturation and cyanosis. Irreversible pulmonary hypertension due to a right-to-left intracardiac shunt with equalization of pulmonary and systemic pressures is known as *Eisenmenger's physiology.* This phenomenon can occur in infancy, particularly with a large ventricular septal defect, but also can occur later in life when the pulmonary-to-systemic shunt ratio chronically exceeds 2:1.

Abnormal Chamber and Great Vessel Connections

Echocardiographic diagnosis is more difficult when there are abnormal connections between the atrium and the ventricles and/or between the ventricles and great vessels. In adults, poor acoustic access may further compromise the examination. However, with a systematic ap-

proach, a correct anatomic evaluation usually is possible.

Since the position of the heart in the chest may be abnormal, the echocardiographer cannot rely on the intrathoracic position of the chambers for correct identification of cardiac anatomy. In *dextrocardia*, the heart is located in the right hemithorax with the apex in the right midclavicular line. With *situs inversus*, there is right-to-left reversal of thoracic and abdominal viscera. *Dextroversion* is a rightward shift in the cardiac apex without mirror-image inversion.

The first step in a systemic examination of complex congenital heart disease is determination of *atrial situs*. The inferior vena cava nearly always drains into the right atrium, allowing correct identification of this chamber by imaging the inferior vena cava from a subcostal approach and following it into the right atrium. Thus the subcostal window often is a useful starting point for examination of a patient with complex congenital heart disease. The left atrium, then, is the "other" atrial chamber, since although the pulmonary veins normally drain into the left atrium, this is not always the case (e.g., partial or total anomalous pulmonary venous return).

The *anatomic right and left ventricles* (Table 15–2) can be distinguished from each other by several features. The anatomic right ventricle has more prominent trabeculation than the left ven-

TABLE 15–2. ECHOCARDIOGRAPHIC FEATURES DISTINGUISHING THE ANATOMIC RIGHT VENTRICLE FROM THE LEFT VENTRICLE

FEATURE	RIGHT VENTRICLE	LEFT VENTRICLE
Atrioventricular valve	Trileaflet	Bicuspid—unless cleft anterior mitral leaflet present
Annulus location	More apical	More basal
Trabeculation	Prominent	Less prominent
Moderator band	Present	Absent
Infundibulum	Present	Absent—fibrous continuity between anterior mitral valve leaflet and great vessel

tricle and has a moderator band. The infundibular region is seen only in the right ventricle, so fibrous continuity of the anterior mitral valve leaflet and the aortic valve occurs only with a normally related left ventricle and aortic root. When the anatomic right ventricle connects to the aortic root, a band of myocardium is seen between the base of the atrioventricular valve leaflet and the great vessel. The atrioventricular valves develop with the appropriate anatomic ventricle, so identification of the mitral valve is another feature that differentiates the left from the right ventricle. Caution is needed if a cleft anterior mitral valve leaflet is present because it may superficially resemble the tricuspid valve. In addition to the number of atrioventricular valve leaflets, the relative positions of the atrioventricular valve annuli are helpful, since the tri-

cuspid valve annulus lies slightly closer to the apex than the mitral valve annulus. Note that ventricular size, shape, and/or wall thickness do not distinguish the two ventricles, since congenital lesions can result in dilation and hypertrophy of either chamber.

After identifying the atrium and ventricles, attention is directed toward the *great vessels*. The aortic root is best identified by following the vessel downstream to image the arch and head-and-neck vessels. Origins of the coronary arteries also may be seen, but anomalous origin of the coronary arteries from the pulmonary artery must be considered. The pulmonary artery is identified by its bifurcation into right and left branches. The position of the great vessels within the thorax and relative to each other often are altered in congenital disease. Normally, the

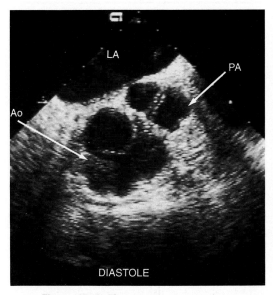
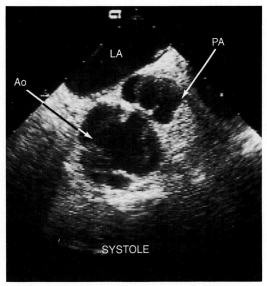

Figure 15–2. Transposed great arteries seen on a transesophageal view with an anterior aorta and a smaller posterior pulmonary artery with a bicuspid valve in a 42-year-old with congenital transposition of the great arteries, pulmonic stenosis, and a ventricular septal defect.

pulmonary artery lies anterior and slightly medial to the aortic root at its origin and then courses posteriorly and laterally, with the right pulmonary artery lying posterior to the ascending aorta. The aortic annulus normally lies posterior to the right ventricular outflow tract, with the aortic root extending medially and anteriorly before turning posterolaterally to form the aortic arch. The normal relationship of the aortic and pulmonic valve planes is approximately perpendicular to each other, with the pulmonary valve slightly more superior within the chest than the aortic valve. With transpositions of the great vessels, these relationships are altered so that the semilunar valves lie in the same tomographic plane, and the aorta and pulmonary artery lie parallel to each other instead of in their normal "crisscross" positions (Fig. 15–2). If the aorta is located anterior and to the left, *L* (for *levo*) *transposition* is present. An anterior and medial (rightward) aorta is termed *D* (for *dextro*) *transposition*.

Most patients with abnormal connections between the cardiac chambers and great vessels have associated abnormalities that require echocardiographic evaluation. These include intracardiac shunts, stenotic and regurgitant lesions, pulmonary hypertension, and ventricular dysfunction. The echocardiographic examination in these patients is facilitated by (Table 15–3)

1. Knowledge of the clinical history, including prior surgical procedures and diagnostic tests.

2. Formulation of specific clinical questions to be answered by the echocardiographic examination.

During the examination, the physician and sonographer work together in:

1. Identifying the cardiac chambers, great vessels, and their connections.

2. Identifying associated defects, and evaluating the physiologic consequences of each defect with appropriate Doppler modalities.

3. Identifying which clinical questions remain unanswered at the end of examination, and proposing appropriate alternate diagnostic tests that can provide answers to these questions.

CONGENITAL DEFECTS SEEN IN ADULTS WITH OR WITHOUT PRIOR CARDIAC SURGERY (Table 15–4)

Congenital Aortic Valve Abnormalities

Although a congenital bicuspid aortic valve is the most common type of congenital heart dis-

---

TABLE 15–3. APPROACH TO ECHOCARDIOGRAPHIC EXAMINATION IN ADULTS WITH COMPLEX CONGENITAL HEART DISEASE

Before the Examination

Review the clinical history

Obtain details of any prior surgical procedures

Review results of prior diagnostic tests

Formulate specific questions

Sequence of Examination

Identify cardiac chambers, great vessels, and their connections

Identify associated defects, and evaluate the physiology of each lesion
   Regurgitation and/or stenosis
   Shunts
   Pulmonary hypertension
   Ventricular dysfunction

After the Examination

Integrate echo and Doppler findings with clinical data

Summarize findings

Identify which clinical questions remain unanswered, and suggest appropriate subsequent diagnostic tests

---

ease (reported to occur in 1 to 2 percent of the general population), the bicuspid valve often is functionally normal until about age 50 to 60 years, when superimposed fibrocalcific changes lead to aortic valve stenosis. Significant regurgitation of a congenital bicuspid valve occurs somewhat less commonly but presents in young adulthood with a diastolic murmur and symptoms of exercise intolerance.

The presentation of significant left ventricular outflow obstruction in a young adult should prompt consideration of abnormalities other than a bicuspid valve—specifically a unicuspid aortic valve, a subaortic membrane, or hypertrophic cardiomyopathy. A unicuspid aortic valve will appear as a thickened, deformed valve with systolic bowing of the valve on 2D imaging. A high parasternal short-axis view may show the eccentric unicuspid opening in systole, even allowing 2D planimetry of the valve orifice (see Fig. 14–17). Doppler echocardiography can be used to determine the transvalvular gradient and valve area as for any type of aortic valve stenosis. Restenosis of the aortic valve in patients who previously underwent surgical valvotomy in childhood or adolescence is common. Restenosis occurs in up to 40 percent of patients a mean of 13 years after open surgical valvotomy.

Congenital subaortic obstruction can range anatomically from a muscular ridge to a thin membrane (Fig. 15–3). Although typically located 1 to 1.5 cm apically from the aortic valve plane, the membrane may be located immediately adjacent to the aortic valve. In either case, a subaortic membrane can be difficult to visualize in adults due to poor acoustic access. The possibility of a subaortic membrane should be considered when high-velocity flow is recorded in the left ventricular outflow tract, but the aortic valve leaflets appear normal. Transesophageal echocardiography may allow direct imaging of the subaortic membrane, especially if multiple image planes are used to identify this thin structure. Conventional pulsed Doppler, high-pulse-repetition-frequency Doppler, and color flow imaging can be extremely helpful from either transthoracic or transesophageal approaches in demonstrating that, in contrast to valvular aortic stenosis, the increase in antegrade velocity and poststenotic flow disturbance occur on the *left ventricular* side of the aortic valve, indicating that subaortic obstruction is present (Fig. 15–4). Coexisting aortic regurgitation may be present due to chronic exposure of the aortic valve leaflets to the high-velocity subaortic flow, resulting in a "jet lesion" on the aortic valve, or (rarely) due to fibrous attachments from the subaortic membrane to the aortic valve leaflets.

Congenital Obstructions to Right Ventricular Outflow

Right ventricular outflow obstruction may be subvalvular (in the muscular outflow tract), valvular, or supravalvular (either in the main pulmonary artery or its major branches). Pulmonic stenosis can occur as an isolated anomaly but more often is part of a complex of abnormalities—for example, tetralogy of Fallot—or is associated with other abnormalities—for example, ventricular inversion.

The level of outflow obstruction can be determined using pulsed Doppler and color flow to identify the anatomic site at which the flow velocity increases and the poststenotic flow disturbance appears. The obstruction itself may be visualized on 2D echocardiography as a muscular subpulmonic ridge; as deformed, doming pulmonic valve leaflets; or as a narrowing in the pulmonary artery. If significant obstruction is present, compensatory right ventricular hypertrophy typically is seen.

The degree of obstruction can be quantitated by Doppler ultrasound using the Bernoulli equation (Fig. 15–5) with the proviso that only an estimate of the total obstruction may be possible if serial stenoses are present. Note that in the presence of pulmonic stenosis, the tricuspid regurgitant jet velocity remains an accurate reflection of the right ventricular to right atrial systolic pressure difference but no longer indicates pulmonary artery systolic pressure. Instead, pulmonary artery systolic pressure can be estimated by (1) calculation of the right ventricular systolic pressure by adding the right ventricular to right atrial gradient (ΔP_{RV-RA} from the tricuspid regurgitant jet) to an estimate of right atrial pressure (P_{RA}), and then (2) subtracting the right ventricular to pulmonary artery gradient (ΔP_{RV-PA} calculated from the pulmonic stenosis jet):

Estimated pulmonary artery systolic pressure

$$= [(\Delta P_{RV-RA}) + P_{RA}] - \Delta P_{RV-PA}$$

The end-diastolic velocity in the pulmonic regurgitation jet also may give useful data on pulmonary artery pressures because it reflects the diastolic pressure difference between the pulmonary artery and the right ventricle (high in patients with pulmonary hypertension, low in patients with pulmonic stenosis and normal pulmonary artery diastolic pressures).

TABLE 15–4. COMMON UNOPERATED CONGENITAL HEART DISEASE SEEN IN ADULTS

CONGENITAL DEFECT	2D ECHO FINDINGS	DOPPLER FINDINGS
Bicuspid aortic valve	Bicuspid valve identified in systole (raphe seen in diastole).	Mild stenosis and/or regurgitation.
Unicuspid aortic valve	Abnormal, deformed aortic valve with systolic doming; sometimes the unicuspid orifice can be imaged.	Aortic stenosis (may be severe) and/or aortic regurgitation.
Subaortic membrane	Membrane from anterior MV leaflet to ventricular septum; TEE may be needed for visualization.	High-velocity signal just proximal to aortic valve; AR due to nonsupport of aortic annulus or to a "jet lesion."
Pulmonic stenosis	Thickened pulmonic valve leaflets with systolic doming, increased a wave on pulmonic M-mode.	Mild pulmonic stenosis (more severe stenosis is recognized and treated in childhood).
Aortic coarctation	Coarctation may not be easy to visualize since descending thoracic aorta goes out of the image plane from SSN; associated with bicuspid aortic valve; highly pulsatile aortic root and akinetic abdominal aorta.	High-velocity systolic flow in descending thoracic aorta with extension of flow into diastole with severe obstruction; nonparallel intercept angle limits quantitation of severity in unoperated patients.
Marfan's syndrome	Dilated aortic root with loss of the sinotubular junction; elongated, redundant anterior MV leaflet; dilation of ascending aorta, arch, and descending aorta may be present.	Aortic regurgitation.
Sinus of Valsalva aneurysm	Dilated, thin sinus with "wind sock" type of projection into adjacent cardiac structures depending on sinus involved.	May have fistula from aorta into RA, LA, RV, or LV depending on cusp involved.
Coronary AV fistula	May not be able to visualize fistula, but coronary sinus may be dilated; proximal coronary artery may be dilated.	Disturbed flow in coronary sinus or in abnormal epicardial echolucent structures.
Ebstein's anomaly	Septal tricuspid valve leaflet is adherent to RV wall, appearing "apically displaced"; apparent RA enlargement (part of anatomic RV is physiologically part of RA); associated with WPW and with right-to-left atrial shunt.	Tricuspid regurgitation.
Myxomatous mitral valve disease	Thick, redundant, prolapsing mitral valve leaflets; LV and LA enlargement depending on severity of MR; tricuspid and aortic valves also may be affected; can be seen in syndrome of polyvalvular dysplasia.	Mitral regurgitation.
Atrial septal defects	Right ventricular and right atrial volume overload with RVE, RAE, and paradoxical ventricular septal motion. Secundum ASD: Absence of interatrial septum in fossa ovalis region best seen on subcostal or parasternal four-chamber view.	$Q_p:Q_s$ can be calculated from Doppler stroke volume measurements in LVOT (or Ao) versus PA. Color flow imaging of left-to-right flow across interatrial septum; IV echo contrast shows some right-to-left shunting.

TABLE 15–4. COMMON UNOPERATED CONGENITAL HEART DISEASE SEEN IN ADULTS
Continued

CONGENITAL DEFECT	2D ECHO FINDINGS	DOPPLER FINDINGS
	Primum ASD: Defect in IAS adjacent to central fibrous body; associated with atrioventricular valve abnormalities (cleft anterior MV leaflet).	Color flow imaging of left-to-right flow across interatrial septum; may have associated mitral regurgitation.
	Sinus venosus ASD: Defect at SVC-RA junction (may be associated with anomalous PVR); TEE helpful for imaging defect; suspect when $Q_p{:}Q_s$ is elevated without clear evidence of secundum or primum ASD.	TEE to visualize site of defect and left-to-right flow with color imaging.
Partial anomalous pulmonary venous return	RVE, RAE, and paradoxical septal motion reflecting right-sided volume overload (may be associated with ASD).	Suspect when $Q_p{:}Q_s >1$ with no evidence for flow across interatrial septum.
Ventricular septal defects	Small membranous, muscular, or outflow defects may be difficult to image; membranous defects may be partially or completely closed (ventricular septal aneurysm) by the septal leaflet of the tricuspid valve.	High-velocity jet from left to right in systole with pulsed or CW Doppler; color flow imaging shows flow disturbance on right ventricular side of the defect; normal PA pressures.
	Eisenmenger VSD: Large defect, often membranous or subaortic, with equal size and wall thickness of LV and RV.	Low-velocity bidirectional flow across the ventricular defect; severe pulmonary hypertension.
Patent ductus arteriosus	Mild LV and LA enlargement; duct itself rarely visualized in adults.	Diastolic flow reversal in the pulmonary artery (typically along the anterior PA wall); diastolic flow reversal in the descending thoracic aorta.
Ventricular inversion (corrected transpositon)	RV-LV reversal; pattern of blood flow is physiologic: RA to LV to PA; LA to RV to Ao. Associated defects are common, including pulmonic stenosis, VSD, heart block, and Ebstein's type anomaly of the inverted tricuspid valve with systemic atrioventricular valve regurgitation.	Normal physiology in absence of associated defects; Doppler findings of pulmonic stenosis, VSD, atrioventricular valve regurgitation when present.
Persistent left SVC	Dilated coronary sinus; absence of inominate vein on SSN view; small right SVC.	Contrast injection from left arm opacifies coronary sinus first, then right atrium.
Hypertrophic cardiomyopathy	Asymmetrically hypertrophied LV with several patterns of involvement; 2D and M-mode signs of dynamic LVOT obstruction.	Dynamic LVOT obstruction; mitral regurgitation; diastolic LV dysfunction.
Tetralogy of Fallot	Large, overriding aorta, VSD, subvalvular or valvular pulmonic stenosis.	High-velocity flow in RVOT and/or across pulmonic valve; bidirectional flow across VSD.

AR = aortic regurgitation, ASD = atrial septal defect, IAS = interatrial septum, LA = left atrium, LVOT = left ventricular outflow tract, LV = left ventricle, MV = mitral valve, PA = pulmonary artery, PDA = patent ductus arteriosus, PVR = pulmonary venous return, RA = right atrium, RAE = right atrial enlargement, RV = right ventricle, RVE = right ventricular enlargement, RVOT = right ventricular outflow tract, SSN = suprasternal notch, SVC = superior vena cava, TEE = transesophageal echocardiography, TGA = transposition of the great arteries, TOF = tetralogy of Fallot, VSD = ventricular septal defect, WPW = Wolff-Parkinson-White (pre-excitation) syndrome.

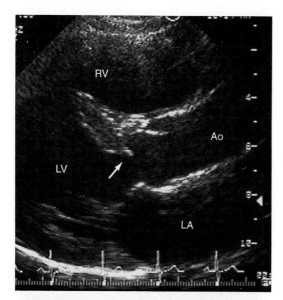

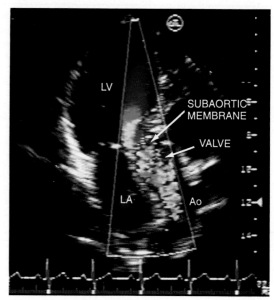

Figure 15–4. Color Doppler in an apical long-axis view in the same patient as in Figure 15–3 showing that the flow disturbance occurs proximal to the aortic valve (*arrow*).

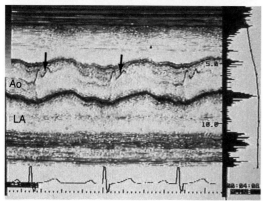

Figure 15–3. Parasternal long-axis 2D view (*above*) and M-mode (*below*) in a patient with a subaortic membrane (*arrow*). Note the early systolic notch on the aortic valve M-mode (*arrow*).

Congenital Abnormalities of the Aorta

Aortic Coarctation

A congenital narrowing in the proximal descending thoracic aorta most often is located just upstream from the entry site of the ductus arteriosus. Less often, postductal coarctation is seen. The coarctation may be relatively discrete, with involvement of only a short segment of the aorta, or may be a long, tubular narrowing. Imaging of the coarctation site is difficult from transthoracic or suprasternal notch windows in adults. From the suprasternal notch approach, the descending thoracic aorta has a tapering appearance, even in normal individuals, due to the oblique tomographic view of the descending

aorta obtained as the descending aorta leaves the image plane. Adults with prior surgical repair of a coarctation may present with restenosis, depending on the specific surgical procedure utilized and the patient's age at the time of repair. For both operated and unoperated coarctations, transesophageal imaging with a long-axis view of the descending aorta may be helpful.

Doppler examination shows an increased velocity across the coarctation and, if the obstruction is severe, persistent antegrade flow into diastole (Fig. 15–6). If elevated, the proximal velocity should be included in the Bernoulli equation for pressure gradient estimation. The jet direction in an unoperated coarctation may be very eccentric, so it rarely is possible to achieve a parallel alignment between the ultrasound beam and jet direction, leading to underestimation of the severity of obstruction. In restenosis of a previously operated coarctation, the jet orientation tends to be more symmetrical, and a parallel intercept angle with correct estimation of the pressure gradient is more likely. In either case, other clinical methods for assessing severity of the coarctation are available (e.g., upper versus lower extremity blood pressure).

Marfan's Syndrome

Marfan's syndrome is inherited in an autosomal dominant pattern with variable penetrance. It is characterized by a specific, but variable, gene defect coding for fibrillin, a component of microfibrils (a key structure in elastic fibers), resulting in musculoskeletal, ocular, and cardiovascular manifestations.

Cardiovascular abnormalities of Marfan's syndrome include dilation, aneurysm formation, and rupture of peripheral arteries, an abnormally redundant anterior mitral valve leaflet, and most important, dilation and dissection of the aortic root. Echocardiography may be helpful in confirming or excluding a diagnosis of Marfan's syndrome in patients with a suspected diagnosis. Examination also is indicated to screen first-degree relatives of an affected individual.

Characteristic echocardiographic findings include dilation of the aortic annulus, aortic root, sinuses of Valsalva, and ascending aorta with loss of a clearly defined sinotubular junction (see Figs. 14–1, 14–6, and 14–7). Aortic annular dilation results in aortic regurgitation and consequent left ventricular volume overload. Aortic dissection occurs frequently and can occur even when aortic dilation is not severe. With an aortic root diameter of more than 55 mm, the risk of spontaneous rupture is high, so many clinicians recommend periodic echocardiographic examination with prophylactic aortic root replacement with a valved aortic conduit when ascending aortic diameter exceeds this limit (see Fig. 14–27).

Sinus of Valsalva Aneurysm

A congenital aneurysm of the aortic sinuses of Valsalva appears as a thin, dilated area that projects into adjacent cardiac structures, often with a fistulous communication depending on which sinus is involved. On 2D imaging, a congenital aneurysm often has a "wind sock" appearance with a long, convoluted, mobile sac of tissue extending from the aortic sinus into adjacent cardiac structures (see Fig. 14–3). This appearance contrasts with the more symmetrical dilation seen in aneurysms due to endocarditis. An aneurysm of the noncoronary sinus projects into the right atrium, the left coronary cusp into the left atrium, and the right coronary cusp into the right ventricular outflow tract. If a fistula is

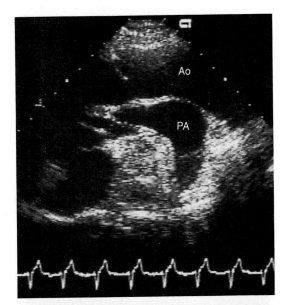

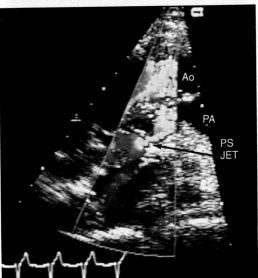

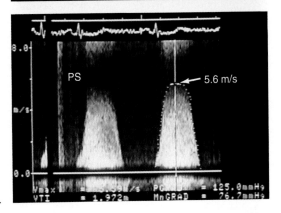

Figure 15–5. 2D parasternal long-axis view (*above*) of the same patent as in Figure 15–2 showing the transposed great vessels. Color flow imaging (*center*) shows an eccentric jet with proximal acceleration across the stenotic bicuspid pulmonic valve. Note the proximal isovelocity surface area. Continuous-wave Doppler from a high right parasternal position (*below*) shows a maximum velocity of 5.6 m/s consistent with a maximum pulmonic stenosis (PS) pressure gradient of 125 mmHg.

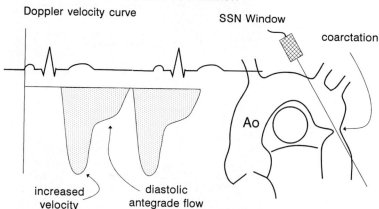

Figure 15-6. Aortic coarctation. From a suprasternal notch (SSN) window, continuous-wave Doppler of the coarctation shows an increased velocity in systole with persistent antegrade flow into diastole. Imaging of the coarctation often is suboptimal in adults.

present, pulsed and color Doppler flow imaging demonstrate a left-to-right shunt with a flow disturbance in the receiving chamber. Continuous-wave Doppler shows a high-velocity systolic and diastolic flow signal.

Coronary Arteriovenous Fistula

A coronary arteriovenous fistula is a rare congenital anomaly that may present in young adults as a continuous murmur. Abnormal communication from a coronary artery to the coronary sinus or right atrium has been described. A coronary arteriovenous fistula is recognized echocardiographically as an abnormal area of dilation with diastolic or continuous flow plus a flow disturbance at the site of entry into the cardiac chamber (Fig. 15–7).

Other coronary artery abnormalities may be diagnosed on echocardiography, particularly when transthoracic or transesophageal images are of high quality, allowing identification of the proximal coronary arteries, such as the origin of the circumflex coronary artery from the right sinus of Valsalva, the origin of the right coronary artery from the left sinus of Valsalva, or the origin of the left main coronary from the right sinus of Valsalva. An anomalous coronary artery arising from the pulmonary artery rarely is diagnosed initially in adulthood because the resulting myocardial ischemia results in significant clinical manifestations at a younger age.

Congenital Regurgitant Lesions

Ebstein's Anomaly

Ebstein's anomaly is characterized by adherence of the basal segments of one (most often the septal) or more of the leaflets of the tricuspid valve to the right ventricular endocardium, resulting in the appearance of apical displacement of the tricuspid valve attachment (Fig. 15–8). The normal difference in the distance from the apex to the tricuspid versus mitral annulus is less than 10 mm. In Ebstein's anomaly, this distance is 10 mm or more. In severe cases, the tricuspid valve may be displaced nearly to the right ventricular apex. In addition, the tricuspid valve leaflets are thickened and malformed. Functionally, tricuspid regurgitation nearly always is present and may be severe. Typically, there is no antegrade obstruction to right ventricular diastolic filling (Fig. 15–9).

Owing to the apical displacement of the tricuspid leaflet insertion, a portion of the anatomic right ventricle physiologically serves as part of the right atrium. This "atrialized" ventricle adds to the appearance of right atrial enlargement, which is augmented by chronic atrial volume overload from tricuspid regurgitation. Ebstein's anomaly may be seen as an isolated anatomic defect, may be associated with an aberrant atrioventricular conduction bypass tract (Wolff-Parkinson-White syndrome), or may be seen in association with other congenital anomalies (e.g., ventricular inversion). Ebstein's anomaly of the anatomic tricuspid valve in a patient with ventricular inversion results in systemic atrioventricular valve regurgitation and chronic volume overload of the systemic ventricle.

Myxomatous Mitral Valve Disease

Like a bicuspid aortic valve, myxomatous mitral valve disease may be silent clinically until late in life, when progressive leaflet changes re-

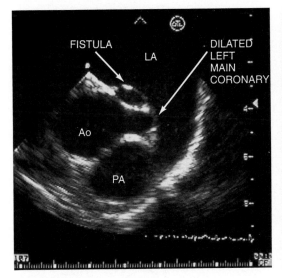

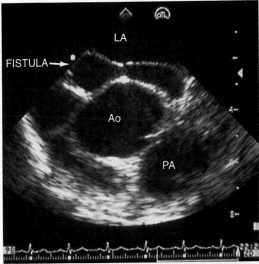

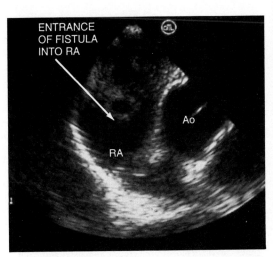

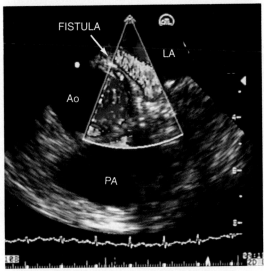

Figure 15–7. Coronary arteriovenous fistula from the left main coronary artery to the right atrium in a 20-year-old woman with a continuous murmur on auscultation. Transthoracic echocardiography showed an abnormal flow pattern in the right atrium. Transesophageal imaging showed a dilated left main coronary artery (*above, left*) with a tortuous channel (*above, right*) leading to an entrance in the right atrium (*below, left*). Color flow imaging shows disturbed systolic and diastolic flow in the fistula (*below, right*).

sult in significant mitral regurgitation and symptom onset. The thickened, redundant mitral valve leaflets of myxomatous disease may result in slowly increasing severity of chronic mitral regurgitation with progressive volume overload of the left ventricle and atrium. Alternatively, chordal rupture can result in acute mitral regurgitation with abrupt symptom onset. Myxomatous involvement of tricuspid and, less often, aortic valves also may be present. Myxomatous mitral valve disease is discussed in detail in Chapter 10.

Atrial Septal Defects

Anatomy

There are three basic anatomic types of atrial septal defect (Fig. 15–10). The most common is a *secundum* defect, in which the central section of the atrial septum (the fossa ovalis) is absent due to failure of the secundum atrial septum to cover the foramen secundum during development.

A *primum* atrial septal defect is absence of the section of the interatrial septum adjacent to the

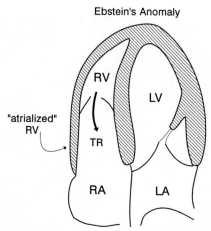

Figure 15–8. Schematic diagram of Ebstein's anomaly showing apical displacement of the tricuspid valve, and "atrialization" of the base of the right ventricle. Tricuspid regurgitation with right ventricular and right atrial enlargement typically is present.

central fibrous body. Developmentally, there is abnormal formation of the septum primum with failure of closure of the foramen primum. Primum defects often are associated with abnormalities of the atrioventricular valves, especially a cleft anterior mitral leaflet. A cleft anterior leaflet can be visualized in parasternal short-axis and long-axis views, demonstrating the cleft and dif-

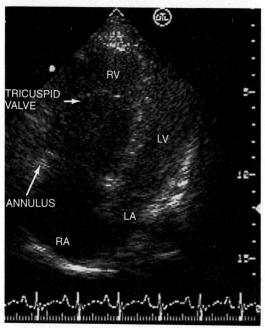

Figure 15–9. Apical four-chamber view of a 42-year-old woman with Ebstein's anomaly showing the apically displaced tricuspid valve (*arrow*) and right ventricular and right atrial enlargement. Color flow imaging showed severe tricuspid regurgitation.

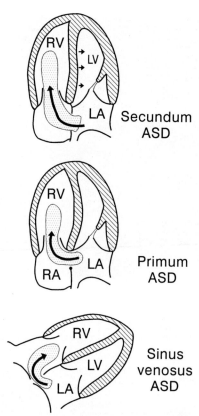

Figure 15–10. Schematic of primum, secundum, and sinus venosus atrial septal defects (ASDs). A secundum atrial septal defect is seen in the midsection of the atrial septum with prominent left-to-right flow on color imaging (*stippled area*). Paradoxical septal motion and right ventricular and right atrial enlargement are present when the shunt is significant. A primum atrial septal defect is located near the atrioventricular connection and may be associated with abnormalities of the atrioventricular valves. A sinus venosus atrial septal defect is located at the base. Imaging may be difficult on transthoracic views but sometimes can be demonstrated from a subcostal approach.

fering motion of the medial and lateral segments of the anterior leaflet (Fig. 15–11). In the long-axis view, lateral to medial angulation of the image plane shows the differing patterns of leaflet motion. The cleft mitral valve may be competent if adequate apposition of the edges of the cleft occurs in systole or may result in mitral regurgitation if closure is functionally inadequate. In a more severe developmental abnormality—atrioventricular canal defect—the entire central fibrous body is absent, resulting in a primum atrial septal defect, a ventricular septal defect, and abnormalities of the atrioventricular valves.

The third type of atrial septal defect is the *sinus venosus* defect. This abnormal communication between right and left atrium is located near the junction of either the superior or infe-

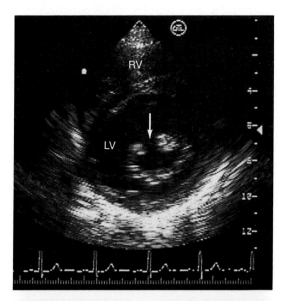

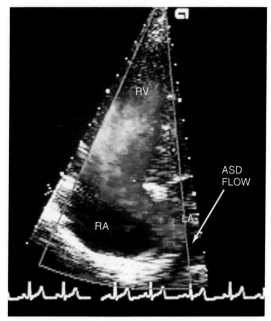

Figure 15–12. Secundum atrial septal defect demonstrates a large color flow area across the central region of the atrial septum (in an apical four-chamber view) into an enlarged right atrium and ventricle.

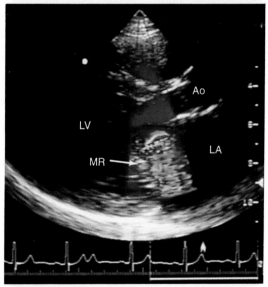

Figure 15–11. Cleft anterior mitral valve leaflet seen in a parasternal short-axis view (*above*). Discontinuity of the anterior leaflet is seen (*arrow*). On color flow imaging in a long-axis view (*below*), an eccentric regurgitant jet with proximal acceleration is present.

Two-Dimensional Imaging

Two-dimensional imaging of an atrial septal defect is most reliable from a subcostal approach so that the ultrasound beam is perpendicular to the plane of the interatrial septum. From apical or parasternal windows, apparent loss of signal from the atrial septum may be due to a parallel alignment between the ultrasound beam and the structures of interest (i.e., no ultrasound is reflected back to the transducer).

Secundum atrial septal defects are seen in the central portion of the atrial septum (Fig. 15–12), and primum defects (Fig. 15–13) are seen adjacent to the annuli of the atrioventricular valves. Imaging of a sinus venosus defect may not be possible on a transthoracic study. However, because the defect is located in the superior and posterior aspects of the interatrial septum, a subcostal approach can visualize the defect in some patients. Transthoracic 2D echocardiography from a subcostal approach has a sensitivity of 89 percent for detection of a secundum atrial septal defect and 100 percent for a primum defect but only 44 percent for a sinus venosus defect. Sinus venosus defects are well visualized from the transesophageal approach (Figs. 15–14 and 15–15).

If an atrial septal defect is associated with a significant left-to-right shunt (Fig. 15–16), right

rior vena cava and the right atrium. Developmentally, it is related to abnormal fusion between the embryologic sinus venosus and the atrium. A sinus venosus defect may be associated with partial anomalous pulmonary venous return. Partial anomalous pulmonary venous return also may be seen as an isolated defect and may not present until adulthood. The anomalous veins can drain directly into the right atrium or into the superior or inferior vena cava.

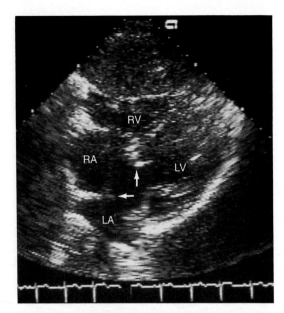

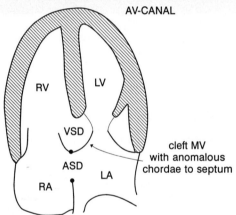

Figure 15–13. Ostium primum atrial septal defect (*above*) in a 20-year-old woman with a complete atrioventricular canal defect seen in a subcostal four-chamber view. Note the intact superior aspect of the atrial septum and the large atrial septal defect (*between arrows*). Schematic of an atrioventricular canal defect in a four-chamber view (*below*).

atrial enlargement, right ventricular enlargement, and paradoxical septal motion consistent with right-sided volume overload (Fig. 15–17) is uniformly present. In fact, evidence for right-sided heart volume overload often is the first abnormality noted during the echocardiographic examination. When evidence for right-sided heart volume overload is present in the absence of a visualized atrial septal defect or other definable cause for volume overload (e.g., tricuspid regurgitation), the possibility of a sinus venosus defect or partial anomalous pulmonary venous return should be considered.

Doppler Examination

With conventional pulsed Doppler or continuous-wave ultrasound, the diastolic/systolic low-velocity flow signal across an atrial septal defect can be difficult to distinguish from other venous flow signals in the right atrium—superior and inferior vena cava inflow patterns or coronary sinus flow. Occasionally, a tricuspid regurgitant jet directed along the interatrial septum results in a confusing flow pattern.

Color flow imaging allows more reliable identification of the atrial septal defect flow based on the spatial distribution of the flow disturbance. However, even with color flow imaging, multiple tomographic image planes are needed for correct identification of the origin of the flow signal.

The subcostal window is optimal for color imaging of flow across the atrial septal defect, since the direction of flow is parallel to the ultrasound beam. Color flow imaging from other windows (including parasternal and apical) also is helpful, since it is the location and timing of the flow disturbance—rather than the absolute velocity of flow—that are diagnostic of the defect in the atrial septum. Color flow imaging shows a broad flowstream from left to right atrium in both diastole and systole with a more prominent diastolic component. With large shunts, the flow across the atrial septum extends across the open tricuspid valve into the right ventricle in dias-

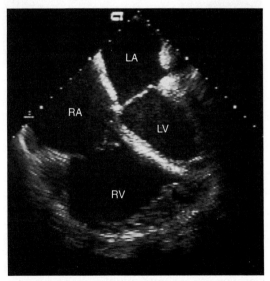

Figure 15–14. Sinus venosus atrial septal defect in a 74-year-old man. Although the transesophageal four-chamber view shows marked volume overload of the right side of the heart, the atrial septum appears intact in this view.

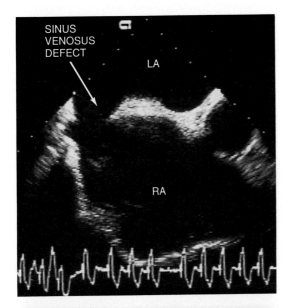

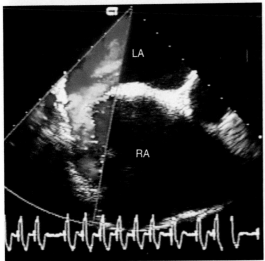

Figure 15–15. In the same patient as in Figure 15–14, the region of the atrial septum just inferior to the superior vena cava is absent (*above*), and color flow demonstrates left-to-right flow across this defect (*below*).

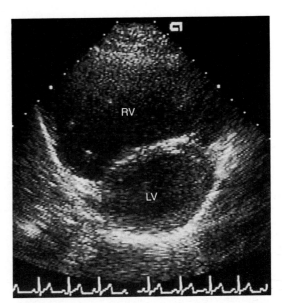

Figure 15–16. Right ventricular enlargement due to a secundum atrial septal defect seen in a parasternal short-axis view.

and flow communication in the superoposterior portion of the interatrial septum. Small secundum defects also are most likely to be detected from a transesophageal approach.

The severity of left-to-right shunting across the atrial septal defect can be quantitated as described above (Fig. 15–18).

Contrast Echo

In a patient with a primum or secundum atrial septal defect, peripheral venous injection of echo contrast material shows passage of microbubbles

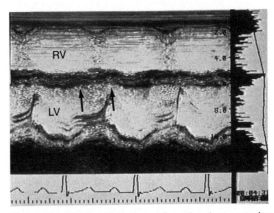

Figure 15–17. Paradoxical septal motion (note anterior motion in systole between arrows) and right ventricular enlargement on M-mode in a patient with a sinus venosus atrial septal defect.

tole. Proximal flow acceleration on the left atrial side of the septum usually is evident. Care must be taken to avoid mistaking superior vena cava flow into the right atrium, which often streams along the interatrial septum, for atrial septal defect flow. This appearance can be particularly misleading in high-volume flow states, such as pregnancy.

Transesophageal echocardiography may be helpful when a sinus venosus defect or partial anomalous pulmonary venous return is suspected. Using a biplane approach, 2D and color flow imaging will identify the abnormal defect

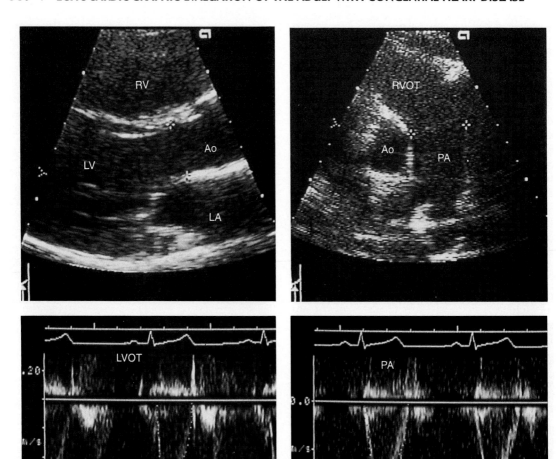

Figure 15–18. In a 23-year-old man with an atrial septum defect (shown in Fig. 15–12), systemic flow (Q_s) is calculated from the left ventricular outflow tract diameter (2.0 cm) and Doppler flow curve (VTI 17.3 cm) (*left*), while pulmonary blood flow is calculated from the pulmonary artery diameter (2.8 cm) and Doppler flow curve (VTI 25.1 cm) (*right*). In this example, Q_s is 54 ml, Q_p is 154, with a Q_p:Q_s of 2.9:1.

across the interatrial septum, even when the shunt is predominantly left to right in direction. The explanation for this observation is that right atrial pressure transiently and briefly exceeds left atrial pressure, allowing passage of a small volume of blood from right to left. This small volume can be visualized when contrast echos from the right atrium appear in the left atrium. Dense contrast in the right atrium also allows visualization of a "negative" contrast jet across the atrial septal defect; that is, the blood flow from the left atrium into the right atrium will appear as an area with no echo contrast.

Contrast echo studies are rarely needed for diagnosis of an atrial septal defect when typical 2D

echo, Doppler, and color flow imaging findings are present. The principle of using echo contrast to identify very small degrees of right-to-left shunting can be utilized to detect a patent foramen ovale as a potential etiology for a systemic embolic event (see Chap. 13).

Post-ASD Repair

With a prior atrial septal defect repair, there may be mild residual right ventricular and right atrial dilatation. More than mild persistent dilation should prompt a search for a residual defect or a leak around the patch repair.

Ventricular Septal Defects

Anatomy

There are four anatomically different types of ventricular septal defects (Fig. 15–19). The most common type is a membranous defect located in the region of the membranous septum immediately inferomedial to the aortic valve and lateral to the septal leaflet of the tricuspid valve. Small membranous ventricular septal defects may close spontaneously during childhood by approximation of the tricuspid valve septal leaflet across the defect. A completely closed defect may be undetectable in adulthood, or a residual anatomic abnormality—a ventricular septal aneurysm—may be visualized at the closure site without evidence of blood flow from the left to the right ventricle. Incomplete closure leads to a persistent, albeit smaller, ventricular septal defect which may be difficult to distinguish from septal aneurysm on 2D imaging and requires Doppler evidence of an abnormal flow communication for diagnosis.

Muscular ventricular septal defects occur at any location in the muscular portion of the septum and may be multiple. When small, imaging the defect may not be possible with a tomographic imaging technique (such as echocardiography) even when multiple image planes are examined.

Inlet ventricular septal defects are the result of failure of complete formation of the central fibrous body. This defect is located inferior to the aortic valve plane, adjacent to the mitral and tricuspid valve annuli. Inlet defects often are associated with other anomalies of the central fibrous body such as a primum atrial septal defect, atrioventricular valve abnormalities, or a complete atrioventricular canal defect.

Supracristal ventricular septal defects are located in the right ventricular outflow portion of the septum (above the crista ventricularis), lateral and just inferior to the aortic valve. These defects are rarely initially diagnosed in adulthood.

2D Echo Findings

As noted above, while large defects may easily be imaged with 2D echo, small defects may be very difficult to demonstrate. Membranous defects are imaged best in a parasternal long-axis view angulated slightly medially (Fig. 15–20). In the short-axis view just below the aortic valve level, the defect is seen in a 10 o'clock position inferior to the right coronary cusp of the aortic valve and adjacent to the septal leaflet of the tricuspid valve. In this view, a supracristal defect is located at the 2 o'clock position, inferior to the left coronary leaflet of the aortic valve and adja-

Membranous VSD

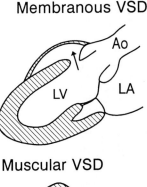

Supracristal VSD

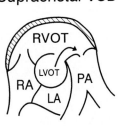

Figure 15–19. Schematic of types of ventricular septal defects (VSDs). A membranous VSD is seen in a medially angulated parasternal long-axis view, immediately adjacent to the aortic valve. A supracristal VSD is seen well in a short-axis view just below the aortic valve with flow from the left ventricular outflow tract (LVOT) into the outflow region of the right ventricle. A muscular VSD can be located anywhere in the muscular portion of the ventricular septum and may be multiple. An inlet VSD is seen in the apical four-chamber view and may be associated with an atrioventricular canal defect.

Muscular VSD

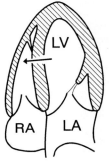

Inlet VSD

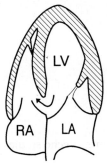

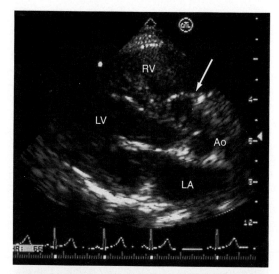

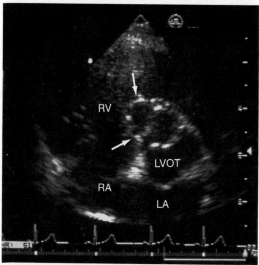

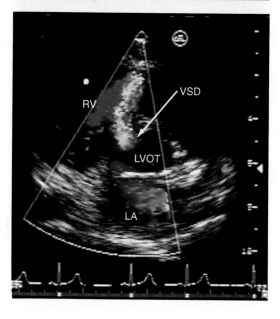

cent to the pulmonic valve. A supracristal defect is imaged in the long-axis plane by lateral angulation of the transducer from the standard long-axis view. Muscular ventricular septal defects may be seen in sequential basal-to-apical short-axis views of the left ventricle or in the apical four-chamber view. Inlet defects are best imaged in the apical four-chamber view or from the parasternal window in a short-axis view at the mitral valve level.

With a ventricular septal defect and a left-to-right shunt, dilation of the left ventricle and left atrium is seen due to volume overload of these chambers. Right ventricular size usually is normal, since the systolic flow across the defect is ejected directly into the pulmonary artery. Left ventricular systolic function typically is preserved because the shunt flow is ejected into the low-impedance pulmonary vascular bed. With large shunts, pulmonary vascular hypertension supervenes, resulting in Eisenger's physiology with right ventricular hypertrophy and dilation (Fig. 15–21).

Doppler Findings

Pulsed or color Doppler flow imaging shows a flow disturbance on the right side of the ventricular septum (with a left-to-right shunt). The presence and location of this flow disturbance are diagnostic even in the absence of a demonstrable defect on 2D imaging. The flow disturbance is detectable in the defect itself with proximal acceleration on the left side of the septum, immediately adjacent to the defect. Conventional pulsed Doppler ultrasound has a sensitivity of 90 percent and a specificity of 98 percent for detection of a ventricular septal defect. The sensitivity of color flow imaging probably is even greater.

Continuous-wave Doppler ultrasound shows a high-velocity left-to-right signal, with the shape of the velocity curve similar to that of mitral regurgitation, as determined by the instantaneous left ventricular to right ventricular pressure differences. In diastole, left-to-right shunting persists at a lower velocity (proportional to the diastolic left ventricular to right ventricular pressure differences) and with the

◄**Figure 15–20.** Small membranous ventricular septal defect with associated ventricular septal aneurysm (*arrow*) seen in a medially angulated parasternal long-axis view (*above*) in a 21-year-old man. In short axis, a deformity (*arrows*) just inferior to the right coronary sinus of Valsalva is seen (*center*). Color flow demonstrates left-to-right flow across this defect (*below*).

shape of the time-velocity curve similar to that of mitral stenosis. Brief reversal of flow may be, but is not always, present during isovolumic relaxation and contraction phases. Both the diastolic flow and brief reversals during the isovolumic periods are low velocity and thus may not be appreciated except at low high-pass filter settings on the Doppler spectral recording. Because this reversal of flow may not occur, intravenous injection of echo contrast material is less sensitive for detection of an intracardiac shunt at the ventricular level than at the atrial level.

Calculation of a pulmonic to systemic shunt ratio rarely is needed in adults with ventricular septal defects because either (1) the defect is small with a small volume of left-to-right shunt or (2) a large defect with a significant shunt in childhood now has resulted in Eisenmenger's physiology with equalization of right and left ventricular pressures. If calculation of a shunt ratio is needed, systemic flow can be calculated in the aorta, and pulmonary flow can be calculated either in the pulmonary artery (if not disturbed by the septal defect flow) or across the mitral valve (pulmonary venous return).

Patent Ductus Arteriosis

A patent ductus arteriosis is difficult to image in adults because of limited acoustic access. However, the chronic volume overload of the left atrium and left ventricle is manifested as dilation of these chambers. Left-to-right flow through the ductus can be detected with either conventional pulsed or color Doppler flow imaging utilizing both parasternal short-axis and right ventricular outflow views of the pulmonary artery (Figs. 15–22 and 15–23). Diastolic ductal flow in the pulmonary artery, typically seen along the lateral wall of this vessel, has a sensitivity of 96 percent and specificity of 100 percent for diagnosis of a patent ductus arteriosus. Recording of flow in the descending aorta, from a suprasternal notch approach, shows holodiastolic flow reversal due to antegrade flow

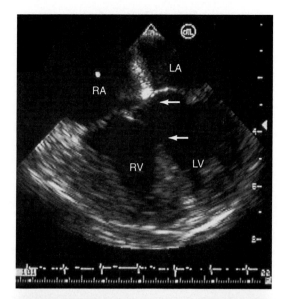

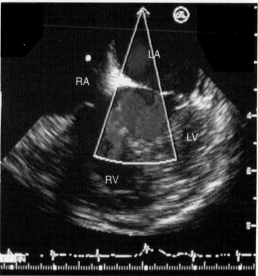

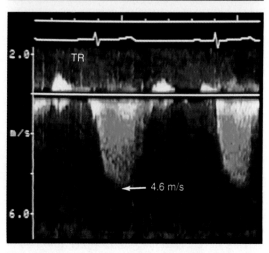

Figure 15–21. Large ventricular septal defect (*between* ▶ *arrows*) in a 32-year-old woman with Eisenmenger's physiology seen on a transesophageal four-chamber view (*above*). Severe right ventricular hypertrophy is present, and color flow (*center*) shows bidirectional flow across the defect due to equalization of right and left ventricular pressures. Continuous-wave Doppler (*below*) of the tricuspid regurgitant jet shows a maximum velocity of 4.6 m/s, confirming that right ventricular pressure is equal to systemic pressure.

Patent Ductus Arteriosus

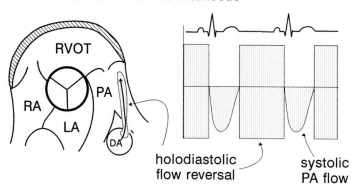

holodiastolic flow reversal

systolic PA flow

Figure 15–22. Schematic of a patent ductus arteriosus. Flow (*stippled area* and *arrow*) from the descending aorta into the pulmonary artery often streams along the lateral wall of the pulmonary artery on color flow imaging. Pulsed or continuous-wave Doppler shows holodiastolic flow reversal in the pulmonary artery. Systolic flow typically is abnormal as well, since aortic pressure exceeds pulmonary artery pressure throughout the cardiac cycle (giving rise to a continuous murmur on auscultation).

into the ductus in diastole. This finding must be distinguished from diastolic flow reversal due to aortic regurgitation, since the two conditions may coexist in adult patients.

Ventricular Inversion

Congenitally corrected transposition of the great arteries (TGA) is more clearly designated "ventricular inversion," since the anatomic right ventricle serves as the systemic ventricle, and the anatomic left ventricle serves as the venous ventricle. Physiologically, the pathway of venous and systemic blood flow is normal in uncomplicated ventricular inversion (Fig. 15–24). Systemic venous blood returns to the right atrium, crosses the mitral valve into an anatomic left ventricle, and then is ejected into the pulmonary artery. Pulmonary venous return to the left atrium crosses the tricuspid valve into an anatomic right ventricle and then is ejected into the aorta. In the absence of associated defects, the diagnosis may be made "incidentally" in adulthood. However, associated defects are common, including ventricular septal defects, pulmonic stenosis, complete heart block, and Ebstein's anomaly of the "inverted" tricuspid valve. Dilation, and eventual systolic dysfunction, of the systemic ventricle is common, although it is unclear whether this is due to the anatomy of the right ventricle being less suited to performing as the systemic ventricle, to inadequate coronary blood flow via the right coronary artery, or to associated systemic atrioventricular valve regurgitation.

On echocardiographic examination, ventricular inversion is recognized by identifying the anatomic ventricles (see Table 15–2) and demonstrating the pathway of blood flow. Associated defects have 2D echo and Doppler findings as described for each abnormality. In addition,

the position of the great vessels is abnormal, with the two semilunar valves lying in the same image plane—best seen in parasternal short-axis views—and with the great vessels parallel to each other—best seen in parasternal long-axis views. Typically, the aortic annulus is anterior and to the left of the pulmonic valve. Ventricular inversion also is associated with dextroversion (apex points toward the right), which makes the echocardiographic examination technically more difficult because the cardiac structures lie directly behind the sternum, limiting acoustic access.

"Incidental" Congenital Anomalies

A few congenital anomalies have no known adverse clinical effects but are important in that, if not recognized, they can be mistaken for pathologic conditions and prompt other (possibly harmful) diagnostic tests. A *persistent left superior vena cava* is seen in a small percentage (0.3 to 0.5 percent) of otherwise normal individuals and in a higher percentage (3 to 10 percent) of patients with other congenital heart abnormalities. Since this vein drains into the coronary sinus, dilation of the coronary sinus is seen on parasternal long- and short-axis views and on an apical four-chamber view angulated posteriorly (see Fig. 13–6). This latter view nicely illustrates the entry of the dilated coronary sinus into the right atrium. The diagnosis can be confirmed (if questions remain) by injection of echo contrast material into the left arm, which will first opacify the coronary sinus and then the right atrium. Injection of echo contrast material into the right arm will opacify only the right atrium. The dilated coronary sinus can protrude into the left atrium, particularly on the parasternal long-axis view, sometimes being mistaken for a left atrial mass.

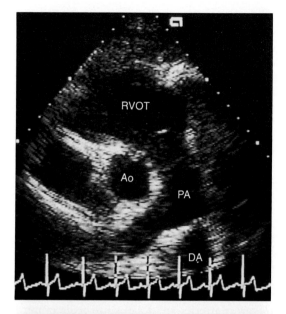

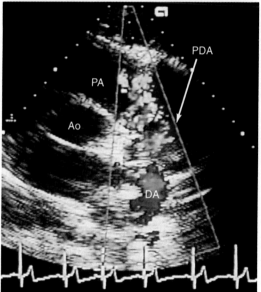

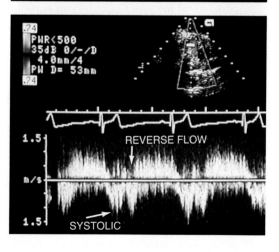

Idiopathic dilation of the pulmonary artery is another uncommon benign abnormality. The diagnosis is made when the pulmonary artery is enlarged but there is no evidence of pulmonic stenosis (which might result in poststenotic dilation) or other congenital abnormalities.

A *Chiari network* is a prominent inferior vena cava valve with fibrous extensions to the crista terminalis and/or coronary sinus valve. These fibrous connections are fenestrated and lax, forming a "network" which shows rapid chaotic motion during the cardiac cycle. On 2D imaging, the appearance of small, echogenic targets moving rapidly in the right atrium suggests this diagnosis.

A *left ventricular web* or *chord* is a bright linear band which traverses the ventricular chamber but is attached to the endocardium at both ends. It appears to represent an "aberrant" mitral valve chordae or a prominent trabeculation of the ventricle. Occasionally, this benign structure is mistaken for the edge of an apical thrombus.

Other Congenital Cardiac Diseases Presenting in Adults

In addition to conditions considered under the category of congenital heart disease, other cardiac diseases in adults are congenital (or genetic) in origin but usually present in adulthood. For example, hypertrophic cardiomyopathy is an inherited disorder (see Chap. 7). Other types of cardiomyopathy may show a familial pattern, suggesting a genetic component. As our knowledge of molecular cardiology expands, other "acquired" diseases may be found to be genetic in origin.

ADULT CONGENITAL HEART DISEASE WITH PRIOR SURGICAL PROCEDURES (Table 15–5)

Classification of Types of Procedures

Numerous palliative and corrective surgical treatments for congenital heart disease have

◄**Figure 15–23.** Patent ductus arteriosus in a 22-year-old asymptomatic man. The parasternal short-axis view shows the pulmonary artery and descending aorta (*above*). Color flow (*center*) and pulsed Doppler (*below*) images show characteristic diastolic flow reversal extending into systole (*arrows*) and disturbed systolic flow in the pulmonary artery.

Ventricular Inversion

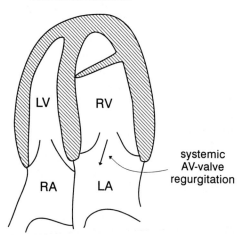

Figure 15–24. Schematic of ventricular inversion. With ventricular inversion (or "corrected" transposition of the great arteries), systemic venous blood returns to the right atrium, passes across the mitral valve into an anatomic left ventricle, and exits the left ventricle into the pulmonary artery. Pulmonary venous return into the left atrium is directed across the tricuspid valve into an anatomic right ventricle (with moderate band) and from there into the aorta. Common associated abnormalities are an Ebstein's-type malformation of the tricuspid valve resulting in systemic atrioventricular valve regurgitation, pulmonic stenosis, a ventricular septal defect, and complete heart block.

been developed since the first closure of a patent ductus arteriosus in 1938. These procedures can be grouped in several categories, as indicated in Table 15–5. The approximate years during which each procedure was performed are shown to indicate which are likely to be encountered in a patient of a given age and to provide a historical explanation of why a patient may have had a particular procedure.

In conditions with low pulmonary blood flow, such as tetralogy of Fallot, transposition of the great arteries, pulmonary atresia, or tricuspid atresia, an intracardiac shunt is created to increase pulmonary blood flow. Shunts may be made from a systemic artery to a pulmonary artery (Blalock-Taussig, Potts, Waterston), from a systemic vein to the pulmonary artery (Glenn), or at the atrial level (Blalock-Hanlon or balloon atrial septostomy). In some cases these shunts are removed ("taken down") at the time of subsequent corrective surgery. Complications of surgical shunts include (1) inadequate pulmonary blood flow due to kinking or closure of the shunt, (2) excessive pulmonary blood flow resulting in pulmonary hypertension, and (3) thrombus formation.

Procedures to close congenital intracardiac shunts—atrial septal defects, ventricular septal defects, patient ductus arteriosus—are conceptually straightforward and may be performed by suturing the edges of the defect (primary closure) or by using a pericardial or synthetic patch. The most common long-term complication of a shunt closure is a residual shunt.

Pulmonary banding is a palliative procedure that creates functional pulmonary stenosis to reduce pulmonary blood flow and "protect" the pulmonary vasculature from irreversible pulmonary hypertension. It is performed in patients with a large left-to-right shunt if definitive repair is not possible or must be delayed. If the degree of banding is not adequate, pulmonary hypertension still may ensue. Distal migration of the band can result in unequal right versus left pulmonary artery obstruction.

Atrial baffle procedures for transposition of the great arteries are designed to redirect intra-atrial flow so that systemic venous return goes to the pulmonary artery (via the anatomic mitral valve and left ventricle) and pulmonary venous return goes to the aorta (via the anatomic tricuspid valve and right ventricle). The 3D anatomy of these baffles is complex and may be difficult to demonstrate on a transthoracic study due to poor ultrasound penetration at that depth. A transesophageal approach improves image quality, but multiple tomographic planes are needed to fully assess the interatrial baffle. Late complications of this procedure include baffle obstruction, baffle leaks, systolic dysfunction of the systemic (anatomic right) ventricle, and arrhythmias. More recently, the great vessel switch procedure has been used to treat patients with transposition. Complications of this procedure are related to reimplantation of the coronary arteries and supravalvular great vessel obstruction at the anastomotic sites.

Procedures to relieve congenital stenotic lesions include aortic coarctation repair; pulmonic, aortic, or mitral valvotomy either with direct surgical inspection or with a percutaneous balloon; and the Konno procedure to relieve left ventricular outflow obstruction. A residual gradient may be present after these procedures, and valvular regurgitation may be induced.

More complex intracardiac repairs that utilize conduits (with or without valves) include (1) the Fontan procedure (right atrial to pulmonary artery), (2) the Rastelli procedure, (3) the Damus-Kaye-Stansel procedure, and (4) the Norwood procedure, as indicated in Table 15–5. When patients with prior surgical procedures for congenital heart disease present for echocardiographic evaluation, more detailed references on congenital heart disease can be helpful in planning, performing, and interpreting the echocardiographic examination.

Tetralogy of Fallot (TOF)

The three primary characteristics of tetralogy of Fallot are a membranous ventricular septal defect, a large aorta that is positioned across the ventricular septal defect ("overriding"), and right ventricular outflow obstruction that may be sub-, supra- or valvular in location (Fig. 15–25). The fourth feature of this tetralogy is right ventricular hypertrophy secondary to outflow obstruction.

Adults with an untreated tetralogy of Fallot are rarely seen due to the high mortality of this condition without surgical intervention. In adults with a repaired tetralogy of Fallot, the ventricular septal defect patch is evident, the aortic root is enlarged, and some degree of residual right ventricular outflow obstruction may be present (Fig. 15–26).

Transposition of the Great Arteries (TGA)

Adults with surgical treatment of TGA present for echocardiographic evaluation either for routine follow-up in the asymptomatic patient or for recurrent cardiac symptoms. Adults with a prior interatrial baffle procedure are most often seen given the more recent introduction of the arterial switch procedure (Fig. 15–27). Echocardiographic evaluation includes identification of the transposed great arteries, correct identification of the two ventricles, evaluation of the blood flow pathway, and evaluation of the intraatrial baffle with transthoracic and transesophageal echocardiography (Fig. 15–28).

Tricuspid Atresia

Evaluation of the adult patient with tricuspid atresia includes assessment of the prior surgical procedures to increase pulmonary blood flow. A complete surgical history is very helpful in directing the echocardiographic examination. Systemic arterial or venous shunts to the pulmonary artery may be difficult to demonstrate if image quality is suboptimal, in which case other tomographic imaging procedures or angiography may be needed. If a Fontan conduit or anasto-

mosis from the right atrium to pulmonary artery is present, it usually can be visualized anteromedially and superiorly to the right atrium (Fig. 15–29).

Truncus Arteriosus

A surgically treated patient with truncus arteriosus will have variable 2D echocardiographic findings depending on the anatomic type of truncus present and the specific repair performed. Again, obtaining a complete surgical history before performing the study is very helpful. The echocardiographic examination then is directed toward the specific clinical question, after demonstrating the basic anatomy and pathway of blood flow in the patient.

LIMITATIONS OF ECHOCARDIOGRAPHY/ ALTERNATE APPROACHES

Calculations of Shunt Ratios

Accurate calculation of shunt ratios by Doppler echocardiography depends on accurate stroke volume determinations at two intracardiac sites. Each of these stroke volume determinations can be affected by several factors, as discussed in Chapter 4. Specifically, both the mean spatial flow velocity and the cross-sectional area of flow must be measured correctly. Flow at each site is assumed to be laminar with a flat flow velocity profile. Furthermore, accuracy depends on a parallel intercept angle between the direction of blood flow and the ultrasound beam. The cross-sectional area of flow typically is assumed to be circular and is calculated from a 2D echo diameter measurement. Small errors in diameter measurement (which is squared in calculating a circular area) translate into large errors in stroke volume determinations. In adult patients, imaging of the diameter of the pulmonary artery often is difficult and thus is the major source of error in Doppler-derived shunt ratios.

Alternate methods for calculation of pulmonary to systemic shunt ratios include (1) cardiac catheterization with measurement of intracardiac oxygen saturations and total body oxygen consumption and (2) first-pass radionuclide estimation from the early recirculation pattern of the time-activity curve.

**TABLE 15–5. COMMON OPERATIONS FOR CONGENITAL HEART DISEASE
SEEN IN SURVIVING ADULTS**

TYPE	PROCEDURE	DESCRIPTION	DEFECTS TREATED	YEARS
Shunts	Blalock-Taussig	Anastomosis of subclavian artery to PA (with or without modification) Conduit (subclavian remains intact)	Reduced pulmonary blood flow (TOF, TGA, pulmonary atresia, tricuspid atresia)	1945–present
	Blalock-Hanlon	Surgical atrial septostomy (largely replaced by percutaneous blade-and-balloon septostomy)	TGA (early pallation), mitral atresia, complex congenital heart disease	1950–early 1980s (occasionally still performed)
	Rashkind balloon	Percutaneous atrial septostomy	TGA	1966–present
	Potts	Descending aorta to left PA	Alternate to Blalock	1946–mid-1960s
	Waterston	Ascending aorta to right PA	Alternate to Blalock	1962–present
	Glenn	SVC to divided right PA (bidirectional = SVC to right PA without isolation from left PA)	Tricuspid atresia, pulmonic atresia, constitutes a portion of a hemi-Fontan	1959–present (1985–present)
Closures	Atrial septal defect (ASD)	Primary or patch closure	ASD with $Q_p:Q_s > 2:1$	1954–present
	Ventricular septal defect (VSD)	Primary or patch closure	Isolated VSD or with other anomalies (TOF)	1955–present
	Patent ductus arteriosus (PDA)	Ligation $+/-$ division of PDA (transcatheter technique 1981)	Patent ductus arteriosus	1938–present
	Endocardial cushion defect repair	Closure of ASD and VSD, repair of atrioventricular valve abnormalities (e.g., cleft mitral leaflet)		
PA banding		PA band to decrease PA flow and pressure	Large left-to-right shunts	1952–present
Atrial baffles	Mustard	Dacron or pericardial baffle directs systemic venous return to PA via LV, pulmonary venous return to aorta via RV	TGA (replaced by arterial switch procedures at many centers)	1964–present
	Senning	RA free wall and interatrial septal tissue used for similar baffle	TGA (replaced by arterial switch procedures at many centers)	1959–1964, 1980–present
Relief of stenosis	Aortic coarctation repair	Various procedures including end-to-end anastomosis, patch enlargement, Gore-Tex graft; balloon dilation for recoarctation	Aortic coarctation	1944–present Balloon dilation 1983–present
	Pulmonic valvotomy	Brock trans-RV approach; direct surgical repair; balloon dilation	TOF, pulmonic stenosis	1948–1960s 1960s–present 1982–present

TABLE 15–5. COMMON OPERATIONS FOR CONGENITAL HEART DISEASE SEEN IN SURVIVING ADULTS *Continued*

TYPE	PROCEDURE	DESCRIPTION	DEFECTS TREATED	YEARS
	Aortic valvotomy	Direct surgical valvotomy	Congenital aortic stenosis	
	Mitral repair	Open commissurotomy	Congenital mitral stenosis	
	Konno procedure	LVOT enlargement by creation of a VSD which is then patched, plus aortic valve replacement	LV outflow obstruction not amenable to valvotomy	1976–present
Great vessel switch	Jatene procedure	Switch of aortic root and PA trunk, coronaries transposed to neoaorta	TGA	1976 (Brazil) 1988–present
Conduits	Fontan procedure	Conduit from RA to PA with prosthetic conduit (+/− valve)	TGA, double-inlet ventricle with pulmonic stenosis, tricuspid atresia	1971–present
	Rastelli procedure	Valved conduit from RV to transsected PA. LV to aorta via VSD and intraventricular patch	TGA + VSD + subvalvular pulmonic stenosis, truncus arteriosus, double-outlet RV	1968–present
	Damus-Kaye Stansel	Supravalvular anastomosis of aorta and PA (functions as aortopulmonary window) to relieve subvalvular stenosis	Irrepairable subaortic obstruction with a double-inlet ventricle	1975–present
	Norwood procedure	Ascending aorta enlarged with pulmonary trunk; Fontan from RV to PA (two-stage procedure)	Aortic valve atresia, hypoplastic left heart	1983–present

AR = aortic regurgitation, ASD = atrial septal defect, IAS = interatrial septum, LA = left atrium, LVOT = left ventricular outflow tract, LV = left ventricle, MV = mitral valve, PA = pulmonary artery, PPA = patent ductus arteriosus, PVR = pulmonary venous return, RA = right atrium, RAE = right atrial enlargement, RV = right ventricle, RVE = right ventricular enlargement, RVOT = right ventricular outflow tract, SSN = suprasternal notch, SVC = superior vena cava, TEE = transesophageal echocardiography, TGA = transposition of the great arteries, TOF = tetralogy of Fallot, VSD = ventricular septal defect, WPW = Wolff-Parkinson-White (pre-excitation) syndrome.

Imaging (Table 15–6)

Two-dimensional echocardiographic imaging in adult patients with congenital heart disease may be limited by poor acoustic access. Even when image quality is acceptable, evaluation of posterior structures may be limited by lateral resolution at the depth of interest. This can be problematic, particularly in the evaluation of posterior conduits, interatrial baffle repair procedures, sinus venous atrial septal defects, or anomalous pulmonary venous return. Transesophageal echocardiography offers improved image quality, especially of posterior structures, and is a useful adjunct to transthoracic imaging in this patient population.

Evaluation of extracardiac anatomy also is difficult. This limits evaluation of the pulmonary artery branches, systemic arterial or venous shunts to the pulmonary artery, and abnormalities of the ascending aorta and aortic arch. Other tomographic imaging techniques are especially helpful in assessing the position of the cardiac structures in the chest and in evaluating mediastinal abnormalities not accessible by ultrasound. Both chest computed tomography (CT) and magnetic resonance imaging (MRI) can be utilized, with the advantage of a wide field of view for both techniques. With MRI, the data can be re-formatted, in an orientation based on the long-axis of the left ventricle, into standard long- and short-axis views, facilitating identification of abnormal structures.

Other limitations of echocardiography are due to the use of a tomographic approach. For example, coronary anatomy cannot be assessed ad-

Tetralogy of Fallot

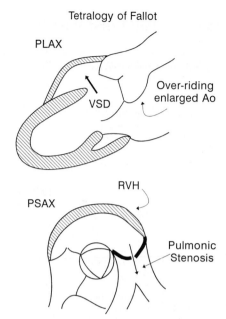

Transposition of the Great Arteries

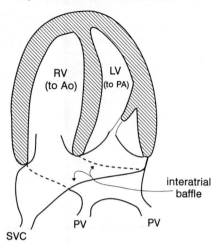

Figure 15–27. Schematic of interatrial baffle repair for transposition of the great arteries which directs systemic venous return to the anatomic left ventricle (and then to the pulmonary artery) and pulmonary venous return to the anatomic right ventricle (and then aorta). With this repair, the anatomic right ventricle serves as the systemic ventricle. Adequate visualization of the interatrial baffle usually requires transesophageal imaging in adults.

Figure 15–25. Schematic of tetralogy of Fallot. Tetralogy of Fallot is characterized by a large ventricular septal defect with an enlarged aorta that spans (or overrides) the defect, pulmonic stenosis (which may be subpulmonic or valvular), and compensatory right ventricular hypertrophy (RVH) (PLAX = parasternal long-axis view; PSAX = parasternal short-axis view).

equately with tomographic techniques. Angiography, with injection of dye into the coronary arteries, followed by cine- or digital radiographic recording is needed. Another example of potential shortcomings of echocardiography

is that multiple ventricle septal defects may be missed unless careful evaluation in numerous tomographic planes is performed. A silhouette technique, such as ventriculography from an angle where the septum forms one of the borders of the ventricular chamber, has a higher reliability for this diagnosis. Limitations of angiography include the risks of contrast dye injection and its cost and invasive nature.

Intracardiac Hemodynamics

While the definitive method for assessment of intracardiac hemodynamics remains cardiac catheterization with direct pressure measurement, much indirect information on intracardiac hemodynamics can be derived from the continuous-wave Doppler signal. Pulmonary artery pressure can be approximated by evaluation of pulmonic regurgitation and/or the tricuspid regurgitant jet. Maximum and mean pressure gradients across stenotic valves can be measured accurately with Doppler techniques. Inferences about the chronicity of regurgitation and the presence or absence of v waves can be made from the shape of the regurgitant velocity curve. Estimates of left ventricular end-diastolic pressure may be possible based on aortic regurgitant velocity at end-diastole, the pattern of

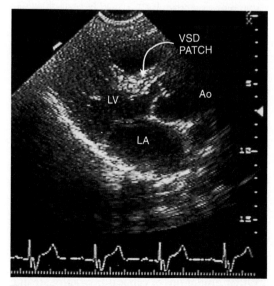

Figure 15–26. A 46-year-old man with repaired tetralogy of Fallot. The overriding aorta and ventricular septal defect patch are seen in the parasternal long-axis view.

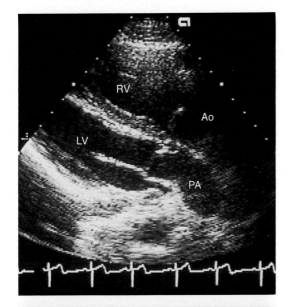

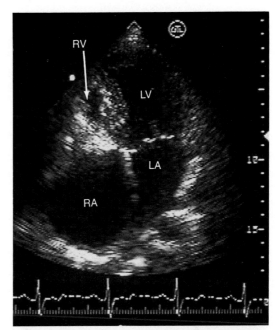

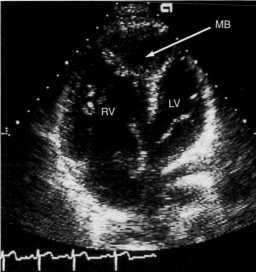

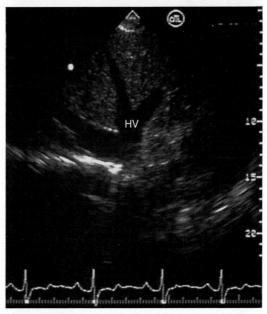

Figure 15–28. Transposition of the great arteries seen in a parasternal long-axis (*above*) and apical four-chamber (*below*) views in a 20-year-old man with an interatrial baffle procedure performed as a child. The *anatomic* right and left ventricles and the moderator band (MB) are indicated. The interatrial baffle is not well seen.

Figure 15–29. Tricuspid atresia in a 25-year-old man with a previous Fontan conduit from the right atrium to the pulmonary artery. The large right atrium, absent tricuspid valve, and small residual right ventricular chamber (connected to the left ventricle via a VSD) are seen (*above*). Subcostal imaging shows severe dilated hepatic veins (HV) due to high right atrial filling pressures (*below*).

left ventricular diastolic filling, or pulmonary venous flow patterns. However, invasive pressure measurements may be needed for appropriate clinical decision making in some individuals.

Integrating the Diagnostic Approach

Whichever diagnostic imaging procedure is performed first in an individual patient—be it echocardiography, catheterization, or an MRI scan—the next step should be to consider the data acquired in terms of both the anatomic and physiologic diagnoses and the certainty that these diagnoses are correct. Then, the remaining important clinical questions should be formu-

TABLE 15–6. ALTERNATE DIAGNOSTIC IMAGING PROCEDURES IN CONGENITAL HEART DISEASE

DIAGNOSTIC TEST	STRENGTHS	WEAKNESSES
Echocardiography (transthoracic, including Doppler)	Detailed 2D anatomy allowing identification of anatomic chambers, valves, and great vessels; blood flow pathway; structural abnormalities Assessment of stenotic and regurgitant lesions by Doppler Detection of intracardiac shunts Assessment of ventricular size and systolic function $Q_p{:}Q_s$ calculations Estimate of PA pressure Noninvasive, no discomfort	Poor acoustic access limits image quality in some individuals Definition of posterior structures is suboptimal $Q_p{:}Q_s$ calculation depends on accurate diameter measurements No direct measures of intracardiac pressures
Transesophageal echocardiography	Excellent image quality, especially of posterior structures Detailed Doppler evaluation of pulmonary veins, interatrial septum atrioventricular valves is possible	Anterior cardiac structures now in far field of ultrasound image Apex may not be visualized Oblique image planes limit quantitative measurements of chamber size Some risk of procedure, plus discomfort to patient
Radionuclide ventriculography	Nongeometric accurate EF determination Detection and quantitation of intracardiac shunts using first-pass time-activity curve	EF less accurate with irregular rhythms (e.g., atrial fibrillation) With abnormal position of the ventricle, it may be difficult to "isolate" LV for accurate EF calculations Limited anatomic data No evaluation of valve function
Computed tomography	Detailed anatomic images if gated to cardiac cycle Excellent for posterior structures, extracardiac vascular abnormalities, and exact position of cardiac structures in the chest	Limited image quality if not "gated" to cardiac cycle May need intravenous contrast injection Radiation exposure Little physiologic data
Magnetic resonance imaging	Detailed anatomic images on gated images Excellent for posterior structures, extracardiac vascular abnormalities, and position related to chest wall Blood has intrinsic "contrast" using different MR imaging sequences Images can be realigned to cardiac major and minor axes Cine-MRI images allow assessment of ventricular function	Tomographic sections at different times in the cardiac cycle Still images provide little data on dynamic cardiac function Research on assessment of valve dysfunction with MRI is in progress Expensive, not portable
Cardiac catheterization	Direct measurement of intracardiac pressures Detection and quantitation of intracardiac shunts Assessment of ventricular size and systolic function Only method that adequately assesses coronary anatomy	Invasive (risks and discomfort) Expensive Requires contrast injection for visualization of structures

EF = ejection fraction, LV = left ventricle, MRI = magnetic resonance imaging, PA = pulmonary artery.

lated and the most appropriate study to answer those questions performed next. When this approach is utilized, the echocardiogram may be the initial test to assess cardiac anatomy and physiology or may be performed only to answer a specific clinical question.

SUGGESTED READING

1. Sahn DJ, Anderson F: Two-Dimensional Anatomy of the Heart. John Wiley and Sons, New York, 1982.
   Useful reference with comprehensive schematic drawings and echocardiographic images for each type of congenital heart disease.

2. Snider AR, Serwer GA: Echocardiography in Pediatric Heart Disease. Year Book Medical Publishers, Chicago, 1990.
   Detailed text with illustrations on the echocardiographic approach to congenital heart disease. Useful reference.

3. Roberts WC: Adult Congenital Heart Disease. F.A. Davis Company, Philadelphia, 1987.
   Textbook with chapters by experts in each area with excellent discussions of functional assessment and clinical syndromes seen in adults with congenital heart disease.

4. Perloff JK: The Clinical Recognition of Congenital Heart Disease, 4th Ed. W.B. Saunders Company, Philadelphia, 1994.
   Single-author textbook with chapters on each of the most common abnormalities. Includes congenital disease both in children and adults.

5. Emmanouilides GG, (ed): Adams' Heart Disease in Infants, Children and Adolescents, 5th Ed. Williams and Wilkens, Baltimore, 1994.
   Comprehensive detailed textbook of pediatric cardiology. Useful reference for descriptions of congenital abnormalities, clinical presentation and management, and surgical procedures.

6. McNamara DG: The adult with congenital heart disease. Curr Probl Cardiol 14:63–114, 1989.
   Excellent review with emphasis on problems unique to the adult with congenital heart disease, categories of cardiovascular dysfunction, and descriptions (with clear illustrations) of operations for palliative or definitive repair of congenital heart disease. One hundred and twenty-six references.

7. Reller MD, McDonald RW, Gerlis LM, Thornburg KL: Cardiac embryology: Basic review and clinical correlations. J Am Soc Echocardiogr 4:519–531, 1991.
   Brief review of cardiac embryology with correlation with clinical syndromes of congenital heart disease.

8. Hagler DJ, Edwards WD, Seward JB, Tajik AJ: Standardized nomenclature of the ventricular septum and ventricular septal defects, with applications for two-dimensional echocardiography. Mayo Clin Proc 60:741–752, 1985.
   Detailed description with illustrations of ventricular septal abnormalities and nomenclature.

9. Hausmann D, Daniel WG, Mugge A, et al: Value of transesophageal color Doppler echocardiography for detection of different types of atrial septal defect in adults. J Am Soc Echocardiogr 5:481–488, 1992.
   In 121 adults with an atrial septal defect, all 6 ostium primum defects were diagnosed on transthoracic imaging (sensitivity 100 percent). Of the 97 secundum defects, 95 percent (54 of 57) of those >5 mm in diameter and 20 percent (8 of 40) of those ≤5 mm in diameter were detected on transtho-
racic imaging. *All were detected on transesophageal study. A sinus venosus defect was diagnosed in only 9 percent (1 of 11) on transthoracic and 100 percent (11 of 11) on transesophageal imaging. Partial anomalous venosus return was missed in all 12 cases on transthoracic imaging and correctly identified in 83 percent (10 of 12) on transesophageal study.*

10. Moller JH, Anderson RC: 1000 consecutive children with a cardiac malformation with 26- to 37-year follow-up. Am J Cardiol 70:661–667, 1992.
    In 997 children with congenital heart disease diagnosed 30 to 40 years ago, 712 are alive, with 632 (89 percent) being asymptomatic without plans for further treatment.

11. Perloff JK (Conference Chairman): 22nd Bethesda Conference. Congenital heart disease after childhood: An expanding patient population. J Am Coll Cardiol 18:311–342, 1991.
    Series of articles describing the outcome, diagnosis, and management of adults with congenital heart disease.

12. O'Fallon WM, Weidman WH (eds): Long-term follow-up of congenital aortic stenosis, pulmonary stenosis, and ventricular septal defect: Report from the Second Joint Study on the Natural History of Congenital Heart Defects (NHS-2). Circulation 87(suppl 2):I1-I126, 1993.
    Reports of several long-term outcome studies of patients with congenital heart disease.

13. Lundstrom U, Bull C, Wyse RKH, Somerville J: The natural and "unnatural" history of congenitally corrected transposition. Am J Cardiol 65:1222–1229, 1990.
    In 111 patients with congenitally corrected transposition, only 9 percent had no associated anatomic abnormalities. The most common associated anomalies were a ventricular septal defect in 81 percent, pulmonary stenosis in 72 percent (valvular or subvalvular), tricuspid valve abnormalities in 33 percent (usually Ebstein's anomaly), atrial septal defect in 11 percent, and a double outlet right ventricle in 11 percent. The median age of survival was 20 years (range 1 to 58 years) with 46 percent having undergone intracardiac repair procedures.

14. Horvath KA, Burke RP, Collins JJ, Cohn LH: Surgical treatment of adult atrial septal defect: early and long-term results. J Am Coll Cardiol 20:1156–1159, 1992.
    Surgical repair of secundum or sinus venosus atrial septal defects was performed in 166 adults (mean age 44 years with 35 percent ≥50 years old) with an operative mortality of only 1.2 percent and a 10-year survival rate of 94 percent. These results emphasize the importance of the echocardiographic recognition of atrial septal defects in adults without a previous diagnosis of congenital heart disease.

15. Driscoll DJ, Offord KP, Feldt RH et al: Five- to fifteen-year follow-up after Fontan operation. Circulation 85:469–496, 1992.
    The 10 year survival after the Fontan operation in 352 patients (mean age at surgery 11 years, range 1 to 42 years) was 60 percent with reoperations necesssary in 29 percent of the study group. The primary congenital lesion was tricuspid atresia in 36 percent, and a univentricular heart in 64 percent. Detailed outcome measures in these patients including recurrent hospitalization, exercise capacity, arrhythmias, and functional class are reported.

16. Murphy JG, Gersh BJ, Mair DD, et al: Long-term outcome in patients undergoing surgical repair of tetralogy of Fallot. N Eng J Med 329:593–599, 1993.
    The 30-year actuarial survival rate for patients with a repaired tetralogy of Fallot was 90 percent of the expected survival rate with excellent functional status after surgery.

Predictors of a poor outcome were older age (>12 years old) at surgical repair, a previous Waterston or Potts shunt procedure, and a higher postoperative ratio of right to left ventricular systolic pressure.

17. Hopkins WE, Waggoner AD: Right and left ventricular area and function determined by two-dimensional echocardiography in adults with the Eisenmenger syndrome from a variety of congenial anomalies. Am J Cardiol 72:90–94, 1993.

    Of 24 adults (age 19 to 45 years) with Eisenmenger's physiology, the 15 patients with a nonrestrictive ventricular septal defect had similar right and left ventricular sizes and preserved right ventricular systolic function. The 9 patients without a ventricular septal defect (Eisenmenger's physiology due to patent ductus arteriosus or atrial septal defect), had severe right ventricular dilation and systolic dysfunction. These discordance patterns of ventricular response to differing shunt locations are reflected in the echocardiographic findings in adults with Eisenmenger's syndrome.

18. Celermajer DS, Bull C, Till JA, et al: Ebstein's anomaly: presentation and outcome from fetus to adult. J Am Coll Cardiol 23:170–176, 1994.

    Of 220 cases of Ebstein's anomaly diagnosed over a 33-year period at 5 London hospitals, 23 (10 percent) initially presented in adulthood. Symptoms at presentation in these 23 patients were arrhythmias (44 percent), heart failure (26 percent), an incidental murmur (13 percent) or other (17 percent). Associated defects were uncommon (only 8 percent) in the adult patients. The severity of Ebstein's anomaly was graded using the four-chamber view at end diastole to calculate the ratio of the area of the right atrium plus atrialized right ventricle compared with the functional right ventricle plus left heart. This severity scale, which ranged from a ratio <0.5 (mild) to ≥1.5 (severe), was a significant predictor of death. Other predictors included fetal presentation and right ventricular outflow tract obstruction.

INDEX

Note: Page numbers in *italics* refer to illustrations; page numbers followed by t refer to tables.